Leadership and Nursing Care Management

Diane Huber, PhD, RN

Associate Professor
The College of Nursing
The University of Iowa, and
Adjunct Director of Nursing
Mercy Hospital
Iowa City, Iowa

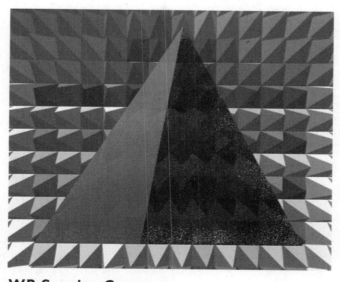

W.B. Saunders Company
A Division of Harcourt Brace & Company

Philadelphia London Toronto Montreal Sydney Tokyo

W.B. SAUNDERS COMPANY

A *Division of Harcourt Brace & Company*

The Curtis Center
Independence Square West
Philadelphia, Pennsylvania 19106

Library of Congress Cataloging-in-Publication Data

Huber, Diane.
    Leadership and nursing care management / Diane Huber. — 1st ed.
        p.   cm.
    ISBN 0-7216-4428-7
    1. Nursing services—Administration.   2. Nursing services—United States—
Administration.   I. Title.
    [DNLM: 1. Nursing Services—organization & administration—United
States.   2. Nursing, Supervisory.   3. Leadership—nurses' instruction.
WY 105 H877L 1996]
RT89.H83   1996
362.1'73'068—dc20
DNLM/DLC   95-42000

LEADERSHIP AND NURSING CARE MANAGEMENT   ISBN 0-7216-4428-7

Printed in The United States of America

Last digit is the print number: 9   8   7   6   5   4   3   2   1

About the Author

Diane Huber, PhD, RN, has published widely and made numerous presentations under her former name, Diane L. Gardner. She is an associate professor at the College of Nursing, the University of Iowa, Iowa City, Iowa, and is one of the core faculty in nursing service administration. In this capacity, she also is an adjunct director of nursing at Mercy Hospital in Iowa City. The adjunct position is a service-education collaborative position designed to link teaching faculty with clinical practice in administration. She teaches leadership and management at the undergraduate level and nursing administration at the graduate level.

Her nursing background includes positions as staff nurse, nursing supervisor, and assistant director of nursing for maternal-child services. Her research and publications are in the areas of nursing service administration and in maternal-child nursing. Her prior work includes research on conflict and career commitment as a member of a research team investigating satisfaction, commitment, professionalism, and turnover among staff nurses that was under the direction of Joanne McCloskey. Diane was part of the team that developed the Iowa Model of Nursing Administration; she has been co-leading a nursing administration research team at the College of Nursing. Her most recent research projects are related to the development of a management evaluation system, the use of nurse extenders (including the 1992 *American Journal of Nursing* survey), and the development of testing of a nursing management minimum data set. She received the 1994 American Organization of Nurse Executives' Research Scholar Award.

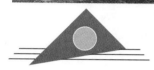

Feature Authors

DEBORAH K. CHARNLEY, MN, RN

Director, Critical Care and Emergency Nursing, Cleveland Clinic Foundation, Cleveland, Ohio

EXEMPLAR: RESTRUCTURING THE ICU LEADERSHIP TEAM

JULIE HENDERSON, BSN, RN

Nurse Manager, PICU/Pediatrics, The Cleveland Clinic Foundation Children's Hospital, Cleveland, Ohio

EXEMPLARS: EFFECTIVE COMMUNICATION; STAFF EVALUATIONS

CATHY LOPEZ HOUSTON, MBA, RN

Analyst, Department of Nursing, Harbor–University of California Los Angeles Medical Center, Torrance, California

EXEMPLARS: SUPPORTING THE PROFESSIONAL STATUS OF NURSES; PATIENT-CENTERED CARE; COMMUNICATING VISION, MISSION, AND VALUES

E. MARY JOHNSON, BSN, RN, CNA

Director, Ambulatory Clinic Nursing, Cleveland Clinic Foundation, Cleveland, Ohio

EXEMPLAR: PERSONAL TOUCHES

ELIZABETH KEMPE, BSN, RN, CEN

Assistant Nurse Manager, Clinical Decision Unit, Cleveland Clinic Foundation, Cleveland, Ohio

EXEMPLAR: MOTIVATING AND PROMOTING STAFF TO TAKE OWNERSHIP OF THE NEW CDU

JoELLEN KOERNER, PhD, RN, FAAN

Vice President, Patient Services, Sioux Valley Hospital, Sioux Falls, South Dakota

JoELLEN KOERNER ENVISIONS EMPOWERMENT AND TRANSFORMATIVE LEADERSHIP; NURTURING THE SELF AND OTHERS

CHRISTINE TASSONE KOVNER, PhD, RN, FAAN

Associate Professor, Division of Nursing, School of Education, New York University, New York, New York

CHRISTINE KOVNER ENVISIONS FINANCIAL MANAGEMENT

DONNA W. MARKEY, MSN, RN

Patient Care Service Manager, Transplant and Surgical Subspecialties, University of Virginia Health Sciences Center, Charlottesville, Virginia

EXEMPLARS: CHANGING THE SKILL MIX; RENEGOTIATING ADVANCED PRACTICE ROLES

JOANNE COMI McCLOSKEY, PhD, RN, FAAN

Distinguished Professor of Nursing, University of Iowa College of Nursing; Adjunct Associate Director of Nursing, University of Iowa Hospitals and Clinics, Iowa City, Iowa

JOANNE COMI McCLOSKEY ENVISIONS PROFESSIONAL COMMITMENT

SHARON E. MELBERG, MPA, RN

Assistant Director, Hospital and Clinics, University of California, Davis, Medical Center, Sacramento, California

EXEMPLARS: DEVELOPMENT AND IMPLEMENTATION OF A PAIN MANAGEMENT PROTOCOL; CREATION OF A DEDICATED AIDS UNIT

LYNNE A. NEZBEDA, BSN, RN, CURN

Nurse Manager, Urology Department, Cleveland Clinic Foundation, Cleveland, Ohio

EXEMPLAR: INSTITUTING A NURSE-MANAGED CLINIC

JIM O'MALLEY, MSN, RN, NP, CNS

Senior Vice President, Nursing Services, Allegheny General Hospital; Associate Dean of Clinical Studies, Duquesne University School of Nursing, Pittsburgh, Pennsylvania

JIM O'MALLEY ENVISIONS TRANSFORMING THE AMERICAN HEALTHCARE SYSTEM; LEADERSHIP TRANSFORMATION; CHANGE . . . MORE CHANGE . . . AND CHANGE AGAIN!

SANDY PIRWITZ, MS, BSN, RN, CIC

Nurse Epidemiologist and Manager of Infection Control, Cleveland Clinic Foundation, Cleveland, Ohio

EXEMPLARS: RELENTLESS INCREMENTALISM; CREATING EXPERT POWER

TIM PORTER-O'GRADY, EdD, PhD, RN, CS, CNAA, FAAN

Senior Partner, Tim Porter-O'Grady Associates, Inc.; Senior Consultant, Affiliated Dynamics, Inc.; Assistant Professor, Emory University, Atlanta, Georgia

TIM PORTER-O'GRADY ENVISIONS DECENTRALIZATION AND SHARED GOVERNANCE

MARGARET SANDVIG, BSN, RN

Nurse Manager, University of Washington, Harborview Medical Center, Seattle, Washington

EXEMPLAR: MOTIVATING AND MENTORING

PAULA SILER, MS, RN

Director, Professional Practice Affairs, Harbor–University of California Los Angeles Medical Center, Torrance, California

EXEMPLARS: SUPPORTING THE PROFESSIONAL STATUS OF NURSES; PATIENT-CENTERED CARE; COMMUNICATING VISION, MISSION, AND VALUES

MARGARET D. SOVIE, PhD, RN, FAAN

Associate Deputy Executive Director and Chief Nursing Officer, University of Pennsylvania Medical Center, Philadelphia, Pennsylvania

MARGARET SOVIE ENVISIONS SHIFTING FROM ILLNESS CARE TO WELLNESS CARE

JOHNESE SPISSO, MBA, BS, RN, CCRN

Assistant Administrator/Patient Care Services, University of Washington, Harborview Medical Center, Seattle, Washington

EXEMPLAR: EMPOWERING THE TEAM

ROXANE SPITZER-LEHMANN, MBA, RN, FAAN, CNAA

Vice President, Managed Care Operations, Medicus Systems Corporation, San Diego, California

ROXANE SPITZER-LEHMANN ENVISIONS THE DIFFERENCES BETWEEN LEADERSHIP AND MANAGEMENT

PETER J. UNGVARSKI, MS, RN, FAAN

Clinical Nurse Specialist, HIV/AIDS; Clinical Director, AIDS Project, Visiting Nurse Service of New York Home Care, New York, New York

PETER UNGVARSKI ENVISIONS THE IMPORTANCE OF NURSING RESEARCH IN HEALTH POLICY

ANDREA WASDOVICH, BSN, BA, RN

Nurse Manager, Clinical Decision Unit, Emergency Department, Cleveland Clinic Foundation, Cleveland, Ohio

EXEMPLAR: MOTIVATING AND PROMOTING STAFF TO TAKE OWNERSHIP OF THE NEW CDU

CONTRIBUTORS TO STUDY QUESTION ANSWERS

PATRICIA RITOLA, MSN, RN

Manager of Maternity, Munson Medical Center, Traverse City, Michigan

JEANNE L. ROODE, BSN, RN, CNA

Director, Neurology/Urology Services; Master's Student at Grand Valley State University, Grand Rapids, Michigan

MARY KAY RUSSELL, MN, BSN, RN

Director, Pediatric Service, Devos Children's Hospital at Butterworth, Grand Rapids, Michigan

LINDA SCOTT, MSN, RN

Adjunct Faculty, Kirkhof School of Nursing, Allendale, Michigan; Doctoral Student at the University of Michigan, Ann Arbor, Michigan

Answers compiled by:

JEAN NAGELKERK, PhD, RN

Associate Professor of Nursing, Grand Valley State University, Grand Rapids, Michigan

Reviewers

Carolyn E. Adams, EdD, RN, CNAA
Associate Professor, Washington State University,
Spokane, Washington

Helen M. Castillo, PhD, RN-C
University of Texas at El Paso College of Nursing and
Health Sciences, El Paso, Texas

Ann E. Cook, PhD, RN
Associate Professor, Columbia College of Nursing,
Milwaukee, Wisconsin

Sheila P. Englebardt, PhD, RN, CNA
University of North Carolina at Chapel Hill, Chapel
Hill, North Carolina

Katty Joy French, PhD, RN
Loma Linda University School of Nursing, Loma
Linda, California

Rita S. Glazebrook, PhD, RNC, ANP
St. Olaf College, Northfield, Minnesota

Roselyn Holloway, MSN, RN
Methodist Hospital School of Nursing, Lubbock, Texas

Marilyn J. Jefferson, MSN, RN
Marian College, Indianapolis, Indiana

Joyce T. Jones, EdD, MSN, MEd, RN
Ida V. Moffett School of Nursing, Samford University,
Birmingham, Alabama

Ruby S. Morrison, DSN, RN
Capstone College of Nursing, The University of
Alabama, Tuscaloosa, Alabama

Giovanna Bisato Morton, EdD, RN
Marshall University, Huntington, West Virginia

Cynthia L. Roach, DSN, RN
Associate Professor, Beth-El College of Nursing and
Health Services, Colorado Springs, Colorado

Marlene K. Strader, PhD, RN
University of Tampa, Joint Commission on
Accreditation of Healthcare Organizations, Tampa,
Florida

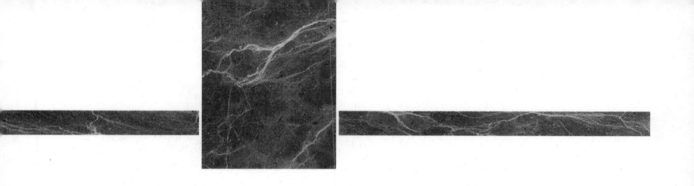

Preface

CURRENT TRENDS IN NURSING LEADERSHIP AND MANAGEMENT

It can be argued that nursing is a unique profession whose primary focus is caring: giving and managing the care that clients need. Thus nurses are both healthcare providers and healthcare coordinators; that is, they have both clinical and managerial role components. *Leadership and Nursing Care Management* adopts the philosophy that there are two components to the nurse's role that can be discussed separately but that in fact overlap. Since all nurses are involved in coordinating client care, leadership and management principles are a part of the core competencies needed by nurses to function in a complex healthcare environment.

The turbulent swirl of change within this country's healthcare industry has provided challenges and opportunities for nursing. As the nursing environment has changed and become more complex, nurses have needed a stronger background in nursing leadership and client care management to be prepared for contemporary and future nursing practice. As nurses mature in advanced practice roles and as the healthcare delivery system restructures at the community level, nurses will become increasingly pivotal to healthcare delivery. Leadership and management are crucial skills and abilities in complex, integrated community and regional networks of healthcare delivery systems that employ and deploy nurses to provide healthcare services to clients and communities.

In the present and future of nursing practice, nurses will be expected to be able to manage care across the healthcare continuum, a radically different approach to the practice of nursing than has been the norm for hospital staff nursing practice. In all settings, including nurse-owned and nurse-run clinics, nursing leadership and management are complementary skills to solid clinical care and client-oriented practice.

There is a discernible trend across the country for hospital nursing services to "decentralize," with the potential of eliminating or changing the nurse manager position and vesting with staff nurses the responsibility for decisions previously made by nurse managers. This movement can become a practical reality only if the knowledge level of staff nurses about essential precepts of nursing leadership and management is enhanced. In addition, nurses expected to make and implement day-to-day management decisions need to know how this knowledge can be practically applied to the organization and delivery of nursing care to clients.

Another trend is to deemphasize acute care hospitalization as the primary modality for healthcare in the United States. As prevention, wellness, and alternative sites for care delivery become more important, nurses will be able to draw on their already rich experiential tradition of practice in these settings. This text reflects this contemporary trend by blending the hospital and non-hospital perspectives when examining and analyzing nursing care, leadership, and management and thus, for example, adopts the convention of "client" instead of "patient." The reader will notice examples from the wide spectrum of nursing practice settings as specific applications of nursing leadership and management principles.

PURPOSE AND AUDIENCE

The intent of this text is to provide both a comprehensive introduction to the field and a synthesis of both nursing leadership and nursing management. It is a research-based blend of practice and theory. It combines traditional management perspectives and theory with contemporary healthcare trends and issues and consistently integrates leadership and management concepts. These concepts are illustrated and made relevant by practice-based examples.

Important legal and ethical aspects of nursing management are integrated throughout the text, as are specific issues related to multicultural diversity. These important themes are thus related to specific leadership and management topics, clearly showing their application to practice, rather than segregated into separate chapters.

The impetus for writing this text comes from teaching both undergraduate and graduate students in nursing leadership and management and from perceiving the need for a comprehensive, practice-based textbook that blends and integrates leadership and management into an understandable and applicable whole.

The main goal of *Leadership and Nursing Care Management* is therefore twofold: to clearly differentiate traditional leadership and management perspectives and to relate them in an integrated way with contemporary nursing trends and practice applications. This textbook is designed to serve the needs of the undergraduate nursing student and the staff nurse or nurse manager who seeks a basic foundation in the principles of coordinating nursing services. It will serve the nurse's need for these principles, whether in relation to client care, peers, superiors, or subordinates. This multiple perspective is especially important because of the return of team-focused approaches and the fading of all-RN staffing.

ORGANIZATION AND COVERAGE

The organizational framework of this book groups the 31 chapters into seven parts. Part I, "The Environment," sets the contemporary context for the practice of nursing management with an overview of nursing administration, the healthcare system, and the nursing profession.

In Part II, "Framework for Leadership and Management," the principles of leadership and management that underlie the rest of the book are clearly laid out.

Part III, "Planning in Nursing Administration," goes into the basic tools that every manager must master: problem solving, decision making, relying on groups and team building, and budgeting and financial management skills (an increasingly essential skill for today's nurse manager).

Perhaps the most profound changes nurse managers see in today's health care environment are reflected in Part IV, "Organizational Design and Governance in Nursing." Many of these changes are taking place at the organizational level, which prompted coverage of organizational design in four chapters, two of which are devoted to organizational structure. If "restructuring" is to be a fact of life, it would seem that the elements of "structure" should first be mastered. Chapter 15, "Delegation," deals with such timely issues as unlicensed assistive personnel. In Part IV, Chapter 14, "Decentralization and Shared Governance," and Chapter 17, "Case Management and Managed Care," are unique presentations of topics that have come to the fore in the recent upheavals in healthcare.

Part V, "Managing Professionals and Their Practice," presents chapters on the skills required to manage professional personnel: communication, motivation, power, conflict, persuasion and negotiation, and staffing and scheduling.

Contemporary developments have also strongly influenced Part VI, "Evaluation and Control in Nursing Administration." Among the chapters that address the most up-to-date trends are "Computer Applications in Nursing Administration," "Quality Improvement and Risk Management," and "Productivity and Costing Out Nursing."

Finally, in Part VII, "Future Perspectives," the reader is asked to look forward to examine the role of the nurse manager in health policy development and to the manager's own career in what promises, at the moment, to continue to be a healthcare system in flux.

Each of the 31 chapters follows a consistent format: concept definitions, theoretical and research background, leadership and management implications, and current issues and trends. This format is designed to bridge the gap between theory and practice and to increase the relevance of nursing leadership and management to the beginning student by showing how the theory translates into behaviors appropriate to contemporary nursing care management.

TEXT FEATURES

In addition to the traditional text features—chapter objectives, chapter summary, and references—this book contains other interesting and effective aids to student comprehension and application.

Study Questions   At the end of every chapter the study questions ask students not only to recall specific information but also to synthesize what they have read. These questions are answered in the Appendix by a panel of students under the direction of Jean Nagelkerk, thus providing the reader with a peer's perspective on the information presented.

Critical Thinking Exercise   Also at the end of the chapters, a situation is presented along with questions that challenge the student to inquire and reflect and to analyze critically the knowledge they have absorbed and apply it to the situation.

Research Notes   These summaries of current research studies are highlighted in every chapter and introduce the student to the liveliness and applicability of the rich literature now being developed in nursing management.

Leadership and Management Behaviors   This table found in every chapter summarizes the applicable behaviors that fall under either leadership or management and identifies behaviors that overlap. This table is designed to help students reflect back on the chapter content in a way that distinguishes leadership from management and that also shows how the two are integrated.

Exemplars   Vignettes presented by practicing nurse managers at some of the nation's leading hospitals introduce the student to the "real world" of nursing management and show how the concepts in the chapter were displayed in true situations. Regardless of the topic, these vignettes all show the creativity and energy that characterize expert nurse managers at the top of their form.

Vision Statements   These statements, by acknowledged national leaders in the field of nursing administration, show the student how a true leader looks and sounds. These leaders graciously agreed to write about their vision of the future of nursing and nursing administration as it relates to the chapter topic for which they wrote. Their voices and their distinguished careers should help inspire readers to build on the knowledge gained from this text, discover their own leadership qualities, and apply these qualities to build a better future for nursing.

TEACHING/LEARNING AIDS

The innovative text is accompanied by two excellent teaching/learning tools. The *Instructor's Manual for Huber: Leadership and Nursing Care Management,* prepared by Jean Nagelkerk, RN, PhD, guides the instructor through each chapter of the textbook with a chapter purpose, objectives, and key terms. It offers discussion questions and critical thinking activities for the classroom, including role playing and other group activities. Each chapter's case studies and related questions facilitate classroom discussion of how concepts in the textbook relate to realistic situations. Using a variety of questions in each chapter, including essay, true/false, matching, and multiple choice, the instructor can evaluate students' comprehension of material in the text. The manual also includes transparency masters that summarize key concepts from each chapter.

The *Study Guide for Huber: Leadership and Nursing Care Management,* also prepared by Jean Nagelkerk, follows the textbook chapter by chapter, condensing key terms, information, and concepts into each chapter's Study Focus. Learning tools and resources such as group activities, self-assessments, case studies, and discussion questions encourage students to explore different roles, responsibilities, and challenges related to nursing leadership and management. Students can test their comprehension of text context with study questions at the end of each chapter. Each chapter also lists suggested supplemental readings.

DIANE HUBER

Acknowledgments

This book is dedicated to my husband, Bob Huber. He made this book a reality and was the text and graphics support behind it. For his love, caring, and support, I am eternally grateful. To my children, Brad and Lisa Gardner, for their enthusiasm and love, I am forever thankful that they are in my life.

To my friend John Folkrod, I am thankful for the constancy of friendship and ideas for examples. To my professional colleagues who inspired me and served as examples of excellence in nursing, I am grateful. To my nursing students, past and future, my thanks for being a source of continual intellectual stimulation and challenge.

I am grateful to Jean Nagelkerk, PhD, RN, of Grand Valley State University, Grand Rapids, Michigan, for undertaking the *Instructor's Manual* and *Study Guide* that accompany this book and also for her oversight of the creation of the study question answers. To the contributors who wrote those answers, the nurse managers who supplied the exemplars, and the illustrious nursing leaders who wrote the vision statements, I offer my sincere thanks for sharing their experience, expertise, and excitement about nursing management.

This book evolved under the tender care of Mr. Thomas Eoyang, Vice President and Editor-in-Chief at W.B. Saunders Company, whose guidance was invaluable. To the excellent staff at W.B. Saunders and Cracom Corporation, a sincere thank you.

DIANE HUBER

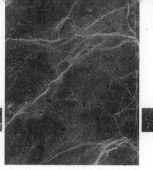

Contents

PART I

THE ENVIRONMENT 1

1 Overview of Nursing Administration 2

2 The Healthcare System 13
Jim O'Malley Envisions Transforming the American
Healthcare System 15

3 Professional Nursing Practice 28
Joanne Comi McCloskey Envisions Professional Commitment 33
Exemplar: Supporting the Professional Status of Nurses—Paula Siler
and Cathy Lopez Houston 35

PART II

FRAMEWORK FOR LEADERSHIP AND MANAGEMENT 49

4 Leadership Principles 50
Exemplar: Empowering the Team—Johnese Spisso 56
Jim O'Malley Envisions Leadership Transformation 73

5 Management Principles 79
Roxane Spitzer-Lehmann Envisions the Differences between
Leadership and Management 80

PART III

PLANNING IN NURSING ADMINISTRATION 103

6 Problem Solving 104
Exemplar: Relentless Incrementalism—Sandy Pirwitz 112

7 Decision Making 120

8 The Use of Groups, Committees, and Teams 144
Exemplar: Instituting a Nurse-Managed Clinic—Lynne A. Nezbeda 149

9 Budgeting and Financial Management 167
Christine Kovner Envisions Financial Management 179

PART IV

ORGANIZATIONAL DESIGN AND GOVERNANCE IN NURSING 189

10 Organizational Culture and Environment 190
    Margaret Sovie Envisions Shifting from Illness Care to Wellness Care . . . 202

11 Organizations, Mission Statements, Policies, and Procedures . . 208

12 Organizational Structure: Concepts 225

13 Organizational Structure: Types 241
    Exemplar: Restructuring the ICU Leadership Team—
    Deborah K. Charnley 252

14 Decentralization and Shared Governance 259
    Tim Porter-O'Grady Envisions Decentralization and
    Shared Governance 270

15 Delegation 278
    Exemplar: Changing the Skill Mix—Donna W. Markey 294

16 Nursing Care Delivery Systems 299
    Exemplar: Patient-Centered Care—Paula Siler and
    Cathy Lopez Houston 308

17 Case Management and Managed Care 318

PART V

MANAGING PROFESSIONALS AND THEIR PRACTICE 333

18 Communication 334
    Exemplar: Communicating Vision, Mission, and Values—Paula Siler
    and Cathy Lopez Houston 344
    Exemplar: Personal Touches—E. Mary Johnson 348

19 Motivation 357
    Exemplar: Motivating and Mentoring—Margaret Sandvig 371

20 Power 381
    Exemplar: Creating Expert Power—Sandy Pirwitz 387
    JoEllen Koerner Envisions Empowerment and
    Transformative Leadership 400

21 Conflict 406
    Exemplar: Effective Communication—Julie Henderson 423

22 Persuasion and Negotiation 431
    Exemplar: Renegotiating Advanced Practice Roles—Donna W. Markey . . 443

23 Staffing and Scheduling 448

PART VI

EVALUATION AND CONTROL IN NURSING
ADMINISTRATION 465

24   Computer Applications in Nursing Administration 466

25   Quality Improvement and Risk Management 481
      *Exemplar: Development and Implementation of
      a Pain Management Protocol—Sharon E. Melberg* 498

26   Management of Change 506
      Jim O'Malley Envisions Change . . . More Change . . . and Change Again! 509
      Exemplar: Creation of a Dedicated AIDS Unit—Sharon E. Melberg 511
      *Exemplar: Motivating and Promoting Staff to Take Ownership
      of the New CDU—Andrea Wasdovich and Elizabeth Kempe* 519

27   Performance Appraisal 529
      Exemplar: Staff Evaluations—Julie Henderson 538

28   Productivity and Costing Out Nursing 547

29   Managing a Stressful Environment 560
      JoEllen Koerner Envisions Nurturing the Self and Others 572

PART VII

FUTURE PERSPECTIVES 577

30   Health Policy and the Nurse 578
      *Peter Ungvarski Envisions the Importance of Nursing Research
      in Health Policy* 582

31   Career Development 592

APPENDIX: ANSWERS TO STUDY QUESTIONS 611

INDEX 659

PART I

The Environment

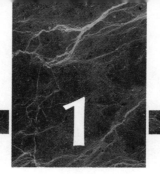

Overview of Nursing Administration

Chapter Objectives

ॐ

describe the study of nursing administration

ॐ

define nursing administration

ॐ

define leadership and management

ॐ

distinguish between leadership and management

ॐ

identify and compare theories and models for
nursing administration

ॐ

exercise critical thinking to conceptualize and analyze
possible solutions to a practical experience incident

*n*ursing is a service profession whose core mission is the care and nurturing of human beings in their experiences of health and illness. Nurses have two basic roles: care providers and care managers. In the United States the acute care medical model in hospitals was traditional. In this illness-focused model, the nurses' care provider role was emphasized. With a shift to managed care, the nurse's care management role has become more prominent.

> The delivery of nursing services involves the organization and coordination of complex activities which include both nursing and nonnursing tasks related to the health care needs of clients. Nursing administrators use managerial and leadership skills to facilitate delivery of quality nursing care (McCloskey, Gardner, Johnson, & Maas, 1988, p. 92).

In nursing administration, the perspective of nursing is combined with the methods of administration in order to manage client care. Nursing has evolved a subfield of the advanced practice of administration as a result of the "glue" phenomenon: nurses not only provide direct care to clients but also coordinate and manage the environment in which all providers deliver client care. Thomas (1983, pp. 66-67) observed:

> One thing the nurses do is hold the place together. . . . My discovery, as a patient first on the medical service and later in surgery, is that the institution is held together, glued together, enabled to function as an organism, by the nurses and by nobody else.

Thus the study of nursing administration is the creative investigation of the intersection of administrative methods with the practice of nursing. It focuses on nursing care management in order to accomplish health outcomes for clients.

DEFINITIONS

here is no uniformly accepted definition of nursing administration, although several have been proposed. Nursing service administration was defined by Arndt and Huckabay (1980, p. 21) as: "the process of setting and achieving objectives by influencing human behavior within a suitable environment." They noted that "determining the collective objectives of a nursing service organization and generating an environment for their achievement, therefore, is the total function of a nursing service administrator." (Arndt & Huckabay, 1980, p. 22).

Arndt and Huckabay (1980) constructed a model of administrative theory for nursing service. The act of administration was considered to be composed of conceptual and physical actions which combined to create a conceptual and physical environment related to both individual and organizational objectives. *Conceptual acts*, such as thinking and making decisions, are manifested in the intellectual processes of planning and organizing. *Physical acts*, such as communicating and implementing programs, are manifested in the doing processes of directing and controlling. Administration was viewed as a composite process made up of the individual components of planning, organizing, directing, and controlling. The nursing service administrator was seen as a composite process specialist, whose prime task was to create a healthy physical, mental, and interpersonal work climate that will induce others to willingly contribute their efforts to achieve the objectives of the institution.

> Nursing administration can be broadly defined as those persons who through their actions within a situational context manage courses of affairs specific to the provision of nursing now and at future times to described populations served by an institution, and in so doing exercise powers given them by the established authorities of

the formally constituted enterprise, the purposes of which are accomplished in whole (Orem, 1989, p. 55).

Orem's (1989) approach differentiated nurse providers who manage the work of client care for persons and groups from nurse managers who manage nursing services for organizations. Orem saw nursing administration as nursing-oriented but embedded within an organizational structure and bounded by vested managerial power.

Scalzi and Anderson (1989, p.137) described one view of nursing administration as "the application of administrative knowledge to nursing to provide quality nursing care." Their new definition, derived from what is called a system view model, is that the practice of nursing administration is:

> The use of the system perspective to maximize system vitality through the assessment and management of system concerns. The system of concern to nursing administration is composed of the nursing and organizational domains and their interface. System vitality comprises quality nursing products and organizational effectiveness (Scalzi & Anderson,1989, p.140).

Hermansdorfer, Henry, Moody, and Smyth (1990) said that nursing administration focuses on the production, distribution, and impact of nursing services and on the practitioners and organizational units responsible for those services. Allison, McLaughlin, and Walker (1991, p. 73) developed a straightforward definition: nursing administration "is responsible for ensuring a reasonable quality of delivery of nursing services. It must also facilitate the work of the nurses in the delivery process in a fiscally responsible way and create an environment that supports professional growth and development."

There is no one accepted definition, theory, or model to describe nursing administration. Commonalities among definitions include: a synthesis of management theory with nursing practice; the use of power and authority to provide quality and effective nursing care; and managing both nursing care and a delivery system in order to generate an environment to achieve an organization's objectives. Thus, for the purposes of this textbook, the various definitions of nursing administration will be synthesized into one definition. The definition of *nursing administration* is: the creative combination of leadership and management knowledge and skill applied to the practice of nursing for the purposes of organizing nursing care delivery, coordinating and managing client care, and creating a positive work climate. Within an organization, nursing administration is concerned with the use of power and authority to provide quality and effective care and with managing both nursing care delivery and a delivery system in order to generate an environment to achieve an organization's goals.

Leadership and management emerge as the two major organizing frameworks for understanding nursing administration. *Leadership* is defined as the process of influencing people to accomplish goals. *Management* is defined as the coordination and integration of resources through planning, organizing, coordinating, directing, and controlling in order to accomplish specific institutional goals and objectives. Thus leadership can occur in any group, whereas management is focused on an organization or institution, usually an employer of nurses.

BACKGROUND

Nursing administration knowledge is derived from three primary sources: nursing theory, management theory, and leadership theory. The two most commonly identified disciplines for nurse managers to synthesize are nursing and management (Stevens, 1979). Dienemann (1989) noted that nursing administration integrates knowledge from nursing and organizational theory to design, implement, and monitor productive nursing delivery systems in organizational contexts.

Knowledge, concepts, and theories useful to nursing administration can be drawn from anthropology, business, economics, education, hospital administration, management science, political science, psychology, social work, sociology, and public health. These other areas likewise might draw useful knowledge, concepts, and applications from nursing administration.

Some theories from the other areas that have been applied to nursing administration include systems theory, bureaucratic theory, economic theory, management theory, organizational behavior theory, conflict theory, structural systems theory, and strategic choice theories (Dienemann, 1989). In an analysis of nursing administration research from 1976-1986, Hermansdorfer et al (1990) found that one third of the nursing administration studies used some perspective in administrative theory. Theories of motivation, role, decision making, leadership, communication, and conflict, applied at the level of individuals, were found to be the administrative theories most often used. These individual-level theories have been the most common focus of nursing administration research. Group level research is more difficult and complex to do.

Meleis and Jennings (1989) found that the theoretical basis of nursing administration relied primarily on managerial, sociological, and psychological frameworks. Nurse administrators appear to use and apply organizational, role, social exchange, change, social, motivational, and general systems theories. The use of business and management models by nurse administrators can be likened to the use of the medical model by nurses to shape clinical practice. The challenge is to develop a synthesis in which nursing care is the focus of both nursing leadership and management.

LEADERSHIP AND MANAGEMENT IMPLICATIONS

Leadership theory, although integral to nursing administration, often is discussed separately from management theory. Their area of overlap may not be clear or explained. The premise of this textbook is that leadership and management are not identical ideas. They are distinct, and yet they overlap (see Fig. 1.1). Both leadership and management will be explored separately in Chapters 4 and 5, and their intersection will be developed within each of the chapters in order to better integrate the two concepts with nursing practice.

Clearly one trend in the nursing administration literature has been to draw from business and management ideas. There is a need for nurses to have a solid foundation of knowledge in care management. This applies at all levels: nurse care provider, nurse manager, and nurse executive. However, the depth and focus of care management roles and skills may vary by level. For example, the nurse care provider concentrates on the coordination of nursing care to individuals or groups. This may include such activities as access to services, direct care provision, referrals, and family support. In contrast, the nurse manager concentrates on the day-to-day administration of services provided by a group of nurses. The nurse executive's role and function concentrates on long-term administration of an institution or program that delivers nursing services.

If the delivery of nursing services involves the organization and coordination of complex activities in the human services realm, then both leadership and management are important elements. Their definitions indicate that they are not isomorphic with each other. Bennis (1989) noted that the leader focuses on people; the manager focuses on systems and structure. Thus while both are processes used to accomplish goals, each focus is different. For exam-

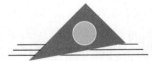 *Leadership & Management Behaviors*

LEADERSHIP BEHAVIORS

- influences people to accomplish group goals
- inspires confidence
- envisions the future
- motivates followers
- guides or leads the way

MANAGEMENT BEHAVIORS

- coordinates resources
- integrates the use of resources
- plans
- organizes
- directs
- controls
- accomplishes specific institutional goals and objectives

OVERLAP AREAS

- plans for goal accomplishment
- motivates and directs followers

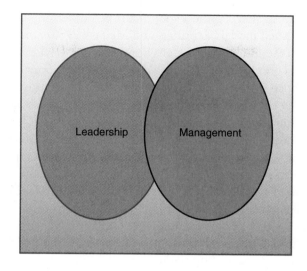

Figure 1.1
The relationship between leadership and management.

ple, a nurse may use leadership strategies or management strategies to motivate others. However, the desired outcome of the motivation is likely to be different. There are, however, similarities between leadership and management in an area of overlap. In the area of overlap, the processes and strategies look similar and may be employed for a similar outcome.

CURRENT ISSUES AND TRENDS

Without an organized nursing administration knowledge base, some may question why nurses are not taught administration in established business colleges (McCloskey et al., 1988). Theories and models help to explain the scientific base for studying nursing administration and its potential contribution to nursing practice. A good model identifies relationships among important variables.

Although there is no one generally accepted theory of nursing administration, there are some examples of available theories and models. Arndt and Huckabay (1980) developed an administrative model within a systems frame of reference. Scalzi and Anderson (1989) proposed a conceptual model of nursing administration called the system view model. Orem (1989) considered her descriptive explanation of nursing administration to be a general theory of nursing administration. In general, however, development of the theoretical basis of nursing administration did not receive much attention until the late 1980s.

There have been several beginning efforts to formulate models for nursing administration (Blair, 1989; Gardner, Kelly, Johnson, McCloskey, & Maas, 1991; Jennings & Meleis, 1988; Johnson, Gardner, Kelly, Maas, & McCloskey,

1991; 1992; Kim, 1988; Scalzi & Anderson, 1989). In one of the first published models, Jennings and Meleis (1988) combined concepts of person, interaction, transition, environment, and health. Kim (1988) proposed a model of administrative knowledge that included nursing requirements, nursing service practice, nursing organization, and the environment. Blair's (1989) model reviews nursing administration knowledge as an overlapping area of nursing with administration. Scalzi and Anderson's (1989) model depicts nursing administration knowledge as an interface of organization knowledge and nursing knowledge within the broader social context. These models attempt to organize the knowledge base of nursing administration. They present a visual display of the relationships among the important concepts related to nursing administration.

Two key features emerge: (1) the degree of integration of clinical nursing and nursing administration knowledge, and (2) a synthesis of nursing and management knowledge. The concept of leadership has not been obvious in these models. Leadership is a subconcept in the Iowa Model: it is one process at the organization level in the systems domain. Thus the Iowa Model has the advantage of lending itself to identifying and explaining both leadership and management concepts.

Figure 1.2 shows the Iowa Model of Nursing Administration (Gardner et al., 1991; Johnson et al., 1991; 1992). Within the context of the larger envi-

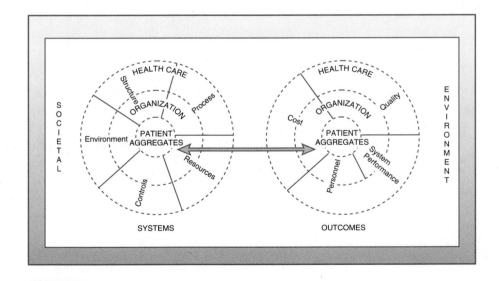

Figure 1.2
The Iowa Model of Nursing Administration. (Reprinted with permission from the NSA Program, The University of Iowa College of Nursing, Iowa City, Iowa.)

ronment, two domains are identified: systems and outcomes. Administrative practice occurs within identifiable systems for the purpose of achieving specific outcomes. Outcomes are necessary to evaluate both systems and managerial effectiveness. Three levels are specified within both systems and outcomes: patient aggregates, organizations, and health care. Thus the Iowa Model addresses the differences among levels when discussing the relationships among important ideas. The Iowa Model incorporates an open systems orientation. As a model, the Iowa Model is useful for identifying nursing administration knowledge and the content of nursing administration practice. Its richness lies in the integration of complex concepts and its comprehensiveness. Both leadership and management subconcepts are included. Research questions can be derived, and the model can be applied to practice for purposes such as evaluation, managing change, and leadership and management education.

RESEARCH NOTE

Source: Gardner, D., Kelly, K., Johnson, M., McCloskey, J., & Maas, M. (1991). Nursing administration model for administrative practice. *Journal of Nursing Administration, 21*(3), 37-41.

Purpose

The purpose of this article was to apply the Iowa Model of Nursing Administration to administrative practice in nursing. The model is displayed, described, and discussed. This research in theory and model development is explained by two examples of the model's relevance to specific practice situations: the use of nurse extenders and discharge planning systems.

Discussion

The Iowa Model of Nursing Administration has the two domains of systems and outcomes within the context of the environment. There are three levels in each domain: patient aggregates, the organization, and the healthcare level. This open systems-type model indicates that interactions flow back and forth between domains and among levels. As a simplified model, this visualization displays, describes, and clarifies important variables and their linkages. It suggests relationships between and among elements and levels of activity.

Application to Practice

The Iowa Model can be used in four ways: as a guide for thinking about nursing administration, as a road map for planning, as a means to facilitate decision making, and as a method of communication about important practice elements and their relationships. Models can be useful for describing, explaining, and predicting outcomes. This model provides a perspective of nursing administrative practice. It can be used to guide decision making and for evaluating change.

SUMMARY

- With a shift to managed care, the care management role of the nurse has taken on a renewed importance.
- Nursing administration is viewed as a combination of nursing leadership and management.
- Leadership and management are separate but overlapping ideas.
- There is no one accepted definition, theory, or model to describe nursing administration.
- Commonalities among definitions include:
  a. a synthesis of management theory with nursing practice
  b. the use of power and authority to provide quality and effective nursing care, and
  c. managing both nursing care and a delivery system in order to generate an environment to achieve an organization's objectives.
- Individual level theories, such as motivation, communication, and conflict, have been the most common focus of nursing administration research.
- Among the fairly recent models, the Iowa Model incorporates both leadership and management subconcepts.

Study Questions

1. Does nursing administration differ from nursing practice? If so, how?
2. Are all nurses managers or is management more properly confined to levels above staff nurses?
3. Are all nurses care coordinators? Is this the same as being a manager?
4. Should a nurse follow a theory of administration as well as a theory of nursing?

Critical Thinking Exercise

Nurse Jones graduated with a BSN. It was tough to find a traditional hospital staff nurse job, but Nurse Jones now has 6 months experience in adult medical nursing. There are rumors of an impending layoff of nurses. Prior layoffs have followed strict seniority criteria. Nurse Jones knows of two openings in other places: one as a charge nurse in a long-term care facility and one as a case manager in ambulatory care. Nurse Jones is considering a job change.

1. What is the problem?

2. What are the key issues?

3. How should Nurse Jones handle this situation?

4. Which roles are nursing administration roles? Why?

5. Is Nurse Jones prepared for a nursing administration role?

6. How can Nurse Jones prepare to interview for the two available openings?

7. What (if any) additional education should Nurse Jones consider?

REFERENCES

Allison, S., McLaughlin, K., & Walker, D. (1991). Nursing theory: A tool to put nursing back into nursing administration. *Nursing Administration Quarterly, 15*(3), 72-78.

Arndt, C., & Huckabay, L. (1980). *Nursing administration: Theory for practice with a systems approach* (2nd ed.). St. Louis: Mosby.

Bennis, W. (1994). *On becoming a leader.* Reading, MA: Addison-Wesley.

Blair, E. (1989). Nursing and administration: A synthesis model. *Nursing Administration Quarterly, 13*(2), 1-11.

Dienemann, J. (1989). Theoretical perspectives in organization science for nursing administration. In B. Henry, C. Arndt, M. DiVincenti, & A. Marriner-Tomey (Eds.), *Dimensions of nursing administration: Theory, research, education, practice* (pp. 159-174). Boston: Blackwell.

Gardner, D., Kelly, K., Johnson, M., McCloskey, J., & Maas, M. (1991). Nursing administration model for administrative practice. *Journal of Nursing Administration, 21*(3), 37-41.

Hermansdorfer, P., Henry, B., Moody, L., & Smyth, K. (1990). Analysis of nursing administration research, 1976-1986. *Western Journal of Nursing Research, 12*(4), 546-557.

Jennings, B., & Meleis, A. (1988). Nursing theory and administrative practice: Agenda for the 1990s. *Advances in Nursing Science, 10*(3), 56-69.

Johnson, M., Gardner, D., Kelly, K., Maas, M., & McCloskey, J. (1991). The Iowa model: A proposed model for nursing administration. *Nursing Economic$, 9*(4), 255-262.

Johnson, M., Gardner, D., Kelly, K., Maas, M., & McCloskey, J. (1992). The Iowa model of nursing administration. In B. Henry (Ed.), *Practice and inquiry for nursing administration: Intradisciplinary and interdisciplinary perspectives* (pp. 91-96). Washington, DC: American Academy of Nursing.

Kim, H. S. (1988). *Nursing knowledge and theory: Implications for nursing administration theories.* Paper presented at the Rockefeller Foundation International Conference on Nursing Administration. Bellagio, Italy.

McCloskey, J., Gardner, D., Johnson, M., & Maas, M. (1988). What is the study of nursing administration? *Journal of Professional Nursing, 4*(2), 92-98.

Meleis, A., & Jennings, B. (1989). Theoretical nursing administration: Today's challenges, tomorrow's bridges. In B. Henry, C. Arndt, M. DiVincenti, & A. Marriner-Tomey (Eds.), *Dimensions of nursing administration: Theory, research, education, practice* (pp. 7-18). Boston: Blackwell.

Orem, D. (1989). Nursing administration, a theoretical approach. In B. Henry, C. Arndt, M. DiVincenti, & A. Marriner-Tomey (Eds.), *Dimensions of nursing administration: Theory, research, education, practice* (pp. 55-62). Boston: Blackwell.

Scalzi, C., & Anderson, R. (1989). Conceptual model for theory development in nursing administration. In B. Henry, C. Arndt, M. DiVincenti, & A. Marriner-Tomey (Eds.), *Dimensions of nursing administration: Theory, research, education, practice* (pp. 137-141). Boston: Blackwell.

Stevens, B. (1979). Improving nurses' managerial skills. *Nursing Outlook, 27,* 774-777.

Thomas, L. (1983). *The youngest science: Notes of a medicine-watcher.* New York: Viking Press.

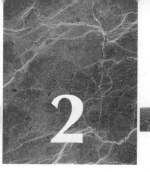

The Healthcare System

Chapter Objectives

☙

define and describe the U.S. healthcare system

☙

identify five types of healthcare organizations

☙

list four ways to differentiate healthcare organizations

☙

review U.S. healthcare costs

☙

analyze factors related to U.S. healthcare costs

☙

explain the role of nursing in the changing healthcare environment

☙

exercise critical thinking to conceptualize and analyze
possible solutions to a practical experience incident

*n*ursing, as an occupation, is embedded within the larger healthcare system. Thus it is important for nurses to understand the larger environment of which nursing is one component. For example, nurses practice and make decisions about nursing care. Yet the larger system impacts directly on nurses' ability to plan and implement care. Health policy and economics are examples of external forces impinging on nursing practice.

DEFINITIONS

asic health and medical care is a pervasive social need. *The healthcare system* is defined as all of the structures, organizations, and services designed to deliver professional healthcare services to consumers.

Weinerman (1971) defined the health services system as all of the activities of a society that are designed to protect or restore health, whether directed to the individual, community, or environment. Fuchs (1966) and Kovner (1990) developed working definitions for health services that included services from personnel engaged in medical occupations, physical plant, capital, and other goods and services (see Chart 2.1). Roemer (1986) noted that every system of health care has five main components: production of resources, organizational structure, management, economic support, and delivery of services. Pyramidal care delivery levels of primary, secondary, and tertiary have been described within the U.S. system of healthcare (Roemer, 1986).

Traditionally, U. S. healthcare has been organized around the physician and the acute care hospital. That is why the above definition equated health service with medical occupations even though not all healthcare is medical care. A triad of client, nurse, and physician became the basis of healthcare delivery, although not all members had equal status. For nursing this has meant that a higher status and greater resources have been devoted to medical care. Nursing has been seen as a medical support service. Clearly, nursing care delivery is the core function or backbone of acute care hospitals.

Today, healthcare is increasingly more complex, and care frequently is delivered by a multidisciplinary team of providers across a continuum of care. Nursing personnel constitute the largest group of healthcare providers in the United States. They are the healthcare personnel who both deliver and coordinate healthcare for clients. Therefore, nurses are poised to be the care providers most prepared for case management roles. As healthcare becomes coordinated and integrated across settings and sites, nurses will need to better understand the larger healthcare system. Five leading types of healthcare organizations were identified by Kovner (1990) as hospitals, ambulatory care, long-term care, home health, and mental health (see Chart 2.2). Identifying and discussing the types of healthcare organizations highlights the broader scope of healthcare services, beyond acute care hospitals, in which clients experience health and illness service delivery. Healthcare organizations can be differentiated in four ways:

1. The focus of care (e.g., surgical, hospice, or maternity)
2. The geographic area served (e.g., community hospital, local Public Health Nursing Agency, regional medical center, or U.S. Public Health Service-national)
3. Ownership category (e.g., public or private)
4. Revenue structure (e.g., incorporated for tax purposes as for-profit or not-for-profit).

The 1990s look to be a time of integration within the healthcare delivery system. Changing reimbursement structures have triggered strategic alliances and networks among hospitals and other health delivery services. Negotiation

Jim O'Malley
Envisions Transforming
the American Healthcare System

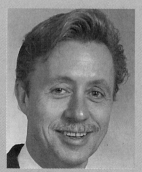

Jim O'Malley

Healthcare reform, along with managed care and capitation, are driving the transformation of the American health care system. The next critical step in redefining the context and structures of our healthcare systems is characterized by a transition from multi-hospital systems to integrated delivery networks. By definition, integrated delivery networks are a series of consensual linkages and partnerships which organize and align risks and rewards for providing healthcare to a defined population over time between providers, hospitals, and payors. As a model, its success is contingent upon creating a shared vision and reaching a high level of cooperation and collaboration among all of its partners in achieving high quality–low cost outcomes.

Integrated delivery networks differ significantly from multi-hospital systems in that they do not own facilities and do not directly employ physicians or other healthcare providers. Networks link providers, facilities, and healthcare plans by collaboratively engaging in direct contracting and sharing financial risk and rewards under capitation. Successful network integration strategies have included (1) developing clinical care protocols to manage resources, (2) sharing of support functions and restructuring of operations to eliminate service redundancy, and (3) linking services and facilities to ensure a continuum of care. Ultimately, networks will need to move away from their loosely aligned organizations and formally consolidate clinical services, facilities, and providers. At best, networks will serve as a cooperative transitional strategy laying the groundwork for the inevitability of large scale mergers.

Jim O'Malley, MSN, RN, NP, CNS, is currently Senior Vice President of Nursing Services at Allegheny General Hospital, a large academic medical center in Pittsburgh, PA. In addition, he is on the faculties of the schools of nursing at the University of Pittsburgh and Duquesne University, where he holds the title of Associate Dean for Clinical Studies.

A nurse practitioner, clinical nurse specialist, and administrator, O'Malley is a recognized leader within the nursing profession. He has extensive operational experience in care delivery redesign, managed care, and the design and implementation of innovative roles for advanced practitioners. He has published and presented widely and serves as editor for *Advanced Practice Nursing Quarterly*. Additionally, he serves on the editorial boards of *Aspen's Advisor for Nurse Executives*, *Nursing Administration Quarterly*, *Topics in Emergency Medicine*, and *Seminars for Nurse Managers*.

for managed care contracts has been a driving force. New integrated healthcare systems have arisen via mergers and acquisitions. Integration is the coordination of work across the various parts of an organization. Using systems theory as a framework, Stichler (1994) defined these *integrated healthcare systems* as interactive and interdependent healthcare units with their own identities and organizational structures that are grouped together, serve a common purpose, and are developed to meet expressed market needs. Thus they are a collection of healthcare providers, work interdependently, and function as an open system to adapt to changes in the healthcare industry and market forces. Financial pressures drive the creation of integrated healthcare systems. Efficiencies can be obtained by a systems approach to strategic planning, quality management, and human resource management. By all accounts, the implementation of these integrated healthcare systems is challenging, threatening, costly in some ways, and difficult overall. Culture, a sense of direction, and the creation of a shared vision are immediate leadership needs. Power, control, and turf issues can be expected to be encountered as systems struggle through the integration process (Stichler, 1994).

All healthcare organizations take their work, the delivery of healthcare services, and structure it into a formal organization that relates the jobs of the workers, the managers, and the support services together in some manner. Each type of organization has a certain structure, and within that structure are prescribed roles. The roles that people have will vary according to the skills that are needed. The skills needed for those roles will vary by level of authority (see Fig. 2.1). For example, the skills needed for the very top level of management require a greater vision and conceptual ability than do the specific technical skills in any field. The opposite is true at the lower levels of the organization. Despite the level, a solid ability to relate well to others is needed

Figure 2.1
Skill mix variance by level of authority. (From Hersey, P., and Blanchard, K. [1993]. MANAGEMENT OF ORGANIZATIONAL BEHAVIOR: Utilizing Human Resources, 6/E. Englewood Cliffs, N.J.: Prentice Hall, p. 8, and from 4/E. Reprinted with permission from the Center for Leadership Studies.)

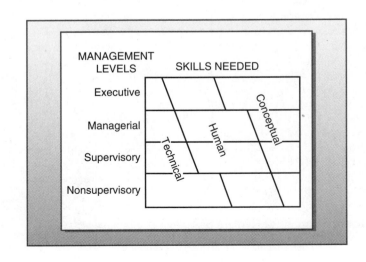

by all members in order to have a smooth running institution (Hersey & Blanchard, 1993).

RESEARCH NOTE

Source: Shindul-Rothschild, J., & Gordon, S. (1994). Single-payer versus managed competition: Implications for nurses. *Journal of Nursing Education, 33*(5), 198-207.

Purpose

The purpose of this critical analysis was to examine the research basis for claims of efficacy in the financing and cost-control approaches of "managed competition" and "single-payer" plans. The history of federal regulation and control of spending on hospital and physician services is reviewed and explained. The impact of regulation and competition on access to and quality of care is examined. Effects on nurses are specifically addressed. Single-payer systems are contrasted to managed competition systems within the framework of a critical approach to the healthcare reform process.

Discussion

The authors indicated that there is a lack of data-based evidence for the superiority of managed competition. Further, under competition there are layoffs of nurses and replacement with unlicensed assistive personnel. Nurses report an increased workload as downsizing occurs more rapidly and predictably. Administrative costs are less in a single-payer system. When administrative costs go up, dollars allocated to nursing go down. Thus nurses are impacted by the structure and financing of healthcare.

Application to Practice

The nursing community needs to be informed and analytical about health reform proposals and policies. Nurses may be disillusioned about the realities of the health reform impacts on healthcare delivery. Financial underpinnings of health reform may increase corporate control over healthcare. Nursing is an easy target, an expendable labor force when healthcare is a commodity in a system dominated by corporate interests and sustained by a select group of powerful providers. Nurses will need to monitor and lobby for successful implementation of a client-oriented system.

BACKGROUND

Healthcare Expenditures

In the 1980s, public attention became focused on the spiraling costs of healthcare. The mid-1980s saw the implementation of a new system of reimbursement, a prospective payment system, for Medicare clients in hospitals. An incentive was created to decrease the number of days of a hospital stay as a way to reduce costs. As Diagnostic Related Groups (DRGs) were implemented in hospitals in the mid-80s, a series of payment reforms were initiated, and cost containment became a necessity for hospitals. As the amount of money spent on healthcare continued to burgeon, physician payment reforms were initiated. The expenditures still grew and began to influence the competitive edge of U.S. businesses because employers bore the cost burden of health insurance benefits for their employees (Castro, 1993). By the early 1990s, the focus of the healthcare crisis expanded to include access to care. A considerable number of U.S. citizens had no healthcare coverage.

The federal government is the third-party payor source for approximately 42% of all expenditures for healthcare (U.S. Bureau of the Census, 1993). As a major financer of healthcare, the U.S. government provides access to care for a substantial portion of the elderly, disabled, and indigent. The majority of expenditures flow from two programs: Medicare and Medicaid. *Medicare* is a program of assistance with healthcare costs for the over-65 elderly and some disabled. It has two parts: Part A covers aspects of hospitalization and some nursing home care; Part B covers physician services. *Medicaid* is a joint federal and state program, administered by the states, designed to pay for indigents' healthcare, including maternal-child and nursing home care; and care for the disabled, blind, and families with dependent children (U.S. Bureau of the Census, 1993) (see Chart 2.3). There is tension in political spheres of influence between desires for expansion in federal healthcare financing and economic pressures for cost control. The very real burden of healthcare costs needs to be paid by someone, but who will do this and how is in dispute.

The published statistical data available from the federal government on healthcare expenditures lags behind the current situation by several years. Thus, although the most "recent" data are several years old, they can still be analyzed for trends and compared to data reported by professional associations. The total U.S. population is estimated to be about 255 million. Total U.S. healthcare expenditures were $751.8 billion in 1991. Large numbers of Americans, approximately 14% of the U.S. population, estimated to be 37 million in 1992, were uninsured. Medicare payments in 1991 were $118.55 billion. Even though approximately $77 billion was spent in the United States in Medicaid payments alone, one in seven Americans was not covered by any type of insurance (U.S. Bureau of the Census, 1993). The costs of healthcare prevent access unless the client is adequately insured, very wealthy, or eligible for government assistance.

The problem of allocation of money for healthcare relates to the total amount of money available and the soaring costs for healthcare in the United States. These problems have been accelerating since the 1970s. For example, in the United States, national healthcare expenditures rose 10.5% in one year between 1989 and 1990, from $602.8 billion to $666.2 billion (U.S. Bureau of

---

CHART 2.3
∽ DEFINITIONS

Medicare
a program of assistance with healthcare costs for the over-65 elderly and some disabled.

Medicaid
a joint federal and state program designed to pay for indigents' healthcare.

From U.S. Bureau of the Census (1993).

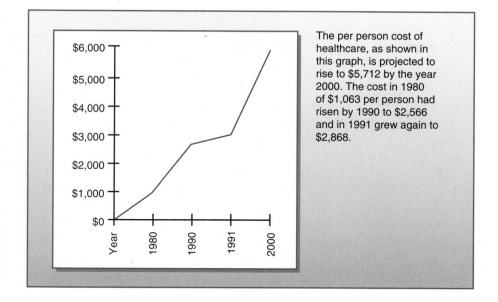

The per person cost of healthcare, as shown in this graph, is projected to rise to $5,712 by the year 2000. The cost in 1980 of $1,063 per person had risen by 1990 to $2,566 and in 1991 grew again to $2,868.

Figure 2.2
Per person cost of healthcare in the U.S. (Data from U. S. Bureau of the Census [1993].)

the Census, 1993). For 1991, healthcare spending rose by 11.4% to reach $751.8 billion, or 13.2% of the gross domestic product (*Hospitals*, 1993a). Outpatient care costs are expected to rise 15.8% annually over the next decade (Bocchino, 1992). Health costs are rising about four times faster than overall inflation (Castro, 1993). As a result, there has been a proliferation of managed care organizations, designed to drive down overall costs.

The per person cost of healthcare in the United States, which was $1,063 in 1980, is projected to multiply by 437% to $5,712 by the year 2000 (see Fig. 2.2). According to statistics compiled by the federal Health Care Financing Administration (HCFA) in 1992, the United States spent about $840 billion for healthcare. That is approximately 14% of the gross national product (GNP). The healthcare industry is clearly a major segment of the U.S. economy.

The prediction is that by the year 2000, healthcare costs in the United States will increase to $1.7 trillion, about 18% of the gross national product. Obviously, this is a lot of money. The statement that there is no money for healthcare is not exactly accurate. There is a substantial amount of money being spent on healthcare. Because the amount spent is rising, more and more of the productive U.S. economy is going into healthcare services. The largest and most recent price increases have been for hospitals. Temporarily, in the mid- to late 1980s, the annual increase in hospital costs was as low as 6%. However, the percent annual increase was 10.9% from 1989 to 1990, and from 1991 to 1992 the annual percentage increase was 8.8%, making hospital costs account for 38.4% of the total national health expenditures (U.S. Bureau of the Census, 1993).

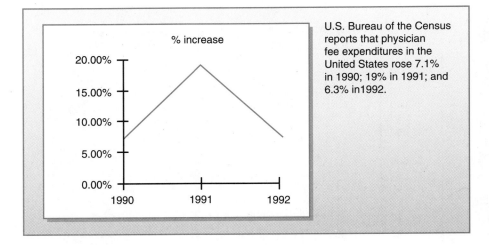

Figure 2.3
Physician fee increases.
(Data from U. S. Bureau of
the Census [1993].)

Physician fees, the second highest category of total expenditures, continue to rise, although at a lower rate of increase (U.S. Bureau of the Census, 1993) (see Fig. 2.3). Physicians' income now has come under the Medicare/Medic-aid/HCFA federal government review program. This review attempts to control, constrain, and increase or decrease certain physician fees based on relative value units. According to a 1992 survey, the direct median annual physician compensation ranged from $101,876 for family practice to $420,090 for cardiovascular surgery specialties (*Hospitals*, 1993b).

Prescription drugs rose 8.4% from 1989 to 1990 and 6.4% from 1991 to 1992. They are the third highest category of total expenditures. However, the rate of price increases, with some drugs doubling or tripling in a five year span, has focused attention on the pharmaceutical industry as a source of rising costs. Clients who have to take medications note that prescription drugs are a major cost item for them. In fact, many clients simply will not take their medication because they cannot afford it. Subsequent complications frequently increase the need for acute care in hospitals. This form of noncompliance is increasingly becoming a nursing care problem. Another rise is nursing home care, which has grown recently to become 8% of national health expenditures (U.S. Bureau of the Census, 1993). In both cases, nurses are challenged in working with clients and families to provide access to needed services and thereby enhance health and coping. Coordinating and managing care delivery are key strategies nurses use.

Nursing Compensation

Costs of nursing care increase as nursing salaries rise. One annual source for nursing salary information has been the *American Journal of Nursing* (Brider, 1991; 1992; 1993). It was reported in 1992 that starting salary rates

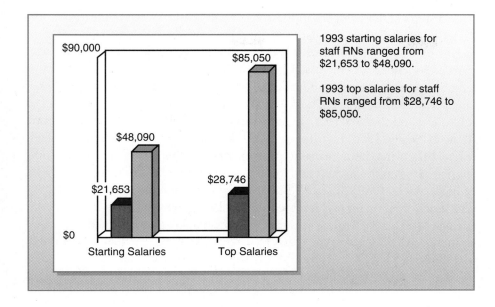

1993 starting salaries for staff RNs ranged from $21,653 to $48,090.

1993 top salaries for staff RNs ranged from $28,746 to $85,050.

Figure 2.4
1993 U.S. nursing salary ranges. (Data from Brider [1993].)

for staff nurses ranged from $21,000 to $45,000. Starting salaries ran highest in San Francisco, Boston, New York, Philadelphia, and Los Angeles. Top rates ranged from $30,000 to over $60,000. The national average salary for all staff nurses in 1992 was $34,462. Staff nurses with some experience typically earned $30-35,000, depending on the size of the institution and its location (Brider, 1992). By 1993, pay gains slowed and hospitals eliminated RN positions (see Fig. 2.4). The 1993 national average salary for all staff nurses was $35,982. The starting average was $27,625; the maximum pay averaged $41,559 (Brider, 1993). Salaries are increasing. Table 2.1 gives some nursing salary comparisons over time (AJN News, 1989; Brider, 1993).

Table 2.1

Average Salaries Paid to All Staff Nurses in the United States

YEAR	AVERAGE ANNUAL SALARY
1977	$12,948
1980	$17,398
1985	$18,750
1988	$28,383
1991	$32,257
1992	$34,462
1993	$35,982

Data from AJN News (1989) and Brider (1993).

Nursing's major compensation problem had been the lack of incentives for career longevity. Starting salaries for new graduates had increased in order to recruit nurses. Yet a nurse who had been in an organization for ten to forty years experienced a compressed salary range. Statistics showed a $7,000 difference between the new graduate and a nurse with four years of tenure. The salary scale was compacted to a $24,000 range between the base salary of a staff nurse and the director of nursing services, a small differential for a career (Cole & Sizing, 1988; Herzlinger, 1989). In one study, the majority of nurses reached their maximum earning potential in less than seven years. The difference between the highest and lowest salaries was 26% (Johnson, Holdwick, & Frederiksen, 1989). In 1992, Brider noted that the University of Texas' 30 year series of salary surveys reported that in 1982 a new graduate started at an average of $16,000, while a senior career nurse made a top salary of $21,000, an increase of 30% across the span of a career. The spread gradually broadened to 35% in 1983; 37% in 1985; 39% in 1987; 49% in 1991; and 51% in 1992. Salaries are tied into healthcare costs, because in a service industry the major cost component typically is the salary and benefits of the employees. Thus nursing salaries and job availability are sensitive to economic pressures from the healthcare system.

Other Cost Factors

Some of the other factors influencing healthcare costs include:
* the aging of the population, changing ethnicity patterns, and increasing chronicity of illness
* government regulation and administrative costs for insurance handling
* lack of practice standardization and defensive medicine
* accelerating use of sophisticated technology, and the equating of quality with high-tech care
* insurance companies had been paying whatever physicians and hospitals asked for, rather than being cost-based for reimbursement
* medical influence: physician fees account for about 20% of medical costs; physician decisions are thought to control about 80% of medical costs; there are increased numbers of physicians with increased specialization, and incomes amounting to about five times that of other professionals (Grace, 1990; Menzel, 1986)
* clients had not been paying the bills directly; however, clients with co-insurance and deductibles now are paying part of the costs
* consumer expectations and lack of health practices
* new diseases and treatments
* cost shifting to capture reimbursement
* overcapacity of hospital beds

Approximately $225 billion a year is being spent on diagnostic testing. Some of these tests are no more than 80% accurate. As consumers begin to bear the burden of rising costs, they are questioning the effectiveness and necessity of these tests. Third party reimbursers question the need for the tests, when, for example, coronary angiography was shown to be inappropriate in 17% of cases (Chassin, Kosecoff, Solomon & Brook, 1987).

There has been little focus on reimbursement for prevention. The focus has been on paying for acute inpatient hospital care. In the past, there was no reimbursement for preventive care, only for illness care. Therefore, where the money is being spent becomes an issue in relation to the costs of healthcare and how to bring them down.

The cost of AIDS care, for example, is projected to be a major factor within the total healthcare economy. One federal researcher estimated the national cost for treating all people with HIV at $10.3 billion in 1992, rising to $15.2 billion in 1995 (*Hospitals*, 1993c).

Reimbursement

How do the bills get paid in healthcare? Two ways: the client pays or a third-party payor takes care of the payment. About 35% of all healthcare costs are paid by the client, and 65% are covered by the third-party payors (U.S. Bureau of the Census, 1993). Third-party payors include private insurers such as Blue Cross and Blue Shield or government programs for the indigent including Title XIX and Medicare or Medicaid. The healthcare system appears to be splitting into four tiers: indigent without any coverage, people on government assistance, people with health insurance, and the wealthy who can afford private healthcare (Grace, 1990).

LEADERSHIP AND MANAGEMENT IMPLICATIONS

The anticipated changes in the U.S. healthcare delivery system appear to offer exciting opportunities for the value of nursing to emerge and be recognized. Since nurses manage and coordinate the environment in which all providers deliver client care, as well as directly providing some of that care, managed care programs will rely on the expertise and actions of nurses. As healthcare delivery changes to emphasize primary care, nursing is poised to become the mainstay of the healthcare delivery system. Thus, this has been identified as the "age of the nurse."

Healthcare forecasters predict that by the year 2000, the principal point of care delivery will no longer be at the acute care hospital. Care will most likely be community-based. If the healthcare delivery system is reformed in this dramatic way, the roles and functions of the nurse will undergo a simultaneous

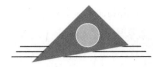 *Leadership & Management Behaviors*

LEADERSHIP BEHAVIORS	**MANAGEMENT BEHAVIORS**	**OVERLAP AREAS**
• understands the healthcare system	• understands the healthcare system	• understands the system
• is knowledgeable about healthcare economics and finance	• is knowledgeable about healthcare costs and charges	• understands the impact of economic and healthcare policies on nursing service delivery
• provides planning and direction for salary equity and workforce skill mix	• administers the salary structure and position control plan	
• guides the organization's human resources policies	• implements human resources policies	
• fosters creativity and innovation	• manages resources and reduces costs	

dramatic change. A de-emphasis on acute medical care creates an environment for nursing's skills to be in demand. Release from the bureaucratic mold initiates new avenues for nursing practice to develop toward a true professional model. The education, preparation, and reward structure for RNs will need to change to ensure the preparation needed to assume practice responsibilities within the changed delivery system.

Leadership in nursing is knowing the group's goals and how to get to the "preferred future." Innovation in the form of fostering creativity and the implementation of new ideas is a key strategy. Nurses have the skills to focus on the care of special populations, such as the elderly, and on community services. Nursing will need to make strides in solving internal problems such as diverse educational levels and in generating research to demonstrate effectiveness.

CURRENT ISSUES AND TRENDS

Consumers are highly sensitized to the huge bills incurred by hospital admissions. Disposable supplies have been cited as a hospital's second largest expense after salaries (Perry, 1994). Further, media publicity identified that the typical hospital bill totals $10,000 and is likely to contain mistakes or overcharges that range from $500 to $700 (Wang, 1992). Auditors hired by insurance companies estimate that two-thirds of all hospital bills contain mistakes in the hospital's favor, with overcharges of 5% to 7% on most bills (see Fig.

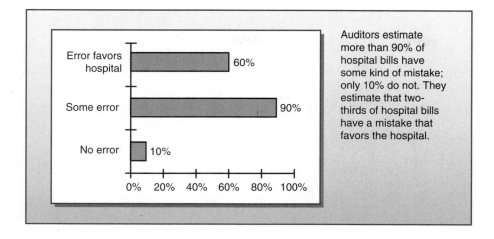

Auditors estimate more than 90% of hospital bills have some kind of mistake; only 10% do not. They estimate that two-thirds of hospital bills have a mistake that favors the hospital.

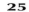

Figure 2.5
Estimated hospital billing errors. (Data from Wang [1992].)

2.5). The most common billing errors were inaccurate, duplicate, or inappropriate charges (Wang, 1992).

Masson (1992) suggested that nurses "count the costs." An awareness of what healthcare services are costing a client helps nurses in their role as client advocates. If baseline bloodwork costs $30, an upper-GI series costs $330, thirty Zantac tablets cost $47, plus the cost of office visits; then a client with a part-time job at McDonald's and no health insurance cannot afford "the best" care. The more practical goal may become "adequate" care, not "the best" care. Today and for the future, the challenges to all who work within the healthcare system will revolve around the triple tensions of access, cost, and quality. Challenges are projected to arise around issues of:

- availability/affordability of care
- effectiveness/outcomes
- regulation
- quality
- balance of service ethics with business profitability
- episodic versus continuum of care
- governance/practice models/human resources management

The twin pressures of cost and access have resulted in a public awareness of and readiness for change. Dramatic changes in healthcare are predicted for the near future under healthcare reform scenarios. The term most commonly identified in relation to medical healthcare reform is "managed competition," sometimes called "managed care" (Enthoven & Kronick, 1989). Under this system, large health plans that offer all necessary health services for a set fee per client per year would be formed. The plans would compete for clients, based on cost and quality. Influence would be brought to bear on employers and employees to choose the least costly plans. The government would cover the unemployed, the elderly, and women and children who are uninsured. Other measures, such as tighter controls on capital for hospitals, are predicted to force collaboration, alliances, cooperatives, and comprehensive health planning through local healthcare networks. The most likely reform plan is aimed at controlling healthcare costs first and then phasing in health coverage for all Americans (AHA, 1993).

SUMMARY

- The healthcare system is comprised of organizations and services designed to deliver professional healthcare to society.
- The five leading types of healthcare organizations each have a certain structure with defined roles.
- Costs in the healthcare sector of the economy have been rising at a dramatic rate, creating a problem of access and payment burdens.
- The rapid increase in costs has created national pressure for reform.
- Nurses have, and continue to play, a key coordinative role that may emerge as crucial as the healthcare delivery system changes.

Study Questions

1. What are the recent and projected developments in healthcare delivery? Are they changing?
2. What developments will challenge nurse leaders and managers the most?
3. Where should nurses focus their vision and energy for the improvement of health services?
4. Does the emphasis on cost containment overshadow nursing's role as a caring client advocate?
5. Should nursing control healthcare costs by slowing or halting nursing salary/benefit increases?

Critical Thinking Exercise

Nurse Smith works in a busy ambulatory care clinic. The organization is very concerned about holding down costs and processing patients rapidly. Nurse Smith is assigned to care for Mrs. Greenjeans, a 60-year-old newly diagnosed diabetic with a blood glucose over 400. She is accompanied by six family members and had to travel a great distance to reach the clinic. She would have come for care sooner, but was afraid of the cost and the time away from work that it took to travel and receive care. Some family members seem confused about what is going on.

1. *What is the problem?*

2. *What are the key issues?*

3. *How should Nurse Smith handle this situation?*

4. *What priorities related to care delivery might be competing?*

5. *What ethical dilemmas might arise?*

6. *What pressures might arise?*

REFERENCES

AJN News. (1989). The nation's RN population now tops 2,000,000; Hospital employment growing at fastest rate. *American Journal of Nursing, 89*(9), 1230.

Bass, B. (1985). *Leadership and performance beyond expectations.* New York: Free Press.

AHA. (1993). Clinton's election to affect health care planners, marketers. *Healthcare Planning and Marketing, 16*(1), 1-2.

Bocchino, C (1992). Transition . . . A time for change. *Nursing Economic$, 10*(6), 432, 434.

Brider, P. (1991). Solid gains behind leaner times ahead. *American Journal of Nursing, 91*(2), 28-36.

Brider, P. (1992). Salary gains slow as more RNs seek full-time benefits. *American Journal of Nursing, 92*(3), 34-40.

Brider, P. (1993). Where did the jobs go? *American Journal of Nursing, 93*(4), 31-40.

Castro, J. (1993). Paging Dr. Clinton. *Time, 141*(3), 24-26.

Chassin, M., Kosecoff, J., Solomon, D., & Brook, R. (1987). How coronary angiography is used. *Journal of the American Medical Association, 258*(18), 2543-2547.

Cole, B., & Sizing, M. (1988). Nurse compensation. *Modern Healthcare, 18*(49), 24-47.

Enthoven, A., & Kronick, R.(1989). A consumer-choice health plan for the 1990s. *New England Journal of Medicine, 320*(1), 30-37.

Fuchs, V. (1966). The contribution of health services to the American economy. *The Milbank Memorial Fund Quarterly, 44*(4), 65-101.

Grace, H. (1990). Can health care costs be contained? *Nursing & Health Care, 11*(3), 125-130.

Hersey, P., & Blanchard, K. (1993). *Management of organizational behavior: Utilizing human resources* (6th ed.). Englewood Cliffs, NJ: Prentice Hall.

Herzlinger, R. (1989). The failed revolution in health care—The role of management. *Harvard Business Review, 89*(2), 95-103.

Hospitals. (1993a). HHS: Health care spending at 13.2% of 1991 GDP. *Hospitals, 67*(4),8.

Hospitals. (1993b). Direct median physician compensation, by specialty. *Hospitals, 67*(2), 12.

Hospitals. (1993c). AIDS tab to grow. *Hospitals, 67*(2), 8.

Johnson, J., Holdwick, C., & Frederiksen, S. (1989). A non-traditional approach to wage adjustment. *Nursing Management, 20*(11), 36-39.

Kovner, A. (1990). *Health care delivery in the United States* (4th ed.). New York: Springer.

Masson, V. (1992). Seven keys to nursing. *American Journal of Nursing, 92*(10), 12.

Menzel, P. (1986). *Medical costs, moral choices.* New Haven, CT: Yale University Press.

Perry, N. (1994). Undercover in a hospital. *Money, 23*(12), 140-145.

Roemer, M. (1986). *An introduction to the US health care system* (2nd ed). New York: Springer.

Stichler, J. (1994). System development and integration in healthcare. *Journal of Nursing Administration, 24*(10), 48-53.

U. S. Bureau of the Census. (1993). *Statistical abstract of the United States* (113th ed.). Washington, DC: U.S. Government Printing Office.

Wang, P. (1992). Here's how to spot mistakes and get a refund. *Money, 21*(3), 138-142.

Weinerman, E. R. (1971). Research on comparative health service systems. *Medical Care, 9*(3), 272-290.

Professional
Nursing Practice

Chapter Objectives

❧

define and describe a profession

❧

define professional, professionalism, and professionalization

❧

compare the criteria for a profession to nursing

❧

analyze service, knowledge, autonomy, and legal and
ethical aspects of professionalization in nursing

❧

relate nursing to a continuum of professionalization

❧

identify barriers to true professional status for nursing

❧

explain influences on nursing as a profession

❧

exercise critical thinking to conceptualize and analyze
possible solutions to a practical experience incident

*i*s nursing a profession? Does the distinction of being recognized as a profession matter, or is it a waste of nurses' energy to fret over this designation?
Quinn and Smith (1987) asserted that nursing's claim that it is a profession is
the source of many major issues in nursing. This is because of nurses' behaviors, societal attitudes, and the type of social institutions that encompass the
practice of nursing. Nursing has been described as an occupational grey area

because some nurses consider themselves to be and act as professionals while others do not; some parts of society treat nurses as professionals while others do not; and in some institutions nurses are autonomous professionals while in others they are dependent, semiskilled employees. This inconsistency creates a problem for classifying nursing either as a profession or as a nonprofessional occupation. Nursing has struggled with elements of large size, diversity of levels of educational preparation, and intra-occupational differences in its quest for the status of full profession.

A profession is comprised of a system of roles that are socially defined. Thus changes in society influence professions. This occurs because professions are social institutions designed to serve some important function and to advance the welfare of society. Professions are said to have a contract with society: society grants professions broad autonomy and prestige. However, this means that there are duties and responsibilities of professions to provide a service and uphold the public's trust.

There are economic and psychological reasons why occupations desire professional status: their members enjoy higher prestige, income, and independence or autonomy over their work (McCloskey, 1981; Quinn & Smith, 1987). Professions have begun to occupy an increasingly important position in the United States as the shift to an information and service society has accelerated. Professions have become an important aspect of the provision of necessary services in highly industrialized and urban societies. Active involvement in a profession and having a professional identity provide individuals with career goals and opportunities for self-actualization and enhanced self-esteem (Stuart, 1981).

Professionalism is important to nurses because it affects the way nurses think about themselves professionally and about their work. Further, professionalism is one antecedent variable postulated as important in causal models of nursing turnover (Price & Mueller, 1981). For a variety of reasons, the movement to professionalize nursing has been important to every generation of nurses (Brodie, 1994).

DEFINITIONS

 profession is defined as a calling, vocation, or form of employment that provides a needed service to society and possesses characteristics of expertise, autonomy, long academic preparation, commitment, and responsibility. Quinn and Smith (1987) defined professions as requiring:

- complex knowledge base
- commitment to the direct benefit of humans

- minimal societal control over practice
- organization within itself for effective control of practice

The word profession is an abstract term, referring to a broad category of an organized occupation. "Profession" is a word that is assigned by society to an occupational group. Law, medicine, and theology are considered to be the traditional full professions (McCloskey, 1981; Miller, 1988; Quinn & Smith, 1987). However, the word professional is used commonly by a variety of people and occupations. For example, there are self-identified professional plumbers, beauticians, and carpenters. Sometimes licensure is confused with professionalism, when it is assumed that one is a professional if one must be licensed by the state. The value of the word professional can be decreased as a variety of groups use it indiscriminately (Wilensky, 1964).

One way of defining a profession is to use a checklist of criteria. There are specific criteria that any occupational group must meet in order to be considered a full profession. This idea originated with Flexner (1910), who identified the criteria for a profession from an analysis of the acknowledged professions of law, medicine, and theology (Parsons, 1986). The use of the word profession technically means that the members of an occupational group have met all the criteria that are generally acknowledged to be necessary to meet the definition of a full profession. This means that the majority of the members have attained an identified level of accomplishment (Davis, 1966; Hall, 1969). Another way of defining a profession is to look at the skill level required to do the work. The difference between a professional and one who is not is the knowledge, expertise, and complexity that is needed in the decision making of an occupation. According to the *International Standard Classification of Occupations* (1990), professionals are at the fourth skill level: education beginning at age 17 to 18, lasting 3 to 4+ years, and leading to a University degree.

There are four terms used in discussing a profession: profession, professional, professionalism, and professionalization. The word *professional* means one who is engaged in a profession. An individual who is professional meets and conforms to the standards of his or her profession. *Professionalism* is defined as the extent to which the individual identifies with a profession and adheres to its standards (McCloskey & McCain, 1987; Price & Mueller, 1981). Professionalism has also been viewed as the degree to which a group directs its own evolution (Fiesta, 1983). *Professionalization* is the dynamic process where occupations such as nursing can be observed changing in the direction of a true profession. It is the process whereby an occupational group moves from non-professional status to professional status, and the group or occupation becomes a profession (Hall, 1968; McCloskey, 1981; Stuart, 1981; Vollmer & Mills, 1966).

BACKGROUND

Is nursing a profession? There have been a variety of conclusions drawn about nursing's professional status (Bixler & Bixler, 1945; 1959; Quinn & Smith, 1987; Sleicher, 1981). Some writers feel nursing has accrued all the external trappings of a profession (Hawkins, 1992), while others view the quest for professionalism as a key element in marginalizing nursing and constraining its knowledge development (Wuest, 1994). The majority of nurses practice nursing as employees of an organization. Nurses consider themselves professional employees. In a complex and highly technological environment such as healthcare today, the work of nursing can be argued to be professional because it requires a high level of expertise and sophisticated decision making.

There may be two ways of viewing professionalism: an external view and an internal view. The external view posits that diversity in educational preparation is problematic for classifying nurses as professional. This is because although discretion and decision making occur, nursing's lack of differentiated practice results in the employer's difficulty in assigning classification as a professional when there are three educational levels equated within one job assignment and when the job assignment does not distinguish among caregivers as to the sophistication of the decision making. Nursing cannot ignore the outside world. It will be difficult for nursing to move along with professionalization until the external view of professionalism is attended to by differentiating nursing practice.

The external view also incorporates the reality of two approaches to labeling professionalism. The traditional way labels law, medicine and the clergy as professions, based on education, knowledge, and service aspects. The other approach is the modern one of looking at occupations as being professions if their practitioners routinely use a level of decision making and judgment with discretion that is usually associated with a baccalaureate education. Nursing has relied on licensure as the basis for professionalism until recently, when nurses began to emphasize their expertise and clinical decision making skills.

In the internal view, nurses see themselves as professionals. As viewed from within the occupation, nurses may see professionalism in one of two ways: (1) from the perspective of professional role orientation, which emphasizes a service orientation or sense of altruism, or (2) from the perspective of personal professional enhancement, which is a focus on personal advancement within the profession. These two internal perspectives relate to Gouldner's (1957) cosmopolitan-local dichotomy. The internal view is less concerned with socially-based labeling of professions.

Criteria for Professionalization

Numerous authors have identified the criteria needed for a profession. Various theorists say there are 2, 5, or 6 criteria that are necessary (see Table 3.1). Hall (1968) considered five attitudinal attributes to be important: the use of the professional organization as the major referent, a belief in service to the public, a belief in self-regulation, a sense of calling to the field, and autonomy. Carr-Saunders and Wilson (1933) identified the formation of associations, sense of responsibility, standards of competence, specialized service, possession of a technique, and fixed remuneration as important characteristics of a profession. Flexner's (1915) landmark list included: formation of a brotherhood, devotion to the larger good, learned character, intellectual activities, technique communicated in an orderly way, and practical activities. Goode (1960) listed the two characteristics of prolonged specialized training in a body of abstract knowledge, and a collectivity or service orientation. Greenwood (1957) listed systematic theory, professional culture, community sanction, ethical codes, and authority as important attributes of a profession. Moore's (1970) list included formalized organization, service orientation, specialized education, commitment to calling, autonomy, and full-time practice.

While authors disagree as to the number and type of criteria, an analysis of the literature reveals that the three most prominent and consistent criteria among all lists can be described as service, knowledge, and autonomy (Carr-

Table 3.1

Comparison of Criteria for Professionalization

CARR-SAUNDERS AND WILSON (1933)	FLEXNER (1915)	GOODE (1960)	GREENWOOD (1957)	HALL (1968)	MOORE (1970)
Formation of associations	Formation of a brotherhood	Prolonged specialized training in a body of abstract knowledge	Professional culture	Use of the professional organization as the major referent	Formalized organization
Sense of responsibility	Devotion to the larger good	A collectivity or service orientation	Community sanction	Belief in service to the public	Service orientation
Standards of competence	Learned character		Ethical codes	Belief in self-regulation	Specialized education
Specialized service	Intellectual activities		Systematic theory	Sense of calling to the field	Commitment to calling
Possession of a technique	Technique communicated in an orderly way		Authority	Autonomy	Autonomy
Fixed remuneration	Practical activities				Full-time practice

Data from Carr-Saunders & Wilson (1933); Flexner (1915); Goode (1960); Greenwood (1957); Hall (1968); and Moore (1970).

Joanne Comi McCloskey
Envisions Professional Commitment

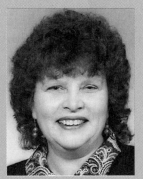

Joanne Comi McCloskey

While we have accomplished much over this century of organized nursing, we are not yet full partners in health care. For me, being a full partner means that for every important decision nursing is present and fairly represented and for every high level committee there is nursing participation. Moreover, for a good number of these decision making bodies, a nurse is the leader. Nursing is always included because we are recognized by others as having essential skills, knowledge, influence, and vision. When we become full partners, more nurses will be independent practitioners able to receive reimbursement for care provided, nursing knowledge classifications will be included in federal and state health care databases, more nurses will hold influential positions of authority both inside and outside of nursing, and nursing's values of patient participation and choice, preventive care and wellness, accessible and affordable health care for all, and time for teaching, counseling, and learning will be an integral part of the health care system.

Some of the students who read this book will become the future leaders of the profession; others will help these leaders accomplish the dream. The future of health care and of nursing is shaped by individuals who are prepared and committed to take action. My hope for the future is that more nurses will prepare themselves for a leadership role. The first essential step is to become committed to a career in nursing. We have a history of individuals choosing nursing for the job security or for a way to practice caring behaviors. These are fine reasons for entering nursing but those who make the maximum contribution develop a commitment to the profession. Developing a commitment means that you think in terms of a career rather than the particular job. Committed nurses continue their education and earn graduate degrees, they read professional literature and subscribe to nursing journals, they belong to the American Nurses Association and the organization of their specialty, they do the jobs they were hired for well and figure ways to give added value to the organizations they work in. Being career-oriented means that your development as a nurse enters into your important life decisions—where to live, whom to marry, when to have children. Career committed individuals do not take time off from work for long periods of time. Having a family and a personal life outside work is possible and healthy but the job, the career, the nursing profession matter. If more of you who read this book take this first step of becoming committed to a career in nursing, then the goal of nursing's full partnership in health care will follow. There is much to be accomplished and an important piece of work is waiting for each of you. Welcome to the profession.

Joanne Comi McCloskey, PhD, RN, FAAN, is a University of Iowa Foundation Distinguished Professor of Nursing, the University of Iowa. She is also Adjunct Associate Director of Nursing at the University of Iowa Hospitals and Clinics. Since 1982, McCloskey has directed the nursing service administration program at the University of Iowa. McCloskey is an active researcher and writer, with many publications on nursing turnover, job performance, and nursing interventions, and has received numerous awards for her teaching and research. She is the editor and author of nine books, among them Current Issues in Nursing, 2nd edition (1994); Nursing Interventions: Essential Nursing Treatments, 2nd edition (1992); and Nursing Interventions Classification (NIC), 2nd edition (1996). McCloskey's current research is on the construction and validation of a taxonomy of nursing interventions. She is co-principal investigator of the Iowa Intervention Project, which is funded by the National Institute of Nursing, NIH.

Saunders & Wilson, 1933; Flexner, 1910; Goode, 1960; Hall, 1969; McCloskey, 1981; Stuart, 1981; Snizek, 1972).

Service

Service means a focus on service to clients, or the care of the sick. Nursing meets service criteria without dispute. Hall (1968) compared results across professions and found teachers, social workers, and nurses strongly professionalized on the belief in service to the public and a sense of calling to the field attributes. Nurses agree on the need for client-oriented service, and in fact, in the original nurse's training, service was the driving focus. The criteria of knowledge and autonomy have been more problematic for nursing to resolve.

Knowledge

Knowledge criteria cover both a systematic body of knowledge and specialized education. A systematic body of knowledge includes both systematic theory and a specialized technique. Education refers to education that is obtained in an institution of higher learning, specifically, colleges and universities. This means a minimum of a baccalaureate degree. As long as a majority of registered nurses do not have a baccalaureate degree at minimum, nursing will not meet the knowledge criterion. There are various routes to becoming a registered nurse: diploma, associate degree, baccalaureate degree programs, and generic master's. A minimum of a baccalaureate degree has been identified as a definitive criterion for being considered professional. This is reflected in established national and international labor standards that identify the baccalaureate as a minimum degree for classification as a professional occupation (*International Standard Classification of Occupations*, 1990).

Exemplar
3.1

Supporting the Professional Status of Nurses

Through the years, the roles of our nursing staff have increased in both complexity and responsibility. Today's healthcare needs require providers with a defined set of characteristics to continue to meet the demands of a highly technological environment with an increasing complexity of illnesses and at the same time balance the psychosocial and caring aspects of the nurse's role. This environment requires caring individuals with tremendous knowledge and expertise coupled with sophisticated decision making.

The composition of the nursing staff at our 553-bed, academic, public, and tertiary medical center consists of diploma, associate, baccalaureate, master's, and doctorally prepared nurses. Although their educational preparation is vastly different, there is a common thread that weaves our nursing staff together. This common thread is the continued affirmation from their practice that nursing is a profession. With job descriptions such as a Clinical Nurse Specialist and Nurse Practitioner, it is apparent that our nurses are continuing to expand their roles to positions requiring a higher level of expertise, greater autonomy, and critical thinking skills—characteristics that support a professional status.

Our organization believes that the nursing profession must also reflect defined behaviors to support its professional status. At our facility, we have identified specific professional role behaviors which we feel reflect the expected behaviors of nurses within our facility. Realizing that behaviors need to be practiced within specific environments,

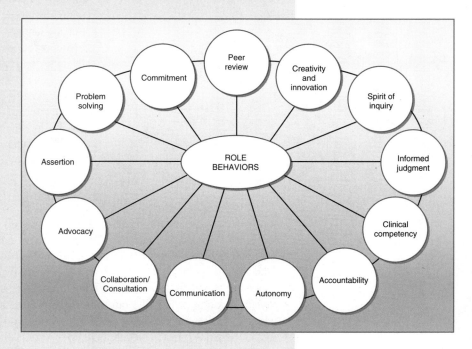

we have also identified the environments where professional nursing practice takes place. It is through the integration of the environments and the behaviors that professional nursing practice is operationalized.

Specific behaviors were identified through a careful review of the literature, existing research studies related to professionalism, and ANA Standards of professional performance. We also conducted work with various nursing groups on our campus and assessed our standing with relation to professionalism. Critical attributes that we as an organization would like to see reflected in the work of our staff resulted in our final selection.

The role behaviors that we identified include commitment, autonomy, accountability, clinical competency, informed judgment, spirit of inquiry, creativity and innovation, peer review, problem solving/leadership, assertion, advocacy, collaboration and consultation, and communication. The professional environments are the patient, nursing unit, nursing peers (network), nursing department, medical center, community and health care industry/professional organizations.

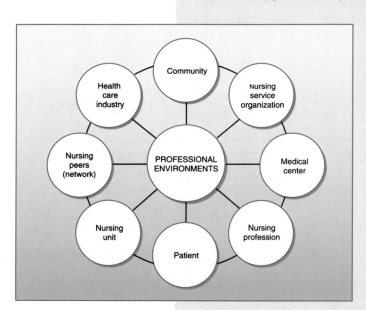

Upon identification of the professional behaviors and environments, the leadership team developed strategies to involve other nursing leaders in defining and describing the behaviors and environments. The nursing leaders comprised nurse managers, clinical nurse specialists, clinical instructors, divisional directors, and a quality improvement coordinator. This team worked for several months identifying the conceptual and operational definitions, as well as organizational factors that currently existed that supported the behavior and expected outcomes that we could observe in our staff.

The task of determining the role behaviors and professional environments broadened our managers' appreciation of professionalism and clearly identified critical behaviors to expect of our staff. The information collected was utilized to create learning opportunities for staff relating to each specific behavior, and recognition and reward systems were created. Nurse recognition nomination forms communicated the behaviors as well as the environments to be assessed relative to the identified criteria. Additionally, our performance evaluation system and standards of clinical nursing practice integrated the previous work.

Specific outcomes achieved include an understanding and acceptance of what professional performance and practice is in our environment. An added result is the expectation that staff participate not only in their unit environment, but also outside of their areas. There was also increased participation on teams and groups that are working on different educational opportunities relating to the behaviors and environments.

The professional status of nurses continues to be reaffirmed by their practice. As a profession, it is clearly important to promote the behaviors that support our status. Nurses must take initiative, be innovative, and continually expand our professional roles. Only then will the grey areas that question the professional status of nurses be eliminated.

PAULA SILER, RN, MS
Director, Professional Practice Affairs
Harbor–University of California Los Angeles Medical Center
Torrance, California

CATHY LOPEZ HOUSTON, RN, MBA
Analyst, Department of Nursing
Harbor–University of California Los Angeles Medical Center
Torrance, California

Despite the great diversity within the ranks of registered nurses as to their level of educational preparation, employers have treated registered nurses as if they were equal and interchangeable. The mixture of nurses with no collegiate educational background within the same job category as those with an associate degree and those with a baccalaureate creates a difficulty for the delineation of nursing as a healthcare profession. While the debate as to the degree of professionalism nursing has as an occupation continues within nursing, outside of nursing there is a different view. It is considered problematic, from a standardized job classification perspective, to confer professional status on an occupational group whose members have less than a baccalaureate degree.

Nurses are the largest group of healthcare workers in this country, and yet nursing has allowed minimal academic preparation for its members compared to other allied healthcare workers. Other groups are raising their standards. For example, it is almost impossible to work in the field of social work without a master's degree. It becomes difficult for nursing to argue for pay equity based on complex decision making and expertise when nurses' educational preparation has not been set at a minimum of a baccalaureate. However, this issue is highly controversial within nursing and is tied into emotional feelings of loyalty, status, and professional identity.

Autonomy and Ethics

In professional terms, autonomy means that the occupational group has control over its own practice. Autonomy is defined as authority and accountability for one's decisions and/or activities. The professional group identifies its ethical codes, policies, procedures, and standards; and thus the group mandates the scope of practice parameters for that group. Autonomy also means that the group has a professional organization to which its members belong. This is Flexner's (1915) idea of a "brotherhood". The American Nurses Association is the professional organization that exists to represent nursing, but its membership represents only about 10% of the over 2 million licensed RNs, over 1.6 million of whom are employed in nursing (Hawkins, 1992). Thus nurses cannot say that they are self-organized as a group to the extent that the general professional organization is not well subscribed to and multiple specialty organizations splinter nursing's representation. Autonomy also means being held accountable and liable for actions. To the extent that nurses are subject to malpractice lawsuits and carry malpractice insurance, nurses are held accountable (see Chapter 12).

There are extensive legal aspects to both nursing practice and nursing management. For example, Nurse Practice Acts exist for each state and govern the legal practice of nursing including delegation and supervision (see Chapters 15, 25, and 31 for further discussion). The legal regulation of nursing via Nurse Practice Acts and related administrative rules comes about because society needs to have safeguards that protect the health and safety of citizens. In regard to health care, the public demands assurance that health care providers, including nurses, are properly prepared and competent to deliver needed services. Thus to practice nursing, the person must hold a valid license issued by the state. Therefore, it is illegal to practice nursing without a license. State licensure confers on nurses autonomy to the limit of legal standards of practice. As professional autonomy and responsibility increase, so does the level of accountability and liability (Aiken, 1994).

The legal aspects of nursing management center around decision making and supervision. Since all nurses retain personal accountability for their own acts and the use of knowledge and skills in the provision of care, personal accountability cannot be assumed by another. Nurse managers keep their own personal accountability for their own specific acts, but they are also accountable for their acts of delegation and supervision (see Chapter 15 for further discussion). Nurse managers carry the major responsibility for developing and upholding the standards of care for the staff. Nurses and nurse managers carry the accountability for the supervision of others who are often unlicensed assistive personnel. Supervision includes monitoring the tasks performed, assuring that functions are performed in an appropriate fashion, and ensuring that assigned tasks and functions do not exceed competency or require a license to perform. Nurse managers use their autonomy to make decisions about practice situations. Nurse managers are accountable for carrying out supervisory responsibilities; proper notification; assessing the competency of staff; training, orientation, and evaluation of staff; reasonable staffing decisions; and monitoring and maintenance of professional treatment relationships with clients, called non-abandonment (Aiken, 1994) (see Chapters 7, 9, 23, and 25 for further discussion of legal aspects of nursing leadership and management, and Chapters 21 and 22 for collective bargaining issues).

The American Nurses Association's (ANA) Social Policy Statement (1980) identified two mechanisms that frame autonomy: the legal regulation of nursing practice via state licensure laws and the professional regulation of nursing practice via standards and ethical codes of practice (see Chapter 31). Ethical codes are guidelines for decision making based on values and standards for conduct (see Chapters 7, 9, 10, 11, 20, 25, and 30 for further discussion of ethical applications to nursing leadership and management).

Ethics is another aspect of autonomy: does the occupational group have a defined Code of Ethics? The American Nurses Association (1980) created and defined nursing's Code of Ethics in 1950, which has been revised since then. The Code of Ethics actually is a mandate for the standards of conduct by its practitioners: it tells nurses how they should act (Viens, 1989). Historically in nursing, ethics referred primarily to etiquette, manners, and morals. Ethical decision making knowledge has developed as nurses balance principles of justice, veracity, beneficence, and non-maleficence. For example, one area of ethics that remains problematic is nurses who refuse, or desire to refuse, to take care of clients with contagious diseases. This is analogous to today's problem in which some nurses desire to refuse to take care of clients with AIDS out of fear of transmission to themselves. As healthcare becomes more technologically complex, the area of ethics in nursing practice has grown. This is seen, for example, in decisions about termination of life support.

In the effort to achieve full professional status, nursing has not yet acquired recognition as a legitimate profession. However, nursing has a Code of Ethics, standards of practice, professional organizations, and a growing body of knowledge. Progress has been made in educational standards, autonomy, research base, and public policy influence.

A Continuum of Professionalization

Overall, the "criteria of a profession" lists resulted in a checklist approach to justifying professional status (Stuart, 1981). However, there is a dynamic process to professionalization as occupations evolve. Therefore, identifying occupations as professions or not is related to degree or amount, rather than being an either-or determination. An alternative approach to professionalization is to view it as a continuum or scale along which an occupation can move. Those elements deemed absolutely necessary for an occupational group to be a profession can be visualized along a continuum, from not applicable to fully possessed. Thus, professionalization can be conceptualized as a continuum, from non-professional to semi-professional to professional, related to the degree to which an occupational group is characterized by the achievement of identified professional criteria. Phrases like "nursing is an emerging or a marginal profession" are all indicative of the idea that nursing is in the process of attempting to move from a semi-professional to a true professional status.

Etzioni (1969) identified the difference between semi-professional and professional occupations. The semi-professions were seen to have less education, a less specialized body of knowledge, less autonomy, and less status than fully professional groups have. Nursing, teaching, and social work were labeled as semi-professional occupations in Etzioni's work.

Nursing has struggled since Flexner's (1910; 1915) ideas took hold to demonstrate that it meets the criteria of a full profession. Meeting all the criteria is assumed to result in society granting full professional status and prestige to nursing. However, nursing is still viewed externally as a part of "medical care," and medical care is considered to be equivalent to all healthcare. Thus nursing becomes invisible. Others may take credit for what nurses actually do. Nursing also may be pitted against medicine in the struggle for full professional recognition.

RESEARCH NOTE

Source: Miller, B., Adams, D., & Beck, L. (1993). A behavioral inventory for professionalism in nursing. *Journal of Professional Nursing, 9*(5), 290-295.

Purpose

The purpose of this research is to describe the Behavioral Inventory for Professionalism in Nursing. The Inventory is an evaluative instrument based on Miller's Model for Professionalism in Nursing. Based on the model, behaviors to demonstrate professionalism in nursing were identified. The original 16-item tool was revised to include 9 categories and a revised scoring system. The revised tool was pilot tested and then used in a mailed sample survey of 1,600 registered nurses which had a 36.6% (N = 586) return rate.

Discussion

The Inventory covers the nine categories of educational background; adherence to the code of ethics; participation in the professional organization; continuing education and competency; communication and publication; autonomy and self-regulation; community service; theory, development, and evaluation; and research involvement. The Inventory has good reported reliability and validity. Professionalism in nursing can thus be measured using a valid and reliable measurement tool.

Application to Practice

The instrument can be used by nurses to provide direction for professional growth and for self-evaluation purposes. Results can indicate to nurses how to achieve a higher degree of professionalism in nursing. Thus the instrument was designed to be evaluative and act as a guide. It is important for nurses to define and delineate the concept of professionalism from a nursing perspective.

Professionalization Barriers

A number of barriers to nursing's achievement of professional status can be identified. Aydelotte (1990) included variability in educational preparation, lack of a strong exclusive knowledge base, and nursing's approach to problem solving as nursing's barriers. The regulation of advanced practice may present another barrier (Dalton, Speakman, Duffey, & Carlson, 1994).

Two of the barriers that have obstructed nursing from achieving true professional status are historical influences that have affected nursing's development. The first is a religious influence derived from a time when nursing was done by individuals in religious orders. The religious influence created some positive values within nursing, as well as some influences that over time became negative. The ideas of subservience, passivity, and obedience historically were part of the socialization into nursing. For example, the idea of unquestioning obedience meant that nurses followed orders and did what they were told. This value defeats the ideas of autonomy, self-regulation, and self-control. Through the religious tradition, nursing also derived the idea of subservience and the motivation of altruism. Altruism means giving selflessly of oneself or of giving service to other human beings. While increasing the public's sense of trust, the concept of altruism has had an economic impact on nursing. The second primary influence on nursing has been the military. Nursing becomes a highly valued service in times of war. The military ethic of discipline likewise transferred the value of unquestioning obedience into nursing practice. While efficient for running an organization, unquestioning obedience defeats autonomy and creativity in problem solving. It thus affects the real and perceived status of nursing as a profession.

Another barrier to nursing has been its traditions. Nurses have neglected to evaluate traditions in nursing to determine if they are still relevant in today's world. For example, the wearing of caps was a tradition. Although few nurses today wear caps, they are still a symbol of nursing as reflected in the public's perception of what represents nursing. Other traditions pervade nursing practice and are ingrained in everyday procedures. For example, despite a focus on including the family in client care, few acute care hospital units do a comprehensive family assessment with an inpatient admission.

Stereotypes have been both negative and positive throughout nursing's history. Florence Nightingale, the lady with the lamp, is nursing's most positive image. The image of the nurse as a prostitute or an alcoholic has been a hindrance as it carried over into the stereotype that nurses have loose morals

(Kalisch & Kalisch, 1978; 1982). Nurses today struggle to improve the public's image of nursing by demonstrating, through research and policy making, nursing's centrality and effectiveness within the healthcare delivery system (Melosh, 1982; Muff, 1982) (see Chapters 18 and 27).

Gender issues also have affected nursing. Although gender per se was not one of the identified professionalism criteria, it turns out that nursing, teaching, and social work are made up of a majority of women workers. Nursing is composed of approximately 95% female workers (AJN News,1993). It is thought that, as women's work has not been valued in society, being a female-dominated profession has been a hindrance in the process of becoming a full profession.

Nurses' attitudes may pose another barrier to professionalism. Hall (1968) analyzed the structural and attitudinal aspects of professionalization and noted that the attitudinal attributes reflect the manner in which practitioners view their work. Looking at nursing historically, there are elements that indicate that nurses appear to behave as an oppressed group. Research indicates that if members of a group act oppressed, they will continue to be oppressed. Oppressed group behavior relates to feelings of powerlessness (Roberts, 1983). However, Hall (1969) felt that a key element in the process of professionalization was public acceptance of an occupation as a profession, not just the level of professional attitudes or fulfilling a set of prerequisites. He found that the place of the occupation in the wider social structure was an additional factor in professionalization. Thus it is not clear what proportion of influence can be attributed to nurses' attitudes versus societal acceptance in nursing's lack of professional status.

LEADERSHIP AND MANAGEMENT IMPLICATIONS

Being a professional nurse involves leadership and management behaviors. Nurses exhibit professional behaviors as a way of demonstrating their value to the organization and in order to foster a positive work climate. An appreciation of nursing's history, coupled with skills in leadership and management, nursing's developing knowledge base, and commitment to the profession are useful for each professional nurse in the work force and also for the profession of nursing as it strives to achieve true professional status. Each nurse can take on a leadership role within nursing. Developing a personal philosophy of nursing will anchor the nurse's leadership activities. Self-awareness based on self-analysis will provide a foundation for professionalism. Each nurse might analyze the following questions: is nursing a profession, and does it matter? This is important because nurses will face issues related to levels of nursing practice and educational standards for practice.

Developments in nursing research have been the most recent trend to increase the professional status of nursing. With research, nurses are able to

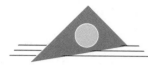 *Leadership & Management Behaviors*

LEADERSHIP BEHAVIORS

- envisions nursing as a full profession
- communicates with nurses about professional attributes in nursing and related issues
- influences nurses to be professional
- guides changes in research, education and practice that improve nursing's professional status
- opens a dialogue to promote nursing as a profession

MANAGEMENT BEHAVIORS

- understands nursing's struggle for professionalization
- plans for workforce diversity
- organizes nursing practice to best utilize professional registered nurses
- directs the work of nurses as professional employees
- manages professional-bureaucratic conflicts

OVERLAP AREAS

- delivers professional nursing practice
- balances professional and bureaucratic role demands

demonstrate the cost effectiveness of nursing outcomes and of advance practice nurses as primary care providers. Each nurse can take responsibility for the leadership activities of research utilization in practice. Nurse managers can promote nursing research and its dissemination and use in practice.

Nurse managers deal with both professional autonomy and job autonomy issues. Professional autonomy is the individual and collective authority and accountability for practicing a profession. Job autonomy is the authority and accountability for one's work. Bureaucratic institutions that employ professionals to do a job demand a measure of control over their work to assure desired outcomes. Professional and bureaucratic values may mesh or clash with each other (Hall, 1968). The idea that there is an inherent conflict between professionals and their employing organizations was proposed by Corwin (1961), Etzioni (1964), and Gouldner (1954), who argued that there is a basic incompatibility between professionals and organizations which is related to divergent authority patterns. The professional authority base is expertise, while the organization uses authority based on hierarchical position. The professional entering an organization is seen as having to choose between commitment to the profession and commitment to the organization (Blau & Scott, 1962; Gouldner, 1957; Wilensky, 1959). Nurse managers can be role models for professional behaviors and encourage the same in others. Nurse managers may find that professionalism plays a part in their interface with administration and in their advocacy of professional issues.

Gouldner's (1957) conceptualization of the cosmopolitan-local construct noted that since the values of the profession and the organization conflict, the professional either becomes a local and accepts the organization's values, or becomes a cosmopolitan and maintains a professional allegiance. However, some authors have noted that organizational professionals may be committed to both their professions and their organizations (Bennis, Berkowitz, Affinito & Malone, 1958; Glaser, 1963). Thornton's (1970) research indicated that professional and organizational commitments can be compatible if the situation within the organization reaffirms principles of professionalism. Both leadership and management strategies will need to be employed in the delicate balancing of professionals with their employing organizations.

CURRENT ISSUES AND TRENDS

Fortunately, the nature of elements that compose criteria for a profession have been changing in nursing over time. Even though there have been changes in the image of nursing and changes related to stereotypes, negative aspects still linger. They are noticeable in the electronic and print media. Media images and stereotypes frequently are degrading, as they do not convey commitment to professional nursing as a career. At worst, media images capitalize on and perpetuate negative stereotypes related to the idea of being a nurse. As a result they affect the attitude of the general public in terms of how the public views nurses. In some cases, the predominant media representations overlook nursing, making it "invisible". For example, the public is unaware, in most instances, about nursing's scholarly works, nursing research, and the achievements of nurses throughout history, particularly in relation to social causes and against social injustice. Nurses also may not realize their heritage. Thus others may lay claim to the caring role and the health promotion and prevention roles of nurses.

In the beginning of U.S. nursing, nurses were a combination of social worker and nurse, because social work did not become an occupation until approximately 1915. For example, Lillian Wald is considered to be one of the greatest humanitarians who ever lived in this country. She was the innovator and creator of public health nursing in this country and developed the Henry Street Settlement in New York City, which is now the Visiting Nurse Service of New York. Yet she is identified as a social worker, not a nurse. Professionalism is enhanced through nurses' knowledge about, advocacy of, and promotion of nursing as a profession.

Appearance is related to professionalism through its effect on image, although not all nurses agree that appearance makes a difference. What makes a difference about appearance? Some nurses rebel against dress codes. Yet appearance gives an impression of competence. Nurses want the client to trust that their nurse will render a high quality of care. However, what nurses prefer to wear and what clients prefer to see nurses wear often do not coincide. Nurses prefer comfortable scrubs; clients prefer a white dress uniform (Barnum, 1990; Kucera & Nieswiadomy, 1991; Magnum, 1991).

There was a time in nursing when nurses were not allowed to wear any make-up or jewelry at all, not even wedding bands, partially in reaction to negative societal views about makeup and jewelry and partially as an infection control mechanism. This was based on the premise that in terms of professionalism, appearance is important. In nursing there are some practical aspects to dress. For example, earrings can be dangerous, particularly if a pierced or drop earring gets caught in equipment. In the management literature, dressing for success is discussed as a tactic related to competence, ability, and power.

Appearance and dress are only one nonverbal strategy designed to convey professionalism in nursing. This is because outward appearances are designed to communicate an image of professionalism. However, there are other important elements for an occupation to address in the quest for societal recognition as a true profession. Miller's (1988) model of professionalism in nursing was visualized as a wheel with the two critical attributes of education in a university setting and scientific background in nursing at the hub. There were eight spokes, each representing related attributes of professionalism that have been identified as essential characteristics for professionalism in nursing. They are adherence to code for nurses; theory development, use, and evaluation; community service orientation; continuing education and competence; research development, use, and evaluation; self-regulation and autonomy; professional organization participation; and publication and communication. Thus the degree of professionalization in nursing would be reflected by how the profession adheres to and exhibits behaviors related to these identified characteristics.

RESEARCH NOTE

Source: Hutchinson, S. (1992). Nurses who violate the nurse practice act: Transformation of professional identity. *Image*, *24*(2), 133-139.

Purpose

The purpose of this descriptive, interpretive research was to explore and describe the experiences of a volunteer purposive sample of 30 nurses who had been accused of violating the Nurse Practice Act in Florida. Data were gathered from phone and in-person interviews. Participant observation occurred at six Board of Nursing meetings and three administrative hearings. Documents were reviewed and analyzed. Data were analyzed by grounded theory method using the constant comparative method.

Discussion

Nurses accused of violating the Nurse Practice Act were found to experience a transformation of professional identity over time. Their ways of viewing themselves, their work, and the profession of nursing were altered. The nurses were found to progress over several years through five phases: being confronted, assuming a stance, going through it, living the consequences, and re-visioning. The author noted that this work presents the dark side of nursing.

Application to Practice

By understanding what happens when there are nursing practice problems, nurses learn more about the parameters of nursing practice. Further, nurses need to learn about the legal aspects of their professional practice, including state statutes and what violations should be reported. The standards and laws that govern or guide practice must be known and understood to be followed. They must be followed as a way to assure the public's safety.

SUMMARY

* Nursing as an occupation has sought full professional status during the 20th century.
* Professionalism is important to nurses.
* "Profession" is a word assigned by society to an occupational group.
* Professions have been defined by using a checklist of criteria.
* Professions can be defined by their placement on a continuum of professionalization.
* There are barriers to nursing achieving full professional status.
* Leadership and management strategies are useful for professional activities.

Study Questions

1. On what basis can nursing argue that it is a profession?
2. How close to a true profession is nursing today? What elements are progressing the fastest?
3. Should nurses put energy into activities of professionalization?
4. What strategy or strategies can nursing use to move nursing's professionalization to full professional status?
5. Should nurses care about image and appearance, and if so, why?
6. What is the most prevalent media stereotype of nurses today? How could this be changed?
7. Do nurses need to act and look professional to give a professional impression?
8. Can you design the "ideal" nursing uniform: one that nurses like, find comfortable and practical, and yet clients can identify with?

Critical Thinking Exercise

Suzanne Thomas, Vice President for Nursing and Healthcare at a large urban teaching hospital, just announced a new strategy for human resources management in nursing. In six months a new policy will go into effect which splits registered nurses into two job categories based on educational credentials. There will be a Staff Nurse I category for all registered nurses who do not have a BSN. There will be a Staff Nurse II category for staff nurses with a BSN or higher degree. The educational criteria are firm, with no equivalency for years of experience or tenure. This policy has created controversy. Some nurses threaten to unionize. Some nurses are seeking BSN program admission information. Some nurses plan to quit or move. Some nurses allege that the policy unfairly favors BSN schools over associate degree or diploma programs. Few are neutral.

1. *What is the problem?*

2. *What are the key issues?*

3. *How should Vice President Thomas handle the situation?*

4. *What values might be in conflict?*

5. *What ethical dilemmas might arise?*

6. *What leadership and management strategies might be helpful?*

REFERENCES

Aiken, T. (1994). *Legal, ethical, and political issues in nursing.* Philadelphia: F. A. Davis.

AJN News. (1993). Enrollments surging in BSN schools; New men's movement into nursing seen. *American Journal of Nursing, 93*(3), 99-100.

American Nurses Association. (1980). *Nursing: A social policy statement.* Kansas City, MO: American Nurses Association.

Aydelotte, M. (1990). The evolving profession: The role of the professional organization. In N. Chaska (Ed.), *The nursing profession: Turning points* (pp. 9-15). St. Louis: Mosby.

Barnum, B. (1990). Wear your designer clothes on duty. *Nursing & Health Care, 11*(9), 484-485.

Bennis, W., Berkowitz, N., Affinito, M., & Malone, M. (1958). Reference groups and loyalties in the out-patient department. *Administrative Science Quarterly, 2,* 481-500.

Bixler, G., & Bixler, R. (1945). The professional status of nursing. *American Journal of Nursing, 45*(9), 730-735.

Bixler, G., & Bixler, R. (1959). The professional status of nursing. *American Journal of Nursing, 59*(8), 1142-1147.

Blau, P., & Scott, W. (1962). *Formal organizations.* San Francisco: Chandler.

Brodie, B. (1994). Nursing's quest for professionalism. In J. C. McCloskey & H. K. Grace (Eds.), *Current issues in nursing* (4th ed.) (pp. 559-565). St. Louis: Mosby.

Carr-Saunders, A., & Wilson, P. (1933). *The professions.* Oxford: Clarendon Press.

Corwin, R. (1961). The professional employee: A study of conflict in nursing roles. *American Journal of Sociology, 66,* 604-615.

Davis, F. (1966). *The nursing profession: Five sociological essays.* New York: John Wiley and Sons.

Dalton, J., Speakman, M., Duffey, M., & Carlson, J. (1994). The evolution of a profession: Where do boards of nursing fit in? *Journal of Professional Nursing, 10*(5), 319-325.

Etzioni, A. (1964). *Modern organizations.* Englewood Cliffs, NJ: Prentice-Hall.

Etzioni, A. (1969). *The semi-professions and their organizations.* New York: The Free Press.

Fiesta, J. (1983). *The law and liability: A guide for nurses.* New York: John Wiley & Sons.

Flexner, A. (1910). *Medical education in the United States and Canada.* Boston: Merrymount Press.

Flexner, A. (1915). Is social work a profession? *School and Society, 1*(26), 901-911.

Glaser, B. (1963). The local-cosmopolitan scientist. *American Journal of Sociology, 69,* 249-259.

Goode, W. (1960). Encroachment, charlatanism, and the emerging professions: Psychology, sociology and medicine. *American Sociological Review, 25,* 902-914.

Gouldner, A. (1954). *Patterns of industrial bureaucracy.* Glencoe, IL: Free Press.

Gouldner, A. (1957). Cosmopolitans and locals: Toward an analysis of latent social roles-II. *Administrative Science Quarterly, 2*(4), 444-480.

Greenwood, E., (1957). *Attributes of a profession. Social Work, 2*(4), 45-55.

Hall, R. (1968). Professionalization and bureaucratization. *American Sociological Review, 33,* 92-104.

Hall, R. (1969). *Occupations and the social structure.* Englewood Cliffs, NJ: Prentice-Hall.

Hawkins, J. (1992). Empowering the new graduate: A renewed professionalism for nursing. *Journal of Professional Nursing, 8*(5), 308-312.

International standard classification of occupations: ISCO-88. (1990). Geneva: International Labour Organization.

Kalisch, P., & Kalisch, B. (1978). *The advance of American nursing.* Boston: Little, Brown.

Kalisch, P., & Kalisch, B. (1982). *Politics in nursing.* Philadelphia: Lippincott.

Kucera, K., & Nieswiadomy, R. (1991). Nursing attire: The public's preference. *Nursing Management, 22*(10), 68-70.

Mangum, S., Garrison, C., Lind, C., Thackeray, R., & Wyatt, M. (1991). Perceptions of nurses' uniforms. *Image, 23*(2), 127-130.

McCloskey, J. (1981). The professionalization of nursing: United States and England. *International Nursing Review, 28*(2), 40-47.

McCloskey, J., & McCain, B. (1987). Satisfaction, commitment and professionalism of newly employed nurses. *Image, 19*(1) 20-24.

Melosh, B. (1982). *The physician's hand: Work, culture and conflict in American nursing.* Philadelphia: Temple University Press.

Miller, B. (1988). A model for professionalism in nursing. *Today's OR Nurse, 10*(9), 18-23.

Moore, W. (1970). *The professions: Roles and rules.* New York: Russell Sage Foundation.

Muff, J. (1982). *Socialization, sexism, and stereotyping.* St. Louis: Mosby.

Parsons, M. (1986). The profession in a class by itself. *Nursing Outlook, 34*(6), 270-275.

Price, J., & Mueller, C. (1981). *Professional turnover: The case of nurses.* New York: Spectrum Publications.

Quinn, C., & Smith, M. (1987). *The professional commitment: Issues and ethics in nursing.* Philadelphia: Saunders.

Roberts, S. (1983). Oppressed group behavior: Implications for nursing. *Advances in Nursing Science, 5*(4), 21-30.

Sleicher, M. (1981). Nursing is not a profession. *Nursing & Health Care, 2*(4), 186-191, 218.

Snizek, W. (1972). Hall's professionalism scale: An empirical reassessment. *American Sociological Review, 37,* 109-114.

Stuart, G. (1981). How professionalized is nursing? *Image, 13*(1), 18-23.

Thornton, R. (1970). Organizational involvement and commitment to organization and profession. *Administrative Science Quarterly, 17,* 417-426.

Viens, D.C. (1989). A history of nursing's code of ethics. *Nursing Outlook, 27*(1), 45-49.

Vollmer, H., & Mills, D. (1966). *Professionalization.* Englewood Cliffs, NJ: Prentice-Hall.

Wilensky, H. (1959). *Intellectuals in labor unions.* Glencoe, IL: Free Press.

Wilensky, H. (1964). The professionalization of everyone? *American Journal of Sociology, 70*(2), 137-158.

Wuest, J. (1994). Professionalism and the evolution of nursing as a discipline: A feminist perspective. *Journal of Professional Nursing, 10*(6), 357-367.

PART II

Framework for Leadership and Management

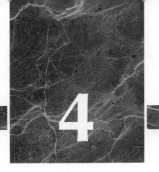

Leadership Principles

Chapter Objectives

❧

define and describe leadership

❧

explain the process of leadership

❧

identify the qualities of leadership

❧

analyze leadership styles

❧

distinguish among theories of leadership

❧

relate followership to leadership

❧

relate leadership to nursing practice

❧

exercise critical thinking to conceptualize and
analyze possible solutions to a practical experience incident

*M*ost nurses have a single focus: how to best take care of clients by diagnosing their health problems and structuring nursing interventions for optimal client outcomes. However, for the registered nurse, nursing
practice is broader than just a focus on taking care of a few clients. The majority of nurses work in bureaucratic organizations and in work groups or
units. Possessing the license of a registered nurse implies certain leadership
skills and requires the ability to delegate and supervise the work of others.
Leadership can be seen as the ability to inspire confidence and support among
followers and those whose competence and commitment produce performance (Kim & Mauborgne, 1992).

Leadership is an important issue related to how nurses integrate the various elements of nursing practice to ensure the highest quality care for clients. There are two critical skills that every nurse needs to possess to enhance professional practice. One is a skill at interpersonal relationships. This is fundamental to leadership and the work of nursing. The second is the skill of applying the problem solving process. This involves the ability to think critically, to identify problems, and to develop objectivity and a degree of maturity or judgment. Leadership skills build on professional, clinical skills: in order to fulfill a nurse's role successfully, interpersonal, organizational, and political skills are needed as well as basic nursing psychomotor skills.

Leadership content in nursing is studied as a way of increasing the skills and abilities needed to facilitate working with people across a variety of situations and to increase understanding and control of the professional work setting. Bennis (1994) made a strong argument for leadership, stating that quality of life depends upon the quality of the leaders. He noted three reasons why leaders are important: the character of change in society, deemphasis on integrity in institutions, and the responsibility for the effectiveness of organizations. Fiedler and Garcia (1987) argued that leadership is one of the most important factors that determine the survival and success of groups and organizations. Thus effective leadership is important in nursing.

DEFINITIONS

There are a number of definitions of leadership. McCloskey and Molen's (1986) definition describes leadership as a process of influencing either individuals or groups to accomplish goals. Key concepts related to leadership are influence, communication, group process, goal attainment, and motivation. Hersey and Blanchard (1993) defined leadership as a process of influencing the activities of either an individual or a group in an effort to achieve goals in a given situation. Burns (1978) noted that leadership occurs when human beings with motives and purposes mobilize in competition or conflict with others so as to arouse, engage, and satisfy motives.

All leadership definitions incorporate the two components of an interaction among people and the process of influencing. Thus, leadership is a social exchange phenomenon. Leadership is influencing people. *Leadership* is defined here as the process of influencing people to accomplish goals. In contrast, management involves influencing employees toward the organization's goals and is focused primarily on organizational goals and objectives. Bennis (1994) listed a number of distinctions between leadership and management. He noted that the leader focuses on people, while the manager focuses on systems and structures. Another distinction is that a leader innovates, whereas a manager administers.

CHART 4.1
↬ DEFINITIONS

Leadership
the process of influencing people to accomplish gains.

Management
the coordination and integration of resources through planning, organizing, coordinating, directing, and controlling in order to accomplish specific institutional goals and objectives.

Leadership Styles
different combinations of task and relationship behaviors used to influence others to accomplish goals.

Followership
an interpersonal process of participation by following.

Empowerment
the act of giving people the authority, responsibility, and freedom to act on what they know.

Management is defined as the coordination and integration of resources through planning, organizing, coordinating, directing, and controlling in order to accomplish specific institutional goals and objectives. Hersey and Blanchard (1993, p. 5) defined management as a "process of working with and through individuals and groups and other resources to accomplish organizational goals." They identified management as a special kind of leadership that concentrated on the achievement of organizational goals. If this idea were visualized, it would be in concentric circles, not as overlapped separate circles.

Leadership is a broad concept and a process that can be related to any group. Grant (1994) noted that leadership, management, and professionalism have different but related meanings:

- *leadership:* guiding, directing, teaching, and motivating to goal setting and for achievement.
- *management:* resource coordination and integration to accomplish specific goals.
- *professionalism:* an approach to an occupation that distinguishes it from being merely a job, and focuses on the ideal of service, follows a code of ethics, and is seen as a lifetime commitment.

A key point to remember about leadership and management is that they are not the same, although they are related and can be integrated at an area of overlap. Related leadership definitions are leadership styles, followership, and empowerment (see Chart 4.1). *Leadership styles* are defined as different combinations of task and relationship behaviors used to influence others to accomplish goals. *Followership* is defined as an interpersonal process of participation by following. *Empowerment* means giving people the authority, responsibility, and freedom to act on what they know; and it means instilling in them belief and confidence in their own ability to achieve and succeed (Kramer & Schmalenberg, 1990).

BACKGROUND

Leadership: Five Interwoven Aspects

Hersey and Blanchard (1993) noted that the leadership process is a function of the leader, the followers, and other situational variables. The leadership process includes the five interwoven aspects of the leader, the follower, the situation, the communication process, and the goals (Kison, 1989). Figure 4.1 shows how these components relate to each other.

The Leader The leader's values, skills, and style are important. The leader's internalized pattern of basic behaviors influence actions and the ability to lead. Leaders' perceptions of themselves and their roles also will make a

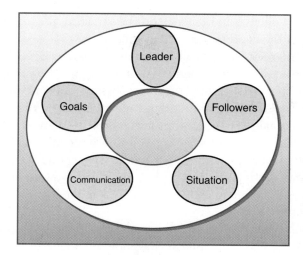

Figure 4.1
Components of a leadership moment.

difference in the leadership situation. The leader's expectations will impact on the followers. Internal forces in a leader that impinge on leadership style are values, confidence in employees, leadership inclinations, and sense of security in uncertainty (Tannenbaum & Schmidt, 1973).

The Follower   Followership is the flip side of leadership. Followers are vital because they accept or reject the leader and determine the leader's personal power (Hersey & Blanchard, 1993). If the leader needs self-awareness, then the followers also must know themselves in reference to their expectations. Situations in which the group is not accustomed to working together or do not hold shared expectations frequently lead to conflict. Groups have personalities that include a discernable level of trust. The leader must assess the readiness level of the group. If the group is knowledgeable and experienced in solving problems, the leadership situation is very different than if the group is not experienced at the task or at working together.

The Situation   The specific circumstances surrounding any given leadership situation will vary. Elements such as work demands, control systems, amount of task structure, amount of interaction, amount of time available for decision making, and the external environment shape the differences among situations (Hersey & Blanchard, 1993). Organizational culture and ethos also are important factors in the situation (see Chapter 10). For example, in one place the culture may resemble one big happy family. For every occasion there is a morale-boosting event. The cultural aspects of that leadership situation are different from an organization where everyone marches to a fast tempo and people seem very busy. Environmental or cultural differences make the leadership situation radically different. Also, the personality styles of both superiors and peers will have an influence on the situation, the work demands, and the amount of time and resources available.

The Communication Process   Communication processes will vary among groups as to the patterns and channels utilized and as to how open or closed the communication flow is. Communicating is basic to influencing. By communication, the leader's vision and message are received by the followers. After choosing a channel, the sender transmits a message. However, the message is filtered through the receiver's perception. Communication is transmitted through both verbal and nonverbal modes. In organizations, there will be unique communication structures. These may be downward, upward, horizontal, grapevines, or communication networks. Communication may be formal or informal (Hersey & Blanchard, 1993).

The Goals   Organizations have goals, and individuals working in organizations have goals. These may or may not be congruent. For example, the goal of the organization may be to decrease costs. In contrast, the goal of the individual nurse may be to spend time counseling and teaching clients because that is what is seen professionally by the nurse as the most important activity. Goals may be in conflict, in which case there is tension and a need for leadership.

Thus all five elements interact within any leadership moment. Nurses can improve their leadership abilities by greater analysis of leadership moments. Hersey and Blanchard (1993) identified three skills needed for leading or influencing:

- *diagnosing:* Diagnosing activities involve being able to understand the situation and the problem to be solved or resolved.
- *adapting:* Adapting activities involve being able to adapt behaviors and other resources to match the situation.
- *communicating:* Communication activities are employed to advance the process in a way that individuals can understand and accept.

Clearly, leadership is a complex process. Nurses need to be aware of the interacting elements in any leadership situation. Critical thinking can be applied to diagnosing and analyzing the five elements, adapting to the situation, and communicating for effectiveness.

Leadership Theories

The three basic phases that occurred in studying leadership theory can be grouped as trait, attitudinal, and situational (Hersey & Blanchard, 1993). The trait approach focuses on certain characteristics of leaders. The attitudinal approach measures attitudes toward leader behavior. The situational approach focuses on observed behaviors of leaders. Research and theory about leadership has a long history. Leadership theories have evolved away from an early focus on the traits or characteristics of the leader as a person because it was not found to be possible to predict leadership from clusters of traits. However, several authors have developed lists of traits common to good leaders (Bass, 1982; Bennis & Nanus, 1985; Yukl, 1981), and interest still remains in the characteristics to look for in good leaders.

Characteristics of Leadership

Bennis (1994) identified a recipe for leadership that contained six ingredients: a guiding vision, passion, integrity (including self-knowledge, candor, and maturity), trust, curiosity, and daring. Leaders arise in a context, and they are said to be "made" not "born". Thus leadership skills can be both taught and learned.

Leaders are active, not passive. The risk-taking element of leadership involves taking action. Leaders engage their environment with behaviors of doing, influencing, and moving. These are action terms. Pagonis (1992) noted that to lead successfully a leader must demonstrate two active, essential, and interrelated traits: expertise and empathy. Leaders are those who talk about adventures into new territory and take the risks inherent in innovation (Kouzes & Posner, 1987).

Leadership involves an element of risk and courage in accepting the role of a leader and moving the group's goals forward. Kennedy's (1956) *Profiles in Courage* clearly demonstrated that courage is one essential leadership element. A leader may see the need to chart a course that is new or unknown, unpopular, or risky because it challenges vested interests who have much to lose. In a way, nursing's struggle for greater economic parity in healthcare is courageous and risky.

Leadership means excellent guidance. It is establishing a vision or a goal, examining where an organization should move, and then determining how the organization can get there (Vestal, 1989). In nursing, for example, leadership has been needed to guide nursing's quest for true professional status.

Leadership confers empowerment. Empowering in nursing leadership means transferring power over clinical practice decisions to staff nurses and enabling them to do what they do best. This process is similar to nurses empowering clients. Leadership also is forward thinking or visionary. A leader needs to articulate a vision as a way to motivate people. Leadership involves elements of vigor and vision and can be understood as a dynamic combination of competence, willingness to take responsibility, and the strength of character to do what is right because it is right.

Empowering the Team

Successful leadership in the current healthcare market requires the ability to create and empower teams that embrace and implement change. Highly motivated and functional nurse managers are essential elements of the organization. Leadership principles that I have employed to create an empowered team include guidance, motivation, recognition, mentoring and the ability to influence change. As an Assistant Administrator in Patient Care Services responsible for Intensive Care Units, Emergency Department, Burn Center and Level I Trauma Center, it is critical to the success of the institution that the nurse managers and I are able to manage in a proactive manner, seek opportunities for growth, implement strategic initiatives, and re-engineer the work force to achieve effective patient care and organizational outcomes.

A recent example that demonstrates this philosophy is the formation of a work group of nurse managers to design and implement a joint venture process between our institution and a local Children's Hospital to achieve Pediatric Level I Trauma Center Designation by the State. Trauma designation remains a politically charged effort, especially in a competitive healthcare environment. Achieving a successful affiliation between the two facilities and subsequent designation required effective coordination of pediatric trauma care along the continuum. The nurse managers in both institutions are responsible for the operation and outcome of the individual patient care areas (ICU's, Acute Care Wards, Operating Room, Post Anesthesia Care Unit, Emergency Department, and Rehabilitation). I designed a work group that consisted of nurse managers from each of the trauma care areas, spanning both institutions. While each facility had a unique mission, the joint venture effort focused on developing a shared vision for pediatric trauma care. The nurse managers' expertise in the specific care needs of the pediatric trauma population was critical to designing a program that met desired outcomes.

As the Chair of this work group, I placed my emphasis on developing the nurse managers to assume responsibility for the institutional requirements, the State guidelines and laws pertaining to trauma care and preparation of their staff for the designation site survey review. They quickly assumed responsibilities and embraced the project by setting goals and monitoring the implementation. I provided oversight coordination and mentoring to challenge each nurse manager to contribute and develop additional expertise in this specialty area. The work group became empowered to identify and design effective care delivery systems that not only met the Level I Trauma requirements, but also improved care. They had struggled with many of these issues in the past and had identified them as frustrations with care fragmentation. They now had a voice and an opportunity to effect change. The nurse managers continued to excel in their motivation and creativity with the project. The nursing and ancillary staff working on the individual units were subsequently given unique opportunities for growth by the nurse managers. Many of the projects were developed and implemented by sub-groups on the units through the leadership and mentoring of the nurse manager. By setting the example and providing support, guidance, assistance, and leadership, by open and direct communication, and by maintaining high standards for performance expectation, I was able to effectively develop and empower this work group and sustain motivation through a 21 month project. As an administrator responsible for the various nurse managers, these abilities were critical processes for me to achieve and maintain.

The project came to fruition by a successful joint venture working relationship between the two facilities and the successful award of Level I Pediatric Trauma Designation by the State. The site survey team reflected its opinion of our process by verifying that all individuals of the healthcare team were knowledgeable and vested in their commitment to pediatric trauma care. While some facilities approach joint ventures at the most senior or executive level, this exercise was completed by mid-level managers with assistance from administration and proved to be the best approach for success. The goals attained charged the group with additional energies and motivation. A successful venture builds confidence. These nurse managers now continue to enthusiastically volunteer to participate in even the most difficult strategic planning groups and assume additional responsibilities to effect change.

JOHNESE SPISSO, RN, BS, MPA, CCRN
Assistant Administrator, Patient Care
 Services
University of Washington, Harborview
 Medical Center
Seattle, Washington

Characteristics like knowledge, motivating people to work harder, trust, communication, enthusiasm, vision, courage, being able to see the big picture, and the ability to take a risk are associated in research findings with important leadership qualities. For example, Bennis and Nanus (1985) studied 90 chief executives from 1978 to 1983, and found that there are two key leadership traits. One is a guiding set of concepts and the other is ability to communicate a vision. Kouzes and Posner (1987) defined five behaviors correlated with leadership excellence: enabling others to act, challenging the process, inspiring shared vision, modeling the way, and encouraging the heart. In one research study concerning what particular clusters of characteristics nurses preferred in their leaders, the top quality was caring, followed by other responses of respectability, trustworthiness, and flexibility (Meighan, 1990). The qualities of leadership that people say they want to see their leaders possess are (Curtin, 1989):

- *visibility:* people want to see their leader and have frequent, casual contacts.
- *flexibility:* people learn from leaders who can "roll with the punches," tolerate ambiguity, and have a sense of personal empowerment.
- *authority:* this is the right to make decisions, give direction, and accept and administer criticism. Authority is recognition granted from below.
- *assistance:* this occurs by serving those who serve, create, or produce, and by creating the environment and resources necessary to do the job.
- *feedback:* people want their leaders to listen to them and give them quality feedback as they go about their particular work.

The eight competencies of leaders synthesized from the literature by Murphy and DeBack (1991) are:

- managing the dream
- mastery of change

- organizational design
- anticipatory learning
- taking the initiative
- mastery of interdependence
- holding high standards of integrity
- exercising broad-perspective decision making

Followers expect that leaders will provide a sense of vision and a sense of direction with standards for achieving the group's goals. Leaders can create an environment positively charged for productivity or allow the followers to languish without direction or mission. It is possible that leaders can create a negative climate that becomes destructive to the group. If the leader plays a major role in creating a group's culture and ethos, then closing down communication, breeding distrust and competition, and neglecting positive motivation can sow the seeds of group disintegration. Thus the characteristics possessed and used by the leader can make a crucial difference in the functioning and effectiveness of any group.

RESEARCH NOTE

Source: Irurita, V. (1994). Optimism, values, and commitment as forces in nursing leadership. *Journal of Nursing Administration, 24*(9), 61-71.

Purpose

The purpose of this grounded theory, four year study of nursing leadership in Western Australia was to develop a theory of leadership that explained how nurses achieved influence on the delivery of healthcare and how they advanced the nursing profession. Data were gathered by 32 semistructured interviews of nurse leaders, participant observation, interviews with others in the system, a demographic data sheet, a questionnaire, and document and literature review. Data were analyzed using ethnography and the constant comparative analysis method.

Discussion

The leadership context was revealed to be predominated by turbulence and disadvantage. Optimizing, the process of making the best of the situation, was used by leaders to cope with the situation. Besides failing to optimize (floundering), there were three progressive levels of optimizing: surviving, investing, and transforming. The level of optimizing reached in a situation depended on the availability of resources and the leader's characteristics of optimism, values, and commitment.

Application to Practice

A model was developed that related optimism, values, and commitment to levels of optimizing. Both levels and focus differed for values and commitment and were related to different levels of optimizing. Thus the factors are interrelated. If excellence occurs under the influence of a good leader, then this is most associated with transformers. Any structures or conditions that sustain optimism, commitment, and strong values appear to be related to outcome levels of optimizing. Work settings can be analyzed for their cultures and environments and the subsequent impact on leadership and outcomes.

Attitudinal Leadership Theories

As leadership theories evolved, leadership came to be viewed as a dynamic process and an interaction among the leader, the followers, and the situation. Hersey and Blanchard (1993) identified a second approach to leadership research that focused on the measurement of attitudes or predispositions toward leader behavior. Occurring mainly between 1945 and the mid-1960s, the attitudinal approaches began with the Ohio State Leadership Studies and included the Michigan Leadership Studies, Group Dynamics Studies, Likert's management studies, and Blake and Mouton's Managerial Grid.

Leader behavior was described on two separate dimensions: (1) initiating structure and consideration in the Ohio Leadership Studies and (2) employee-orientation and production-orientation in the Michigan Leadership Studies. These terms are similar to authoritarian or task, and democratic or relationship ideas of the leader behavior continuum. The Group Dynamics Studies highlighted goal achievement (similar to task) and group maintenance (similar to relationship) elements of leadership behavior (Cartwright & Zander, 1960). Likert (1961) studied high performance managers to develop an understanding of a general pattern of management. He found that close supervision was less associated with high productivity. High productivity was associated with clear objectives and transmitting an idea about what is to be accomplished to the subordinates, then giving them the freedom to do the job. He described a continuum of management styles, called System 1 through System 4, from no trust in subordinates through condescending confidence, substantial but not complete confidence, to complete trust and confidence in subordinates. This parallels the task to relationship continuum.

Blake and Mouton (1964) used task and relationship concepts in their grid. Five types of leadership or management styles, based on concern for production (task) and concern for people (relationship), emerged:
- *impoverished:* this style uses minimal effort to get the work done
- *country club:* this style uses attention to effect satisfying relationships
- *task:* this style strives for efficiency in operations
- *middle of the road:* this style works on balancing the necessity to accomplish the task with maintaining morale
- *team:* this style promotes work accomplishment from committed people and interdependence through a common stake, leading to trust and respect.

Hersey and Blanchard (1993) noted that the Blake and Mouton's (1964) conceptualization tended to be an attitudinal model that measured the values and feelings of managers, whereas the Ohio State model included both attitudes and behaviors and focused on leadership.

Situational Leadership Theories

A third phase of leadership theories grew out of contingency theories that postulated that organizational behavior is contingent upon the situation or environment. Situational leadership theories focus on the frequency of observed behaviors in order to make predictions. Thus no one leadership style is optimal in all situations. The nature of the situation needs to be considered. Styles can be chosen to match the situation (Hersey & Blanchard, 1993).

LEADERSHIP STYLES

Leadership styles are defined as different combinations of task and relationship behaviors used to influence others to accomplish goals. They are sets or clusters of behaviors used in the process of effecting leadership. Hersey and Blanchard (1993) said that leadership styles are the behavior patterns exhibited in influencing the activities of others, as perceived by those others. There are different styles that evoke variable responses in different situations. The way people influence others through actions taken and the perspectives of other people is related to leadership efforts and constitutes leadership style. The two major leadership terms are task behavior and relationship behavior. Thus, a leader's leadership style is some combination of task and relationship behavior. Hersey and Blanchard (1993) defined these terms as follows:

- *task behavior:* the extent to which leaders organize and define roles, explain activities, determine when, where, and how tasks are to be accomplished, and endeavor to get work accomplished.
- *relationship behavior:* the extent to which leaders maintain personal relationships by opening communication and providing psychoemotional support and facilitating behaviors.

Tannenbaum and Schmidt (1973) suggested that a leader might select one of seven behavior styles arrayed along a continuum. The continuum ranges from democratic to authoritarian, or subordinate-centered to leader-centered. Their work suggested that there are a variety of leadership styles (see Fig. 4.2). Essentially, however, there are three distinct leadership styles or points along the continuum: authoritarian, democratic, or laissez-faire (Tannenbaum & Schmidt, 1958; 1973; White & Lippett, 1968), although some individuals are able to integrate all three styles and flexibly match to the situation.

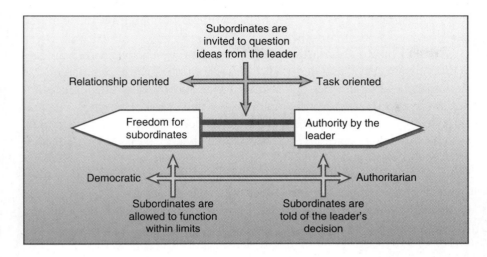

Figure 4.2
Continuum of leader behavior.

Authoritarian This style is reflected in primarily directive behaviors. Techniques and activity procedures are determined by the leader and dictated to followers. Decisions of policy are made solely by the leader. Leaders tell the followers what to do and how to do it. This style emphasizes a concern for task. Authoritarian leaders are characterized by giving orders. Their style can create hostility and dependency among followers. It may stifle creativity and innovation. However, this style can be very efficient, especially under a crisis.

Democratic This style implies a relationship and person orientation. Policies are a matter of group discussion and decision. The leader encourages and assists discussion and group decision making. Human relations and teamwork are the focus. The leader shares responsibility with the followers by involving them in decision making. The current nursing literature emphasizes how important teamwork is in nursing. For example, continuous quality improvement implies interdisciplinary teamwork. The democratic style moves slower than an authoritarian style. Group consensus needs to be considered. Further, the needs of the disenfranchised minority groups need to be balanced. Intergroup cohesion is needed with this style. The challenge of the democratic style is to get people with different professional backgrounds, personal biases, and ego-psychic needs together to focus on what the problem is and how can it be fixed.

Laissez-faire This style promotes complete freedom for group or individual decisions. There is a minimum of leader participation. This style, as defined, may seem apathetic to some. Because the style is premised on non-interference, there may never be a clear decision formulated. The laissez-faire style is a decision, conscious or otherwise, to avoid interference and let events take their own course. The leader is either permissive to foster freedom or is inept at guiding a group. This style has advantages with groups of independent care providers working together.

One style is not necessarily better than another. Each style has advantages and disadvantages. The styles should vary according to the appropriateness of the situation with reference to an evaluation of effectiveness. Flexibility is important to effectiveness. For example, a nurse prefers to operate in a democratic style. Suddenly, however, a code situation occurs. The nurse must rapidly switch from a democratic to an authoritarian style. Some democratic leaders cannot vary their style sufficiently to handle crisis situations. On the other hand, in a staff meeting, an authoritarian leader may be ineffective with a group of professionals. The basic need is for self-awareness and to know the group's ability and willingness before examining the situational elements and choosing a leadership style.

Fiedler's Contingency Theory

As situations become more complex, leadership becomes more difficult. Fiedler (1967) developed a Leadership Contingency Model. He classified group situational variables of leader-member relations, task structure, and position power into eight possible combinations, ranging from high to low on the three major variables. Leader-member relations refers to the type and quality of the leader's personal relationships with followers. Task structure refers to how structured the group's assigned task is. Position power refers to that power conferred on the leader by the organization as an integral component of the assigned job. Fiedler examined the favorableness of the situation from the perspective of the leader's influence over the group. The most favorable situation occurs with good leader-member relations, high task structure, and high position power. The least favorable situation occurs when the leader is disliked, has an unstructured task, and has little position power. Using Fiedler's model, group situations can be analyzed to determine the most effective leadership style.

Fiedler (1967) examined which style (task- versus relationship-oriented) would be most effective for each of eight situations. A key general principle is that the need for task-oriented leaders occurs when the situation is either highly favorable or very unfavorable. A task style is needed for the situations on the extremes, whereas a relationship-oriented style is needed when the situation is moderately favorable.

For example, a staff nurse goes into a nursing unit meeting not wanting any extra assignments but wanting some of the ongoing problems solved. If there is a reasonably good relationship with the leader, then the leader should use a high-relationship style with the nurse. The leader should use selling, convincing, encouraging, and motivating strategies. The leader should make the nurse feel good about his/her ability to accomplish a task, to provide something of quality, and to work together with other people. If, however, the staff nurse's mind is closed about any changes, or if passive-aggressive or subversive actions occur, then the leader needs be more directive. A possible reaction might be to give the nurse an assigned task. On the extremes of highly favorable or highly unfavorable situations, leaders need to use task-oriented behavior to get the work moving. In the middle of the continuum, a high relationship style is needed.

In situational leadership theory, leadership in groups is never a static circumstance. The situation is subject to change. In a very difficult situation, relationships may be the leader's preferred emphasis. However, if interpersonal relationships are not an immediate problem or the group is on the verge of collapse, then what is needed is strong authoritative direction to get the group moving and accomplishing. For this situation, the task-oriented leader is a more effective match between leader and job. But groups do not remain static. Groups move back and forth through stages. When the problem no longer is the need to just get the group moving but includes solving numerous interpersonal conflicts, a relationship-oriented leader is better matched to the situation. Eventually, as the situation moves along, a relationship-oriented leader can become less effective. This occurs because once the group becomes less conflictual, individuals may begin to coast, and positive motivation may be lost as individuals become apathetic. Once again, a task-oriented style is called for: someone who can challenge individuals with the continuing motivation that they need to continue to produce. Because of the factor of constant change, maintaining good leadership is complicated for any group. One way to foster effective leadership is to evaluate leaders according to Fiedler's (1967) contingency model and then use this information to increase leaders' awareness of their natural style tendency: relationship-oriented or task-oriented. Fiedler's measure for leadership style is the Least Preferred Coworker (LPC) scale (Fiedler & Chemers, 1984). The LPC is an 18-item semantic differential scale that is the personality measure of Fiedler's Contingency Model (Fiedler & Garcia, 1987).

Favorable or unfavorable situations are determined in part by the receptivity of the followers, but also are determined by whether the larger environment is positive or negative. An example of an unfavorable situation in nursing might be if a nurse's job is to lead and manage a hospital's critical care area with serious morale problems. The nurse may have a master's degree yet soon discovers that a majority of the followers have a diploma from the School of Nursing run for many years by that hospital but now defunct. Both educational and experiential backgrounds are likely to differ and possibly clash between leader and followers. The task is to change the environment, yet the nurse discovers that this work group has maintained its traditions over a long period of time. That is an unfavorable situation and a leadership challenge.

Fiedler's (1967) theory suggested that the best leadership style under unfavorable circumstances is task-oriented.

Hersey and Blanchard's Tri-Dimensional Leader Effectiveness Model

Hersey and Blanchard (1993) developed the Tri-Dimensional Leader Effectiveness Model. First, a two-dimensional model was constructed in which task behavior and relationship behavior were displayed on a grid from high to low and divided into four quadrants: high task, low relationship; high task, high relationship; high relationship, low task; and low task, low relationship (see Fig. 4.3). Hersey and Blanchard (1993) said that these quadrants represented four basic leadership styles: telling, selling, participating, and delegating. As applied to the continuum of authoritarian versus democratic styles, telling would be authoritarian, and delegating would be democratic. In the middle are the two styles that draw from both: the selling and the participating leadership styles. Selling is a little more authoritarian than participating, and participating is a little more democratic than authoritarian, but both are mixed styles.

In order to choose an appropriate style, the leader needs to be knowledgeable about the readiness of the followers. This leads to the third dimension of effectiveness (see Fig. 4.4). Effectiveness is defined as how appropriately a given leader's style interrelates with a given situation. Hersey and Blanchard (1993) described the third dimension as the environment in which a leader operates and which interacts with the leader's style.

Overlaid on the basic grid is a continuum of readiness ranging from low to high. Readiness has two aspects: ability and willingness. Job *ability* is predicated on the amount of past job experience, job knowledge, problem solving ability, ability to take responsibility, and ability to meet deadlines. This forms

Figure 4.3
Hersey-Blanchard two-dimensional model of leadership. (From Hersey, P., and Blanchard, K. [1993]. MANAGEMENT OF ORGANIZATIONAL BEHAVIOR: Utilizing Human Resources, 6/E. Englewood Cliffs, N.J.: Prentice Hall, p. 128, and from 4/E. Reprinted with permission from the Center for Leadership Studies.)

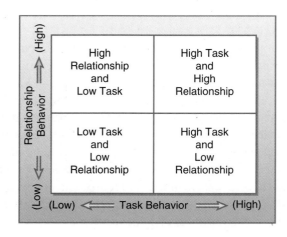

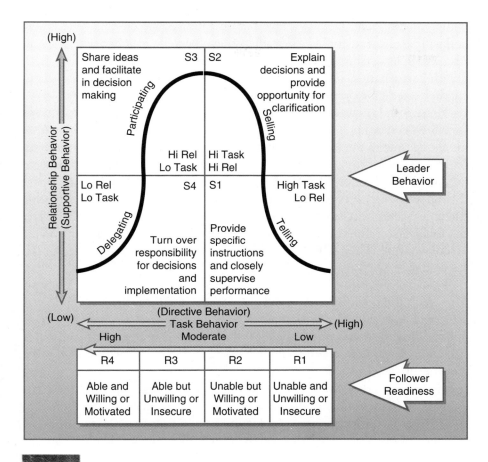

Figure 4.4
Hersey-Blanchard Situational Leadership® model. (From Hersey, P., and Blanchard, K. [1993].
MANAGEMENT OF ORGANIZATIONAL BEHAVIOR: Utilizing Human Resources, 6/E.
Englewood Cliffs, N.J.: Prentice Hall, p. 186, and from 4/E. Situational Leadership® model is a
registered trademark of the Center for Leadership Studies, Escondido, California. Reprinted with
permission from the Center for Leadership Studies.)

a composite of the ability to do the job. The other part of readiness is psychological *willingness*. Psychological willingness means being willing to take responsibility and have a positive attitude toward accepting the obligation to complete a task. Psychological readiness is manifested by willingness to take some risk and by accepting the job requirements. It includes achievement motivation, wanting to do well, persistence, a work attitude, and a sense of independence. These things create a willingness to take on and complete a job. Hersey and Blanchard (1993) combined ability and willingness into 4 levels of readiness. Level 1 is unable and unwilling or insecure. Level 2 is unable but willing or confident. Level 3 is able but unwilling or insecure. Level 4 is able and willing or confident. These readiness levels can be matched with the corresponding leadership styles of level 1 with telling, level 2 with selling, level 3 with participating, and level 4 with delegating. Thus readiness assessment can help predict appropriate leadership style selection.

Hersey and Blanchard (1993) emphasized the readiness of followers. Readiness can be applied to a work group. Have the members worked together for a long time in the job, or are they new employees? The culture is more solidified in a work group that has worked together for many years on a particular unit. The leader's leadership style would have to take into account where the followers are in terms of their readiness as a critical factor for determining the style to choose. Using leadership theory, leaders assess themselves, look at the followers' readiness, and assess the situation as to whether it is favorable or unfavorable. Then a telling, selling, participating, or delegating style is selected.

For example, telling is an appropriate leadership style to use with followers who are at the novice level, as well as in other situations where the followers are not able or willing. For example, a nurse is appointed the chair of a committee. First the nurse might undertake a leadership analysis to figure out if this group needs high relationship behaviors. If they do not know each other and the situation is politically charged, then the nurse leader needs to help people become comfortable with each other. If the nurse leader is a task-oriented person, then a high-relationship person may need to be called upon to assist the group process so that it is facilitated and becomes effective.

One currently accepted view of organizational behavior describes leadership as situational or contingent and concerned with what produces effectiveness. Hersey and Blanchard (1993) noted that the common themes include: the leader needs to be flexible in behavior, be able to diagnose the leadership style appropriate to the situation, and be able to apply the appropriate style. Thus, there is no one best way to influence others nor one best style. Situational leadership is a synthesis of the interplay among task behavior, relationship behavior, and the readiness of the followers.

Transactional and Transformational Leadership

Burns (1978; Dunham & Klafehn,1990) broadened the concept of leadership styles to look at political and revolutionary leaders. Burns identified two types of leaders: the transactional leader and the transformational leader.

A *transactional* leader is defined as a leader or manager who functions in a caretaker role and is focused on day-to-day operations. They survey their followers' needs and set goals for them based on what can be expected from the followers.

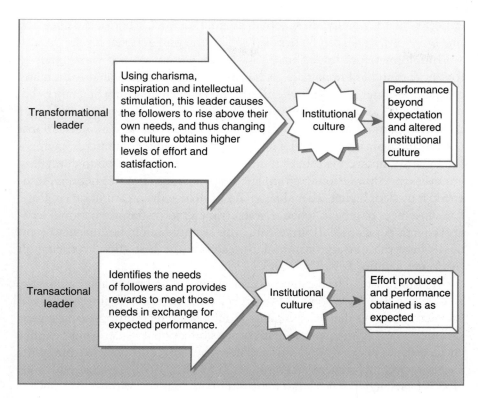

Using charisma, inspiration and intellectual stimulation, this leader causes the followers to rise above their own needs, and thus changing the culture obtains higher levels of effort and satisfaction.

Transformational leader

Institutional culture

Performance beyond expectation and altered institutional culture

Identifies the needs of followers and provides rewards to meet those needs in exchange for expected performance.

Transactional leader

Institutional culture

Effort produced and performance obtained is as expected

Figure 4.5
Transactional and transformational leadership.

A *transformational* leader is defined as a leader who motivates followers to perform to their full potential over time by influencing a change in perceptions and providing a sense of direction. Transformational leaders use charisma, individualized consideration, and intellectual stimulation to produce greater effort, effectiveness, and satisfaction in followers (Bass & Avolio,1990). Figure 4.5 distinguishes between transactional and transformational leadership.

The transactional leader is more often found. The transactional leader approaches followers in an exchange posture: with the purpose of exchanging one thing for another, such as a politician who promises jobs for votes. Burns (1978) said that transactional leadership occurs when the leader takes the initiative in contacting others for the exchange of valued things. Therefore, transactional leadership occurs like a bargain or contract for mutual benefits and to aid the individual differences of both the leader and follower. Key characteristics are contingent rewards and management-by-exception. Expected effort and expected performance are the outcomes. The transactional leader works within the existing organizational culture and is an essential component of effective leadership (Bass & Avolio, 1990). In nursing, an example would be the exchange of a salary for the services of a nurse to provide care (Barker, 1991). Another example occurs when a leader offers release time to entice staff to do quality assessment or committee work. Change of degree, the first order of change, can be handled well at the transactional level.

Transformational leadership occurs when persons engage with others so that leaders and followers raise each other to higher levels of motivation and ethical decision making (Burns, 1978). Instead of emphasizing differences between the leader and the followers, transformational leadership emphasizes collective purpose and mutual growth and development. Transformational leadership augments transactional leadership by being committed, having a vision, and empowering others in order to heighten motivation in a way that attains extra effort beyond performance expectations. Transformational leadership is used for higher order change and to change the organization's culture. Circumstances of growth, change, and crisis call forth transformational leaders (Bass & Avolio, 1990). In nursing, the example would be "magnet hospitals" where the nursing organizations facilitate the best effort in their staff (McClure, Poulin, Sovie, & Wandelt, 1983).

Transformational leadership is a concept useful and applicable to nursing. The finding that leadership quality is a key element in developing a culture of excellence among magnet hospitals is important for nursing management (Kramer, 1990). Organizations with a transformational leader would exhibit characteristics like pride and satisfaction in the work, enthusiasm, team spirit, a sense of accomplishment and satisfaction (Barker, 1990). Bennis and Nanus (1985) identified four activities for transformational leadership:

- creating a vision
- building a social architecture that provides meaning for employees
- sustaining organizational trust
- recognizing the importance of building self-esteem

Three factors underlie effectiveness as a transformational leader: individual consideration, charisma, and intellectual stimulation (Bass, Waldman, Avolio, & Bibb, 1987; McDaniel & Wolf, 1992). In one comparative study, nurse executives' transformational scores were found to be higher than those of general managers (Bass, 1985; Dunham & Klafehn, 1990). Other research has been done to test transformational leadership theory in nursing (see Research Note). Transformational leadership qualities appear to be better suited to the work of professionals. Nurses can learn about transformational leadership and work to set up structures to facilitate it in practice.

In summary, to be effective, leadership styles need to be matched to the situation. Styles of leadership range from authoritarian to permissive to democratic, and from transactional to transformational. The individual nurse's task is to figure out what environments s/he functions best in and is most comfortable with, or where s/he most likely will succeed. This facilitates placement for success and a better match between leader and follower.

RESEARCH NOTE

Source: McDaniel, C., & Wolf, G. (1992). Transformational leadership in nursing service: A test of a theory. *Journal of Nursing Administration, 22*(2), 60-65.

Purpose

The purpose of this research was to test transformational leadership theory in one nursing service with one executive, nine midlevel managers, and 46 staff RNs. The descriptive comparative survey explored whether a site with transforming leaders also exhibits work satisfaction and retention among staff nurses. Leadership was measured by the Multifactor Leadership Questionnaire, satisfaction with work was measured by the Work Satisfaction Scale, and turnover was collected from monthly reports.

Discussion

The leadership scores showed a cascading effect, where followers exhibit similar leadership qualities but of a lesser score than the leader. There was a statistically significant difference between transformational and transactional scores, favoring transformational. Overall work satisfaction scores were above average and highly correlated. The turnover rate was low. The findings of positive leadership, high work satisfaction, and low turnover appear to support the transformational theory.

Application to Practice

Leadership has been identified as important for establishing a culture of excellence. Individual consideration, charisma, and intellectual stimulation are key characteristics of effective transformational leaders. Transformational leadership qualities are reported in successful nurse executives and are argued to be more suited to the work of professionals. Transformational leadership is related to work satisfaction, higher productivity, and lower turnover. Nursing leaders can learn about and practice qualities of transformational leadership. Creating structures to support transformational leadership can provide a competitive edge to an institution.

FOLLOWERSHIP

Pagonis (1992) noted that by definition leaders do not operate in isolation. Instead, leadership involves cooperation and collaboration. The basic nature of leadership is interactive and involved with the interpersonal relationships among leaders and followers. Therefore, cooperation and collaboration between leader and followers and between followers and leader enhance the group's effectiveness.

Followership is an interpersonal process of participation by following. The importance of followership is emphasized because leadership requires the presence of followers. The relationship between the leader and the followers defines leadership. The corollary to leadership is followership, or helping to get the job done. A good leader clearly needs good followers (Brakey, 1991). Bennis (1994) noted that there are three things that followers need from leaders: direction, trust, and hope. With these three elements in place, followers are empowered in their participation efforts.

It may be that as nurse leadership becomes recognized as a vital element in meeting future challenges, nurse followership will assume a greater importance in practice. At one level, the nurse functions as a leader within the nurse-client relationship and within the framework of care management. However, within nursing, the staff nurse often is viewed as being at the level of a follower within the nursing organizational hierarchy. Murphy (1990) reviewed Kelley's (1988) model of five categories of followers and applied them to nursing. "Sheep" are followers who lack initiative, sense of responsibility, and critical thinking. "Yes-people" lack enterprise and yield to the opinions, will, or decisions of others. "Alienated" followers are capable of independence and critical thinking but appear passive because they resist open opposition. The result is frustration and disillusionment. "Survivors" never make waves or take risks; they check which way the wind is blowing. "Effective" followers have initiative and think for themselves. They manage themselves well and are responsible and well balanced. They are competent and committed. Effective followers are an asset to be nurtured, developed, and valued. Effective followers contribute to success in organizations.

Guidera and Gilmore (1988) stated that the enlightened follower incorporates the cohesiveness of collective group thought without being afraid to be candid or to criticize objectively. Self-awareness is an important aspect of both leadership and followership. Self-assessment tools are available to assist nurses in awareness of leadership and followership behaviors. One example is the LEAD instruments developed by Hersey and Blanchard (1993). Other instruments include the Leader Behavior Description Questionnaire-LBDQ-12 (Stodgill, 1963), the Least Preferred Coworker Scale (Fiedler & Chemers, 1984; Fiedler & Garcia, 1987), the Leadership Practices Inventory (Kouzes & Posner, 1988), the Multifactor Leadership Questionnaire-MLQ (Bass & Avolio, 1990), the Self-Assessment Leadership Instrument (Smola, 1988), and several training instruments (*University Associates Instrumentation Kit*, 1987).

A related leadership-followership concept is a psychological idea called the Pygmalion effect or self-fulfilling prophecy. It is related to theories about expectations. If the leader holds and communicates clearly an expectation that the group will perform well, group members are bright and motivated, and they will work in positive ways, then those expectations are likely to be fulfilled. If the leader holds and communicates an expectation that the group is not capable and unmotivated, the leader is likely to get the kind of response back that was expected. Therefore, leaders should have positive assumptions about followers' potential (Hersey & Blanchard, 1993). This self-fulfilling prophecy is manifested through leadership styles and in the communication of the leader's attitudes. Leader expectations are thought to interact with leadership styles to result in managerial behavior (Getzels & Guba, 1957). The manager's value system, confidence in subordinates, leadership inclination, and feelings of security influence their leadership style (Tannenbaum & Schmidt, 1973) and are transmitted to the followers in both verbal and nonverbal ways. It is in the dynamic interaction between leaders and followers that leadership results in productivity and other outcomes.

LEADERSHIP AND MANAGEMENT IMPLICATIONS

Leadership is a key element in operating successful groups and organizations. Leadership is a key resource for the improvement of nursing services. Five practices have been found common to most exceptional leadership achievements (Kouzes & Posner, 1990): (1) challenging the process by searching for opportunities, experimenting, and taking risks, (2) inspiring a shared vision by envisioning the future and enlisting the support of others, (3) enabling others to act by fostering collaboration and strengthening others, (4) modeling the way by setting an example and planning small successes, and (5) encouraging the heart by recognizing contributions and celebrating accomplishments. Nurse leaders can read, learn, and practice leadership skills. For example, the five practices identified through research as being associated with exceptional leadership can serve as an assessment guide for leadership situations. Further, they can form the basis for strategic plans and activities to improve a given nursing work environment. Individuals can use this information for self assessment.

As nurses work in a rapidly changing practice environment, leadership is important because it affects the climate and work environment of the organization. It affects how nurses feel about themselves at work and about their jobs. By extension, then, leadership is thought to affect organizational and individual productivity. For example, if nurses feel goal-directed and that their contributions are important, then they are more motivated to do the work. Important for the professional practice of nurses is how they feel about themselves and how satisfied they are with their jobs. Both aspects have implications for how well nurses are retained and recruited. Leadership cannot be overlooked because leaders function as problem finders and problem solvers. They are people who help everyone else overcome obstacles.

Leadership in nursing is a key element to the profession because of a number of factors. First, it is important to nurses because of the size of the profession. Nurses are the largest single healthcare occupation and one that is mov-

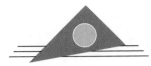 *Leadership & Management Behaviors*

LEADERSHIP BEHAVIORS

- show followers how to think about old problems in new ways
- treat followers as unique individuals
- stimulate critical thinking
- inspire followers
- demonstrate expertise and empathy
- are visible to followers
- are flexible
- provide assistance and feedback (coaching)
- communicate a vision
- establish trust
- motivate the group to achieve goals
- promote innovation and risk taking
- empower followers
- master change
- mentor followers
- are creative & innovative

MANAGEMENT BEHAVIORS

- make decisions
- communicate
- plan and organize
- manage changes
- motivate followers

OVERLAP AREAS

- exercise broad-perspective decision making
- communicate to followers
- motivate followers

ing from semi-professional status toward that of a full profession. In order to have society confer full professional status, nursing needs to be able to demonstrate the expertise, the creativity, and the knowledge base to match the complex environment in healthcare. Pressures, including costs, in the healthcare environment are rapidly thrusting nurses into leadership roles.

Second, nursing's work is complex, often conducted in complex settings. Tremendous changes in nursing have occurred in the last 25 years. These are changes in philosophy, knowledge base, technological complexity, ethical dilemmas, and impacts from societal pressures. Thus leadership is needed to guide and motivate the group toward positive achievements for better client care.

Third, nurses enter nursing by licensure but from a variety of educational preparations. A baccalaureate degree does not automatically confer advanced leadership skills. However, without this academic degree at minimum, nursing as a profession is disadvantaged. Thus nurses will need strong leadership to resolve the interprofessional dilemmas derived from educational diversity and the related issues of professionalization and being attractive providers to clients. For example, each nurse will need to develop leadership skills in relating to peers who have a different educational background and value system. Nurses will need to settle questions of educational preparation for entry into practice. Nursing needs strong leadership for public policy advocacy on behalf of nursing as a profession and for its own growth and advancement in the provision of cost-effective client care.

Jim O'Malley Envisions Leadership Transformation

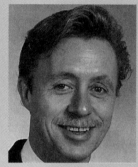

Jim O'Malley

The array of rapid and complex changes in the provision of healthcare services is redefining both healthcare and healthcare leaders. Nursing leaders, in an effort to manage the cost-quality agenda, are initiating changes to reposition their organizations for a successful future. The crisis in healthcare challenges leaders to reevaluate the culture of management. As new definitions of what it will take to successfully manage healthcare emerge, the need and the pressure to develop effective executives has never been more critical. Understanding that executive leadership has always been more of an art than a science, that successful executives are self-made and ultimately accountable for their own development, provides the underpinnings for the important work at hand. As the turbulent healthcare world has become increasingly dynamic, complex, interdependent, and unpredictable, it is no longer possible for any of us to have it all figured out.

We need to take our responsibility for developing and cultivating those who will follow us very seriously. Finding and mentoring those who have a passion for creating vision, an ability to live in the future, and a flair for culture building is perhaps the most significant of our contributions. Although small in number, potential transformational leaders can be found at all levels of an organization. We might do well to begin to import new talent from the arts as well as from the other service industries. Leaders make things happen, get things done, and shake things up—which may be the reason why we don't have more of them.

Jim O'Malley, RN, MSN, NP, CNS, is Senior Vice President of Nursing Services at Allegheny General Hospital, Pittsburgh, Pennsylvania. See page 15 for the complete biographical note.

CURRENT ISSUES AND TRENDS

Looking at the demographic profile of nursing in the United States gives a clue about nursing followership. The average age of a licensed, registered professional nurse in the United States was 43 years old in 1992 (Rosenfeld, 1994). This implies that nurses are going to have to look at how nursing is structured and organized, since nursing is not a young person's profession, on average, any more. The bulk of nursing's population is advancing each year in average age (Rosenfeld, 1994). Therefore, roles, deployment, and work force utilization in nursing may need to shift to accommodate nursing demographics.

The direction of current trends indicates that by the year 2000 there will be major changes in nursing practice demographics. The number of diploma nurses is decreasing, there are fluctuating enrollments in nursing schools, and there are only small increases in the number of men and minorities. There are more advanced practice nurses being prepared as programs spring up and as primary care becomes emphasized.

Only about 10% of nurses belong to the American Nurses Association (ANA), which is the organization that speaks for nursing at the national level. This is a problem for leadership and followership in nursing. The reality of there being 2 million plus nurses licensed with few belonging to the major organization that speaks for nursing reflects a potential dilution of the power of the profession. The individual nurse who is not a member is cut off from participation in the collective and information that can help them in their practice. However, there are many specialty groups in the nursing profession. The specialty groups have organized into a national organization of specialty groups in nursing, the Nursing Organizations Liaison Forum (NOLF), and are linked with the ANA through the Tri-Council for Nursing. At the national level the many nursing groups have banded together so that when there are issues and a need to act from one position, nursing can speak with a united voice.

With the advent of healthcare reform, nurses will adopt new roles; therefore, nurses need knowledge and skill in leadership to be successful in these new roles. Nurses who have had primarily followership roles will be challenged to assume leadership roles in the future. For example, one trend sweeping across healthcare in hospitals in this country is continuous quality improvement (CQI) (see Chapter 25). CQI is a philosophy that emphasizes changing the structure and environment within an organization so that the people at the lowest level can solve work problems free of barriers or hindrances and thereby improve the total quality within the whole organization. Empowerment of workers and the use of multidisciplinary teams are implemented to improve quality. The implication for nursing is that CQI will place the nurse more directly into the primary caregiver and gatekeeper roles. This will require the ability to have leadership skills and acumen in group process.

Under conditions of healthcare reform, turbulence, and change, ethical leadership becomes crucial. There are consequences to the changes being undertaken toward the goal of containing costs. For example, hospitals are closing, merging, and downsizing. Nursing services have been targeted in this process. Nurses will find themselves in positions of both formal and informal leadership when ethical issues arise. There may be questions of advocacy for both clients and nurses. For example, must nursing be targeted for downsizing? When downsizing occurs, how are justice, fairness, respect for persons, and preventing harm handled? How are scarce nursing resources allocated and advocated? What institutional mechanisms help or hinder ethical decision making (Aroskar, 1994)? How nurses incorporate ethics into their leadership styles and decision making affects nurses, nursing, and the delivery of client care.

SUMMARY

- Effective leadership is important in nursing.
- Leadership principles can be learned through education and practice.
- Leaders must know themselves and their followers, the situation, the communication process, and goals, and be flexible enough to make necessary adaptations.
- Leaders are those who innovate and take the risks inherent in new approaches.
- Effectiveness means matching leadership behaviors to the environment and then adapting within that environment.
- Leaders who never vary their style are probably ineffective some of the time.
- Leadership involves a concern for task and a concern for people.
- Good leaders need good followers.

Study Questions

1. How would you describe a leader? Identify one person who personifies leadership.
2. What are the important qualities of leadership?
3. What is the best way to learn leadership skills?
4. Who are the leaders in nursing?
5. Can you be a leader in nursing?
6. What leadership moments happen in groups?
7. What is a good follower?
8. What is your favored leadership style? Followership style?

Critical Thinking Exercise

Nurse White is a well-respected and long-tenured nurse in her work group. She is often called on to orient new staff. Physicians routinely call upon her expertise. One resident was overheard to say that he hoped Nurse White was scheduled to be on when he was because the shift went better. Nurse White has a diploma in nursing as her highest educational credential. However, she was an ICU nurse in Vietnam during the Vietnam War and has worked in an ICU setting ever since then. The nurse manager of Nurse White's unit has called the staff together for a meeting. Many changes, such as requiring a minimum of a BSN for certain positions, have been occurring in this hospital and there are persistent rumors of unionization activities. Nurse White believes unionization is unprofessional, but she has a strong empathy for the pressure on staff nurses. The nurse manager asks Nurse White to chair a group discussion for input about what should be done if a layoff became necessary. All eyes turn toward Nurse White.

1. *What is the problem?*

2. *What are the key issues?*

3. *How should Nurse White handle the situation?*

4. *What should Nurse White do first?*

5. *What leadership style would be most appropriate in this situation?*

6. *What leadership and management strategies might be helpful?*

REFERENCES

Aroskar, M. (1994). The challenge of ethical leadership in nursing. *Journal of Professional Nursing, 10*(5), 270.

Barker, A. (1990). *Transformational nursing leadership: A vision for the future.* Baltimore: Williams & Wilkins.

Barker, A. (1991). An emerging leadership paradigm: Transformational leadership. *Nursing & Health Care, 12*(4), 204-207.

Bass, B. (1982). *Stogdill's handbook of leadership.* New York: The Free Press.

Bass, B. (1985). *Leadership and performance beyond expectations.* New York: Free Press.

Bass, B., & Avolio, B (1990). *Transformational leadership development: Manual for the Multi-factor Leadership Questionnaire.* Palo Alto, CA: Consulting Psychologists Press.

Bass, B., Waldman, D., Avolio, B., & Bibb, M. (1987). Transformational leadership and the falling dominos effect. *Group and Organizational Studies, 12*(1), 73-87.

Bennis, W. (1994). *On becoming a leader.* Reading, MA: Addison-Wesley.

Bennis, W., & Nanus, B. (1985). *Leaders: The strategies for taking charge.* New York: Harper & Row.

Blake, R., & Mouton, J. (1964). *The managerial grid.* Houston, TX: Gulf Publishing.

Brakey, M. (1991). Are you a good follower? *Nursing 91, 21*(12), 78-81.

Burns, J. (1978). *Leadership*. New York: Harper & Row.

Cartwright, D., & Zander, A. (Eds.). (1960). *Group dynamics: Research and theory* (2nd Ed.). Evanston, IL: Row, Peterson.

Curtin, L. (1989). Things unattempted yet. *Nursing Management, 20*(7), 7-8.

Dunham, J., & Klafehn, K. (1990). Transformational leadership and the nurse executive. *Journal of Nursing Administration, 20*(4), 28-34.

Fiedler, F. (1967). *A theory of leadership effectiveness*. New York: McGraw-Hill.

Fiedler, F., & Chemers, M. (1984). *Improving leadership effectiveness: The leader match concept* (2nd ed.). New York: John Wiley & Sons.

Fiedler, F., & Garcia, J. (1987). *New approaches to effective leadership: Cognitive resources and organizational performance*. New York: John Wiley & Sons.

Getzels, J., & Guba, E. (1957). Social behavior and the administrative process. *The School Review, 65*(4), 423-441.

Grant, A. (1994). *The professional nurse: Issues and actions*. Springhouse, PA: Springhouse.

Guidera, M., & Gilmore, C. (1988). In defense of followership. *American Journal of Nursing, 88*(7), 1017.

Hersey, P., & Blanchard, K. (1993). *Management of organizational behavior: Utilizing human resources* (6th ed.). Englewood Cliffs, NJ: Prentice-Hall.

Kelley, R. (1988). In praise of followers. *Harvard Business Review, 66*, 142-148.

Kennedy, J. (1956). *Profiles in courage*. New York: Harper & Brothers.

Kim, W., & Mauborgne, R. (1992). Parables of leadership. *Harvard Business Review, 70*(4), 123-128.

Kison, C. (1989). Leadership: How, who and what? *Nursing Management, 20*(11), 72-74.

Kouzes, J., & Posner, B. (1987). *The leadership challenge*. San Francisco: Jossey-Bass.

Kouzes, J., & Posner, B. (1988). *The leadership practices inventory*. San Diego, CA: Pfeiffer & Company.

Kouzes, J., & Posner, B. (1990). *Leadership practices inventory (LPI): A self-assessment and analysis*. San Diego, CA: Pfeiffer & Company.

Kramer, M. (1990). The magnet hospitals: Excellence revisited. *Journal of Nursing Administration, 20*(9), 35-44.

Kramer, M., & Schmalenberg, C. (1990). Fundamental lessons in leadership. In E. Simendinger, T. Moore, & M. Kramer (Eds.), *The successful nurse executive: A guide for every nurse manager* (pp. 5-21). Ann Arbor, MI: Health Administration Press.

Likert, R. (1961). *New patterns of management*. New York: McGraw-Hill.

McCloskey, J., & Molen, M. (1986). Leadership in nursing. *Annual Review of Nursing Research, 5*, 177-207.

McClure, M., Poulin, M., Sovie, M., & Wandelt, M. (1983). *Magnet hospitals: Attraction and retention of professional nurses*. Kansas City, MO: American Nurses Association.

McDaniel, C., & Wolf, G. (1992). Transformational leadership in nursing service: A test of theory. *Journal of Nursing Administration, 22*(2), 60-65.

Meighan, M. (1990). The most important characteristics of nursing leaders. *Nursing Administration Quarterly, 15*(1), 63-69.

Murphy, D. (1990). Followers for a new era. *Nursing Management, 21*(7), 68-69.

Murphy, M., & DeBack, V. (1991). Today's nursing leaders: Creating the vision. *Nursing Administration Quarterly, 16*(1), 71-80.

Pagonis, W. (1992). The work of the leader. *Harvard Business Review, 70*(6), 118-126.

Rosenfeld, P. (1994). *Profiles of the newly licensed nurse: Historical trends and future implications* (2nd ed.). (Pub. No. 19-2530). New York: National League for Nursing Press.

Smola, B. (1988). Refinement and validation of a tool measuring leadership characteristics of baccalaureate nursing students. In O. Strickland & C. Waltz (Eds.), *Measurement of nursing outcomes* Vol 2 (pp. 314-366). New York: Springer.

Stodgill, R. (1963). *Manual for the Leader Behavior Description Questionnaire-Form XII: An experimental revision*. Columbus, OH: Ohio State University.

Tannenbaum, R., & Schmidt, W. (1958). How to choose a leadership pattern. *Harvard Business Review, 36*, 95-101.

Tannenbaum, R., & Schmidt, W. (1973). How to choose a leadership pattern. *Harvard Business Review, 51*(3), 162-180.

University Associates Instrumentation Kit. (1987). San Diego, CA: University Associates.

Vestal, K. (1989). Increasing resourcefulness: The key to declining resources. *Nursing Economic$, 7*(4), 204-207, 230.

White, R., & Lippitt, R. (1968). Leader behavior and member reaction in three social climates. In D. Cartwright & A. Zander (Eds.), *Group dynamics: Research and theory* (3rd ed.) (pp. 318-335). New York: Harper & Row.

Yukl, G. (1981). *Leadership in organizations*. Englewood Cliffs, NJ: Prentice-Hall.

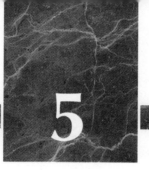

Management Principles

Chapter Objectives

❧

define and describe management and nursing management

❧

explain the management process

❧

discuss the nature of managerial work

❧

analyze the roles a manager plays

❧

identify ways to manage difficult personalities

❧

analyze time management

❧

relate management concepts to nursing leadership and management

❧

review legal aspects of management

❧

exercise critical thinking to conceptualize and analyze
possible solutions to a practical experience incident

*l*eadership and management are equally important processes. Since their focus is different, their importance varies according to what is needed in a specific situation. They are overlapping, but distinct ideas. However, some have viewed them as almost identical or very similar. For example, Hersey & Blanchard (1993) felt that leadership was a broader concept than management. They described management as a special kind of leadership. This view would pose management as a subpart of leadership, not as a distinct concept.

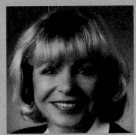

Roxane Spitzer-Lehmann

Roxane Spitzer-Lehmann Envisions the Differences between Leadership and Management

Competent leadership and management are critical elements for success in any organization, whether a nursing department or an entire health care corporation or hospital. Would that these two components were easily distinguishable; unfortunately, they are not. The core components of leadership and management are circular, dynamic, and interrelated. In management the requirements may be to manage a particular process, whereas leadership's role is to assure that the right process is being managed, or the right problem being solved, while focus is kept on the outcome.

The best way to describe leadership and management is to describe those core components necessary to achieve desired outcomes: vision, passion, and execution. Simplistically, the concept of vision is a necessary and common element of leadership. It is an unwavering belief and commitment to the goal, whereas the concept of execution may be described as a management function. An even more simplistic distinction would define leadership as the strategic element (long-range vision and planning), whereas management is the operations function (getting it done). This latter distinction has great applicability to the practice of nursing and supports the notion of the registered professional nurse as the strategic leaders while others execute the plan.

Leaders, however, are often called on to fulfill managerial functions and should be capable of doing so. Managers must develop strengths first in understanding the passion necessary to get the job done and then the ability to communicate the vision.

Across the fine line that distinguishes leadership and management, successful people cross back and forth based on the situation and need. This ability is one of the major hallmarks of the knowledge-based worker, the registered professional nurse.

Roxane Spitzer-Lehmann, PhD, MBA, MA, RN, FAAN, is a professor at the schools of nursing and business and is Associate Dean for Practice and Operations of Community Clinics, Vanderbilt University, Nashville, Tennessee. Dr. Spitzer-Lehmann was formerly Vice President, Managed Care Operations, Medicus Systems Corporation, and CEO, Managed Care Operations, San Diego, California. She is on the faculty of the School of Business at the University of Colorado-Denver in the Executive Program in Health Administration, the School of Business Administration at United States International University, and the schools of nursing at the University of Southern California and Texas Technical University. Dr. Spitzer-Lehmann is also the editor of *Nursing Management Desk Reference* and the journal *Seminars for Nurse Managers*, both published by W.B. Saunders Company, as well as the author of several books and numerous articles on nursing management and health care.

Bass and Avolio (1990) distinguished transactional leadership from transformational leadership. They noted the parallels between what they call transactional leaders and traditional descriptions of managers. Transformational leaders, however, reflected the "strong forces" of leadership. Transactional leaders, or in this case really managers, focus on maintenance of the quality and quantity of performance, reduction in resistance to change, and the implementation of decisions in a specific situation. By contrast, increasing effort, leaps in performance, changing group values and needs, creating innovative ideas, and improving quality are the foci of transformational leaders. In their model, the transactional process occurs first and appears to be essential to effective leadership. It would appear that transactional leadership is another name for management functions and that this theory sees management as a process leading to expected outcomes (see Chapter 4).

Under conditions of maintenance and stability, transactional management appears to be needed. For growth, crisis, or change, transformational leadership is a component of effectiveness. Thus management and leadership do not appear to be identical. The focus of each is different. It is possible that management is focused on task accomplishment and leadership is focused on human relationship aspects. They may be sequential, and they are interrelated. There is a "grey area" in which there is overlap as to the focus of their outcomes. This overlap occurs where the two processes are integrated or synthesized to accomplish goals and where the same strategies are employed even though the goals may differ.

DEFINITION

Management is defined as the coordination and integration of resources through planning, organizing, coordinating, directing, and controlling in order to accomplish specific institutional goals and objectives (see Chart 5.1). Another definition of management is a process by which organizational goals are met through the application of skills and the use of resources. The leadership definition emphasizes actions that influence toward *group* goals; the definition of management focuses on *organizational* goals. The achievement of organizational goals through leadership and manipulation of the environment is management. In a systems approach to management, the inputs would be represented by human resources and physical and technical resources. The outputs would be the realization of goals (see Fig. 5.1). Koontz (1961) concluded that management is the art of:

- getting things done through and with people in formally organized groups
- creating an environment in an organized group where people can perform as individuals, yet cooperate to attain group goals

---

CHART 5.1
↪ DEFINITIONS

Management
the coordination and integration of resources through planning, organizing, coordinating, directing, and controlling in order to accomplish specific institutional goals and objectives.

Nursing Management
the coordination and integration of nursing resources by applying the management process in order to accomplish nursing care and service goals and objectives.

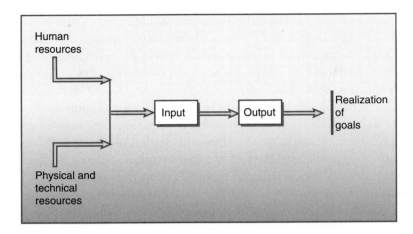

Figure 5.1
Systems view of management.

- removing blocks to performance
- optimizing efficiency in effectively reaching goals.

Thus management is a separate function with a specific purpose and related roles. Management is central to the work of nursing. *Nursing management* is defined as the coordination and integration of nursing resources by applying the management process in order to accomplish nursing care and service goals and objectives.

BACKGROUND: THE MANAGEMENT PROCESS

An organization can be any institution. Working to achieve an organization's goals would involve some process of management. The principles that guide the process of management need to be identified. A Frenchman named Fayol (1949) reasoned that management could not be taught because of the lack of basic principles. Physics can be taught because of Newton, and geometry can be taught because of Euclid. To understand the management process, therefore, he formulated the principles that created a basis for management practice. Fayol (1949) said that managers perform unique and discrete functions: they plan, organize, coordinate, and control. Thus managers of nurses do the work of management, while nurses do the work of nursing (Organizational Dynamics, 1975).

The four steps of the management process are planning, organizing, coordinating or directing, and controlling (Fayol, 1949). These functions comprise the scope of a manager's major effort. The management process is a rational, logical process based on problem solving principles (see Fig. 5.2).

At the lowest levels of an organization, employees are hired for some technical or professional skill. In highly technical, constantly changing fields (such as nursing), it takes nearly all of a nurse's time to be technically compe-

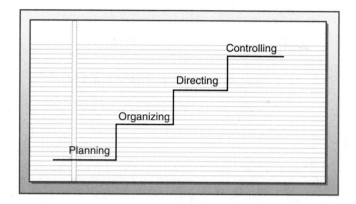

Figure 5.2
Four steps of the
management process.

tent. Yet for a middle manager, only a part of the work time can be spent being technically competent. The other part is spent doing management: planning, coordinating, directing, and controlling the work of nurses. With advancement to the highest nurse executive level, the job change inevitably
results in the nurse executive's becoming the least competent technician because the job demands an increasing focus on management and leadership activities. These are normal organizational dynamics. They occur because management is a discrete function. Part of the task is to link the top of the
organization to the bottom and vice versa, in a two way street. The bottom
also has to know what the top is doing and recognize the fact that managers
do management while technicians do their work; together the group accomplishes individual and organizational goals (Organizational Dynamics, 1975).
This view highlights the value of investing in administrative infrastructure.
Managers in nursing perform discrete and important functions that provide an
environment to facilitate delivery of client services. Mintzberg (1994) described this managing as blended care.

Mintzberg (1994) compared management as cure, which is intermittent
and interventionist, with management as care, which is continuous and involved. Management as care is thought to be more effective. In this modality,
nurses are postulated to be able to move more easily and naturally into management because of nursing's roots in caring. Mintzberg noted that in this
sense nursing is management, as contrasted to medicine as cure. Clearly, nursing's original role was caring for patients. Care management is one of nursing's
emerging roles, as compared to nursing's care provision role.

In nursing, the management process is focused on the human element, or
the management of human resources. It is in this dynamic and interactive
process that the work of nursing is accomplished. Nurse managers balance two
competing needs: the needs of the staff related to growth, efficiency, motivation, morale, and accomplishment and the needs of the employer for produc-

tivity, quality, and cost-effectiveness. Desired outcomes include staff satisfaction and productivity (Kepler, 1980).

RESEARCH NOTE

Source: Mintzberg, H. (1994). Managing as blended care. *Journal of Nursing Administration*, 24(9), 29-36.

Purpose

The purpose of this research is to develop and enhance a new model of managerial work. The new model is based on a review and integration of identified managerial work roles, visualized in concentric circles. The model was tested in a research project on managerial work. One head nurse of a hospital unit in Canada was observed and described during one working day. Roles of leading, linking, controlling, and doing were analyzed and reported. Conclusions were drawn about effective management styles.

Discussion

Mintzberg's classic work on management roles goes back to 1973 and his *The Nature of Managerial Work*. This new model moves from a list approach to an interactive model approach. At the center of the model is a person in a job who creates a frame. The frame is manifested by an agenda of issues and work schedules. Above this core are three levels through which work can take place: information, people, and action. Roles pervade the levels depicted by circles. The research methodology was participant observation, designed to assess the usefulness of the model and identify role behaviors and styles. "Caring" management described this head nurse's management style. It is a kind of blended care that is practiced out in the open and standing up. It resembles a craft style of management.

Application to Practice

This female head nurse administered continuous care. There was a natural rhythm, flow, and blending of the component parts of the Mintzberg model. Thus the doing activities are interwoven with the leading and communicating activities. Mintzberg comments on gender and style research and his observations in healthcare. He comments on the differing perspectives of physicians and nurses regarding good care management. The two professions care differently and in complimentary ways, yet, they need to work out ways to collaborate to the clients' benefit. This article emphasizes how management, like nursing, can be a caring type of work. In a sense, nursing is management.

Planning

Planning is defined as determining the long and short term objectives and the corresponding actions that must be taken to achieve these objectives (see

Chart 5.2). Steiner (1962, p. 28) described planning as "the conscious determination of courses of action to achieve preconceived objectives." Planning can be detailed, specific, and rigid or broad, general, and flexible. Planning is deciding in advance what is to be done and when, by whom, and how it is to be done. Hersey & Blanchard (1993) described planning as involving the setting of goals and objectives and developing "work maps" to show how they are to be accomplished.

The two types of planning are (Levenstein, 1985):
- *strategic planning:* more broad-ranged, this means determining the overall purposes and directions of the organization.
- *tactical planning:* more short-ranged, this means determining the specific details of implementing broader goals.

Levenstein (1985) identified three errors that can create planning flaws:
- errors of fact: the plan is based on misinformation.
- errors in assumption: the plan is based on wrong assumptions.
- errors of logic: the plan is based on faulty reasoning.

Planning flaws carry over into organizing, directing, and controlling activities.

An alternative conceptualization to the model of planning that views it as an orderly, top-down sequence is the model proposed by Hayes-Roth and Hayes-Roth (1979). Their idea was that opportunistic planning approaches were used to face complex planning tasks. Planners, under conditions of complexity, pursue whatever seems opportune or promising at the time. A plan becomes multi-directional and develops by increments. This may appear chaotic compared to systematic planning, but leads to better plans in complex task situations.

Planning is a process that is heavily dependent upon the decision making process. Part of planning is choosing among a certain number of alternatives. Thus, in nursing, the manager often has to balance the needs of clients, staff, administrators, and physicians. Since resources are limited, planning involves an analysis of how to best proceed under the given constraints (Kepler, 1980).

The planning process is intimately involved with establishing objectives. Fayol (1949) identified planning as examining the future and drawing up a plan of action. Activities involved include the laying out of the work to be done, determining the use of resources, and establishing the standards for evaluation. Levenstein (1985) argued that the role of the nurse manager as planner is critical to the successful functioning of the institution and the care of clients. This is because the plan of care is shaped and reshaped with nursing input and then implemented by the nursing staff. Thomas (1983) noted that the institution is held or glued together by the nurses, enabling it to function. The nurse is engaged in a constant mental planning operation when deciding what specific things are to be accomplished for the client.

CHART 5.2
⌒ DEFINITIONS

Planning
determining the long and short term objectives and the corresponding actions that must be taken to achieve these objectives.

Organizing
mobilizing the human and material resources of the institution to achieve organizational objectives.

Coordinating
motivating and leading personnel to carry out the desired actions.

Controlling
comparing the results of work with predetermined standards of performance and taking corrective action when needed.

Organizing

Organizing is defined as mobilizing the human and material resources of the institution to achieve organizational objectives. Fayol (1949) noted that organizing was building up the material and human structures. Authority, power, and structure are used for influence. The goal is to get the human, equipment, and material resources mobilized, organized, and working. Organizing so that the goals and objectives can be accomplished includes establishing some relationship between the workers and the environment. The first step is to organize the work; then the people are organized; finally the environment is organized.

Organizing closely follows the planning process. They are sometimes referred to together: planning and organizing. Organizing encompasses activities designed to bring together an array of various resources including personnel, money, and equipment, in a manner that is the most effective for accomplishing organizational goals. Therefore, the essence of organizing is the integration and coordination of resources (Hersey & Blanchard, 1993).

Organizing also can be thought of as a process of identifying roles in relationship to each other. Thus organizing becomes activities related to establishing a structure and hierarchy of job positions within a unit or department. Responsibilities would be assigned to each job position. The complexity of this aspect of organizing is related to the size of the organization and the number of employees and jobs. For nurse managers, the activities of budget management, staffing, and scheduling are all organizing activities which are interrelated and tied to role relationships (Kepler, 1980). Organizing in nursing also relates to other human resources and personnel functions such as orientation and staff inservice development. Examples of how nurses organize nursing include committees and bylaws. Organizations organize by establishing a structure such as a hierarchy with divisions or departments.

Directing

Coordinating or *directing* is defined as motivating and leading personnel to carry out the desired actions. Motivation is a complex activity, yet motivating and leading personnel to carry out the actions needed to achieve the objectives is a critical managerial responsibility. Fayol (1949) identified activities of binding together, unifying, and harmonizing the activity and effort of various personnel as part of coordinating or directing.

Motivation often is included with activities of directing others, along with communicating and leading. Motivating is a major strategy related to determining the subordinates' level of performance and thereby to influencing how effectively the goals of the organization will be met. The amount of employee effort able to be influenced by motivation is thought to be from 20% to 30% at bottom to 80% to 90% at top (Hersey & Blanchard, 1993).

On a day-to-day basis, coaching is used as a technique to direct and moti-vate subordinates. While working through assigned staff members, the man-ager delegates activities and responsibilities. The function of directing in-volves actions of supervising and guiding others within their assigned duties. The use of interpersonal skills is required to delicately balance the need to di-rect and supervise with the need to create and maintain a motivational cli-mate (Kepler, 1980).

Within nursing there is a legal aspect to the managerial directing function. In some state licensing laws, supervision is a defined legal element of nursing practice. Delegation and supervision are viewed legally as a part of the practice of nursing. Thus nurses have a specific need to know and understand this scope of practice. Managers carry responsibility and accountability for the quality and quantity of their supervision. Nurses also are becoming more cognizant of the importance of their role as care coordinator. Nurse managers carry the added re-sponsibility and accountability for the coordination of groups of nurse providers.

Controlling

The controlling aspect of the managerial process may appear at first to carry a negative connotation. However, when used in reference to manage-ment, the word control does not have the same meaning as being manipula-tive toward others. Controlling is ensuring that the proper processes are fol-lowed. Fayol (1949) called this the activity of seeing that everything occurs in conformity with established rules. In nursing the term evaluation is used to re-fer to similar actions and activities. Control or evaluation means ensuring that the flow and processes of work, as well as goal accomplishment, proceed as planned. *Controlling* is defined as comparing the results of work with prede-termined standards of performance and taking corrective action when needed. This means ensuring that the results are as desired, and if not up to standards, then taking some action to modify, remediate, or reverse the variances.

The management function of controlling involves the feeding back of in-formation about the results and outcomes of work activities, combined with activities to follow-up and compare outcomes with plans. Appropriate adjust-ments need to be made wherever outcomes vary or deviate from expectations (Hersey & Blanchard, 1993). In nursing, when a critical path is used to track client care, the variances are analyzed and corrected as a function of manage-rial control. The controlling function of management has been described as a constant process of re-evaluation to see if what is currently occurring meets needs, plans, and standards as well as to identify where improvements might be a benefit (Kepler, 1980).

In summary, by using the four steps of the management process, goals can be accomplished by and through other people. These managerial functions primarily are aimed at the productivity element of an organization. For nursing, within a human services industry, managerial skills are employed to enhance the utilization of human resources (Kepler, 1980).

MANAGEMENT IN ORGANIZATIONS

The Nature of Managerial Work

Lewin (1947) said that the behavior of human beings is a function of individual psychology, needs patterns of people, and the environment in which they work. Behavioral theory and its applications to the management of people focuses on organizing and processing work and accomplishing organizational objectives at a targeted minimum cost and minimum waste. The responsibility for doing that lies with management. Managers manage people and the environment. One view of management identifies the manager's behavior, role, and situation created for people to work in as causing the followers' behavior.

Mintzberg (1973, 1975) reformulated Fayol's ideas about the nature of managerial work. His synthesis of research findings about managers in general revealed the following:

* Managers work at an unrelenting pace at activities characterized by brevity, variety, and discontinuity. Managers are strongly action-oriented.
* Managers handle exceptions and perform regular work such as ritual and ceremonial duties, negotiation, and processing of soft information linking the organization to its environment.
* Managers prefer oral communication, especially telephone calls and meetings.
* "Judgment" and "intuition" describe the procedures managers use to schedule time, process information, and make decisions.

Zaleznik (1992) noted that managerial culture emphasizes rationality and control: a manager is a problem solver. He noted that it takes neither genius nor heroism to be a manager. What is needed is persistence, tough-mindedness, hard work, intelligence, analytical ability, tolerance, and goodwill. Drucker (1954) outlined three jobs of management:

* managing a business enterprise
* managing managers
* managing workers and work.

The skills needed by nursing service managers include conceptual or thinking skills, technical skills in nursing methods and techniques, and group and human relations skills (Katz, 1955).

Mintzberg (1975) described the manager's job in terms of ten roles or sets of behaviors. Derived from the formal authority and status of the position are three interpersonal roles: figurehead, leader, and liaison. Being the nerve cen-

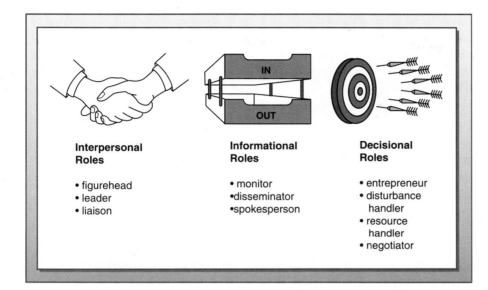

Interpersonal Roles

- figurehead
- leader
- liaison

Informational Roles

- monitor
- disseminator
- spokesperson

Decisional Roles

- entrepreneur
- disturbance handler
- resource handler
- negotiator

Figure 5.3
Mintzberg's ten managerial roles. (Data from Mintzberg [1975].)

ter of the organizational unit, information processing is a key part of the role. Informational roles are monitor, disseminator, and spokesperson. Information is the basic input to decision making. The decisional roles are entrepreneur, disturbance handler, resource allocator, and negotiator (see Fig. 5.3). He suggested a number of important managerial skills:

- developing peer relationships
- carrying out negotiations
- motivating subordinates
- resolving conflicts
- establishing information networks and disseminating information
- making decisions in conditions of extreme ambiguity
- allocating resources

If management is important to achieving organizational goals, then the skills, abilities, functions, actions, and strategies used by managers to manage are important to know and understand. Kepler (1980) suggested that the managerial skills to be mastered are processes of understanding, communication, and effective use and manipulation (through selective use of rewards and punishment) of personnel.

Mintzberg (1994) elaborated his earlier work on the nature of managerial work by expanding it to an interactive model of managerial work. The model uses concentric circles. At the core is a person who is in a job. The person has some unique set of values, experiences, knowledge, and competencies. The combination of the person and the job creates a frame composed of the job's purpose, the person's perspective about what needs to be done, and selected strategies for doing the job. The frame can range across two continnua: from vague to very specific, and from person-selected to externally imposed. The frame results in an agenda of work issues and time scheduling. Placed at the center of the figure, these elements form the core of the job of a manager. Managerial roles and behaviors at this level include conceiving the frame and scheduling the agenda.

Growing out of the core are three concentric circles from abstract to concrete. They are called the information, people, and action levels of managerial work. At the most abstract level, the manager processes information and uses it to drive the action. At the next level, the manager works with people to encourage work activities. At the most concrete level, the manager manages the action.

At the information level, the associated managerial roles are communicating information and controlling by using information to control the work of others. At the people level, the managerial roles are leading and linking. Leading involves encouraging and enabling individuals by mentoring and rewarding, groups by team building and conflict resolution, and the whole organization by building a culture. Linking roles involve relating to the external environment by building networks of contacts and acquiring information from the environment to transmit back to the unit. At the action level, the associated managerial role is called doing or supervising. Behaviors include doing, handling disturbances, and negotiating (Mintzberg, 1994).

Mintzberg's (1994) interactive model provides a visual display of a way of thinking about managerial work and associated roles and activities. The model could be used as a basis for self-assessment and could be applied to specific managerial jobs. Nurses who strive to apply the concepts to their managerial work could use the model to examine and analyze managerial styles, behaviors, and roles. Nurses as managers manage people (clients, themselves, and other staff or providers) and the environment of client care delivery. An understanding of the management process and the roles related to the work of a manager can assist nurses to improve their personal effectiveness and their organization's productivity.

Other Aspects of Management

The understanding of management as a unique and discrete function in organizations can be advanced by examining a manager's work, job, and roles. There also are common management-related issues that can be explored. Two frequently occurring issues will be briefly overviewed: managing difficult people and time management.

Managing Difficult People

Although it seems negative to dwell on the dark side of human nature, in reality managers are challenged by persons who exhibit negative attitudes and behaviors. These negative predispositions occur for a variety of reasons, all related to the complexity of human beings. Lewin (1947) believed that the behavior of humans was some blend of individual psychology and need patterns with the work environment. Individuals have needs and expectations as do organizations. The two sets of needs and goals may clash rather than mesh. The manager directly faces this common situation.

All human working environments experience the management problem of working with difficult people. Lewis-Ford (1993) offered the following categories to describe such people:

- **Sherman tanks:** abusive, abrupt, and intimidating, they charge down on you with a tremendous show of power.
- **snipers:** hostile-aggressive, they use innuendos and digs to take pot-shots at people.
- **exploders:** they suddenly break into temper tantrums to get their way.
- **bulldozers:** they are condescending know-it-alls who are competent but do not easily entertain other people's judgments.
- **balloons:** they like to be in the know but are full of hot air. They range from braggarts to tyrants.
- **clams:** they react to any disagreeable situation by closing down. They use silence as a weapon.
- **negative nabobs:** they are negative, naysayers, and skeptical pessimists.
- **complainers:** they whine and find fault with everything. They want you to fix it for them.
- **stallers:** they agree with plans only to let you down by doing nothing to realize them.

Appeasement generally does not work with people who are negative. While it would be preferable for there to be a change in the behavior toward a positive predisposition, this may not be possible for the manager to effect, especially if the behavior is long-standing and has been rewarded in the past.

Lewis-Ford (1993) recommended a two-pronged management approach. The approaches are (1) grand tactics for immediate challenge to peace and dignity, and (2) long range strategies.

Grand tactics
- calm down and get control of yourself.
- lower your voice to calm the other person.
- choose your ground—is this a difficult person or a difficult situation?
- guard your perspective and avoid taking the behavior personally.
- never cry or whine.

Long-range strategies
- assess and categorize difficult people as a way of cognitively understanding them.
- validate this assessment with others.

- plan a strategy for each category.
- practice the strategy.
- prepare yourself psychologically prior to interacting with difficult people.

Some behavior may be so disruptive to the group that it needs to be corrected through discipline. However, some behavior arises secondary to stress, as a coping mechanism. The manager's interpersonal skills are tested by people who exhibit difficult behavior.

TIME MANAGEMENT

With things changing so much, people feel that they never have enough time to meet all the job demands. The one area individuals have control over and can change is themselves. Technology often is not the limiting factor in work output for nurses; the individuals are through their unique abilities and limits on time. Although each person has the same amount of time per day or week, how that time is used makes all the difference (Parker, 1986).

Perceived excessive time demands coupled with the inability to fulfill them create stress. Time is a scarce and valuable resource. When there is more demand than can be met, rationing is needed. The first step is to treat time as a unique resource that needs to be carefully managed. The second step is to identify the reality of the situation surrounding time demands and do an analysis of the situation and the individual's responses and patterns. Clearly, in most hospitals today, there are not enough nursing resources for the existing workload. The nursing management systems do not have under their control either workload or latitude in decisions controlling resources. This leaves managerial decision opportunities limited to prioritization (Manthey, 1988; Veninga, 1982).

Manthey (1988) discussed the staffing and scheduling difficulties that seem to be perennial in nursing service. Fluctuating workloads, scheduling systems, float pools, austerity programs, and "pulling" nurses from area to area are inadequate to match the right person with the right skills at the right time to the workload demands. This leaves the staff nurse struggling with a myth that help is coming and with the gap between what should be done and what is possible. This dilemma translates into what do you do when there is more work than time available? The nurse may decide what to do but may not have the autonomy to decide what not to do. Autonomy means decision control over the kind and degree of service a client will receive. It involves a conscious decision about what will and will not be done when there is more work than available time. Control over time use is a key aspect of professional nursing practice.

Time needs to be managed. The source of time demands can be identified through analysis. First, a list of all activities and their time usage can be logged for a designated time period. This can be tabulated as to the percentage of time absorbed by each activity. This analysis reveals how time is being spent.

The objectives, whether personal or organization, that need to be met by the allocation of time are then compared to the actual time spent. Priorities need to be set based on the basic purpose of the work to be done. Dalston (1990) identified an overall strategy for effective time management that encompassed four tasks: internalizing the need for change, identifying time expenditures, organizing tasks, and minimizing distractions (see Chart 5.3).

Organizing tasks is a process of reshaping activities to implement a system for accomplishing desired activities. The focus is on tasks. One method is to keep a "things to do" list to keep track of the pool of necessary tasks. However, this habit of deriving a "to do" list can become a compulsion. Rather, the "to do list" activity can be used as an analysis vehicle to help delete unnecessary tasks, identify tasks to delegate, break down tasks into subunits, and select daily tasks (Dalston, 1990).

Minimizing distractions is a process of identifying and modifying time robbers and the misuse of time. The primary causes of time mismanagement are (Veninga, 1982):

- wasted effort
- unproductive meetings
- a crisis orientation.

A fourth area, common in nursing, is interruptions. There are many tips and techniques for time management: signs saying "thank you for not disturbing me," mechanisms to screen or control telephone interruptions, setting a timer to keep phone calls short, analyzing meeting attendance, blocking time, prioritization, and delegation. The greatest time savers are (Parker, 1986):

- setting goals
- specifying priorities
- planning.

Failure to consciously control time expenditure through identification, review, analysis, and then prioritization leads to waste of time and constant crises. Routine crisis creates stress. Prevention through planning and time management avoids the stress of routine crisis. Individuals can change themselves, set priorities, delegate, and eliminate time wasters. This frees up time and energy to cope with change and to be more productive.

It can be argued that all nurses are managers. Staff nurses are the employees at the most critical point in fulfilling the purpose of the organization: they

---

CHART 5.3
❧ STRATEGIES FOR EFFECTIVE TIME MANAGEMENT

- Internalize the need for change
- Identify time expenditures
- Organize tasks
- Minimize distractions

Data from Dalston (1990).

are in close and frequent contact with the client, and they coordinate the delivery of health care services.

The American Organization of Nurse Executives (AONE) (1992) noted that the nurse manager is defined as a registered nurse holding 24-hour accountability for the management of a unit(s) or area(s) within a healthcare institution. The nurse manager's role includes managing human, fiscal, and other resources needed to manage clinical nursing practice and client care: this is central to effective, quality client care. The role of the nurse manager is complex and encompasses multiple responsibilities such as (AONE, 1992):

- management of clinical nursing practice and client care delivery
- management of human, fiscal, and other resources
- development of personnel
- compliance with regulatory and professional standards
- strategic planning
- fostering interdisciplinary and collaborative relationships

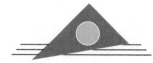 *Leadership & Management Behaviors*

LEADERSHIP BEHAVIORS

- is visible
- communicates a vision
- motivates followers
- seeks out new resources
- evaluates outcomes

MANAGEMENT BEHAVIORS

- coordinates client care
- plans daily operations
- makes assignments
- sets goals for subordinates
- hires staff
- responds to needs/desires of subordinates as long as the work is accomplished
- exchanges rewards for work effort
- manages resource allocation
- monitors work and quality processes
- takes corrective actions
- counsels subordinates
- manages change
- handles conflict situations
- communicates among levels

OVERLAP AREAS

- exercises broad-perspective decision making
- communicates
- motivates subordinates
- evaluates process and outcomes

Management has been described as a discipline that uses a set of tools to achieve desired outcomes. It becomes nursing management when the desired outcomes are nursing goals. If management occurs at all levels of nursing, then the nursing profession needs methods for assisting nurses to develop competence in management (Genovich-Richards & Carissimi, 1986).

Using a conceptual framework of three domains of nursing management behaviors, client care management, operational management, and human resources management, Genovich-Richards and Carissimi (1986) described the use of a management assessment center technique. Seven key areas—leadership ability, decision making skill, analytical ability, organizational ability, group performance skill, and personal characteristics such as sensitivity, flexibility, competitiveness, and self-awareness—were the focus of an intensive one day session using exercises, simulations, and management activities for practice. A management assessment center technique is one tool that nurses can use to develop individuals and enhance their managerial skills and abilities. It could become a staff development or inservice program. It could be used for growth and self-assessment for staff who desire or contemplate advancement along a nursing administration career track.

Legal Aspects of Management

The managers of any healthcare organization are responsible to the policy making body for the organization. The managers also hold an obligation to comply with the laws of society at local, state, and national levels. Managers are responsible for ensuring that laws are adhered to both in the actions of management itself and also in the actions of those employees who assist the managers in carrying out the mission of the organization. Concern for the law involves three general areas: personal negligence in clinical practice, liability for delegation and supervision, and organizational liability related to employment issues.

Activities of clinical client care carry corresponding legal accountability and risk. Errors do happen. Some lead to injury to a client. At minimum, nurses have an ethical obligation to nonmaleficence or to do no harm to clients. This duty is discharged in part by remaining competent in knowledge and skills and the standards of practice. Nursing negligence occurs when nurses' actions are unreasonable given the circumstances, fail to meet the standard of care, or the nurse fails to act and causes harm. Harm can arise from acts that are unintentional, such as omissions or negligence, or harm can come from acts that are intentional, such as defamation, invasion of privacy, assault and battery, false imprisonment, or intentional infliction of emotional distress (Aiken, 1994).

Four elements of negligence are required for malpractice: a duty owed to the client such as to render nursing care, breach of duty, proximate cause or causal connection to the nurse, and damages. Common clinical practice areas of negligence and/or liability include the general areas of treatment, communication, medication, and monitoring/observing/supervising/surveillance. Examples of common negligence allegations in nursing malpractice suits include patient falls, use of restraints, medication errors, burns, equipment injuries, retained foreign objects, failure to monitor, failure to ensure safety, failure to take appropriate nursing action, failure to confirm accuracy of physician's orders, improper technique or performance of treatments, failure to respond to a patient, failure to follow hospital procedure, and failure to supervise treatment (Aiken, 1994).

Over and above personal liability for clinical practice, nurses and nurse managers have accountability and liability for their acts of delegation and supervision. The ethical and legal aspects of delegation and supervision liability are discussed in Chapters 9 and 15. Nurses and nurse managers both carry an obligation to report incompetent practice that occurs at any point in the care delivery process (see Chapter 27). Nurse managers have a duty to train, orient, and evaluate the ability of nursing staff to perform specific functions and tasks. Healthcare organizations have a duty to monitor the competence and ability of nursing and medical professionals and to inquire about their credentials (Aiken, 1994). Both nurses and nurse managers have a duty to follow policies and procedures when reasonable. Nurse managers are advised to carefully review policies and procedures, including the language used, in order to more closely adhere to legal and ethical parameters. Clearly, management in nursing practice means that nurses must fulfill obligations and duties both to clients and to the organization. This means using knowledge, skill, and decision making abilities to reduce the incidence of negligence and malpractice by employees as a way to reduce harm to clients and legal risk to the organization. As the primary care coordinators, nurses need to manage the environment of care delivery. Assuring staff competence and reporting incompetent practice are key activities. For example, in nursing, legal and ethical issues arise when a nurse is impaired by substance abuse. The overall consideration is protecting the client from harm. Confronting suspected abuse must be done carefully. However, when an incident occurs, the nurse manager has a responsibility to intervene.

Organizations are constrained by specific laws related to employment issues. While the various healthcare providers and their employing organizations have specific legal and ethical obligations to clients, such as informed consent and the Patient Self-Determination Act of 1990, organizations carry specific legal and ethical obligations toward employees. The employer has an obligation to provide a safe and secure care delivery environment (Aiken, 1994). For example, the Occupational Safety and Health Administration's (OSHA) rules and regulations must be operational. As a branch of the U.S.

Department of Labor, OSHA has become involved with issues related to protecting healthcare workers from exposure to blood and body fluid-borne pathogens. The major pathogens of concern are Hepatitis B (HBV) and the virus that causes AIDS (HIV). By enforcing universal precautions among healthcare workers, the principle idea is to prevent the transmission of the pathogens from worker to client or client to worker, thus providing a safer work environment. Guidelines from the Centers for Disease Control (CDC) were adopted by OSHA. The mandates include use of universal precautions, employer provision of protective equipment, inspection procedures, and risk management of potentially exposed employees. The employer incurs the costs of HBV vaccine, protective equipment and supplies, and exposure prevention and management. OSHA uses the mechanisms of surprise inspections and steep fines to enlist compliance.

Employment decisions are subject to liability for wrongful failure to hire, wrongful failure to advance and wrongful discharge. Title VII of the U.S. Civil Rights Act of 1964, the Age Discrimination and Employment Act (ADEA) (1967), and the Americans With Disabilities Act (ADA) (1990) are some of the specific pieces of federal legislation that impact on hiring and employment. In addition there are other federal statutes, U.S. Constitution mandates, and state and municipal laws which prescribe and proscribe various actions that are part of or relate to the employment process.

The Equal Employment Opportunity Commission (EEOC) is a federal agency that enforces many of the federal mandates concerning discrimination. There are other federal agencies, including funding agencies, that also have enforcement responsibilities in this area. Most states and many municipalities also have antidiscrimination enforcement agencies, and some laws provide the individual employee with the opportunity to bring private litigation through the courts.

The antidiscrimination statutes, in general, were designed to protect employees from discrimination in the workplace when it is based on race, color, religion, gender, pregnancy, national origin, age, or physical or mental disability. In some cases discrimination based on some of these characteristics is legally acceptable if it is based on what the law describes as a Bona Fide Occupational Qualification (BFOQ). The use of BFOQs to justify discrimination is usually defined in very narrow fashion. Two examples of gender discrimination in employment which can be justified as a BFOQ is for "wet nurse" and "sperm donor."

Management policies and procedures must be in compliance in the areas of hiring, performance appraisal, management of employees with problems, and termination (Aiken, 1994). Lawsuits also have formed the basis for the standards to be met for the termination of employees. Discharges may occur for lack of adherence to employer-established policies or standards, "good cause" per institutional policy, illegal activity, assault, insubordination, or excessive absenteeism. Written notice and the reasons for termination avoid misunderstandings and show justice through due process procedures. Careful documentation is important. If the employee is a member of a protected group, the employer may be required to submit formal justification for the termination (Aiken, 1994).

The various legal and ethical considerations of nursing management span client, provider, and employer rights and obligations. Both nurses and their employing organizations are responsible for knowing and following the various applicable laws and regulations. Inservice education can increase knowledge and awareness. Nurse managers will need to manage the environment of nursing care to ensure client safety, provider justice and safety, and organizational compliance with the law.

CURRENT ISSUES AND TRENDS

The classic notions of management and managerial work were developed in a socio-political era of industrialization and bureaucratization. Currently in business and industry, competitive pressures and economic forces are compelling corporations to adopt new flexible strategies and structures. Organizations are being urged to become leaner, more entrepreneurial, and less bureaucratic. This has created levels of complexity and interdependency.

The result has altered conventional ideas and realities of managerial work, including shifts in roles and tasks. Traditional sources of power are eroding and some motivational tools are less effective. The erosion of power from hierarchical positions is perceived as a loss of authority and may create confusion about how to mobilize and motivate staff (Kanter, 1989). Kanter (1989) noted that in a leaner and flatter corporation there are many more channels for action, and managers have to work synergistically with other departments. Managers' strategic and collaborative roles become more important as they serve as integrators and facilitators, not as watchdogs and interventionists.

Drucker (1988) used the hospital, the university, and a symphony orchestra as models for organizations evolving in today's society. As healthcare reconfigures, healthcare delivery settings will likely be knowledge-based organizations composed primarily of specialists whose performance is directed by organized feedback from colleagues, clients, and headquarters. Nurses' roles may change, but their need for managerial competence will remain. Nurses are well prepared to serve as integrators and facilitators of client care. Thus nurses appear to move easily into management and blend care into management for effectiveness (Mintzberg, 1994).

New managerial ideas include crossfunctional teams, self-managed work groups, and the networked organization (Freedman, 1992). They are derived from theories of chaos (Gleick, 1987) and complexity (Waldrop, 1992). Gleick's (1987) theory of chaos, derived from a study of meteorology, noted that minute changes can lead to drastic alterations in the behavior of a natural system. In nature, simple actions of independent components can combine to produce extremely complex behaviors, even in the absence of any central control or intelligence. Called complex adaptive systems (Waldrop, 1992), these systems are self-managed, capable of engaging in cooperative behavior, use feedback for learning and self-organizing, and operate with flexible specialization. Applied to human organizations, the organization is viewed as a kind of living organism, not as a machine. This requires a holistic approach to the overall behavior of a system. The manager's job becomes one of revealing and handling the largely hidden dynamics of complex systems (Freedman, 1992). Senge (1990) noted that managers must be designers who create learning processes that make self-organization possible. Nurses will be challenged to blend their unique skills and abilities into the managerial work of evolving organizations. Nursing's focus on caring and integration are key healthcare assets.

In the midst of an environment characterized by change, the manager's job becomes challenging. For example, planning is a function that seems to require stability and the ability to predict and project into the future. Learning and adapting are important abilities in a changeable environment. Interactive planning has been suggested as an approach to planning in complex situations and changing environments (Ackoff, 1981; Foust, 1994). Interactive planning takes a developmental approach. Problems are viewed as interrelated. Interactive planning principles emphasize the importance of participation among participants, a nonlinear view of relationships called systems thinking, and a focus on creating a desired future outcome. Interactive planning can contribute to effective care planning and to effective care management by nurses (Foust, 1994).

RESEARCH NOTE

Source: Laschinger, H., & Shamian, J. (1994). Staff nurses' and nurse managers' perceptions of job-related empowerment and managerial self-efficacy. *Journal of Nursing Administration*, 24(10), 38-47.

Purpose

The purpose of this research was to test Kanter's Structural Theory of Organizational Power in a nursing population. The link between perceived job empowerment and managerial self-efficacy in executing management role competencies was explored. A descriptive survey design was used with a proportionate random sampling of full-time staff nurses and a convenience sampling of first-line managers in one Canadian teaching hospital. The sample included 112 staff nurses (53%) and 27 nurse managers (79%). The instruments included managerial competencies and self-efficacy questionnaires. Data analysis included descriptive and inferential statistics.

Discussion

Staff nurses' empowerment scores were in the moderate range, while managers' scores were significantly higher. Nurse manager self-efficacy scores were high, with the highest scores for mentor and facilitator roles. The nurse managers (first-line) perceived the least self-efficacy in the broker role, which requires political acumen and networking skills. Manager perceptions about job empowerment were significantly associated with their perceptions of managerial self-efficacy. Managerial self-efficacy further was related to organizational conditions of work effectiveness, including power and opportunity.

Application to Practice

The results add support to Kanter's theory that power is a key structural aspect that affects organizational behavior and attitudes, thus work effectiveness. Power is defined as efficacy, or the ability to get things done. Power comes from the ability to access and mobilize support, information, resources, and opportunities within a job. With sufficient power, tasks can be accomplished. Power and opportunity vary with organizational level, and differential access interferes with maximum work effectiveness. Nurse managers can provide staff nurses with opportunities for growth and increased power through lines of information, support, and supplies or resources. Powerful managers empower their staff by association. Increased nurse empowerment can improve client care and maximal staff performance.

SUMMARY

- A manager's job is to coordinate and integrate resources.
- Classical management theory defined the management process as planning, organizing, directing or coordinating, and controlling.
- Mintzberg described ten roles managers play.
- Mintzberg evolved a model of managerial work that elaborated on managerial roles.
- Managers are challenged by people who exhibit difficult behaviors.
- Managers are challenged to manage time as a scarce resource.
- All nurses are managers; they coordinate and deliver health services to clients.
- Classic ideas have given way to a new understanding of management based on theories of chaos and complexity.
- As institutions adopt new flexible strategies and structures, managerial roles and tasks are being reconfigured. Nurses have valuable related skills.

Study Questions

1. Which is more important: leadership or management?
2. Why is management important to a nurse?
3. Are middle managers going to become obsolete?
4. How do Mintzberg's ten roles differ for nurses at different positions in a hierarchical bureaucracy?
5. Is it easier for nurses to change to a new managerial role than it is for other types of healthcare workers?

Critical Thinking Exercise

Nurse Tom Black was promoted to the position of Ambulatory Care Manager six months ago. He is just now beginning to feel comfortable in the position. One ongoing challenge he faces is the conflict generated by several physicians who bitterly complain that the nurses in the ambulatory clinic are inexperienced, unavailable, and never know what is going on. Nurse Black is a strong promoter of primary nursing, shared governance, and total quality management, which have been instituted in the clinic. He spends long hours in his office doing detailed planning and organizing. He works on the budgeting and facilities planning projects which often necessitate meetings outside of the Ambulatory Clinic. Today Nurse Black had just felt a swell of pride in the new revenue figures from the Clinic's last quarter that he had just seen, when a physician darkened his door to complain about the nurses and his pager beeped to announce a crisis on the Clinic floor.

1. What is the problem(s)?

2. How should Nurse Black handle the situation?

3. What should Nurse Black do first?

4. What management role would be best suited to this situation?

5. What leadership style might be most effective?

REFERENCES

Ackoff, R. (1981). *Creating the corporate future*. New York: John Wiley & Sons.

Aiken, T. (1994). *Legal, ethical, and political issues in nursing*. Philadelphia: F. A. Davis.

AONE: American Organization of Nurse Executives. (1992). The role and functions of the hospital nurse manager. *Nursing Management, 23*(9), 36-38.

Bass, B., & Avolio, B. (1990). *Transformational leadership development: Manual for the Multifactor Leadership Questionnaire*. Palo Alto, CA: Consulting Psychologists Press.

Dalston, J. (1990). Effective time management: Techniques and guidelines. In E. Simendinger, T. Moore, & M. Kramer (Eds.), *The successful nurse executive: A guide for every nurse manager* (pp. 75-90). Ann Arbor, MI: Health Administration Press.

Drucker, P. (1954). *The practice of management.* New York: Harper & Row.

Drucker, P. (1988). The coming of the new organization. *Harvard Business Review, 68*(1), 45-53.

Fayol, H. (1949). *General and industrial management.* London: Pitman & Sons.

Foust, J. (1994). Creating a future for nursing through interactive planning at the bedside. *Image, 26*(2), 129-131.

Freedman, D. (1992). Is management still a science? *Harvard Business Review, 70*(6), 26-38.

Genovich-Richards, J., & Carissimi, D. (1986). Developing nurses' managerial competence. *Nursing Management, 17*(3), 36-38.

Gleick, J. (1987). *Chaos: Making a new science.* New York: Viking Press.

Hayes-Roth, B., & Hayes-Roth, F. (1979). A cognitive model of planning. *Cognitive Science, 3,* 275-310.

Hersey, P., & Blanchard, K. (1993). *Management of organizational behavior: Utilizing human resources* (6th ed.). Englewood Cliffs, NJ: Prentice-Hall.

Kanter, R.M. (1989). The new managerial work. *Harvard Business Review, 69*(6), 85-92.

Katz, R. (1955). Skills of an effective administrator. *Harvard Business Review, 33*(1), 33-42.

Kepler, T. (1980). Mastering the people skills. *Journal of Nursing Administration, 10*(11), 15-20.

Koontz, H. (1961). The management theory jungle. *Academy of Management Journal,* December, 174-188.

Levenstein, A. (1985). Planning. *Nursing Management, 16*(9), 54-55.

Lewin, K. (1947). Frontiers in group dynamics: Concept, method, and reality in social science; social equilibria and social change. *Human Relations, 1*(1), 5-41.

Lewis-Ford, B. (1993). Management techniques: Coping with difficult people. *Nursing Management, 24*(3), 36-38.

Manthey, M. (1988). Who owns a staff nurse's time? *Nursing Management, 19*(9), 22-24.

Mintzberg, H. (1973). *The nature of managerial work.* New York: Harper & Row.

Mintzberg, H. (1975). The manager's job: Folklore and fact. In M. Matteson and J. Ivancevich (Eds.), *Management classics* (3rd ed.) (pp. 63-85). Plano, TX: Business Publications.

Mintzberg, H. (1994). Managing as blended care. *Journal of Nursing Administration, 24*(9), 29-36.

Organizational Dynamics. (1975). *The evolution of management theory: Part 1.* [Videotape]. Burlington, MA: Organizational Dynamics.

Parker, B. (1986). Taking control: Making time work for you. *CE MGR 6539.* Durham, NH: Health and Sciences Network.

Senge, P. (1990). *The fifth discipline: The art and practice of the learning organization.* New York: Doubleday.

Steiner, G. (1962). Making long-range company planning pay off. *California Management Review, 4*(2), 28-41.

Thomas, L. (1983). *The youngest science: Notes of a medicine watcher.* New York: Viking Press.

Veninga, R. (1982). *The human side of health administration: A guide for hospital, nursing, and public health administrators.* Englewood Cliffs, NJ: Prentice-Hall.

Waldrop, M. (1992). *Complexity: Life at the edge of chaos.* New York: Simon & Schuster.

Zaleznik, A. (1992). Managers and leaders: Are they different? *Harvard Business Review, 70*(2), 126-135.

PART III

Planning in Nursing Administration

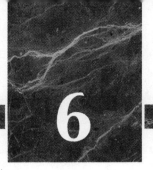

6

Problem Solving

Chapter Objectives

∾

define and describe problem solving

∾

distinguish among the six steps of the
problem solving process

∾

apply the problem solving process to nursing practice

∾

compare strategies for problem solving

∾

relate leadership and management to problem solving

∾

exercise critical thinking to conceptualize and analyze
possible solutions to a practical experience incident

*n*urses make decisions and choices all the time. Assessment, diagnosis, planning, intervention, and evaluation of outcomes constitute activities of clinical problem solving and decision making. Nurses are in a human service profession that requires decisions in response to client problems, such as what treatments or actions are to be performed. Benner (1982) said that there are five stages that nurses go through between novice and expert levels of competence. The five levels are novice, advanced beginner, competent, proficient, and expert. Like the different levels of competence, nurses grow and evolve over time in professional experience and skill at problem solving in nursing. Problem solving is a basic skill, useful for nurses as they manage both their personal and professional lives.

DEFINITIONS

A *problem* is defined as a deficit or surplus of something that is necessary to achieve one's goals (see Chart 6.1). Having identified a problem, the next step is to discover why the deficit or surplus exists and to decide where to look for the cause (Johnson, 1990). Luft (1970) defined *problem solving* as the process that attempts to identify obstacles that inhibit accomplishment of a specific goal. Ackoff (1974) noted that successful problem solving requires finding the right solution to the right problem. The specific problems selected for solution as well as the way they are formulated as problems appear to be related to an individual's philosophy and world view more than to science and technology.

Problems exist where goals need to be attained and there is uncertainty about the appropriate solution (Lancaster & Lancaster, 1982). Beyers (1991) noted that problems present opportunities for decision making and change. She defined a problem as something that needs to be fixed. The logical extension of this would be that problem solving is the process of fixing something that needs to be fixed.

> **CHART 6.1**
> ∽ DEFINITIONS
>
> **Problem**
> a deficit or surplus of something that is necessary to achieve one's goals.
>
> **Problem Solving**
> the process that attempts to identify obstacles that inhibit accomplishment of a specific goal.
>
> Data from Johnson (1990) and Luft (1970).

BACKGROUND

Problem solving activity has been conceptualized from two points of view; individual or clinical problem solving and managerial problem solving. Both have emphasized rational-logical thought processes. At the level of an individual, problem solving is viewed as intimately related to how the individual processes information. In nursing and medicine, a concern about accuracy and effectiveness has placed an emphasis on diagnostic reasoning and clinical decision making. Problem solving becomes more complex for managers in organizations (see Fig. 6.1). It may be more difficult to acquire a broad range of information. Frequently, groups are involved in problem solving, so there is a greater need for interaction, a slower process, and a need for consensus. Problems may be solved at the best possible level, as opposed to an ideal level (see also Chapter 7).

Problem solving as a process can be linked to the nursing process and the change process. A model has been proposed by deChesnay (1983). Within the arena of problem solving and decision making, some situations produce problems (a difficulty), others create problems in which conflicts arise (a dilemma), and yet others become problems in which the solution appears not to have a logical path (a paradox). The complexity of decision making and the psychological impact increase as the situation moves along a hierarchy from difficulty to paradox. Thus, problems can be categorized by their level of complexity. The

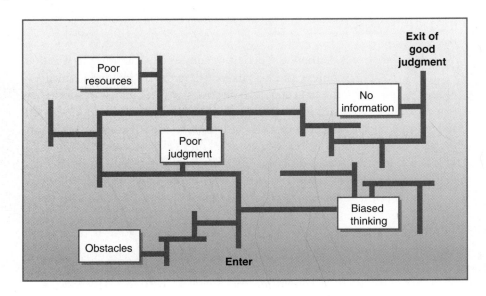

Figure 6.1
The problem solving maze.

nursing process and the change process can then be applied to round out a model of problem solving. The problem can be framed as either an individual's problem or a system's problem. The evaluation of the outcome of problem solving involves an assessment of effectiveness. If the problem is resolved, the problem solving process would be judged as effective. It would be judged ineffective if the problem stayed the same or worsened (deChesnay, 1983).

Managing a difficulty, dilemma, or paradox may require different strategies. A difficulty is only a minor problem. A dilemma results from the combination of a difficulty plus conflict. For example, a minor problem occurs when two competing values arise. One example occurs in cultural differences such as when professional value structures clash with the value structure of the client. A paradox is a situation where there is no logical solution to the problem (deChesnay, 1983). In practice, paradoxes are found commonly within ethical issues.

Newell and Simon (1972) defined human problem solving as information processing. Information processing behavior is dependent on the characteristics of the problem solver and the task. In nursing, the concepts of clinical decision making and nursing informatics are discussed in relation to problem solving as information processing (see Chapters 7 and 24).

Holzemer (1986) noted that a controversy exists regarding the underlying cognitive structures or styles of clinical problem solving. The study of physicians' medical problem solving uncovered five theories of problem solving (Elstein, Shulman, & Sprafka, 1975; Holzemer, 1986). Thus there may be various ways that professionals organize their thinking and problem solving processes. In his research, Holzemer (1986) found that nurse practitioners adopted a common style: a generic problem solving style that focused on the management of the client. The nursing process also is a generic problem solving strategy widely applicable in nursing practice. It is possible that professional socialization and educational patterns influence professionals toward a similar problem solving pattern. This may or may not be beneficial to the profession.

Many organizational interactions occur around the need to identify, define, and solve problems. Individuals appear to have a relatively stable personality-related problem solving style. It appears that problem solving styles have an influence on how well people are able to work together. Further, the personality style relates to how an individual acquires, stores, retrieves, and transforms information (Kirton, 1989). Thus there may be a relationship between problem solving style and effectiveness in any given situation. Like leadership style, no one style is optimum. The effectiveness of a style would be situational and determined by what was appropriate to the circumstances. The Kirton Adaption-Innovation Theory (Kirton, 1989) identified two problem solving styles: adaptors and innovators. Adaptors seek solutions to problems in tried and accepted ways. They are focused on resolving problems rather than finding them. They rarely challenge rules and are methodical, reliable, and efficient. Innovators are the opposite. They seek solutions to problems in original, creative, and challenging ways. They discover problems and avenues for solution. They question current practices and promote changes. Organizations in a stable steady-state of maintenance may tend to prefer adaptors. Organizations in a growth state or undergoing a rapid rate of change or crisis may tend to prefer innovators (Adams, 1994). Problem solving style can be measured by either the Kirton Adaption-Innovation Inventory (KAI) (Kirton, 1976; 1989) or by Hersey and Natemeyer's (1988) Problem-solving and Decision-making Style Inventory, which measures the extent to which an individual engages in directive or supportive behavior. Although there are different ways of thinking about problem solving styles, an analysis of personal style increases a nurse's self-awareness and knowledge about alternative ways of acting on problems. See Chapter 7 for more discussion of innovation.

RESEARCH NOTE

Source: Adams, C. (1994). The impact of problem-solving styles of NE-CEO pairs on nurse executive effectiveness. *Journal of Nursing Administration*, 24(11), 17-22.

Purpose

The purpose of this research was to test whether problem solving styles of nurse executive and chief executive officer pairs differ and whether this difference also influences the effectiveness of the nurse executives. Nurse executive effectiveness is dependent upon support from the chief executive officer. The problem solving styles of the pair affect nurse executive tenure. A descriptive comparative research design using a mailed questionnaire was used with 66 (73%) pairs from 66 mostly rural hospitals. Problem solving styles were measured by the KAI. Effectiveness was measured by the LEAD instrument.

Discussion

The mean score for the nurse executives was 103.3, in the innovative range. The mean score for the chief executive officers was 107.5, also in the innovative style range. Analysis showed that the chief executive officers were significantly more innovative in style than the nurse executives. Of the 66 pairs, 17 had adaptor nurse executives with innovative chief officers; 5 had innovator nurses with adaptor chief executives. The results indicated that problem solving styles of the pairs did not significantly influence nurse executive effectiveness.

Application to Practice

The predominantly innovator problem solving styles of top administrators in hospitals may reflect the current turbulent environment. A disparity in nurse executive to chief executive officer problem solving styles can influence the relationship between them and impact on the nurse's effectiveness. It is possible that the differences in style can influence effectiveness in joint problem solving situations, with ramifications that ripple down to the staff level. An assessment of style allows for self-awareness and the potential to modify behaviors.

The Steps of the Problem Solving Process

The steps of the problem solving process are listed somewhat differently from each other in various literature sources. However, the general framework is similar. The problem solving process is closely related to the scientific process, and thus the nursing process and the research process. There are six basic steps that form the general framework of the problem solving process (see Chart 6.2):

1. *Gather information.* The problem solver cannot overestimate the critical importance of this first step. Too often people start the problem solving process without having spent enough time gathering information about the problem. It is important to remember to start by gathering as much input and information as possible from a variety of sources. Shortening the information gathering process to save time may cause difficulty later on. The input information must then be analyzed.

2. *Define the problem.* Having gathered as much information as possible, the problem solver should work to be able to state the problem in a phrase or a short sentence. This means identifying a very specific definition of the problem, usually stated directly as, The problem is. . . . Reducing this definition to a written sentence or two is the difficult intellectual task of problem clarification. There are people who are very insightful about defining problems. How-

CHART 6.2
∾ SIX STEPS OF PROBLEM SOLVING

1. Gather information
2. Define problem
3. Develop solutions
4. Consider consequences
5. Make decisions
6. Implement & evaluate solutions

ever, it is important for problem solvers to analyze all the available information in order to have a full perspective of the problem. This is the most complex step in that it involves a process of careful clarification.

3. *Develop solutions.* Notice that the word solutions is plural. A problem suggests more than one alternative solution (Lancaster & Lancaster, 1982). One very basic idea is that people have choices, and, therefore, problems have solutions. It may be that in the whole array of multiple solutions to any problem, none of them are particularly enticing. However, there are always solutions or multiple options to any given problem situation. Expanding the ability to look at problems as always having a potential for multiple solutions is a key conceptual element in dealing with problems. It helps to avoid knee-jerk reactions that occur when identifying the problem without careful deliberation. It may be enticing to short-cut the time and energy involved with careful problem analysis and to grab an easily available solution.

4. *Consider the consequences.* This should be done carefully for each alternative solution. The first action is to list the potential consequences. This is a critical thinking stage. It requires a broad perspective that includes all potential consequences. The problem solver's values will play a role in the analysis and evaluation of the consequences. For example, a consequence seen as very negative by one person may be perceived as less so by another.

5. *Make a decision.* This is the decisive action stage. At some point analysis needs to be brought to closure and a decision made. There are a variety of techniques for decision making (see Chapter 7).

6. *Implement and evaluate the solution.* This is the action and feedback stage. The results of the problem analysis and decision making cognitive processes now culminate in the direct action determined as necessary to be taken. This may require risk and courage. Periodic checks on effectiveness need to occur and then be fed back into the problem solving process. Some people can never seem to get to the end of the steps. For example, they cannot seem to generate solutions. Observe your colleagues. Are they problem identifiers? Some people never will be able to identify what the problem is. Some people can easily figure out what the problem is, but then cannot get beyond problem identification. Are individuals solution generators or are they locked into preformed ideas, a form of "hardening of the concepts"? If they are able to generate solutions, are they then able to move into the risk-taking step of making a decision and implementing a solution?

Some questions to ask during problem solving include:
- What specifically is the problem?
- Why, how, and to whom is it a problem?
- Why should anything be done about it?
- What are the facts and what do they mean?
- What are the possible solutions?

- Which solutions are acceptable?
- What is the ideal or preferred solution?
- What is the best solution?
- Will it work? Is it worth doing?
- Is it the right thing to do?

How does this work in nursing practice? Perhaps a nurse announces that there is a problem. The above questions might be asked of the nurse as a clarification process. What are the facts, what do the facts mean, and what kind of solution should be sought? Is the optimum or ideal solution desired, or is it best to look for a solution that is just adequate? Is any solution that comes along acceptable? What are the possible solutions, what is the best solution? Will it work and is it worth doing?

When diagnosing a problem, try to ferret out all of the facts, then separate the facts from interpretation and determine the scope of the problem. The nurse will need to make a deliberate effort to separate facts from interpretation. Facts and interpretation are not always in consonance. Facts can have multiple interpretations because of the phenomenon of human perceptions. One person's interpretation of facts may or may not be consonant with the known facts, and may or may not be an appropriate interpretation. Therefore, determine what happened in detail. The interpretation can be applied later.

Finally, determine the magnitude and scope of the problem. For example, problems can have an urgency difference that distinguishes among them and allows for prioritization. The problem can be assessed for how urgent and how immediate it is:

- A potential problem can emerge at any time. It is just sitting there like a time bomb and can emerge spontaneously.
- An actual problem is occurring in real time and needs prompt action.
- A critical problem is highly urgent and needs crisis intervention.

The continuum of time ranges from "the problem is not happening but it could" to "an immediate crisis is unfolding." The urgency and the importance of action can be two variables plotted against each other and displayed on a grid (Covey, 1990). This is useful as an analysis tool. The first consideration is to decide if the problem is important. The problem then can be analyzed as to its urgency. It may be important but not urgent, or it may be urgent but not important. When this activity is applied to nursing situations, it can give some guidance in terms of the prioritization of time, especially when competing demands are made on an individual regarding the immediacy and impact of a problem (see Fig. 6.2).

Managers use urgency and importance assessments when they attempt to manage their scarce time resources. This is a time management technique (see also Chapter 5). For example, a typical morning might bring many requests

Setting	Immediacy		Impact	
	Low High		Low High	
A Hospital floor nurse finds that a cleaning person just finished vacuuming a room and the cord is stretched across a walkway in a(n):				
• **empty office at night**	(1) 2 3 4 5		1 2 (3) 4 5	
• **nursing station during a weekday**	1 2 3 4 (5)		1 2 (3) 4 5	
• **ambulatory outpatient geriatric clinic**	1 2 3 4 (5)		1 2 3 4 (5)	

Setting	Immediacy		Impact	
	Low High		Low High	
A Community Health Nurse Manager reviews a pile of new mail, including:				
• **a memo about Information Services' daily news summary sheet**	(1) 2 3 4 5		(1) 2 3 4 5	
• **a letter from a sales representative announcing a sale of needed equipment**	1 2 (3) 4 5		1 2 3 (4) 5	
• **a client's complaint letter alleging negligent care**	1 2 3 4 (5)		1 2 3 4 (5)	

Figure 6.2
Activity prioritization.

that arrive simultaneously to the nurse manager. There might be the need to prioritize the following: committee minutes to prepare, phone or e-mail messages to return, the need to get the staffing schedule finalized, a sick call-in that has to be replaced, and a report about a patient or family complaint to handle. A similar phenomenon occurs when staff nurses have multiple requests for their time and attention from their multiple clients. A time and urgency rating schema can be used as a way of sorting out competing demands and planning and organizing for effectiveness.

Exemplar 6.1

Relentless Incrementalism

What a dilemma our Infection Control Department was faced with when, in response to the national increase in tuberculosis, the Centers for Disease Control (CDC) published new guidelines on the need for increased frequency of PPD skin testing of *all* hospital employees. Even though our facility is very big (1000 beds and over 10,000 employees, including physicians), our employee health services at the time were quite meager. We had 1.0 FTE occupational health nurse (OHN) who skin-tested employees on a very irregular basis and was also conducting pre-employment health evaluations, hearing and vision screenings. We were asking her to do what must have seemed insane, not to say impossible—apply and read a skin test on every single employee and physician at least once a year, and on some employees as often as every six months. Even though our geographic area had a low incidence of tuberculosis, we

needed to heed these new guidelines. Compliance with CDC guidelines is not required, per se, but generally they have the weight of law and are considered by both infection control and legal experts to be the community standard.

If this problem was to be solved, it would require cooperation and critical thinking of both clinical and managerial personnel. As expected, the response to our entreaty was a polite but adamant refusal based on unavailable staff. We recommended to hospital administration that more staff be recruited, but we did not have the authority to demand it. This was obviously going to be an obstacle that inhibited accomplishment of a goal that we saw as very important from a medical and a legal viewpoint.

Our Director of Quality Management had recently shared with us a concept called "relentless incrementalism." Simplistically, this means when a goal must be reached, you

keep "nudging" the obstacles until they move out of your way, adopting the philosophy that while you may only make very small progress at one time, you simply never give up.

In retrospect, we used this notion more serendipitously than deliberately or consciously. Although the odds of our success initially seemed insurmountable, we believed strongly that what we proposed simply had to be done.

We invited several key players (i.e., management and physician personnel from Occupational Medicine [OM]) to an Infection Control Committee (ICC) meeting and asked them to bring a copy of the current PPD skin testing policy. We distributed the CDC guideline at the meeting and slowly led the committee members through it, comparing and contrasting it with our current practice in all aspects, not just employee skin testing. When it came time to discuss that aspect, it was clear that this wasn't something we were proposing just because it seemed like a good idea.

It was never our intent to suggest how compliance with the guideline be accomplished. Our role was to be aware of and facilitate compliance with various standards. We maintained this position throughout the problem-solving process and I believe it worked in our favor.

A few weeks after the ICC meeting, we received a draft of a new policy from OM. They had found a way to free the OHN's time sufficiently to, within one year, begin annual skin testing of those employees at highest risk of tuberculosis exposure. We commended this action, but reiterated our original request. Again, we were told that staffing wasn't sufficient. We were patient, but continued our pursuit.

Approximately one year after our initial request, we invited OM management personnel back to another ICC meeting to present an update on the progress of the skin testing program. This time, they had put another plan into place that, within that year, would put them in total compliance with our original request and the federal guidelines.

It took two years, but our patience and relentless move forward in small incremental steps finally paid off. Within four years of our original request, a total of 3.5 OHNs manage the employee PPD skin testing program, and by working together and networking with other professionals in similar situations, they devised time-saving and inventive ways to get the job done, thus improving the quality and quantity

of all of the services they provide. While the original dilemma may have taken a long time to be resolved, it was apparent to us that there was a great deal of careful deliberation, rather than a knee-jerk response, which resulted in everyone's goals being met.

It must be remembered that this was not an urgent or emergency issue—there was no evidence of increased transmission of tuberculosis in our facility. Had there been, the concept of "relentless incrementalism" would likely not have been successful in meeting anyone's needs.

SANDY PIRWITZ, RN, BSN, MS, CIC
Nurse Epidemiologist and Manager of Infection Control
Cleveland Clinic Foundation
Cleveland, Ohio

Strategies for Problem Solving

The third basic problem solving step is to develop solutions. It is helpful to think of all problems as having multiple potential solutions and to systematically consider all options or strategies available. There are a number of different strategies available to resolve problems. Strategies used by nurses and nurse managers for problem resolution are shown in Figure 6.3.

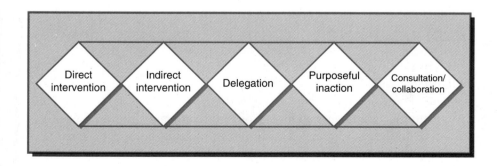

Figure 6.3
Strategies for problem solving.

Direct Intervention This is carrying out some direct physical or verbal activity in order to intervene in a situation and resolve a problem. Problem solvers themselves are directly involved in the actions taken to implement a resolution when they use direct intervention. This is a strategy of personally doing.

Indirect Intervention Being at the center of a communications and operations network, the nurse manager may use interpersonal skills to work around the sides of the problem: for example, getting disputants to talk to each other as a way of indirectly intervening. Negotiation, conflict resolution, persuasion, and confrontation are all examples of indirect intervention where interpersonal skills are used to work through other people in order to help them solve their own problems. The nurse manager does not carry out the actions of resolution, rather action is taken to influence others to resolve the problem. Nurses use this strategy with clients and their families.

Delegation This is assigning certain responsibilities and tasks to others. It is used to solve the problem of workload distribution. Delegation occurs frequently in nursing and is associated with care delivery systems, the use of nurse extenders, and differentiated practice (see Chapters 15 and 16).

Purposeful Inaction There are some times when a problem will go away during the course of time if little attention or emphasis is placed on it. Purposeful inaction is a conscious decision not to act. It may be thought of as "watchful waiting". It is a tricky decision to know when intervention is absolutely called for and when it may be that purposeful inaction or benign neglect is more likely to allow the problem to go away with time. Inaction may be advantageous in certain situations.

Consultation or Collaboration This is finding a peer and exchanging information and ideas. This strategy increases the available knowledge resources as input for analysis in problem solving. It is associated with strategies related to networking and coordinating with others.

If there are multiple potential solutions to problems, then a review and analysis of the possible strategies for problem solving can be helpful to identify options. Leaders and managers may want to try out new strategies to increase personal and professional effectiveness.

LEADERSHIP AND MANAGEMENT IMPLICATIONS

In practice, nurses find that they are solving many types of problems including large, small, explosive, political, fun, sad, and ordinary day-to-day problems. Think about problems faced by the typical college student: perhaps it was planning a wedding, handling a difficult roommate, or finding adequate child care. Individuals are faced with many problems, both in personal and professional arenas.

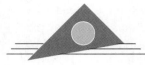 *Leadership & Management Behaviors*

LEADERSHIP BEHAVIORS	**MANAGEMENT BEHAVIORS**	**OVERLAP AREAS**
• influences group and individual problem solving activity	• acts to resolve problems	• uses problem solving processes and techniques to accomplish goals
• inspires others to solve problems	• plans for projected organizational deficits and surpluses	• motivates individuals and groups to problem solve
• envisions creative alternatives to problems	• organizes the environment to decrease problems	
• motivates the group to innovate in response to identified problems	• directs individuals in problem resolution	
• models good problem solving behavior	• delegates tasks and responsibilities	
• networks with nurse colleagues	• controls levels of conflict	

In their professional work, nurses use a level of expertise in problem solving that goes beyond lay care and home remedies: nurses use a more complex and sophisticated level of knowledge and skill in providing health and illness care. The essence of professional practice is the utilization of expertise to solve problems for *clients*. Nurses need to be licensed, considered professional, and have autonomy for practice because nurses make decisions based on nursing expertise. Clients report that an expert nurse makes all the difference in their therapy, care, and psychosocial well-being. What nurses do in decision making involves applying specialized expertise in solving problems for clients.

Nurse managers, as an extension of nursing care, also find themselves faced with problems pressing for a decision. Some problems have to be solved in a short turn-around time and without the benefit of contemplation: for example, how to staff the next shift, or what to do with budget constraints. In their budget process, nurse managers solve problems and make decisions about capital equipment, staffing, and the allocation of scarce resources. The nurse manager's job, then, involves the utilization of expertise to solve problems *in the work environment*. Leadership and management in nursing practice are intimately involved with setting up a work environment including the climate, the culture, the leadership style, the level of morale, and the task structure that allows nurses to function at the highest levels. Decisions that are made by nurses include the structuring of the work environment and allocation of scarce resources. Both are challenges to problem solving skills. With an emphasis on participatory decision making and shared governance in nursing, the ability and willingness of staff nurses to participate in problem solving is a leadership and management issue. Research has indicated that some staff nurses may prefer to defer to their superiors and avoid personal responsibility (Schmeiding, 1990). It is unclear whether this is a personality flaw of individuals or whether it is coping or reinforced behavior that is situationally specific.

Experience and skill in problem solving, like ability at interpersonal relationships, is an elemental skill for nurses. For leadership and management in nursing, developing both interpersonal and problem solving skills are two key foundations for successful practice.

CURRENT ISSUES AND TRENDS

In the leadership and management of nursing practice, problems can arise spontaneously, be chronic, or recur in cycles. For example, one recurring nursing practice management problem is the concern over alleged unsafe nursing practices due to low RN staffing. The strategies adopted to solve this problem vary from individual to group action. In one example, an anonymous writer in an oncology nursing position described the frustration that led to resignation from her position (Name Withheld, 1993). In another example, *AJN News* (1993) reported the efforts of California nurses to solve similar problems by writing staffing ratios into the health code.

Economic interests are at the heart of the clash between nurses who feel stretched thinner and thinner, and healthcare institutions that are responding to reimbursement pressures. In the California case, nearly 500 nurses responded by letters and testimony to the health department to cite declining levels of staffing, problems with floating, and allegations of substandard and unsafe nursing care they experienced. Subsequently, this issue has been investigated at the national level by a federal task force of the Institute of Medicine of the National Academy of Sciences of the U.S. Department of Health and Human Services. There are arguments being presented both for and against federally set nurse-patient staffing ratios (*AJN Newsline*, 1994) (see Chapter 23 for more on staffing).

Problem Solving Teams

Current nursing literature emphasizes the use of problem solving teams as a leadership and management strategy designed to improve productivity and effectiveness. A team-based problem solving method is designed to improve the participation and empowerment of key decision implementers. Dailey (1990) described a nine step problem solving procedure for problem solving teams:

1. Identify the features of the care problems.
2. Determine the perceptions of the most important facets of the problem.
3. Determine the underlying causes of the problem.
4. Conduct a baseline audit to assess magnitude.
5. Construct an action plan.
6. Implement the action plan.
7. Pilot test the action plan after briefing employees.
8. Create indicators and track the solution's effectiveness.
9. Publicize problem solving results.

This might serve as a checklist for problem solving teams as they tackle a project. The nine step procedure for teams incorporates the six basic steps of the problem solving process, then expands on them. The extensively interpersonal nature of teams creates some unique challenges for the problem solving process. For example, more time may be needed to reach consensus. More communication may be required to solve problems. In nursing, some organizations use problem solving teams as a way of placing focused effort on systems problems and thereby improving quality. For example, a team may focus on reviewing and standardizing the forms used for documentation (see Chapter 8 for more on work teams).

SUMMARY

- ❧ Nurses need skills in problem solving.
- ❧ A problem is a deficit or surplus of something.
- ❧ Problem solving is a process of coming to a solution for the problem.
- ❧ The nursing process is a generic problem solving process for nursing.
- ❧ The steps of the problem solving process lead to logical analysis and strategy selection.
- ❧ There are multiple strategies for solving problems.
- ❧ Both leaders and managers use problem solving skills.

Study Questions

1. How can problem solving be used in nursing practice?
2. Identify a problem you are dealing with now. What is your feeling about this problem? How do you approach it psychologically?
3. Do you tend to respond emotionally or logically to a problem?
4. What strategy do you tend to use for problem solving? Are there other strategies to try?
5. How does problem solving relate to leadership?
6. How does problem solving relate to management?

Critical Thinking Exercise

Jane June is a shift supervisor on the "graveyard" shift at a busy local hospital. The adult ICU is usually a busy place, but tonight has been hectic. Jane was paged STAT to the ICU when a code blue was called on a patient with a serious GI bleed. The code was going badly when Jane suddenly noticed that one of the ICU nurses was missing. After the code crisis calmed down and she was no longer needed for assistance, Nurse June began to look for the missing nurse. At the freight entrance Nurse June observes the missing ICU nurse strolling into the hospital with a male friend.

1. *What is the problem?*

2. *Why is it a problem?*

3. *What are the key issues?*

4. *What should Nurse June do first?*

5. *How should Nurse June handle this situation?*

6. *What problem solving style should Nurse June use?*

7. *What leadership and management strategies might be useful?*

REFERENCES

Ackoff, R. (1974). *Redesigning the future.* New York: John Wiley & Sons.

Adams, C. (1994). The impact of problem-solving styles of NE-CEO pairs on nurse executive effectiveness. *Journal of Nursing Administration, 24*(11), 17-22.

AJN News. (1993). Fighting staff cuts, California RNs push for enforceable patient ratios. *American Journal of Nursing, 93*(1), 81, 84.

AJN Newsline. (1994). Nurses demand disclosure of hospital staffing levels. *American Journal of Nursing, 94*(12), 61, 64.

Benner, P. (1982). From novice to expert. *American Journal of Nursing, 82*(3), 402-407.

Beyers, M. (1991). Guest editorial. *Nursing Administration Quarterly, 15*(4), viii-x.

Covey, S. (1990). *The seven habits of highly effective people: Restoring the character ethic.* New York: Simon & Schuster.

Dailey, R. (1990). Strengthening hospital nursing: How to use problem-solving teams effectively. *Journal of Nursing Administration, 20*(7/8), 24-29.

deChesnay, M. (1983). Problem solving in nursing. *Image, 15*(1), 8-11.

Elstein, A., Shulman, L., & Sprafka, S. (1978). *Medical problem solving.* Cambridge: Harvard University Press.

Hersey, P., & Natemeyer, W. (1988). *Problem-solving and Decision-making Style Inventory: Perception of self.* Escondido, CA: Leadership Studies, Inc.

Holzemer, W. (1986). The structure of problem solving in simulations. *Nursing Research, 35*(4), 231-236.

Johnson, L. (1990). The influence of assumptions on effective decision-making. *Journal of Nursing Administration, 20*(4), 35-39.

Kirton, M. (1976). Adaptors and innovators: A description and measure. *Journal of Applied Psychology, 61*, 622-629.

Kirton, M. (1989). *Adaptors and innovators: Styles of creativity and problem solving.* London: Routledge.

Lancaster, W., & Lancaster, J. (1982). Rational decision making: Managing uncertainty. *Journal of Nursing Administration, 12*(9), 23-28.

Luft, J. (1970). *Group process.* Palo Alto, CA: Mayfield Publishing.

Name withheld. (1993). Unsafe nursing. *American Journal of Nursing, 93*(1), 15-16.

Newell, A., & Simon, H. (1972). *Human problem solving.* Englewood Cliffs, NJ: Prentice-Hall.

Schmeiding, N. (1990). A model for assessing nurse administrators' actions. *Western Journal of Nursing Research, 12*(3), 293-306.

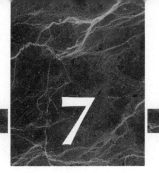

Decision Making

Chapter Objectives

❧

define and describe decision making

❧

differentiate decision making from problem solving

❧

identify ten steps to follow for decision making

❧

explain decision making situations

❧

review administrative decision making models

❧

compare decision making strategies

❧

review ethical decision making in nursing leadership and management

❧

relate decision making to leadership and management

❧

relate perception, creativity, and innovation to decision making

❧

exercise critical thinking to conceptualize and analyze
possible solutions to a practical experience incident

*d*ecision making is one specific subset of problem solving. For any problem solving process, there may be a time separation between the problem solving and the decision making. Decision making is a vital component of problem solving. It is a behavior, the critical mental action that is taken. Decision making may or may not be the result of an immediate problem. Decision making is not a passive term. The purpose of decision making is to identify a course of action (Schaefer, 1974). Within the larger concept of problem solving, there is the specific action of making a decision. Ideally what is desired is a high level of effectiveness. This means that more decisions turn out good than turn out bad. The quality of decision making relates to "vigilant information processing" (Janis & Mann, 1977).

Decision making can be thought of as a process with identifiable steps. Nurses make decisions in personal, clinical, and organizational situations and under conditions of certainty, uncertainty, and risk. There are a variety of decision making models and strategies. Nurses' control over decision making may vary as to amount and place in the process. Awareness of the components, process, and strategies of decision making contributes to effectiveness in nursing leadership and management decision making.

DEFINITIONS

 rainger (1990) called decision making the act of choosing. Veninga (1982) described decision making as the process of converting information into action. *Decision making* is defined as a behavior exhibited in making a selection and implementing a course of action from among alternatives (see Chart 7.1). It may or may not be the result of an immediate problem. The problem solving process is initiated as the result of an immediate problem. Decision making, however, may occur some time later. Decision making also may be the result of opportunities, challenges, or leadership initiatives as opposed to being triggered by an immediate problem. The process of selecting one course of action from among alternatives forms the basic core of the definition of decision making. As a corollary to responsibility, making decisions means realizing the consequences ahead of time (McKenzie, 1985). In any decision the conscious presence of both the end to be accomplished and the means to be used are involved (Barnard, 1982).

There are five core elements to decision making:
- the identification of a problem, issue, or situation
- the establishment of the criteria to be used to evaluate potential solutions
- a search for alternative solutions or actions
- the evaluation of the alternatives
- the selection of a particular alternative

> **CHART 7.1**
> ∾ DEFINITION
>
> **Decision Making**
> a behavior exhibited in making a selection and implementing a course of action from alternatives. It may or may not be the result of an immediate problem.

These can be summarized as the three phases of deliberation, judgment, and choice (Schaefer, 1974). Nurses use deliberation, judgment, and choice in managing client care. Nurse managers use these three phases in managing resources and the environment of care delivery. Management of decision mak-

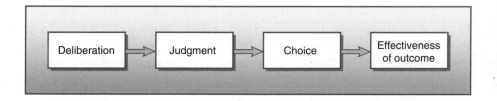

Figure 7.1
Core elements of decision making.

ing involves an evaluation of the effectiveness of the outcomes that result from the decision making process (see Fig. 7.1).

Another way of looking at problems in order to determine the appropriate decision strategy is to ask: "who owns the problem?" Is it an individual's problem or is it a system's problem? This is a process of framing the problem. The determination of where ownership of a problem lies indicates whether to approach the problem individually with the person or by a group strategy such as problem solving or creativity techniques (deChesnay, 1983). In nursing and healthcare, quality improvement techniques emphasize the framing of problems as systems' problems and the subsequent use of group problem resolution strategies. For example, nurses may encounter a "difficult" client. Framing this as a systems problem would lead the nurse to decide to use intervention strategies like staffing adjustments, environmental restructuring, and teaching or counseling the family. Framing this problem as an individual's problem would lead to a decision to counsel the individual to change their habits or approaches toward the client.

BACKGROUND

The basic elements of problem solving and decision making can be summarized into two parts:

1. *Identifying the problem:* The antecedent activities of decision making are those of problem solving and are directed at gathering facts. Decision making assumes that problem solving activity has been going on at some point in time, but it is still vital to identify very specifically the nature of the problem that the decision making is to address. Then the criteria that will be used to evaluate potential solutions need to be pre-determined.

2. *Decision making:* Once the situation is identified, the next activity is to determine what outcome is desired and what criteria need to be met when there is a solution generated. The desired outcome may be a variety of end states, such as ideal, short-term, or covering up the situation. It may be that what is desired is for the problem to go away forever; or simply to make sure that all involved in this problem are satisfied with the solution and get some benefit; or to obtain an ideal solution. It may be that a quick decision is de-

sired, and there is not a concern about researching the aspects of the problem or allowing for participation in decision making.

Ten steps to follow in decision making are (Wren, 1974):

1. Become aware of the situation.
2. Investigate the nature of the situation.
3. Determine the objective of the solution.
4. Determine alternative solutions.
5. Weigh the consequences and relative efficiency of each alternative solution.
6. Evaluate or pilot test various alternatives.
7. Select the best alternative solution.
8. Implement the decision. Communicate it and train those who will carry it out.
9. Evaluate the solution at intervals to determine if it was the best solution and if it is still solving the problem.
10. Correct, change, or withdraw the solution if evaluation indicates it is no longer appropriate.

Thus, decision making steps are similar to the steps of the problem solving process. However, they form a specific subset. Decision making itself is a critical process and thus is examined separately. Nurses exhibit leadership in care delivery and management when they use expertise to make decisions on behalf of clients' care needs.

Decision Making Situations

The situations in which decisions are made may be personal, clinical, or organizational (see Fig. 7.2). Personal decision making is a familiar part of everyday life. Personal decisions range from multiple small daily choices to time management and career or life choices.

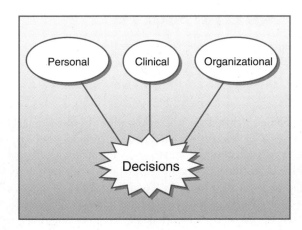

Figure 7.2
Decision making situations.

Clinical decision making in nursing relates to quality of care and competency issues. Clinical decision making, also called clinical problem solving, clinical judgment, or the nursing process, is defined as a series of decisions made by the nurse in interaction with the client (Tanner, 1987). In nursing, clinical decision making is made difficult due to unclear, changing, and overlapping areas of practice in medicine and nursing, increasing complexity of clinical practice, and multidisciplinary (joint or team) approaches to decision making (Prescott, Dennis, & Jacox, 1987). The process of diagnostic reasoning used in medicine has been refined into a general four step model and found to apply to nursing: attending to initially available clues (signs and symptoms), activating hypotheses that may explain the initial cues, gathering data to rule in or out hypotheses, and evaluating hypotheses in light of each new clue until a diagnosis is accepted (Elstein, Shulman, & Sprafka, 1978; Tanner, Padrick, Westfall, & Putzier, 1987). The major nursing practice decisions are judgments about a client problem (diagnosis) and nursing actions (interventions) for the selected diagnosis (Grier, 1984). Clinical decision making is the foundation of nursing practice, the criterion to judge expertise, and the differentiation between professional and technical nursing personnel (Hughes & Young, 1992).

Organizational decision making is choosing options directed toward the resolution of organizational problems and the achievement of organizational goals (Kerrigan, 1991). For example, the purpose of decision making in nursing might be to coordinate nursing care to deliver optimal client outcomes while controlling cost. Etzioni (1989) noted that the traditional model for business decisions was rationalism. However, as information flow becomes more complex and faster paced, a new decision making model based on the use of partial information not fully analyzed is evolving. He calls it "humble decision making." It arises in response to the need to make a decision when there is too much data and too little time.

RESEARCH NOTE

Source: Feldman, C., Olberding, L., Shortridge, L., Toole, K., & Zappin, P. (1993). Decision making in case management of home healthcare clients. *Journal of Nursing Administration*, *23*(1), 33-38.

Purpose

The purpose of this study was to examine the decision making of public health nurses as it related to maintaining or terminating nursing services to clients. The research questions investigated the common decision elements and the differing characteristics of cases maintained versus terminated. A retrospective record review of 633 records and nurse providers was done. A descriptive survey of 33 nurses also was done using vignettes to elicit decision making behaviors. The setting was one health department's community nursing division.

Discussion

The authors use Hansen and Thomas' (1968) model of decision maker variables in public health nursing. The three interacting variables are decision maker variables like attitudes, beliefs, age, and education; situational variables like client characteristics of medical diagnoses, mental status, and support system; and contextual variables like agency policies and organizational structure. In this study, chi-square analysis on variables from the record review showed a relationship between assignment of home health aides and arthritic or orthopedic medical diagnosis with cases remaining open longer. In three client scenarios where expected client outcomes were not being achieved, common themes emerged around client/nurse safety, the appropriate role of the nurse, and ethical/legal factors. Safety and noncompliance were factors identified as influencing decisions to maintain or terminate services.

Application to Practice

There were distinct differences between what was actually being done in case management and what the nurses' beliefs were about how cases should be managed. Agency policies may not be clear or not consistently followed. This makes it difficult to evaluate client outcomes. An audit or record review may need to be done regularly. Further, the roles of the nurse became blurred with those of a social worker, especially in protective cases. The nurse's role could be more clearly defined and the agency's expectations of staff relative to termination could be more clearly delineated in order to better evaluate outcomes and control costs.

Administrative Decision Making

Nurses manage care and make decisions under conditions of certainty, uncertainty, and risk. For example, if research has shown that selection of a specific nursing intervention under prescribed conditions is highly likely to produce an outcome, then the nurse in that situation faces a condition of certainty. An example would be the prevention of decubitus ulcers by frequent repositioning. If little knowledge is available or if the specific situation is more complex or variant from the usual, then the nurse faces uncertainty. Risk situations occur when there is a threat of harm to clients. Conditions of risk also occur commonly in relationship to the administration of medications, crisis events, infection control, invasive procedures, and the use of technology in nursing practice. Further, these conditions also apply to the administration of nursing care delivery, where decision making is a critical function.

Conditions of uncertainty and complexity are common in nursing care management. Overlapping, unclear, and changing roles for nurses create complex decision making situations. Further, the use of multidisciplinary and interdisciplinary teams to make client care decisions increases the complexity of clinical decision making for nurses (Prescott, Dennis, & Jacox, 1987).

Janis and Mann (1977) described four types of administrative decision making strategies. These include satisficing, incrementalism, mixed scanning, and optimizing. *Satisficing* has the goal of selecting a course of action that is "good enough." *Incrementalism* is slow progress toward an optimal course of action. *Mixed scanning* combines the stringent rationalism of optimizing with the "muddling through" approach of incrementalism into a conglomerate of substrategies. *Optimizing* has the goal of selecting the course of action with the highest payoff (maximizes). Limitations of time, money, or people may prevent the decision maker from selecting the more deliberative and slower process of optimizing. Still, the decision maker needs to focus on techniques that will enhance effectiveness in decision making situations.

La Monica and Finch (1977) noted that effective decisions = f (quality × acceptance × time). Thus, these three components can be analyzed together based on a specific situation. The effectiveness of a decision is contingent upon the specific circumstances. For high quality, low acceptance situations, the best choice is to seek an expert. For high acceptance situations, the best choice is to involve the staff. When both components are high, bringing appropriate experts together with the staff who will implement the decision is the best strategy.

Vroom and Yetton (1973) proposed a managerial decision making model that identified five managerial decision styles on a continuum from minimal subordinate involvement to delegation. Their model is a contingency approach which assumes that situational variables and personal attributes of the leader influence leader behavior and thus can affect organizational effectiveness. To diagnose the situation, the decision maker examines seven problem attributes: the importance of the quality of the decision, the extent of sufficient information/expertise, the amount of structure to the problem, the extent to which acceptance/commitment of followers is critical to implementation, the probability that an autocratic decision will be accepted, the motivation of followers to achieve the organizational goals, and the extent that conflict over preferred solutions is likely. Five diagnostic questions guide the decision process. The decision process is arrayed on a decision tree. The decision maker uses the diagnostic questions to work through the decision tree to the end result of one of five decision styles (Hersey & Blanchard, 1993). The decision styles range from autocratic to delegatory/participative. Thus there are a range of decision making styles available. The choice of style is dependent on the situation for effectiveness. Use of this model increases the probability of effective decision making style choice. La Monica and Finch (1977) and Taylor (1978) applied this model to nursing via the analysis of case studies.

Continuum of Control Over Decision Making Actions

Decisions can be thought of as resulting in action. This occurs over a series of sequential steps (see Fig. 7.3). The five steps of the process are (1) col-

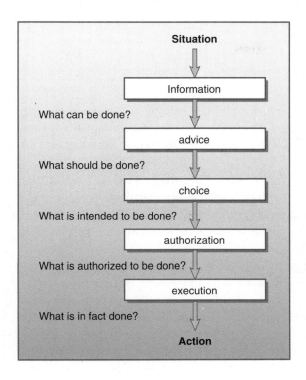

Figure 7.3
Continuum of control over the decision process. (Adapted with permission from Mintzberg, H. [1983]. *Structure in fives: Designing effective organizations.* Englewood Cliffs, NJ: Prentice Hall, p. 100.)

lect information, (2) process information into advice, (3) make the choice, (4) authorize the implementation, and (5) execute what is done. The end result, action, is controlled by more than simply making a choice. Outside influences can exert power or control over any of the steps of the decision process, thereby exerting power over the whole process (Mintzberg, 1983; Paterson, 1969). This idea is helpful to keep in mind as nurses use decision making with their clients in managing care and with situations in their work setting in coordinating nursing services delivery (see also Chapter 14).

Individuals can improve personal decision making by expanding their perspective about what determines their choices and how they make decisions. In order to improve this understanding, individuals can review recent decisions in their own lives, for example, deciding among financial alternatives. In considering some of the decisions which seem, in retrospect, to have been good decisions, they can analyze the process which was followed to arrive at the decision. What decision style was used? Was it fast and impulsive, or slow, methodical, and analytical? Was much time spent in gathering information? Did the decision maker follow a gut feeling or use rationality and logic? Was a very specific, logically structured decision process utilized? The greater the number of possible choices within a range of behavior and thinking, the more likely are the chances of making a good decision (Grainger, 1990). Personal decision making also can be improved by an examination of which steps in the decision making process are subject to the influence, power, or control of the individual.

Decision Making Strategies

There are various strategies used for problem solving and decision making. Strategies reflect time and mental structure variations; for example, fast, slow, impulsive, intuitive, or logical. The following are formal decision making strategies.

Trial and Error This means a "shoot-from-the-hip" or dart-throw type of solution is put into effect. A solution that seems attractive is chosen and simply tried out. Those managers who utilize trial and error as the usual strategy for decision making often are seen as ineffective. They are perceived as poor problem solvers.

Pilot Projects This strategy involves experimentation with limited trials. Pilot projects or limited trials are used to experiment by trying out a solution alternative on a limited basis to see if there are going to be major problems and to reduce risk. Pilot project strategies may resemble research projects.

Problem Critique This occurs in a one-on-one situation where, for example, a nurse manager sits down with a staff person and the two people dialogue about the problem. The purpose is to critique the problem and thereby determine what the facts are, what the problem is, and what potential solutions might be used.

Creativity Techniques These include brainstorming sessions, Delphi, and nominal group techniques, where a group gathers for free thinking exercises (Van de Ven & Delbecq, 1974). They are a way of solving problems especially suited to a complex problem that appears to have no good solution. Creativity techniques are used as a way to generate solutions, ideas, and thoughts by approaching the problem with freedom from pre-formed bias.

Decision Tree This is a graphic model (see Fig. 7.4). It shows the options, outcomes, and risks to be anticipated. A decision tree starts to the left and flows right. A question or problem is posed and the possible options become nodes branching away. Thus decision paths can be traced through option points and beyond. For example, a very simple decision tree might start with the question "Are you committed to becoming a nurse?" The answer to that question is yes or no. Depending on the answer to that question, the corresponding path is followed as mapped out on the decision tree. The tree enables visualization of the alternatives and the consequences. It helps with decision making through analysis and clarity (Hamilton & Kiefer, 1986).

Decision trees and algorithms are utilized for protocols for therapy administration. The advantage is to be able to analyze mapped alternatives, both positive and negative. For example, Willey (1989) developed a decision tree

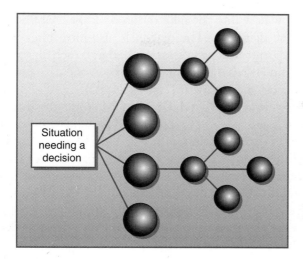

Figure 7.4
Decision tree outline.

model of high tech beds and mattress overlays for clients who are immobilized. The initial question was "Can the client be turned?" Different paths are selected if that answer is no as opposed to yes. The tree leads to an analysis of which beds and mattresses would be the best for a given immobility diagnosis. Critical paths are similar to decision trees and algorithms. Critical pathways are descriptions of the protocol for critical or key incidents that must occur in a predictable or timely order to keep the expected outcomes, length of stay, and overall costs appropriate and within diagnosis-related groups (DRG) allotted time frames (Thompson, Caddick, Mathie, Newlong, & Abraham, 1991). They are developed as a part of managed care or case management nursing care models (Mosher, Cronk, Kidd, McCormick, Stockton, & Sulla, 1992; Thompson et al., 1991). They are developed to incorporate multidisciplinary perspectives in order to display and track the client's entire expected course of treatment and expected outcomes. Variances are identified immediately and managed by the case manager (see Chapter 16).

As nursing evolves in sophistication and knowledge base to better identify nursing diagnoses and array the nursing interventions that match those nursing diagnoses, the use of decision trees may provide a useful way to display the linkages of interventions to diagnoses.

Fish Bone or Cause and Effect Chart   Fish bone charts are graphic figures used to help identify the possible causes of production problems. They resemble the figures used to diagram sentences. They are used in business and industry to clarify the production process and indicate possible points for improvement. The figures flow from left to right, with a horizontal line through the middle that ends with the outcome, product, or end result indicated to the far right side. On the horizontal line is placed the main process. Diagonals above and below flow into the main horizontal line. All feeder processes are indicated by the diagonals. The diagonals also have lines branching off of them which indicate other processes that feed into each diagonal. Flow charts, control charts, and fish bone diagrams have been popularized within Deming's approach to quality management (Aguayo, 1990).

Group Problem Solving and Decision Making In this technique the leader calls the group together to discuss and participate in solving a problem. The leader invites participation, either in the problem identification or the problem resolution part of the decision making process (see Chapter 8).

Cost-Benefit Analysis This is a formal balancing of driving and restraining forces. In this technique an individual will make a list of the benefits or positive factors that are supporting an affirmative decision. Also, a list of the detriments or negatives that are supporting a negative decision is compiled. These lists should be written down so that they can be arrayed visually (see Fig. 7.5). The process of writing out the elements helps to organize decision making. Counselors use this technique to help people with difficult personal life decisions. In the nursing practice setting, when the nurse needs to balance the utilization of scarce resources, a pro-con or cost-benefit analysis helps to clarify the elements inherently related to the problem and to facilitate subsequent decision making.

Worst-case Scenario This technique is found to be especially helpful for risky decisions. Risky decisions frequently but not always relate to the use of money or prestige. In this technique the "worst case," or what is the absolute worst thing to occur if everything that could go wrong did go wrong, is determined. The worst case is outlined for each alternative that might be foreseen.

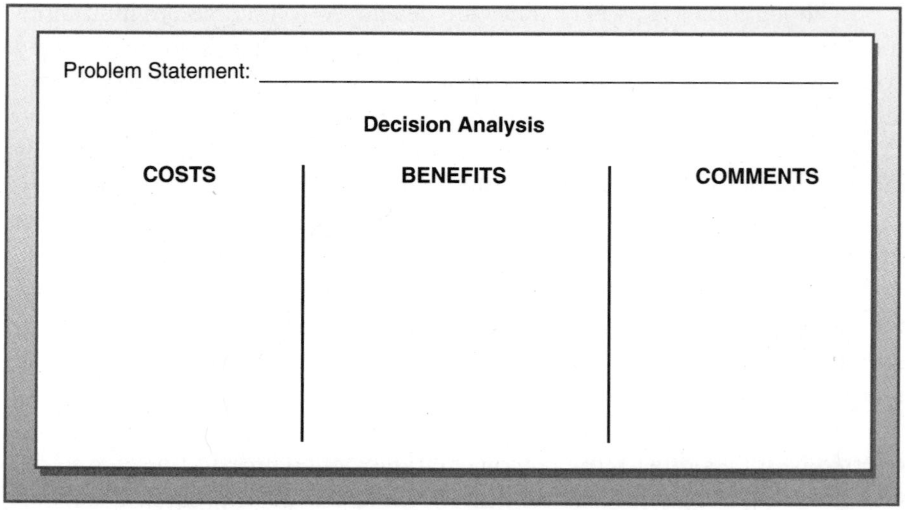
Problem Statement: ______________________

Decision Analysis

COSTS	BENEFITS	COMMENTS

Figure 7.5
Cost-benefit analysis form.

Then the alternative with the better result given when, or if, everything possible did go wrong is selected. So the "lesser of all of the evils" if money or reputation is on the line is chosen. Thus by determining what is the absolute worst that could happen and working backwards from that scenario, the decision maker chooses the best alternative under the situation to minimize potential anticipated risk of damage.

In the arena of decision making strategies, there also are sophisticated and computerized forecasting techniques such as linear programming models and mathematical techniques that assign a probability to each possible outcome. They are elaborations of decision tree models and are used for decision analysis (Grier, 1976). A computation of the statistical probabilities from certain knowns can be performed. These models use computers to calculate outcomes. They are used in forecasting and for sophisticated policy analyses (Baumann & Deber, 1989).

Information Processing

The core of professional nursing practice is nursing expertise applied to problem solving and decision making about client care and care management. Nursing decisions are based on data, therefore, the collection, classification, storage, retrieval, and analysis of data (called information processing) is an area of knowledge related to both problem solving and decision making. Nursing informatics, information systems, and computers in nursing are key words to describe this knowledge domain (Grier, 1984). Clearly, nurses need to acquire and use data for decision making. For example, requests for funding or policy change need to be accompanied by hard data.

Nursing's data have been described as being "invisible" since they are not clearly identified, defined, collected, or used (Grier, 1984). Lack of standardized definitions and measures decreases the comparability of data, and ultimately the quality of administrative decisions. Standardized data sets, including one for nursing management, are under development to alleviate this gap in nursing's data (Huber, Delaney, Crossley, Mehmert, & Ellerbe, 1992). Further discussion of these topics can be found in Chapters 6 and 24.

ETHICAL DECISION MAKING

There are a variety of factors that influence nurse decision making. Time, resources, and values all play a part. Values are derived from generational, religious, and cultural sources. They are conscious or unconscious attitudes, beliefs, biases, and feelings that influence thoughts and behaviors. Thus they influence decision making. Values may influence what is perceived and what are identified as alternatives in decision making. For example, ethical decision making occurs in nursing as nurses face conflicts between ethical principles in clinical client care situations or as resource allocation decisions are made. In complex situations, values and ethics may enter into the decision making process. Rational-logical decision making is one method for arriving at an administrative decision; ethical decision making is a second alternative (Botter & Dickey, 1989; Gordon, Murphy, Candee, & Hiltunen, 1994).

Values are strongly held beliefs or attitudes that are thought to be freely chosen, enduring, and forming a foundation for standards and actions. Value systems provide human beings with a structure for resolving conflicts and making decisions. The closer people are to having a similar culture, experiential background, and needs dispositions, the closer their value systems will harmonize because values are culturally derived in many instances (Scalzi & Nazarey, 1989).

Three value sets have been identified: personal, professional, and organizational. For example, a nurse may hold a personal value related to caring in nursing care. The ANA's Code for Nurses is an example of a professional value set. Cost containment or making a profit may be organizational value sets. Clashes of value sets lead to conflict (Scalzi & Nazarey, 1989).

Value structures form a context that surround and guide both personal lives and professional work situations. Strong values influence thoughts and actions. Leadership occurs within human interpersonal relationships, and thus values impinge on leadership. In one study, nurse leaders expressed fundamental values related to caring and concern for clients and the delivery of quality care, to investing in developing staff members, and to commitment to organizational and professional goals. Transforming leaders exhibited total commitment, determination, and a high level of persistence in achieving designated goals. Optimism and strong values may encourage high levels of optimizing outcomes (Irurita, 1994).

Values, however, also can lead to conflict. Ethical conflicts and paradoxes occur in both clinical practice and within the context of nursing leadership and management. Research and discussion about ethical issues in clinical nursing practice are more common than research and discussion about ethical dilemmas in nursing leadership and management (Camunas, 1994). A variety of practice situations raise ethical issues or concerns. Berger, Seversen, and Chvatal (1991) investigated the frequency with which registered nurses encountered specific ethical issues. The five ethical issues encountered most frequently were both clinical and administrative issues. In order of reported frequency, they are inadequate staffing patterns, prolonging life with heroic measures, inappropriate resource allocation, dealing with situations in which patients were discussed inappropriately, and dealing with colleagues' irresponsible activity. Encountering inadequate staffing frequently or very frequently was reported by 71% of the 52 respondents from one hospital. Issues related to prolonging life were reported more frequently by ICU nurses; issues related to the allocation of personnel resources were reported more frequently by administrators. The resources used to help with ethical issues were reported as consultations with nursing colleagues and own personal values. The authors (1991, p. 519) noted that nursing is a "clinical art with moral overtones." Further, they characterized nursing practice as being (1991, p. 519) "carried out in a bureaucratic setting constrained by institutional policies, where there is a great potential for a clash between professional cultural values and corporate values."

Specific examples of nurses' ethical dilemmas include the practice of pulling or floating nurses to areas in which they are not cross-trained and increasing the patient-to-nurse ratio to greater and greater limits. Nurse managers may be asked to reduce expenditures by leaving specialty areas like labor and delivery uncovered when no clients are present. Organizations may refuse to purchase equipment or provide support services on off-shifts. Home visits may be refused if reimbursement cannot be captured. Time for teaching and counseling clients may be denied via staffing practices. Nurses may experience responses of "there is no money" for nursing care needs while the hospital takes over the space occupied by nursing services offices to renovate for a new physicians' lounge and private dining room. Nurses may face the problem of other healthcare providers reading and discussing a client's medical record without appropriate authorization. A nurse manager may be presented with a request from a physician to deploy a hospital nurse to the physician's private practice office to help with clients.

There are several key concepts that underlie decisions about what is right and wrong in situations where an individual has to make a choice between equally unfavorable alternatives. *Autonomy* refers to the client's right of self-determination and freedom of decision making. *Beneficence* means doing good for clients and providing benefit balanced against risk. *Fidelity* means being loyal and faithful to commitments and accountable for responsibilities. *Justice* is the norm of being fair to all and giving equal treatment, including distributing benefits, risks, and costs equally. *Nonmaleficence* means doing no harm to clients. *Veracity* is the norm of telling the truth and not intentionally deceiving or misleading clients (Aiken, 1994; Beauchamp & Childress, 1994). Table 7.1 displays examples of ethical principles and nursing management examples.

Ethical decision making models and processes can form the basis of decision making strategies for ethical dilemmas. Following the problem solving approach, Aiken (1994) outlined a five step ethical decision making process. The first step is to collect, analyze, and interpret as much information as possible about the dilemma. The second step is to state the dilemma as clearly as is possible. The third step is to list and consider all possible courses of action to choose among. The fourth step is to analyze the advantages and disadvantages of each course of action. The final step is to make a decision.

Table 7.1

Ethical Decision Making in Nursing Management

ETHICAL PRINCIPLE	EXAMPLE
Autonomy	Decentralization and nursing shared governance are instituted so that nurses make decisions about client care and nursing practice.
Beneficence	Continuing education opportunities are provided and paid for so that nurses can fulfill mandatory and competency requirements.
Fidelity	Adequate support services are provided to nursing and administration is supportive of nursing's professional activities.
Justice	Fair wages and promotion systems are in place and followed in practice.
Nonmaleficence	Universal precautions are enforced for blood-borne pathogens exposure to prevent client and employee harm.
Veracity	Honest performance appraisals of weaknesses are discussed to stimulate awareness and improvement.

Crisham (1985) developed a model for analysis and resolution of nursing ethical dilemmas. It was designed to make the moral and ethical decision making process explicit by linking judgment, choice, and action and by considering alternatives in view of moral principles. Called the MORAL model, Crisham's (1985) five steps are massage the dilemma by defining and describing conflicts and interests, outlining options by brainstorming to discover alternative solutions, reviewing criteria and resolving the dilemma, affirming a position and acting on the judgment, and looking back to evaluate the effectiveness of the process. Crisham (1985) described the MORAL model as a research-based tool useful for analysis and resolution of nursing ethical dilemmas because of the use of the nurse's experience of a dilemma, the formulation of the nurse's position based on moral principles, and the development of encouragement to act on commitment. Scherb (1995) described the application of the MORAL model to an analysis of a cross-section of schools of nursing's Hepatitis B policies covering student nurses. Schools of nursing are not mandated to cover student nurses for Hepatitis B. The vaccine is expensive, yet student nurses are vulnerable to exposure. The steps of the MORAL model can be applied to an analysis of explicit policies to highlight areas for augmentation and revision.

Any clash of professional and organizational values will surface in nursing management decisions. In one national survey of 315 nurse executives, the majority (94%) reported encountering ethical dilemmas in daily administrative decisions (Camunas, 1994). The issues presenting ethical dilemmas can be categorized as staffing, client care, and personnel. The major conflict occurs between the nurses' professional values related to providing high quality client care and the fiscal responsibilities embedded in their administrative position. The greatest ethical conflict for the majority of subjects was in making decisions about staffing. Financial constraints restricted the use of more skilled, educated, and experienced nurses. The severity of the fiscal restrictions resulted in some respondents voicing a concern about client safety and the institution's ability to provide a minimal level of safe care. Further, about half of the sample reported feeling pressure to compromise their personal standards in order to achieve organizational goals. Clearly, organizations define and control situations in which decisions are made. An organizational climate that supports ethical decision making will include mechanisms to balance cost, quality, and ethical values (Camunas, 1994).

The outcome of an ethical dilemma is that a decision or decisions may need to be made. At issue often are what decisions are needed, who makes the decisions, and how the decisions should be made (Capuzzi, 1994). One major fundamental healthcare ethical dilemma is how to make decisions between humanistic caring for all people and cost containment needs. Ethical decision making is needed under conditions of scarce resources and the rationing of services. Clearly, ethics has an area of overlap and interface with politics (Aroskar, 1987). Thus nurses may become involved in health policy aspects and controversies as they find themselves needing to work through the ethical dilemmas embedded in nursing practice and the delivery of nursing care to client populations.

RESEARCH NOTE

Source: Biordi, D. (1993). Nursing error and caring in the workplace. *Nursing Administration Quarterly, 17*(2), 38-45.

Purpose

The purpose of this study was to explore how nurses categorize their errors and use caring as an underlying ethic to error identification and management. Nursing mistakes can be seen as breaches of the work group's care standards. The methods used were a one year participant observation study of nurses on two units of one midwestern tertiary hospital. The units had 60 nurses and almost complete RN staffing. The nurses represented a diversity of educational backgrounds. The results were used to build a theory about nursing work organization, ethics, and caring.

Discussion

An act, its seriousness, its regularity, or its location can have different meanings at different times and not consistently be labeled an error. Nursing error is a breach of either nursing content or nursing role identity. Nurses' sense of error was shaped by a variety of circumstances, all of which included the centrality of caring, the necessity of full disclosure, and the need for moral remorse or an attempt to repair or reverse the error. Nurses also felt the need for no surprises and held an expectation that all calls for help would be answered. Errors were individual or collective. There were three major and progressively intense categories of error: technical error, or the honest error of technique; judgmental error, or the honest error of role content; and normative error, or breach of honesty, trust, or responsibility.

Application to Practice

Mistakes happen. Nurses try to control or manage the results to identify and control consequences. Informal control is exercised by the standards embedded in practice. Formal control mechanisms include quality control and incident reports. Mistakes reveal what nurses are willing to risk. Analysis of nursing error allows for better interpretation of the true basis for an error and the likely consequences. Issues of risk and choice arise. Decision making occurs in relation to whether an act is a technical, judgmental, or normative error and as to what sanctions are applied to each category.

LEADERSHIP AND MANAGEMENT IMPLICATIONS

Decision making is a central component of leadership and management activity. Leadership decision making focuses on choices made to advance the group's goals. Management decision making focuses on coordinating, integrating, and allocating scarce resources to accomplish organizational goals. Therefore, the focus of leadership and management decision making is related more to the nurse's role as care coordinator than the role of caregiver.

Decision making skill is valued in nursing practice as evidenced by the construction of RN licensure examination questions related to decision mak-

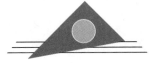 *Leadership & Management Behaviors*

LEADERSHIP BEHAVIORS	MANAGEMENT BEHAVIORS	OVERLAP AREAS
• inspires followers to make decisions	• makes decisions about resource allocation	• uses decision making strategies to accomplish goals
• communicates desired values for decisions	• motivates subordinates to come to consensus	• assists individuals and groups to make decisions
• motivates followers to be creative and innovative	• plans day-to-day operations	• makes decisions
• models decisive actions	• resolves selected problems	
• develops strategic plans	• organizes the work	
• influences followers to make autonomous decisions	• evaluates productivity	
	• takes corrective action	

ing skills of the nurse. What would the nurse do first? How much would the nurse do, versus sharing the decision with the client or vesting the decision totally with the client? Clinical decision making skills can be focused and enhanced by the use of critical paths. Nurses can and do use decision making in all aspects of care management.

Nurse managers face decisions about budgeting, future planning, buying equipment, staffing implementation, and day-to-day tactical management of the nursing service unit. Nagelkerk and Henry (1990) identified two types of executive decisions: (1) routine and operational and (2) nonroutine and strategic. Routine decisions about daily operations are made most often and carry minimal to moderate risk. Step-by-step rational approaches can be used. Nonroutine decisions about novel situations or complex problems involve high risk and a dynamic set of decision activities using intuition and political knowledge.

An important activity related to managerial decision making is the setting of priorities. This is done for time management and to ensure that the most important activities are completed. Delegation is a tool that is used to distribute the workload. Manthey (1988) discussed the issue of who owns a staff nurse's time. Her premise was that nursing resources are insufficient for the existing workload, thus making the time of an RN one of the scarcest resources in healthcare. Workload factors are not under the control of the nursing department, resulting in uncontrollable fluctuations. Further, multiple influences are brought to bear: hospital and healthcare administrators desire greater productivity to take better care of more clients with less cost; clients desire more nursing time and attention; physicians desire flexibility with their schedules to ease their job; and nurse managers desire nursing time to be spent when scheduled and dedicated to the work assigned. Since nearly everyone lays claim to staff nurses' time, the answer to what do you do when there is more work than time available is prioritize. Manthey (1988, p. 24) noted that "the concept of autonomy in a service profession involves decision making about the kind and degree of service a client will receive." The decision uses a complex professional reasoning process about the need and the resources available. Autonomous decision making includes deciding what will *and* will not be done if there is more work than time available. Empowerment results from nurses being enabled to control the use of their time to meet clients' needs.

Nurses make decisions all of the time. Nursing decisions are not trivial; many of these decisions are critical to the client. It may be that decisions are made by virtue of a natural personality style, in response to the latest research literature, or from reading some article. For example, reading that engaging in trust allows the client to relax and, therefore, have better outcomes might become the basis for alterations in the nurse's future care of clients. Decision making may have been a spontaneous, intuitive occurrence. Nevertheless, the nurse makes a choice as to how to approach each client. It is a choice as to how to engage others, how much to personalize or not personalize, how much to use the literature, and how much to use one's experiencing of other people. Client care has been described as being like an orchestra that is made up of individual members, which, when properly directed, comes out with a symphonic sound.

When is a mistake a failure? Nurses make decisions under conditions both of uncertainty and risk. It is part of the human condition to make mistakes. Sometimes an error in judgment results in harm or death. However, when a mistake has been made, the nurse manager makes a decision as to how to approach corrective action. Some adopt the attitude that it is wrong or bad to make mistakes. The person may be labeled as at fault and subjected to negative or punitive corrective action. The natural response is to avoid, deny, or become defensive. The person may experience anger, lowered self-esteem, and blocks to positive learning (Kowalski, 1992).

For some managers, mistakes are viewed as learning experiences. The focus is on what was learned and what corrections need to be made. If the manager asks what could be done differently next time and emphasizes the error as a component of learning, then a sense of responsibility and learning from the experience is instilled (Kowalski, 1992).

CURRENT ISSUES AND TRENDS

New forms of nurse decision making activities include the development of critical pathways and the development of national standards and guidelines. As mentioned earlier in decision trees, critical paths are one component of managed care or case management. They identify key events of care and expected timeframes. Their advantages include streamlined charting (if computerized), outcomes assurance and quality assessment facilitation, and improved client teaching and inter-shift communication. Critical pathways demonstrate the intersection of clinical decision making with administrative decision making; the same tool works to facilitate both goals.

The development of national standards and guidelines have been stimulated by quality improvement and effectiveness initiatives in healthcare. Regulatory agencies have established programs to promote the development of national standards and guidelines as a way of enhancing quality of care related decision making and reducing variance in professional practice patterns. The Joint Commission on Accreditation of Healthcare Organization's (JCAHO) Agenda for Change has promoted the identification and use of appropriate, measurable clinical indicators in nursing. These indicators are to be quantitative measures to monitor and evaluate the quality of care. For example, the occurrence of medication errors, self-extubations of clients on ventilators, or well prepared clients at discharge are indicators that can be quantified, for example, by the number of medication errors divided by the number of doses dispensed (Scholz, 1990; Williams, 1991).

Disciplines and specialties promulgate standards and guidelines for their own practice. When there is overlap between and among specialties, a multidisciplinary approach results in a more comprehensive way to meld divergent practices and intertwined policies. For example, there are different perspectives about how pain should be managed. The individual nurse is responsible and accountable for decisions about intervention strategies. These decisions control pain and impact financial aspects such as length of stay and cost of care.

The Agency for Health Care Policy and Research (AHCPR), the federal agency with responsibility for health services research, has launched an initiative to develop multidisciplinary clinical practice guidelines for selected significant and broadly applicable problems that have a wide variation in decision strategies, a research base, and cost implications of care (Jacox, Ferrell, Heidrick, Hester, & Miaskowski, 1992). Clinical practice guidelines on management of acute pain, urinary incontinence, pressure ulcers, cataracts, and depression have been developed and disseminated. Nurses have been involved actively in the development of these guidelines. It is suggested that, in the future, unsubstantiated deviation from these extensively developed and research-based guidelines may be considered failure to act as a reasonable and prudent nurse. Thus, knowledge about problem solving methods and decision making skills are essential nursing activities to be learned and developed.

Perception and Innovation: Tools for Decision Making

Perception is a powerful influence on problem solving and decision making. Perception is defined as an individual's filtering and interpretation of events. It is how the person sees what is going on (Kramer, 1994). Perception is influenced by such elements as culture, values, and biases. Perception can cloud objectivity and rationality. Perception can diminish creativity and the range of options identified for decision making, or it can be a vehicle to open up routine or automatic decision responses.

Perception affects how problems are viewed and what actions are determined to be the "best" solutions. There have been many problems that have been defined as unsolvable or for which only one solution path has been identified. However, creative solutions can be an outcome of changing the perception of what is a failure. One example is the glue that did not stick and the development of Post-It Notes by 3-M. Post-It Notes were the result of an inspiration by Art Fry in 1974. Fry was sitting in his church with a hymnal book that he kept flipping back and forth. He started thinking how wonderful it would be if there could be some paper with glue that did not stick so he could mark the hymnal pages. Meanwhile, a scientist in Research and Development at 3-M had been experimenting with glues in the research lab and had come up with a glue that did not stick. Obviously the scientist had thought the "glue" was a total failure, and it was shelved. Fry came to the lab with his idea for something that would really work if there was a glue that didn't stick. Thus the concept for Post-It Notes was developed. It took Fry a little while to convince 3-M to manufacture them, but they were overwhelmingly successful ("Post it Notes," 1990). Now it is hard to imagine clerical work without them.

The need for creativity and innovation in healthcare is with us, and it is an urgent need. Creativity and innovation can be used as modes of decision making for the purpose of expanding available actions. See Chapter 6 for a discussion of the Kirton Adaptation-Innovation Theory. Drucker (1986) urged that innovation be a purposeful, systematic activity. He noted that systematic innovation meant monitoring the seven sources for innovative opportunity: the unexpected; incongruity; innovation based on process need; changes in the industry structure or market structure; demographics (population changes); changes in perception, mood, or meaning; and new knowledge. Healthcare in the United States will benefit from nurses who take basic knowledge, employ critical thinking, refuse to see abnormal or different paths as failure, and apply creativity to nursing's needs. A pressing need right now is for people who can adapt technology to nursing's productivity gaps. For example, computers, bar coding, robotics, and communications technology are areas that could be creatively engineered to make technology work for nurses.

For example, one nurse at a tertiary hospital had a 69-year-old woman client who refused to accept a bandage. The woman said she was tired of fooling with bandages since it was hard to get them started when they had to be picked at with fingernails. It hurt her skin. Thinking about bandages and skin care in the elderly, the nurse developed and patented a band-aid designed for ease of pull from the end. Her innovation was generated from a genuine and practical client concern (Anderson, 1989). Clearly, creativity can be fostered in nursing. Reframing problems and encouraging inventors are key strategies. Nurse managers play an important leadership role in stimulating innovation instead of accepting the status quo. Creating an environment that is "safe" or where mistakes are viewed as learning experiences enables and encourages creativity and innovation.

SUMMARY

- Decision making involves the act of choosing and implementing a course of action from among alternatives.
- Decision making may or may not be the result of an immediate problem.
- The core phases of decision making are deliberation, judgment, and evaluation.
- Decision making is a process with identifiable steps.
- Decision making situations are personal, clinical, or organizational.
- There are a variety of administrative decision making models.
- There are different decision styles and strategies.
- Nurses and nursing care managers face ethical dilemmas.

- The essence of professional practice is the application of expertise to solve problems for clients.
- Nurses make decisions all the time.
- Professional autonomy includes decision making about what will and will not be done for clients.
- Perception and innovation are influences and tools for decision making.

Study Questions

1. What is your typical or preferred decision style?
2. How does clinical decision making differ from managerial decision making?
3. How are problem solving and decision making related in nursing?
4. What important decisions do nurses make? Which ones do they collaborate on?
5. What strategies work best for clinical decision making? For managerial decision making?
6. How can information processing help nurse decision making?
7. What resources are available to assist with ethical decision making?
8. What creative or innovative ideas do you have?

Critical Thinking Exercise

Jerald May was recently made a nurse manager on a large medical-surgical nursing unit. He is eager to be a successful leader and manager. He has been carefully reviewing the OSHA standards and guidelines in preparation for his task of revising hospital policies pertaining to OSHA regulations on protection against TB. However, he has some concerns. He is wondering if the hospital should exempt certain employees from being fitted for and wearing HEPA masks. Two situations have arisen: male employees with beards and other employees with a medical condition such as asthma that make wearing the mask extremely uncomfortable because of the tight fit. Nurse May is pondering the problem.

1. *What is the problem?*

2. *Why is it a problem?*

3. *What are the key issues?*

4. *What should Nurse May do first?*

5. *How should Nurse May handle this situation?*

6. *What decision making strategy should Nurse May use?*

7. *What leadership and management strategies might help?*

REFERENCES

Aguayo, R. (1990). *Dr. Deming: The American who taught the Japanese about quality*. New York: Carol Publishing Group.

Aiken, T. (1994). *Legal, ethical, and political issues in nursing*. Philadelphia: F. A. Davis.

Anderson, C. (1989, July 29). Little invention avoids big ouch. *The Iowa City Press-Citizen*, p. 1.

Aroskar, M. (1987). The interface of ethics and politics in nursing. *Nursing Outlook, 35*(6), 268-272.

Barnard, C. (1982). The environment of decision. *Journal of Nursing Administration, 12*(3), 25-29.

Baumann, A., & Deber, R. (1989). The limits of decision analysis for rapid decision making in ICU nursing. *Image, 21*(2), 69-71.

Beauchamp, T., & Childress, J. (1994). *Principles of biomedical ethics* (4th ed.). New York: Oxford University Press.

Berger, M., Seversen, A., & Chvatal, R. (1991). Ethical issues in nursing. *Western Journal of Nursing Research, 13*(4), 514-521.

Botter, M., & Dickey, S. (1989). Allocation of resources: Nurses, the key decision makers. *Holistic Nursing Practice, 4*(1), 44-51.

Camunas, C. (1994). Ethical dilemmas of nurse executives: Part 1. *Journal of Nursing Administration, 24*(7/8), 45-51.

Capuzzi, C. (1994). The Oregon model of decision making and its implications for nursing practice. In J. McCloskey & H. Grace (Eds.), *Current issues in nursing* (4th ed.) (pp. 711-717). St. Louis: Mosby.

Crisham, P. (1985). Resolving ethical and moral dilemmas of nursing interventions. In M. Snyder (Ed.), *Independent nursing interventions* (pp. 25-43). New York: John Wiley & Sons.

deChesnay, M. (1983). Problem solving in nursing. *Image, 15*(1), 8-11.

Drucker, P. (1986). *Innovation and entrepreneurship: Practice and principles*. New York: Harper & Row.

Elstein, A., Schulman, L., & Sprafka, S. (1978). *Medical problem-solving: An analysis of clinical reasoning*. Cambridge, MA: Harvard University Press.

Etzioni, A. (1989). Humble decision making. *Harvard Business Review, 67*(4), 122-126.

Gordon, M., Murphy, C., Candee, D., & Hiltunen, E. (1994). Clinical judgment: An integrated model. *Advances in Nursing Science, 16*(4), 55-70.

Grainger, R. (1990). Making better decisions. *American Journal of Nursing, 90*(6), 15-16.

Grier, M. (1976). Decision making about patient care. *Nursing Research, 25*(2), 105-110.

Grier, M. (1984). Information processing in nursing practice. *Annual Review of Nursing Research, 2*, 265-287.

Hamilton, J., & Kiefer, M. (1986). *Survival skills for the new nurse*. Philadelphia: Lippincott.

Hersey, P., & Blanchard, K. (1993). *Management of organizational behavior: Utilizing human resources* (6th ed.). Englewood Cliffs, NJ: Prentice-Hall.

Huber, D.G., Delaney, C., Crossley, J., Mehmert, P., & Ellerbe, S. (1992). A nursing management minimum data set: Significance and development. *Journal of Nursing Administration, 22*(7/8), 35-40.

Hughes, K., & Young, W. (1992). Decision making: Stability of clinical decisions. *Nurse Educator, 17*(3), 12-16.

Irurita, V. (1994). Optimism, values, and commitment as forces in nursing leadership. *Journal of Nursing Administration, 24*(9), 61-71.

Jacox, A., Ferrell, B., Heidrich, G., Hester, N., & Miaskowski, C. (1992). Managing acute pain: A guideline for the nation. *American Journal of Nursing, 92*(5), 49-55.

Janis, I., & Mann, L. (1977). *Decision making: A psychological analysis of conflict, choice, and commitment*. New York: Free Press.

Kramer, M. (1994). Perception & community: Seeing what we need to see. *Change, 26*(5), 50-51.

Kerrigan, K. (1991). Decision making in today's complex environment. *Nursing Administration Quarterly, 15*(4), 1-5.

Kowalski, K. (1992). From failures to major learning experiences. *MCN, 17*(1), 9-10.

La Monica, E., & Finch, F. (1977). Managerial decision making. *Journal of Nursing Administration, 7*(5), 20-28.

Manthey, M. (1988). Who owns a staff nurse's time? *Nursing Management, 19*(9), 22-23.

McKenzie, M. (1985). Decisions: How you reach them makes the difference. *Nursing Management, 16*(6), 48-49.

Mintzberg, H. (1983). *Structure in fives: Designing effective organizations*. Englewood Cliffs, NJ: Prentice-Hall.

Mosher, C., Cronk, P., Kidd, A., McCormick, P., Stockton, S., & Sulla, C. (1992). Upgrading practice with critical pathways. *American Journal of Nursing, 92*(1), 41-43.

Nagelkerk, J., & Henry, B. (1990). Strategic decision making. *Journal of Nursing Administration, 20*(7/8), 18-23.

Paterson, T. (1969). *Management theory*. London: Business Publications, Ltd.

Post-it notes: A product that's stuck for 10 years. (1990, February 11). *The Des Moines Register*, p. 12X.

Prescott, P., Dennis, K., & Jacox, A. (1987). Clinical decision making of staff nurses. *Image, 19*(2), 56-62.

Scalzi, C., & Nazarey, P. (1989). Value conflicts in nursing administration. In B. Henry, C. Arndt, M. DiVincenti, & A. Marriner-Tomey (Eds.), *Dimensions of nursing administration: Theory, research, education, practice* (pp. 583-591). Boston: Blackwell.

Schaefer, J. (1974). The interrelatedness of decision making and the nursing process. *American Journal of Nursing, 74*(10), 1852-1855.

Scherb, C. (1995). *Need for improved Hepatitis B policies in schools of nursing: an ethical analysis*. Unpublished paper. Iowa City, IA: The University of Iowa.

Scholz, D. (1990). Establishing and monitoring an endemic medication error rate. *Journal of Nursing Quality Assurance, 4*(2), 71-74.

Tanner, C. (1987). Teaching clinical judgment. *Annual Review of Nursing Research, 5*, 153-173.

Tanner, C., Padrick, K., Westfall, U., & Putzier, D. (1987). Diagnostic reasoning strategies of nurses and nursing students. *Nursing Research, 36*(6), 358-363.

Taylor, A. (1978). Decision making in nursing: An analytical approach. *Journal of Nursing Administration, 8*(11), 22-30.

Thompson, K., Caddick, K., Mathie, J., Newlon, B., & Abraham, T. (1991). Building a critical path for ventilator dependency. *American Journal of Nursing, 91*(7), 28-31.

Van de Ven, A., & Delbecq, A. (1974). The effectiveness of nominal, delphi, and interacting group decision making processes. *Academy of Management Journal, 17*(4), 605-621.

Veninga, R. (1982). *The human side of health administration: A guide for hospital, nursing, and public health administrators*. Englewood Cliffs, NJ: Prentice-Hall.

Vroom, V., & Yetton, P. (1973). *Leadership and decision making*. Pittsburgh: University of Pittsburgh Press.

Willey, T. (1989). High-tech beds and mattress overlays: A decision guide. *American Journal of Nursing, 89*(9), 1142-1146.

Williams, A. (1991). Development and application of clinical indicators for nursing. *Journal of Nursing Care Quality, 6*(1), 1-5.

Wren, G. (1974). *Modern health administration*. Athens, GA: University of Georgia Press.

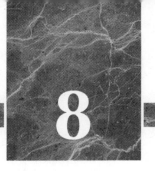

The Use of Groups, Committees, and Teams

Chapter Objectives

∞

define a group

∞

distinguish among the aspects of group interactions

∞

explain the reasons why people join groups

∞

compare advantages and disadvantages of using groups in organizations

∞

distinguish among the points on the continuum
of group decision making power

∞

define and explain committees

∞

analyze the leader's function in committee work

∞

distinguish among three types of meetings

∞

discuss constructive group members

∞

describe the types of disruptive group members

∞

define and analyze work teams

∞

exercise critical thinking to conceptualize and analyze
possible solutions to a practical experience incident

*N*urses do not do their work in isolation. In many nursing care delivery settings, nurses function in a work group environment or as a part of a team. There are some occupations in which people work in relative isolation from other people, but that is not the reality of the work of nursing. As healthcare restructures and becomes more complex, a greater value will be placed on high performing and cohesive work groups. This is because complexity and cost control factors in the environment have encouraged the use of interdisciplinary work teams. Therefore, nurses need to learn how to function constructively in group situations.

In nursing, group process theory relates to both how to be therapeutic with clients and how to work as an employee embedded within an organization that is often large and complex. Nursing has at its core both a caring and a coordinative function. The nurse's coordinative role is at the central hub of all client care information; for example, nurses collect, process, and integrate the initial assessment, laboratory data, the tracking of all the therapeutic interventions for the client, and often are at the bedside for surveillance of minute-by-minute changes. For example, if pain medications are given in a hospital, the nurses track whether or not that intervention has worked, whether or not alternative pain strategies might be needed, and what psychological reaction the client might have. Clients and families note that a physician may visit once a day on a hospital unit and not capture the fine distinctions of change in a client's condition. The nurse is involved more intimately and proximately than any of the other healthcare givers in managing the total healthcare of the client. Therefore, understanding and developing skill in group process and group dynamics is essential within the context of leadership and management in nursing because of the group functioning and coordinative aspects of nursing practice.

Nurses have to work collaboratively, not only with other nurses and their nurse manager, but also with people who do not share the same professional background, such as the administrative structure of the organization, other providers, the supply department, or the legal staff. The swirl of interpersonal and collaborative activities shape the essence of nursing practice. Therefore, as the environment of healthcare becomes more collaborative, nurses will need strong group process and interaction skills in order to communicate clearly with a variety of healthcare workers.

DEFINITIONS

group is defined as any collection of interconnected individuals working together for some purpose (see Chart 8.1). Group interactions are composed of the following elements (Book & Galvin, 1975) (see Fig. 8.1):

CHART 8.1
❧ DEFINITIONS

Group
any collection of interconnected individuals working together for some purpose.

Committee
a relatively stable and formally composed group. A subset of a group.

Team building
the process of deliberately creating and unifying a group into a functioning work unit so that specific goals are accomplished.

Some data from Farley and Stoner (1989).

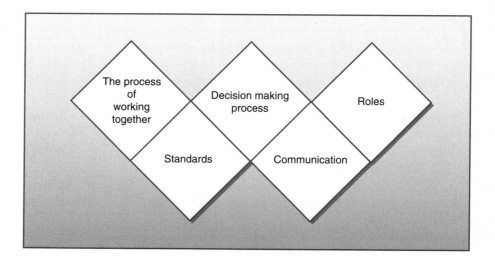

Figure 8.1
Group process elements.
(Data from Book and Galvin
[1975].)

- the *process* that the group undergoes to reach outcomes. This relates to the unique way the group interrelates and begins to work together. The leader can assess group process through observation: what is the process that this group goes through in accomplishing its task?
- the *standards* that regulate the group's behavior. This relates to the specific values and norms that are chosen for group processing. Which are chosen, which are discarded?
- the process of *problem solving or decision making* that the group adopts. Does the group solve problems? How are decisions made?
- the *communication* that occurs among group members. What are the internal patterns and styles of communication among group members? To whom does the group communicate? Do they report as a subcommittee to a full committee? What are the internal and external modes of communication for group input and output?
- the *roles* that are played by each member. Group roles are discussed later in this chapter. It is important to remember when assessing group interactions that roles in the group are not always clearly established by the leader. In fact, sometimes the leader will intentionally leave unspoken, even in response to an inquiry, the type of authority delegation that is taking place. This may be done to allow the group to make its own way through group process. It will be the participants' role in such situations to recognize this non-statement as such and to read the group dynamics to reach a conclusion. In this situation, each group member is allowed to select a group role that suits them.

Groups tend to go through a series of stages. Farley and Stoner (1989) identified these as orientation, adaptation, emergence, and working. The orientation stage occurs when the group first forms and begins to relate to each other and the task. The group needs to develop trust and define boundaries in order to establish involvement and identification. The second stage of adaptation occurs as the group begins to develop a team identity and differentiate roles. The group needs a facilitative structure and climate to maximize its processing and in order to develop roles, rules, norms, and a common language. The third stage of emergence occurs as control issues arise. Disputes, disagreements, confrontations, alliances, and power struggles mark this stage of determining control over the group in order to emerge with a more consolidated identity. The final stage of working occurs when conflict and dissention dissipate and the group achieves greater cohesion through negotiation. The group is now focused on decision making and productivity. The stages may overlap and are not necessarily sequential. The group leader pays attention to the stage of the group as a way of monitoring the group's development and progress. For example, the leader may need to be more alert to the need to personally intervene in the orientation stage than in the working stage.

BACKGROUND

Why People Join Groups

The reasons why people join groups include such things as a desire to satisfy psychological drives and primary needs. Group participation can be desirable to individuals for a variety of reasons. For example, interaction with people and a sense of self-achievement may result from participating. Psychological satisfaction can be derived from making a contribution, being with people, or producing goal accomplishment through group participation. Groups provide an outlet for affiliation needs: to make friends or meet people. There are a number of ways in which groups at all levels fulfill socialization and friendship needs. The following are some reasons why groups would be established in organizations:

- Group activities can create a sense of status and esteem.
- Groups allow an individual to test and establish reality.
- Groups function as a mechanism for getting a job done.

Thus in nursing, the formation of groups occurs for one of two reasons: to provide a personal or professional socialization and exchange forum or to provide a mechanism for work accomplishment. Groups can be social, professional, or organizational in purpose.

Advantages of Groups

There are some advantages to group work. For example, groups are one vehicle for solving problems. Veninga (1982) identified five major advantages of group problem solving over individual problem solving:

- *Greater knowledge and information:* Obtaining a broader and wider range of knowledge and experiences creates a higher quality input into group problem solving. The insights of one member can stimulate the thinking of others (Beachy & Biester, 1986).
- *Increased acceptance of solutions:* If there is a decision to be made in an organization, people can get together in a group to talk about it so that the people themselves are more committed to the decision.
- *More approaches to a problem:* Complex problems typically are more manageable when a number of minds are blended together to address the problem. The advantage includes blending and complementing individual learning and problem solving styles to capitalize on strength through diversity.
- *Individual expression:* Groups allow for individual expression, and in organizations specifically, there may be few mechanisms for expression of individual perspectives. Sharing information and getting input is done best in groups (Veninga, 1982). Sometimes groups allow people to express themselves, for example, if they are anxious about a change or if morale is low.
- *Lower economic costs:* If the group is functioning in a positive and a constructive manner, the use of a group can be less expensive than the use of individual effort to accomplish a task. Group decision making is cost effective if it saves time. For example, when a group meets together for one session as opposed to the leader meeting multiple times with multiple individuals, time is saved by the leader and possibly by the group members. Further, cost effectiveness may occur through the division of labor (Beachy & Biester, 1986).

It is imperative that the purpose of the group be established and assessed when the group is part of a larger organization. This means that all members need to have a clear definition of the work of the group. The leader needs to disseminate this information or the followers need to ask for clarification. Then

Table 8.1

Committee Cost Analysis

MEMBERS	SALARY/HOUR	BENEFITS/HOUR	NO. OF HOURS	COST
Nurse 1	$15.00	$6.00	1	$21.00
Nurse 2	$15.00	$6.00	1	$21.00
Physician	$100.00	N.A.	1	$100.00
Nurse Manager	$22.00	$8.80	1	$30.80
				$172.80 Grand Total per hour of meeting

evaluation of the stated purpose should occur periodically. Is it a functioning group? Is it accomplishing the task to which it was assigned? If not, should the group be disbanded? Sometimes if the work output of a group of nurses is analyzed, the meetings appear to be very costly endeavors. For example, when the number of hours spent by all committee members is multiplied by their individual hourly salary and fringe benefit cost and added together to compute a committee total, the sum of costs for the group may be astounding (see Table 8.1). This is another reason for attending to how well the group is functioning.

A well-tuned and functioning group is positive for an organization. Often such a group is less expensive and time consuming in terms of solving problems. Participation and involvement in a group decision typically results in individuals being more committed to a decision, even if there is disagreement.

Exemplar 8.1

Instituting a Nurse-Managed Clinic

The changes in healthcare require proficient utilization of resources. Nurses today must actively seek out opportunities to make changes in ways that will favorably impact their work and patient care. Although we do not always have a say in whether or not to change the way we work, we have a choice in the way we respond to change. The use of groups to solve efficiency problems is one manner in which to bring about effective and efficient change.

One treatment option for advanced prostate cancer patients is monthly hormone therapy. This treatment blocks the body's utilization of testosterone, thereby "starving" the prostate of testosterone and stopping cancer growth. These patients require monthly treatment for the rest of their lives. The population of these patients in our clinic

had grown such that the volume was unmanageable. It was evident that a change was required.

Each nurse had her own case load of patients seen each month. The norm was that no matter what the nurse was doing when her patient arrived for his appointment, she would quit what she was doing and proceed to see her patient. This method of patient care management was adequate until additional physicians were added to the department and an extraordinary increase in all areas of clinic activity occurred. There was a large increase in procedures, treatments, and clinic visits. The fact that the patient's primary nurse would "drop" whatever she was doing when her patients arrived, became incredibly disruptive to patient flow in all areas of the clinic. It was obvious that a new method of patient care management was needed.

There was a long history of "each nurse has her own patients" to overcome; it was the norm for years. Resistance was expected in changing this norm and instituting a new one. Although most nurses realized the difficulties with the current system, some had fears. In order for the change to be effective, these fears had to be addressed and all had to participate in the process of defining and implementing the change.

A series of staff meetings was held to address the problem. It was important that the entire staff was present so that all could participate, voice opinions, and identify fears and uncertainties. With everyone joining in with suggestions, more ideas with which to work were produced. The Clinical Nurse Specialist (a nurse with a Master of Science in Nursing degree) who specialized in urologic oncology was invited to attend the meeting. She had a long history of working with the group when there were difficult patient situations. She also was a former Head Nurse and her management experience was invaluable. She supported the need for a change.

The manager presented the idea of the need for a change and asked the group for suggestions. Ideas were voiced and were augmented by other members until the concept of an innovative nurse-managed clinic, where the bulk of the ninety patients would be seen on a single day, came about. Monday, the day of least patient activity in the clinic, was chosen. The entire concept was a direct result of seeking member involvement; the finalized idea was better than any *one* person's idea. Now that the basic concept of a nurse-managed clinic had been identified, it was time to address the nurses' concerns about this clinic. These fit into three main categories: adequate patient follow-up, decreased patient satisfaction, and the loss of the nurse-patient relationship. All these concerns involved giving up "control" of the patient care and trusting other staff to maintain the quality care each nurse gave. In the past, each nurse maintained her own case load and had direct control over her patient's care. Each nurse also enjoyed close interpersonal relationships with patients in her case load.

The group discussed the fact that adequate follow-up was crucial because if the patient missed a dose of his medication, the cancer could spread. Each nurse had previously used her own method of scheduling follow-up, and it became obvious that standardization was now essen-

tial. This was addressed by standardizing what was documented each visit, including follow-up appointments, by use of a rubber stamp.

Decreased patient satisfaction was another concern. It was evident that patients enjoyed having one nurse to call with questions and rapport had developed. This concern, however, also contained the fact that nurses might lose relationships with patients and their families that had developed. It was feared that patients would be deeply dissatisfied if they had a different nurse at each monthly visit—"After all, these *are cancer* patients and they have special needs." The group discussed these fears and agreed that, if at all possible, patients should have only two or three nurses that they see in hopes of maintaining rapport and trust. This concern was addressed by assigning each nurse a day of the week to see patients. Because the hormone injection was given every twenty-eight days, patients had the opportunity to schedule their visit on the same weekday each month. This compromise also allowed nurses to maintain some of her relationships with patients and their families.

Implementation took about six months. Nurses had to change their concept of patient care but so did the patients. It was each nurse's responsibility to discuss the new care management system with her case load and move the patient's appointments to Monday, the chosen day of the new clinic. Surprisingly, few patients resisted.

It is now three years since the change was instituted. It is safe to say that the change "has stuck." The

number of hormone therapy patients is now over 200 per month. The original clinic structure still remains with the largest number of patients being seen on Monday. A standardized documentation and assessment system has removed the concern of poor follow-up and standardized the tracking of worrisome patient systems.

Patients are more educated about their disease because the same assessment questions are asked each visit. Patients call with early changes in status, preventing permanent sequelae. Patients usually see one of three nurses when they come for the monthly visit. Some physicians have changed their follow-up of these patients from twice a year to once a year, evidencing their trust in the nursing staff's ability to assess patients and identify problems. A file card system has been implemented to give the nurse immediate access to patient symptoms and information when patients telephone and the patient record is not available. Patient satisfaction has been monitored in a quality assurance study with the result of 100% of patients being "satisfied" or "very satisfied" with their nursing care. This study is repeated bi-annually.

Involving members in change helps both members and management. Members benefit because they are involved in what affects their work. Management benefits because involvement tends to reduce resistance and increase ownership of the change.

LYNNE A. NEZBEDA, BSN, RN, CURN
Nurse Manager, Urology
Cleveland Clinic Foundation
Cleveland, Ohio

Disadvantages of Groups

Group decision making can be derailed at a number of points in the process. The three disadvantages commonly noted about group decision making are the potential for premature decisions, individual domination, and disruptive conflicts (Veninga, 1982).

Premature Decisions The disadvantages of group work include the fact that decisions can result from pressure. Once a majority vote is taken, there is an element of pressure on the minority as a result of psychological dynamics related to the pressures for group acceptance and conformity in groups. It may be difficult to be a "devil's advocate" or to adopt the role of bringing alternative critique points to the group for consideration because of a concern about being socially accepted. For example, derision and humiliation can occur if members react with strong negative opinions. This response will stifle further input.

Individual Domination Some of the disadvantages of groups relate to the possibility of dominating or argumentative members who obstruct the group process. They make it an unpleasant experience for all involved. In a sense, they sabotage the work of the group. If the group is not functioning well or the members will not adhere to the task of the group because of socializing, avoiding the task, or not preparing themselves, then it becomes costly and time consuming to work out interpersonal dynamics instead of progressing forward on the group's task.

Disruptive Conflicts When one position is felt to have an adverse effect on some group member or members, or if people feel threatened, conflicts usually emerge. Conflicts are accelerated in a competitive environment, as members vest in their own position. Conflicts may also occur over personality differences, differences of opinion, or clashes of values.

· · ·

Group work can be, and typically is, a very slow process. It takes more time for a group to arrive at a decision than if one person makes the decision. Sometimes there are strategic administrative decisions in which it is necessary that a problem not be solved too quickly. Perhaps it is known that legislation affecting nursing may change in the next six months, yet there is a related pressing problem needing group input. It would be counterproductive to reach a quick solution and then have to go back and re-do it. Perhaps there is no money to solve the problem, even though it is a pressing one. In these circumstances, a group may be asked to study the issue as a way of stalling for time.

Effective Meetings

Meetings are common occurrences. To maximize the benefits of a meeting, work should be done to structure the meeting for effectiveness. To manage effective meetings, meetings should be analyzed as to the purpose for which they are organized. There are several purposes for meetings (Jacobs & Rosenthal, 1984). First, there is the meeting held for *information dissemination*. For example, the designated leadership person calls the group together to let them know that a command has come down to cut the budget by ten percent due to fiscal retrenchment. A meeting is called to disseminate information about what is happening and provide time for questions and answers. Perhaps there has been an organizational change, such as the decision that one unit is going to be consolidating with another unit, or that a new building is being planned.

Second, there is the meeting held for the purpose of *opinion seeking*. The purpose of the meeting in this instance is open dialogue to solicit group opinions and ideas on specific topics or issues. This purpose does not imply that decision making is the prerogative of the group. Seeking opinions is an input strategy and may be used only for gathering data or testing group reactions. For example, an opinion seeking meeting may be called to invite input on equipment purchases for budget requests.

Third, there is the meeting held for the purpose of *problem solving*. The purpose of the meeting is to solicit help in clarifying, analyzing, and solving a specific problem. This type of meeting is more action oriented. Group participation in decision making is encouraged. For example, group problem solving or unit meetings may be called to discuss ways to solve problems related to disruptive or manipulative clients.

There are several team-related functions of group meetings that can contribute to effectiveness. For example, a meeting provides a structure to facilitate a sense of identity and to define a team. A meeting is a forum for updating shared knowledge among a team. A meeting reinforces the collective goals and objectives of the team. Further, a meeting can create a sense of commitment to group decisions. A meeting can be an opportunity for a manager to be perceived as a leader. However, a meeting will be a waste of time for all concerned unless there is a clear understanding of what the meeting is intended to achieve (Jay, 1982).

Beachy and Biester (1986) discussed restructuring meetings toward effective group management. As nursing department meetings became unmanageable, one organization developed a questionnaire to survey the group and evaluate the meetings. Aspects such as the cost/benefit ratio of attending meetings, group process, decision making, and relevancy of agenda items were examined for individual member's feelings about effectiveness. The group then discussed ideas for restructuring the meetings. Active participation was seen as being the essence of effective meetings. Certain elements of time management, group process, and decision making related to effectiveness in meetings (Beachy & Biester, 1986).

Jay (1982) outlined guidelines for conducting meetings. For example, in a meeting held to achieve specific objectives, each agenda item can be identified as being for information (example: progress reports), for development (example: new policy or strategy plan), for implementation (example: formulating a detailed action plan), or for change within the organization (example: changing documentation forms that multiple user groups use). Identifying on the agenda the category of each item helps to clarify and focus the group discussion.

The leader of the group can facilitate meeting effectiveness by preparing and dealing with both the task and the people involved. The leader needs to listen carefully, process the interactions, control the flow, and keep the meeting directed toward accomplishing the objectives. The ideal size of a group is four to seven people, with 12 being the outside limit (Jay, 1982). Members should be carefully selected for best input. The leader needs to start on time and be alert to seating positions. The leader can facilitate effectiveness by controlling the compulsive talkers, drawing out the silent members, protecting the junior members, encouraging the clash of ideas, discouraging the clash of personalities, avoiding the squashing of creative ideas, and closing on a note of achievement (Jay, 1982) (see Chart 8.2 for a checklist for leading effective meetings). Without thought and preparation, people go into a meeting with their own biases and perspectives; they may not be tuned in to how to be productive within a meeting. In a negative situation, do individuals choose to participate in a way that will assist or enhance the process by making constructive suggestions as to how it could be done better?

Group Decision Making

There is a continuum of decision making power that may be vested in a group (see Fig. 8.2). A committee will have certain powers, tasks, and functions, as well as certain parameters or latitude in terms of how far to go in making a decision. There are four different points on the continuum of authority for decision making.

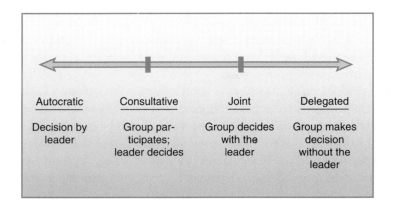

Figure 8.2
Range of decision powers.

On one end of the continuum is an *autocratic decision procedure* where the leader will make the decisions. There are no majority votes honored. There is input, perhaps, but not necessarily a vote. For example, in certain legislative committees the chairperson may or may not be able to put forth legislation or block a bill. It may be the case that there is an autocratic leader who controls the power, and the committee exists for the sake of appearance. This type of committee is set up for other reasons than making participative decisions.

A *consultative decision procedure* occurs when decisions involve subordinate participation, but the leader makes the final decision alone. Thus it is one step away from authoritarian or autocratic decision making. The subordinates may make certain decisions that must then go to the leader, chairperson, or head of the group, who makes the final decision. There is more participation with this procedure, but the ultimate decision is not under the control of the group members.

Some decision procedures result in *joint decision making*. In this procedure the entire group decides, whether by two-thirds vote or a simple majority. In a joint decision procedure, the subordinates have as much influence as the leader. The leader has one voice, one vote. The leader can use persuasion, but when it comes down to the final vote, the leader's vote is equivalent to any other member of the group. This is categorically different from the leader making the decision with group input.

Finally, on the far end of the decision continuum is the *delegated decision procedure*. This occurs when the committee chair or group head allows participants to make the decision. For example, in true self-scheduling, the leader may set up the basic patterns, but the staff actually decide what schedule they will work. The true test of a delegation decision procedure is if the committee head or group leader does not override the followers' decision. Technically, the leader would not have the authority to veto or override. If it is truly a delegation situation, the leader would go forward with the approach that is the choice of the group. The leader becomes the advocate and the spokesperson, but not the decision maker. Hersey & Blanchard (1993) labeled these same four decision procedures as authoritative, consultative, facilitative, and delegative decision making styles. They related the four decision making styles to their situational leadership theory.

When participating in groups, it is advisable for the followers to determine who has the authority to make decisions. Knowledge about what type of group it is and what delegation or decision procedures can be anticipated is critical to participation. Do not go into a group and assume that delegation is the decision procedure rule in effect. Anger is a byproduct of a committee that assumes that a delegated decision is theirs to make, yet the leader has a different idea.

Committees

An essential part of the staff nurse's role is to be involved in committee and group work. Work is accomplished through people, and the coordination of care is furthered through committee actions. Previously the nurse manager or the nursing administrator participated on most committees. This type of arrangement did not necessarily provide the highest quality input because the nurses at the caregiver level often are the people with reliable information about a given problem, especially regarding client care problems. With the changes in healthcare delivery, it is becoming essential that the staff participate in groups and committees. It also is important to the nurses' job satisfaction and autonomy to have an avenue of participation open in which to participate directly in the solving of problems.

Some people dislike committees because they dislike the time involved and because they are frustrated with the psychodynamics of group process and decision making. However, committees are a mainstay of organizations and can be an important way to make changes that are necessary in clinical practice. Developing the knowledge of committee workings should facilitate the process of being a more effective nurse.

DEFINITION

A *committee* is a relatively stable and formally composed group (see Chart 8.1). Committees are a subset of groups. They are a specific type of group in that they are stable, meet periodically, and have an identified purpose that is part of the organizational structure. There is a mechanism for maintaining and selecting members. Typically, committees have official status and sanction within an organization, for example, a policy committee or a quality assurance/improvement committee. There is some mechanism for recommending or implementing the group's decisions. Committee structures are preferable in two kinds of situations:

- when each member's input is needed in order to attain a certain goal. For example, a committee may be set up to implement self-scheduling or start a new program to benefit clients. If the work cannot be done alone, or there is a need to have everyone's agreement, then a committee is probably appropriate.
- situations in which diverse representation facilitates implementation of proposed activities. To have a diverse group of people provide input in order to get the job done, a committee should be created. For example, a multidisciplinary products committee could be established to develop a process in which there would be a review of products before a large amount of purchasing was done. This avoids the nurses at the bedside

finding themselves using products that are potentially unsafe, unusable, and thereby more costly.

Several types of committees are found in organizations. These include standing committees. Standing committees, as the name implies, are a constant, ongoing part of the organizational mission, performing critical and essential functions that must be done. For example, policy committees are standing committees because there always are policies to write and review. The same is true for quality assurance/improvement, because quality improvement activities will never be completed.

Contrasted to a standing committee is the task force, also called design groups or ad hoc committees. This is a committee that has developed in response to some emergent or immediate need. A need arises, a group is formed. A task force is not part of the organizational core mission. It is formed in response to a specific circumstance that arises or to study a specific problem. The committee is expected to disband when the issue is resolved. An example is a search committee to replace a clinical specialist.

There are some groups or committees that are organized based on organizational position or job position in an organized unit. For example, all of the nurse managers may belong to a group of nurse managers or a charge nurse council. Because of holding the position of nurse manager, the individual will belong to that committee.

There are multidisciplinary interdivisional committees. A multidisciplinary committee includes participants from several divisions or specialties. The participants may all be from within the institution or from both in and outside the facility. They often are used to coordinate and eliminate boundary conflicts. Some examples are a products committee, a risk management committee, or a medical liaison committee where there are nurses and physicians who work together collaborating to reduce interprofessional conflicts.

When asked to be on a committee as a unit representative, it is advisable to explore the nature and characteristics of the committee. Determine the powers that are delegated to this particular committee, remembering that this delegation may be formal or informal. Determine who is on the committee and whether you have a positive or negative relationship with the other members. Are the people on the committee highly motivated, are they task or relationship people, and what might be the committee politics? Determine the feedback mechanisms and the committee's productivity. What kind of track record does this committee have? Have they done anything in the last year besides meet? Or are they a dynamic committee that is productive? The characteristics are important for the nurse to understand before beginning to participate. Preparation for followership enhances personal and committee productivity.

LEADERSHIP AND MANAGEMENT IMPLICATIONS

The Leader's Function

The leadership and management role in groups and committees includes inspiring members to participate, preparing critical questions, developing agendas and background materials, and guiding the long-range strategy. Leaders and managers address questions such as what is the task, how will this task be accomplished, how many meetings will it take, how much effort has to go into it, how can the tasks be divided up, and how can they be delegated? This is a planning, coordinative, and tracking function. A good leader puts in the time and effort to get all the members prepared, so that when they come to the meeting they know what the issues are and are familiar with the background of the task to be accomplished. The leader facilitates the group coming to some agreement about rules for decision making, length of discussion, when to vote, and the process through which the task is completed efficiently and effectively. Nurses may find that the group leader role challenges them to plan, organize, coordinate, and evaluate the work of the group.

The duties of chairperson include preparation of the physical environment. Comfort and convenience engineering is part of the leader's responsibility in terms of preparing an environment that is conducive to people being satisfied, productive, positive, and working together. The worst case situation occurs when members have to sit in an uncomfortable chair in a room that is too cold, too hot, or too noisy because of construction; when members cannot hear or talk to other people; or when the technology does not work. Consider

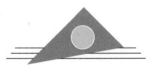 *Leadership & Management Behaviors*

LEADERSHIP BEHAVIORS

- enables group members to participate
- communicates enthusiasm and vision of group goals
- motivates followers to accomplish group goals
- models constructive group participation
- inspires team collaboration
- facilitates constructive group roles
- monitors group process

MANAGEMENT BEHAVIORS

- plans committee agenda and task accomplishment
- organizes a team
- delegates group work and assigns tasks
- arranges support services
- communicates through reporting structure
- handles conflict situations

OVERLAP AREAS

- communicates to further the group's productivity
- monitors the group's movement toward goal accomplishment

how to facilitate group work through host/hostessing functions related to breaks, food, and fluids. It is human nature for members to be more relaxed and productive in comfortable surroundings.

A leader has a responsibility to prepare and motivate participants. The participants' responsibility is to read and be prepared, show up on time, and attend to the task at hand. As a leader, prepare an agenda with handouts and background materials, and distribute this to the members with enough time to read it. The better prepared the members are, the more they can participate, increase the quality of decisions, and be more effective.

The leader's preparation activities include reviewing the status of agenda topics as part of preparing the agenda. Questions to ask include:
- Where are we?
- What else needs to be done?
- What supporting materials might help the committee?
- Who should be invited?

A leader who comes to the meeting and distributes a handout for a quick look before a vote violates the participants' ability to think through what is being presented. This may be done as a tactic to avoid thorough deliberation by pressuring for the immediacy of a vote, but more often this behavior results from disorganization or lack of attention to leader responsibilities.

Constructive Group Members

Lancaster (1981) identified both group building roles and group maintenance roles. Group *building* roles include initiator, encourager, opinion giver, clarifier, listener, and summarizer. Group *maintenance* roles include tension reliever, compromiser, gate keeper, and harmonizer. The group building roles concentrate on relationship functions more than task functions; the group maintenance roles focus more on task functions than relationship functions.

One positive way to handle meetings is to identify, utilize, and structure in a facilitator. Ideally this should be the group leader. A facilitator conducts the meeting ensuring that everyone has the opportunity to speak, maintains the focus of the meeting, and controls the problem participants.

Also needed is a group recorder. The task of taking minutes may need to be delegated to a clerical support person (if possible) if group members are adverse to taking on the task of recording outcomes. However, a recorder who is a group member technically should do more than just take minutes. They should be in tune to the group processing and to the inputs and roles of group members and help keep the group on time. The recorder can provide feedback to the facilitator in terms of how to improve the process.

Finally, group members are needed. Group members in this instance means active participants, each with an equal status in the meeting. The three components of a facilitator, a recorder, and group members contribute to the design of a positive working group.

Disruptive Group Members

Another role that the group leader must assume is that of process controller. The leader must be observant about group member actions and be prepared to control or redirect disruptive behaviors. Following are the types of disruptive group members encountered (Jacobs & Rosenthal, 1984):

Compulsive Talkers   The leader needs to identify individuals who are compulsive talkers and consider how they can be constrained. One suggestion is to thank them for their input and then ask to hear from others on that same topic before they speak again, as a way of guiding and opening up the meeting to be more effective.

Non-talkers   The nontalkers are the quiet ones. The leader can ask them to write down and submit their ideas, or ask to hear their thoughts on the matter at hand. The leader can specifically ask them questions to draw them out and thereby open up a broader range of group input.

Interrupters   The leader has to control the interrupter because the interrupter is demonstrating a lack of self-control. The interrupter can be a problem in groups because the person who is interrupted feels violated and wonders why they are not given the courtesy of finishing a thought and having their full input considered. The leader needs to control and redirect the interrupter.

Squashers   These people try to squash an idea before it is even developed. Suggestions about processes or procedures that have not been proven or even tried are much easier to criticize than are facts or opinions. Persons who are adverse to change may have a litany of reasons as to why a potential solution would never work or why this proposed project simply cannot or should not happen. These are people who do not want to take a personal risk or undergo the personal effort of making a change, so it is easier to squash everything to maintain the status quo. Especially during brainstorming sessions, the leader has to be alert to and have a method for containing the squasher. The leader may choose to handle the negative input for a certain amount of time and then move the group beyond it. One method to move the group is to direct an equal amount of time to exploring the positive benefits and potentials of the proposal.

Busy Bodies   These are people who really are not committed to the group's work. They frequently arrive late, leave early, take personal messages during the meeting, never read the agenda, are passive-aggressive, and simply want to show up for a few minutes for the purpose of appearances but not contribute any effort. They are meeting their needs by showing up, but they are not contributing to the ongoing group work or the task at hand. The leader needs to find creative mechanisms to engage the busy bodies, perhaps by giving them a concrete assignment with accountability. They may need to be released from the group or placed in an advisory role.

•   •   •

Thus the nurse leader can take an active role in structuring group work for positive processing and effective outcomes. One way is to control the flow to modulate disruptive group members without humiliating them. Another way is to structure in positive and constructive group roles among members. The leader's vision, enthusiasm, interpersonal relationship skills, and empowerment of followers all facilitate group effectiveness.

RESEARCH NOTE

Source: Jensen, D. (1993). Interpretation of group behavior. *Nursing Management, 24*(3), 49-54.

Purpose

The purpose of this case study was to assist one group to overcome the frustration that was generated by ineffective behavior and to provide a clear visual diagram of group and leader behavior. Eight group members completed the Systematic Multiple Level Observation of Groups (SYMLOG) questionnaire, which contains 26 items and factors into the three bipolar dimensions of influence (up or down and active or passive) social distance (positive or negative and friendly to unfriendly) and control (forward or backward and controlling to noncontributing). The setting for this case study was one metropolitan community center agency serving homeless street people.

Discussion

Using the SYMLOG instrument, group members and the leader rated themselves and the other group members. The results were plotted on an x-y axis field diagram that combined all of the interactions. The result was a visual diagram clearly depicting the perceived behaviors of individual members and of the group as a unit. The diagrams present how the group was working at one specific point in time. The group perceived the leader as passive, negative, and backward; the opposite of a goal-directed group leader. The group itself was the opposite of a positive, forward, task-oriented group.

Application to Practice

The SYMLOG instrument can be used to plot a visual diagram of group behavior in three dimensions: influence, social distance, and control. Leaders may be surprised to discover how group members perceive their behavior and how they "come across" to others. This tool provides feedback and awareness of the perceptions of behavior as a first step for change. If leaders deny ineffective behaviors, change is very difficult. Leader behavior problems ideally should be identified before followers exhibit signs of stress.

Work Teams

Team building is defined as the process of deliberately creating and unifying a group into a functioning work unit so that specific goals are accomplished (Farley & Stoner, 1989) (see Chart 8.1). A team was defined by Katzenbach and Smith (1993, p. 45) as "a small number of people with complimentary skills who are committed to a common purpose, performance goals, and approach for which they hold themselves mutually accountable." The complementary skills that are needed, in the right mix, to do the team's task fall into three categories: technical or functional expertise, problem solving and decision making skills, and interpersonal skills. To assess and strengthen team performance, Katzenbach and Smith recommended an analysis of each of their six basic elements of teams: small in number, adequate levels of complementary skills, a truly meaningful purpose, specific goal(s), clear working approach, and sense of mutual accountability (see Chart 8.3). Katzenbach and Smith plotted five discrete points along a team performance curve: a working group where there is no incentive to form a team, a pseudo-team that has no common purpose or set of goals, a potential team where significant incremental performance is needed, a real team that fits their definition, and a high-performance team that outperforms other teams and has members deeply committed to each other's growth and success. The greater the performance, the greater the advantage to the group and the organization.

Sovie (1992) noted that care and service teams are the new imperative in healthcare, as a matter of survival. High performance teams are essential to an organization's efficiency and effectiveness. Previously, teamwork was not an explicit performance expectation or organizational value. However, it seems clear now that collaboration and teamwork are essential to achieving quality of work outcomes and cost control in client care.

Performance in teams is linked to productivity, but the direct applicability to the delivery of nursing care remains an issue (Sheafor, 1991). Schmeiding's (1990) research indicated that many staff nurses may prefer dependence on their hierarchical superiors. Clearly, some nurses are not motivated, prepared, or inclined to assume a high level of personal responsibility for decision making in client care coordination and work group administration. This has implications for leadership and management of professional nurses and for decentralization and shared governance.

Nurse leaders need to learn how to manage in a team-centered environment; staff nurses need to learn how to be effective team players (Sovie, 1992). Interactive leadership is needed to create a group identity. Participatory management; sharing power and information; and generating trust, mutual respect, and enhanced self-worth are seen as key elements in successful performance teams. Teamwork begins with members who are well prepared and personally competent. Teamwork then includes shared ownership and decision making (Sovie, 1992). Nurses may begin with experiences on client

CHART 8.3
↩ TEAM PERFORMANCE CHECKLIST

- Small in number
- Adequate levels of skills
- Meaningful purpose
- Specific goal(s)
- Clear working approach
- Sense of mutual accountability

Data from Katzenbach and Smith (1993).

care teams and then be exposed to executive interdisciplinary teams (Farley & Stoner, 1989).

Group process is a framework to understand team development (Farley & Stoner, 1989). Sovie (1992) identified four essential components of high-performing teams: roles, activities, relationships, and the environment. This means that teams will need to incorporate positive roles among the members. They will need to be able to focus their activities toward productivity. Their relationships need to become cohesive. The team needs a facilitative and supportive environment in which to work through the task and relationship elements. Management of team building and team performance includes skill in the process of conflict management. Diverse backgrounds and varying views result in the potential for differences, conflicts, turf battles, and office politics. The leader's repertoire will include strategies of conflict resolution, empowerment, collaboration, and coordination. Sovie (1992, p. 97) called the manager "a gatekeeper at the critical boundary of team and organization" who has to keep communication, objectives, and needs flowing both ways. Diplomacy, negotiation, and power-based strategies or alliances may be employed in team building (Farley & Stoner, 1989). For further discussion of work teams see Chapters 12 and 18.

CURRENT ISSUES AND TRENDS

Groups and committees are used as a vehicle to promote innovation and change in organizations. One example in nursing is the institution of research-based nursing practice by using a planned change process and a research utilization committee to facilitate the process of research utilization in nursing (Horn Video Productions, 1989). Groups and committees take advantage of several creativity techniques in order to heighten both the content and process of group work. Since perceptions and biases may cloud individuals' ability to generate creative ideas or solutions, the techniques of brainstorming, Delphi survey, or nominal group technique (NGT) can be employed (Van de Ven & Delbecq, 1974). Brainstorming is the encouragement of the generation of large numbers of diverse ideas, free from critique or labeling in regard to practicality or feasibility. A Delphi survey technique employs sequential rounds of questionnaires to collect the judgment and opinions of experts on a topic. It often is used for prioritization purposes. The NGT (Van de Ven & Delbecq, 1974) avoids social exchange contamination by following a process of silently gathering ideas in writing, round-robin feedback from group members to identify ideas, clarifying and evaluating each identified idea, and individually voting on priority ideas. The group decision is derived mathematically.

An example of a nationwide group approach to problem solving in nursing is the American Nurses Association's Tri-Council. For a long time one of the problems of organized nursing has been the fact that nurses have not spoken with one unified voice. Despite there being over 2 million people in this country licensed as registered nurses, nursing had not unified to speak on issues of healthcare policy, acquiring resources for nursing, or responding to the larger profession's needs and directions. There are four core groups that comprise the Tri-Council: the American Nurses Association (ANA), the National League for Nursing (NLN), the American Organization of Nurse Executives (AONE), and the American Association of Colleges of Nursing (AACN).

There also is an organization of specialty groups in nursing called the Nursing Organizations Liaison Forum (NOLF). These groups coalesced around the issue of registered care technologists (RCTs), a proposal put forth a number of years ago by the American Medical Association (AMA) to solve nursing's shortage problems. The AMA proposed to start RCT programs to train ancillary workers licensed by medicine, but overseen by nurses, to take care of medical orders. Organized nursing's responses included the Tri-Council's strategies to address the nursing shortage. This was an example of groups working together. The Tri-Council is a group of groups in which representatives of large nursing organizations link together to tackle some national professional problems. It is a good example of how the group process can be used positively and constructively, and how much clout can be generated by working together and speaking in unity.

Another example of groups and committees is total quality management (TQM) programs. Continuous quality improvement (CQI) methods such as TQM are gaining momentum as methods for addressing problems in hospitals related to cost and quality (Sovie, 1992). To restructure or reconfigure the work so that it is less costly and produces a higher quality service is the goal (see also Chapter 25).

Total quality management is a concept that comes from the work of Deming (Aguayo, 1990; Darr, 1989). Deming was an industrial psychologist who was hired by Japan after World War II to make Japan a major economic force. For years he was ignored in the United States. His ideas emphasized moving decision making to the worker level. The worker who is closest to actually producing the work is the one with the greatest knowledge and the greatest potential for solving production problems. Deming further recommended work group problem solving teams. Problems, in Deming's methodology, are defined as systems problems. By contrast, a common way of thinking about problems is to look for an individual to blame. The result of systems thinking is to capture the energy of teams to tackle systems problems.

With Continuous Quality Improvement (CQI) and TQM, changes are occurring in healthcare organizations such that staff nurses are being asked to participate more on multidisciplinary teams. In an organization that looks at problems as systems problems, the next step is to acknowledge that anyone involved in that part of the system is involved in solving the problem. The TQM method is a way of coordinating client care and solving problems through interdisciplinary committees and groups with people of equal status. Nurses find these practices revolutionary when they actually are put into place because few nurses have experienced being on a committee in which they are truly co-equal in terms of status and role with a physician or hospital administrator. Thus it is important for nurses to be prepared for multidisciplinary group or team work and to be skilled in team participation and leadership.

The strategy behind TQM is to bring together interdisciplinary collaborative groups. This means that if there is a problem in client care, the physicians, nurses, ancillary staff, and any other direct caregivers are involved. They get together and collaborate about problems with the client care delivery system and how these problems can be fixed. The person with the most expertise in that problem area is the person who takes the leadership role. To establish co-equal peers regardless of status and to utilize expertise and responsibility is a very different way of looking at work that has implications in terms of how nursing practice may change. It also means nurses are going to be involved more substantially in groups, committees, and teams. See Chapter 18 for further information on work teams and Chapter 25 for further discussion of TQM and CQI.

SUMMARY

- Nurses are involved in groups.
- Group interactions are composed of process, standards, problem solving, communication, and roles.
- Groups tend to go through a series of stages.
- People join groups to fulfill primary needs and psychological drives.
- There are both advantages and disadvantages to the use of groups in organizations.
- Meetings can be structured for effective group participation.
- The purpose of a group meeting may be for information dissemination, opinion seeking, or problem solving.
- Decision making power in groups is delegated along a continuum from none to all.
- A group may be formally structured into a committee, or a relatively stable group, to accomplish an organizational goal.
- The committee leader has certain tasks and responsibilities to perform in managing the group toward productivity.
- One leadership role is to control disruptive group members.
- Group participation probably will be an increasingly large part of the nurse's role in practice due to team building strategies and the devel-

opment of multidisciplinary work groups in complex organizational structures.

Study Questions

1. Does nursing need to be structured into work groups for effective client care delivery?
2. What motivates an individual to join a group?
3. What are the significantly different elements between social groups and organizational groups? What elements are similar?
4. How is leading a group like the nursing process? The management process?
5. What team building strategies are used in nursing? How can this process be improved?

Critical Thinking Exercise

Organize into a small group. The group is to select a leader for the group. Take a few minutes to do this, then a process recorder is to be selected or appointed. The leader's role is that of a Head Nurse/Nurse Manager at Our Lady of Sorrow Community Hospital. The leader has just been informed that (s)he must cut two nurse jobs immediately. This will be part of an immediate RIF (reduction in force) at the hospital to meet some very serious financial reversals. In order to accomplish the task the leader has called together your group (the nurses of the unit). The leader has the task of deciding how to cut the nursing personnel budget and must now lead your group to develop a plan while preserving a sense of teamwork. The process recorder is to prepare a summary of the group's work and report as requested.

1. *Observe the process the group uses to select its own leader. Did everyone try to avoid selection? Was someone an enthusiastic volunteer? How long did it take?*

2. *What method was used to select/appoint a process recorder? What power strategy was used to make this decision?*

3. *What is the problem identified in the task?*

4. *What did the group leader do to handle the situation?*

5. *What should the group leader do to handle the situation?*

6. *How did group members respond to the task?*

7. *What leadership and management strategies might be effective?*

8. *What could the leader and followers consider changing in the situation?*

9. *How did group members feel about what happened?*

REFERENCES

Aguayo, R. (1990). *Dr. Deming: The American who taught the Japanese about quality*. New York: Carol Publishing Group.

Beachy, P., & Biester, D. (1986). Restructuring group meetings for effectiveness. *Journal of Nursing Administration, 16*(12), 30-33.

Book, C., & Galvin, K. (1975). *Instruction in and about small group discussion*. Falls Church, VA: Speech Communication Association.

Darr, K. (1989). Applying the Deming method in hospitals: Part I. *Hospital Topics, 67*(6), 4-5.

Farley, M., & Stoner, M. (1989). The nurse executive and interdisciplinary team building. *Nursing Administration Quarterly, 13*(2), 24-30.

Hersey, P., & Blanchard, K. (1993). *Management of organizational behavior: Utilizing human resources* (6th ed.). Englewood Cliffs, NJ: Prentice-Hall.

Horn Video Productions. (1989). *Research utilization: A process of organizational change*. [Videotape] Ida Grove, IA: Horn Video Productions.

Jacobs, B., & Rosenthal, T. (1984). Managing effective meetings. *Nursing Economic$, 2*(2), 137-141.

Jay, A. (1982). How to run a meeting. *Journal of Nursing Administration, 12*(1), 22-28.

Katzenbach, J., & Smith, D. (1993). *The wisdom of teams: Creating the high-performance organization*. New York: Harper Collins.

Lancaster, J. (1981). Making the most of meetings. *Journal of Nursing Administration, 11*(10), 15-19.

Schmeiding, N. (1990). A model for assessing nurse administrators' actions. *Western Journal of Nursing Research, 12*(3), 293-306.

Sheafor, M. (1991). Productive work groups in complex hospital units: Proposed contributions of the nurse executive. *Journal of Nursing Administration, 21*(5), 25-30.

Sovie, M. (1992). Care and service teams: A new imperative. *Nursing Economic$, 10*(2), 94-100.

Van de Ven, A., & Delbecq, A. (1974). The effectiveness of nominal, Delphi, and interacting group decision making processes. *Academy of Management Journal, 17*(4), 605-621.

Veninga, R. (1982). *The human side of health administration: A guide for hospital, nursing, and public health administrators*. Englewood Cliffs, NJ: Prentice-Hall.

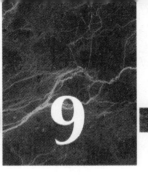

9

Budgeting and Financial Management

Chapter Objectives

∾

define and describe financial management

∾

define and describe a budget

∾

identify three general types of budgets

∾

distinguish between direct and indirect costs

∾

define and differentiate a performance budget from a traditional budget

∾

compare the stages of a typical budgetary process

∾

analyze cost awareness as related to nurse decision making

∾

analyze ethical and legal financial management considerations

∾

explain costing out nursing services

∾

exercise critical thinking to conceptualize and analyze
possible solutions to a practical experience incident

*b*udgeting and financial management concepts are important and under-
emphasized in nursing practice. For a long time nursing has focused its
attention on clinical client care. Yet at all levels of care, the allocation of

scarce resources is an important client care consideration. Nurses carry a major role in the implementation-level decisions about care provision and supplies and equipment usage that carry financial ramifications. Nurses evaluate equipment for purchase and use. Nurses comprise a major element of the personnel budget of a healthcare facility. A basic working familiarity with budgeting and financial management concepts can help nurses make better decisions, communicate with financial management staff, and lobby for scarce resource allocation for nursing.

The management of client care involves a focus on clinical care delivery, quality of care, human resources management, and financial management. Budgeting and financial management are focused on money as a strategic resource. The control over money significantly impacts on the control over nursing practice and nursing care delivery by posing opportunities and constraints. As nurses carry responsibility and accountability for care management, program management, and service delivery, they will need concurrent expertise in and control over budgeting decisions and fiscal management.

DEFINITION

inancial management is defined as a series of activities designed to allocate resources and plan for the efficient operation of an organization (see Chart 9.1). Financial management occurs in four phases: budgeting, recording, reporting, and evaluating. The overall goal of financial management is to meet the total financial needs of an organization (Johnson & Carpenter, 1990). The two major financial statements for the overall organization are the balance sheet and a statement of revenues and expenses (nonprofit organization) or an income statement of profit and loss (for profit organizations). Both are used to understand and analyze the organization's financial status. Operational decisions follow, as do reports to controlling or interested bodies such as Boards of Directors or Trustees, banks, investors, and the Internal Revenue Service (IRS) (DeBoer, 1990).

There is uncertainty and risk associated with cash flow and other forces that impact on the ability to meet the organization's financial needs. Thus the managerial process of planning is linked closely with financial management. Operational plans, or programs and plans for the day-to-day provision of services, are based on an assessment of the organization and its environment. Then a plan for the future provision of services and long-range survival is derived. *Strategic planning* is a process of assessing the organization and its departments or divisions. Strengths and weaknesses are explored and analyzed. Opportunities and external threats are identified and critiqued. External forces are considered and their impacts are projected in relationship to the organization. A strategic plan results in strategy formulation. For example, a

---

CHART 9.1
⌇ DEFINITIONS

Financial Management
a series of activities designed to allocate resources and plan for the efficient operation of an organization.

Strategic Planning
a process of assessing an organization and its departments or divisions.

Budget
a written financial plan aimed at controlling the allocation of resources.

Expenses
the costs of activities undertaken in an organization's operations.

Revenues
income or amounts owed for purchased services or goods.

Capital Budget
tracks purchases of capital assets (i.e. buildings, land, and equipment).

Cash Budget
tracks cash receipts and cash disbursements.

Expense Budget
tracks expenditure of resources or costs paid (i.e. wages, benefits, and maintenance costs.

Data from Finkler and Kovner (1993); Johnson and Carpenter (1990).

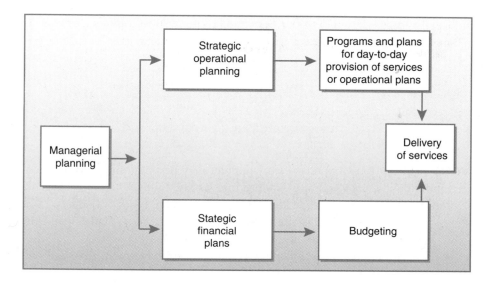

Figure 9.1
Process of managerial and strategic planning.

hospital may need to consider falling occupancy/census trends. Rural hospitals may need an analysis of reimbursement and cost structures. A community health agency may need to plan for shifts in federal health policy such as Medicare waivers that would threaten their core service delivery (Johnson & Carpenter, 1990; Smith, Mahon, & Piland, 1993).

Budgeting is the planning function of financial management. The budget translates operational plans into monetary terms. Strategic and operational plans are implemented by and through people. Budgets become devices for benchmarking performance and outcomes and for controlling actions (Johnson & Carpenter, 1990) (see Fig. 9.1).

A *budget* is a written financial plan aimed at controlling the allocation of resources (see Chart 9.1). A budget is both a planning and an evaluation tool useful for financial management. It is used to manage programs, plan for goal accomplishment, and control costs. Goldsmith (1981) defined a budget as a statement of expected expenses and revenues over a specific period of time. *Expenses* are defined as the costs or prices of activities undertaken in the organization's operations. *Revenues* are defined as income or amounts owed for purchased services or goods. Total operating expenses are the result of summing the costs of all resources used to produce services. Total operating revenues are the result of multiplying the services provided by the charges for the services. Income is the excess of revenues over expenses, or revenues minus expenses, for a given time (Johnson & Carpenter, 1990) (see Chart 9.2). A budget becomes a financial timetable and plan for the organization, which is translated into monetary terms. However, an alternative viewpoint sees a budget as a political document that results from a complicated bargaining process. The output is a financial document, although the budgetary process varies

Chart 9.2 ∾ CALCULATING TOTAL OPERATING EXPENSES, REVENUES, INCOME

Total Operating Expenses = Cost of Resources (1) + Cost of Resources (2) + . . .

$$\text{Total Operating Revenues} = \frac{\text{Service Provided (1)}}{\text{X Charge}} + \frac{\text{Service Provided (2)}}{\text{X Charge}} + \ldots$$

Income = Revenues – Expenses

among organizations. Expenses, for example, may be program-based or itemized individually, on a separate expense line, as line items.

Finkler and Kovner (1993) identified seven general types of budgets:

- The *operating budget* is the plan for the organization's daily operating revenues and expenses and usually applies to a single year.
- A *long-range budget* is a plan, often called a strategic plan, that looks at goals and purposes over a span of three, five, and sometimes ten years.
- A *program budget* analyzes a specific program, one that is planned for the future or one that is in existence and requires evaluation; a program budget often cuts across departments and across years.
- The *capital budget* tracks the acquisition of capital assets, or long-term investments, such as buildings, land, or equipment—things that provide useful service beyond the year they are first acquired or put in use.
- *Product-line budgets*, a recent development in response to the institution of diagnosis-related groups (DRGs) and pressure from health maintenance organizations (HMOs) and preferred provider organizations (PPOs), look at the revenues and expenses associated with a defined group of patients, such as those with a common diagnosis.
- The *cash budget* tracks the monthly cash receipts and cash disbursements.
- A *special purpose budget* is prepared for a program or activity that was not previously planned or budgeted.

For nurses, the primary budgets related directly to the delivery of nursing services are the capital budget and the operating budget. The capital budget is the budget plan specific to major purchases meeting or exceeding the organization's specific definition of a capital expense. The operating budget covers a specific period, called a fiscal year, and is the budget plan for day-to-day service delivery operations. It includes historical or trend data, expenses, and revenues. It may be subdivided, for example, into salaries and nonsalary expenses (Smith, 1988). Another component of the expense budget is the personnel or salary budget, a major focus of effort and energy in nursing financial management.

Nurses primarily are concerned with direct, indirect, and supply costs. Direct costs include elements like nursing time. Johnson (1989) defined *direct costs* as all costs that can be traced to a specific unit or activity. Direct costs have been described as "hands on" costs (McCloskey, 1989). Direct costs may be computed as the amount of time spent with the client times a salary and fringe benefit factor.

Johnson (1989) defined *indirect costs* as all costs that cannot be directly traced to one unit or client. Indirect costs have been described as "other" costs (McCloskey, 1989). Indirect costs may be computed to include all of the overhead costs, for example, lights, administrative costs, building maintenance, and books and supplies used by the staff.

In a review of 73 studies on costing out nursing services, Eckhart (1993) found that there was no consistency in the definitions of direct and indirect nursing costs. Authors frequently did not clearly define the activities being included in direct nursing care. For example, the placement of overtime, orientation, education, and nursing administration costs varied among methods of calculation. Eckhart's recommended standardized definition for direct nursing care is the hourly wages for only the personnel providing "hands on" patient care. Indirect costs should be a constant value generated specifically for each facility and include all supportive services required to provide direct nursing care. Total nursing costs include both direct and indirect nursing costs. Eckhart's opinion is that overhead, housekeeping, and dietary costs are not nursing costs. Therefore they should not be figured in nursing expenses. Thus a standardized definition of nursing costs is needed and would aid in calculation of costs.

Taking a cost accounting perspective, Jones (1994, p. 4) defined direct costs as "those costs that can be identified with the production of a specific product or service." This would include all costs traced directly to the objective of delivering care to clients. Thus salaries, supplies, and pharmaceuticals would be considered direct costs. She defined indirect costs as (1994, p. 4) "costs that cannot be traced to a specific cost objective." Indirect costs include costs allocated from support services (e.g. housekeeping, dietary) and general hospital overhead (e.g. utility costs, insurance, and administrative salaries). Full costs mean direct plus allocated indirect costs. Full costs are used in setting rates and negotiating with third-party reimbursers. Jones noted that the nurse manager's two major issues in relation to indirect and overhead costs are accuracy and control. Accuracy relates to whether specific costs included in the total amount of indirect costs may actually belong to specific services or departments. Thus the indirect costs figure may be inaccurate. The control issue relates to the nurse's ability to control the total unit budget while being given the responsibility to meet cost control goals. Parts of the budget, such as indirect costs, may not be under the nurse's control. Thus nurses need to be alert to whether the aspect of the budget they do not control is expanding faster than the aspects under their direct control. If the aspects they do not control are expanding rapidly, then those areas need to be uniquely identified and strategies employed for specific cost control in the targeted areas.

The nurse needs accurate information about how costs are allocated and what specific costs go into their own budgets. One piece that often is missing is accurate and reliable data. Lack of standard definitions robs nurses of reliable data for cost comparisons. Yet data form the basis of many management decisions. The data need to be accurate and reliable and attached to the costs incurred in the delivery of care to a specific client.

One factor to take into account when estimating costs and budgets is how intensely a client absorbed nursing time. This factor is called intensity. For example, there is a difference in the intensity of direct care between a client who is comatose and one who is ambulatory. Consequently the direct cost generated by the client should be greater for a comatose or highly dependent client (see Chapter 23 for more on intensity).

Johnson (1989) noted that the allocation of supply costs is not standardized. Supplies and equipment sometimes are apportioned directly. For example, for each time a specific piece of equipment, topper sponge, alcohol swab, catheter, or a piece of IV tubing is used, it is attributed to an individual client. Sometimes the supplies and equipment are rolled directly into the client's charges. Sometimes they are considered to be general supplies. Many times small incidentals like alcohol swabs, topper sponges, and tape are the kinds of general supplies for which there would be a unit budget and each client would be charged a certain flat percentage of the total yearly budget, which is broken down and divided by the number of clients as an overhead cost. The nurse needs to know how the organization allocates supply costs in order to be able to make budgetary and financial management decisions.

RESEARCH NOTE

Source: Varricchio, C. (1994). Human and indirect costs of home care. *Nursing Outlook*, 42(4), 151-157.

Purpose

The purpose of this article was to explore what is known about the human and indirect costs associated with home care for cancer clients. The outcome was to formulate questions for further research on the effects of these costs on clients and caregivers. Human costs are psychosocial, physical, and health burdens for clients, caregivers, and families. Indirect costs are financial expenses of providing care at home and not calculated in insurance reimbursement, but paid out of pocket. Both the type and source of care needed directly influence quality of life, burdens, and costs.

Discussion

The author reviewed and analyzed literature that addressed sources of human and indirect costs in home care of clients with cancer. Variables contributing to these costs were isolated and analyzed. The type and source of care needs clustered into four areas: diagnostic or assessment, psychosocial, teaching, and physical functional limitations. Care needs related to formal medical care, formal nonmedical care, and informal care needs. Cancer is described as an expensive illness. Beyond direct costs, there are indirect costs related to psychological and health-related burdens. The costs are borne by caregivers, families, and spouses.

Application to Practice

One aspect of public healthcare policy is the availability, costs, and access to home healthcare services. Costs and quality outcomes of home care are influenced by acuity of medical status, support given to caretaker, the individual situation, and the resources needed for the caregiver to provide care. Among the important questions for further research are, when is home care appropriate, what resources are needed, and what are the real and hidden costs?

BACKGROUND

Nursing comprises the single largest expense in most healthcare organizations (Smeltzer & Hyland, 1989). This occurs because nursing comprises a large personnel component and controls a large share of supplies and equipment. As healthcare generally faces strict fiscal constraints, both staff nurses and nurse managers will need to have knowledge and skill in anticipating financial fluctuations and trends and in making bold decisions based upon rapid management information. Staff nurses primarily will be handling day-to-day financial and budgetary decisions. Nurse managers are more involved with strategic or long-range financial planning and decision making.

Strategic financial planning in nursing includes immediate cost control measures, clinical manager accountability, a method for budget preparation, and inservice or staff development programs to update clinical managers' financial skills (Smeltzer & Hyland, 1989). Further, there appears to be a relationship between strategic planning in the nursing department and financial outcomes such as net income and operating margin in rural hospitals. Managerial strategies, strategic planning, and cost containment efforts add value to and affect financial performance. Thus nursing services are strategically critical to hospitals (Smith, Mahon, & Piland, 1993). Demonstration of these effects strengthens nursing's position in any complex bargaining over scarce resources.

Healthcare Financial Strategies

Goldsmith (1981) described four elements of healthcare finance: taxes, philanthropy, operating finances, and capital financing. Operating finances include revenues and expenses. Healthcare organizations face special issues related to the cost of regulation; cost containment, avoidance, and reduction; and how to allocate costs in order to maximize reimbursement.

Cost containment, avoidance, and reduction strategies are employed to prevent further escalation in the overall costs of healthcare. Goldsmith (1981) noted that typical problems faced by healthcare organizations include cash shortages, overstaffing, poor utilization of present staff, low productivity, and equipment breakdowns. Strategies employed to tackle these problems include paperwork improvements, productivity enhancements, scheduling alternatives, and training. Organizations also focus on better planning, coordination of personnel actions, and developing and maintaining standardized systems and processes. The budgetary process is one system for planning and controlling resource allocation.

The Budgetary Process

Each institution will establish standard budgetary formats and processes. Three basic types of budget formats are traditional, zero-based, and performance.

Traditional budgets identify expenses to be tracked. In nursing, the most common expense items are salaries, benefits, supplies, and equipment. A major nursing expense clearly goes for salaries; they are estimated to be 40% to 70% of the budget by Goldsmith (1981) and 90% of the budget in most nursing departments by Smeltzer and Hyland (1989). Other expenses include overhead, administrative, and educational costs.

Zero-based budgeting is a form of budgeting where the entire budget is rebuilt from zero each year or each budget cycle. The traditional approach takes the previous year's budget as the status quo and builds up from there. With zero-based budgeting, all expenses are rejustified each year. This challenges thinking and forces justification, but has the disadvantage of requiring a considerable amount of work (Goldsmith, 1981). Zero-based budgeting emphasizes the consideration of alternative means of providing the same service or program. It provides a method for a sophisticated analysis of these alternatives (Finkler & Kovner, 1993).

Finkler (1991) defined a *performance budget* as a budget for the activities of a cost center. Traditional budgets focus on the objects of spending, such as salaries, supplies, or equipment costs. A performance budget is focused on the activities of the unit, such as direct care, indirect care, or quality improvement activities. Performance budgeting incorporates specific objectives and the financial resources associated with each activity. The result is to quantify the financial impact of many activities and, thereby, make an assessment of resource investment.

A typical budgetary process follows four distinct stages (Goldsmith, 1981):
1. dissemination of instructions
2. preparation of the first budget draft
3. review and adjustment
4. appeal

It is at stage 3, review and adjustment, that the art of negotiation is employed. At the top levels of management budgetary requests are collated, thinned, and coordinated. In many organizations the final budget must be approved by the governing board or Board of Directors. Therefore, a strong defense for any item or program may need to be prepared.

Nurse managers may find that budgeting involves the utilization of multiple separate financial forms. These include:

- the cash budget
- the general expense (operating) budget
- the labor or personnel budget
- the capital equipment budget

The two key components for budgeting include some *volume measure* and some *cost measure*. The volume measure is an activity standard based on the unit of service or workload measure adopted by the institution. This may be bed occupancy (per day), acuity level, number of visits, number of deliveries, or nursing care hours per patient day. For a hospital, the traditional measure was the census or the number of patient days. The cost measure may be some salary figure, such as the nurses' average salary or wage rate. Smeltzer and Hyland (1989) described a "flexible" budget that changes with volume and is based on a formula that used direct care hours and wage dollars in the calculation. Their major budgetary factors included patient days, nursing care hours per patient day, nonproductive time, training time, historic overtime, average wage rates, average registry expense, and percentage of staff mix.

The various component statistics used for budgeting have both advantages and disadvantages. For example, an average value reduces a large volume of data to a representative number, but it is skewed by outliers and does not tie activity to an individual client. Thus individual client variability may be lost in the aggregate. Some fine but important discriminations may be lost or distorted by the size of the group being aggregated. Volume measures are only one indicator of activity and may not capture aspects important to the delivery and management of nursing services. The question is, what variables are critical and basic for nurses to have to manage nursing care? These would comprise a Nursing Management Minimum Data Set (Huber, Delaney, Crossley, Mehmert, & Ellerbe, 1992).

RESEARCH NOTE

Source: Kitz, D., McCartney, M., Kissick, J., & Townsend, R. (1989). Examining nursing personnel costs: Controlled versus noncontrolled oral analgesic agents. *Journal of Nursing Administration, 19*(1), 10-14.

Purpose

The purpose of this research was to evaluate the costs associated with different pharmaceutical therapy regimens on nursing personnel costs. The authors examined nursing labor costs that resulted from using controlled (schedule II-

III) and noncontrolled (schedule IV) oral analgesic agents in one 698 bed teaching hospital with annual admissions of 23,000 adult patients. Industrial engineering and cost accounting techniques were used to compute costs via identified task activities. The process was to identify nursing units, describe the tasks, identify unique tasks, measure nursing personnel time, and assign dollar values to nursing time. Three nursing units were analyzed.

Discussion

The average number of patients per day on the three units who took controlled oral analgesic agents was multiplied by 365 and then by the additional nursing labor costs for administration of controlled oral analgesic agents for a total yearly additional nursing labor cost. For each task, labor costs were greater for controlled agents due to greater administration and storage activities. The additional costs for administering controlled oral analgesic agents averaged $1.31 per patient day. The additional inventory control storage costs were $2.20 per unit per day. For their average of 72 patients per day, the nursing labor expenses amounted to $34,426.80 per year for administration tasks.

Application to Practice

By analyzing what actually occurred in practice, it was found that additional nursing labor costs were incurred by the use of controlled oral analgesic agents over noncontrolled agents. Clearly, patient care practices by physicians affect nursing labor costs. However, what the article does not point out is that the facility's medication administration system and processes might also contribute to costs and need reanalysis. With fixed rate or capitated reimbursement, such costs become a financial liability. Thus accurately documenting the actual components of a task contributes to analyzing costs. For example, assessing and including inventory control activities such as investigating incorrect narcotic counts (not done in this study) better reflects the important components of nursing personnel time that contribute to costs. Costs may be reduced by changing physicians' prescribing patterns or by interdisciplinary educational programs about therapy choices, reimbursement mechanisms, and costs.

LEADERSHIP AND MANAGEMENT IMPLICATIONS

With a trend to decentralization of decision making, the nurse manager's role includes increasing accountability for financial management of the work unit. With a trend toward the elimination of middle managers, nurses will assume this accountability and responsibility. The smallest functional unit that generates revenues and expenses is called a *cost center*. Some units generate direct revenue or charges, while others (e.g. administration) generate expenses but no direct revenue.

A charge is generated for the purpose of acquiring income for the healthcare organization. There is a difference between the charge and the actual

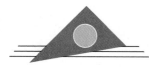 *Leadership & Management Behaviors*

LEADERSHIP BEHAVIORS	**MANAGEMENT BEHAVIORS**	**OVERLAP AREAS**
• determines resource requirements for the group	• plans the budget	• determines resource requirements
• guides a visionary justification of resources	• organizes the needed resources	• motivates expanded knowledge about financial aspects
• analyzes expenditures	• organizes budget justification	
• uses creativity to strategize and negotiate for the group's resource needs	• implements the unit budget and budget processes	
• motivates the group to increase financial knowledge	• controls expenses	
• influences the group to find innovative ways to do things better	• determines resource requirements within organizational constraints	
• finds new sources for resources	• evaluates technology	
• creates a financially savvy work environment	• motivates subordinates to learn about budgeting	

cost, just as there is when purchasing a piece of clothing from a department store. The *charge* is defined as the price asked for services or goods. The *cost* is defined as the amount required as payment for producing the service. *Profit* is defined as the money gained as excess of charges over outlay costs in producing a service. For example, a healthcare facility may bill a client for $5.00 for the use of a vial of sterile saline when it cost the hospital $1.00 to purchase and process the purchase. The difference is profit.

Nursing traditionally was included as part of the room charge and not separated from hospital-based hotel functions like housekeeping, support services, and dietary. Thus the actual costs of care and the revenue captured from nursing effort are in effect "invisible." Research has uncovered the fact that physicians bill for services provided by nurses. In 1989, Ott, Griffith, and Towers found that nurses perform many of the services for which physicians are being reimbursed. An examination of the Current Procedural Terminology (CPT) codes revealed that nurses perform many of the services listed, yet the CPT coding system acknowledged only physicians as providers of all the coded services. Nursing services were not a factor in payment review fee schedules except as a part of a physician's practice costs (Griffith & Fonteyn, 1989; Griffith, Thomas, & Griffith, 1991). Nurses were encouraged to identify explicitly the value of the nursing component involved in each physician service, since others appeared to be capturing revenue for what nurses actually do. Nurses do and coordinate client service delivery. Therefore, they contribute to both costs and charges. Nursing needs to examine ways to capture its contribution to revenues and profit and then communicate and negotiate on this basis. For example, if a respiratory treatment generates a charge when a Respiratory Therapist delivers it but not when done by a nurse, then the perception of nursing's value in an organization may be affected in subtle ways.

Since most nurses traditionally had not captured fee-for-service as reimbursement, nursing was considered to be a cost, not a revenue source. When nursing captures costs and can bill for nursing services, revenue streams can be identified. Unless nursing can accurately capture its costs, nurses really do not know the actual costs of nursing care. Therefore, nurses would not be able to compare the charge for care that may appear on the client's bill as a room charge, and the cost of that care, consisting of such elements as nursing salaries, fringe benefits, and nursing supplies that are not billed separately to the client. It is possible for nursing to then be disadvantaged in negotiations for scarce resources.

Overall, both nurses and nurse managers have seen their role expand in scope and importance as empowerment, innovative change, shared governance, and cost containment have occurred. The nurse's role in financial management has grown in concert with these changes. Jones (1993) noted that nurse managers' financial management efforts are directed at determining resource requirements; being able to justify resources; evaluating technology; and holding down expenses for staff, supplies, and equipment. Similarly, staff nurses' financial management efforts can be directed at contributing data and rationale for resource needs and practicing cost awareness in nursing care delivery. Thus nurses at all levels need awareness and knowledge about the basics and techniques of financial management. Leaders and managers can motivate personnel to expand their knowledge base and can model savvy financial management while planning, organizing, implementing, and controlling money and resources.

Cost Awareness

In trying to improve client care by improving managerial and clinical decisions in nursing, there is a need to be cost conscious in practice (Gardner, 1992). The costs to clients from "what it is that nurses do" is a social and professional concern. The two major themes for nursing practice into the next millennium are cost and quality. The questions that will be asked are, what is the cost, and will this provide high quality care? The cost variable relates to decision making (see Chapter 7). Cost certainly is not the only consideration

Christine Kovner Envisions Financial Management

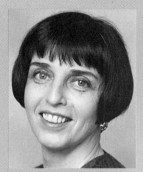

Christine Kovner

Future managers will require nurses in all healthcare organizations and at all levels of these organizations to have financial knowledge. Nurses will face decisions about allocating scarce health resources among their possible uses. Direct care nurses will face decisions such as determining how much time to devote to a patient related activity, the need for sterile gloves compared to unsterile gloves, and how much linen to use. Nurse-managers will continue to be concerned about resources they control such as their own time and that of their staff, supply use, and also cost-effective risk management.

Nurses should understand the basic finances of their organizations and where their unit's budget, including their salaries, fit into the organization's financial operations. Nurses should understand the benefit derived from their nursing activities. Although many nurses think that the escalation of cost-consciousness is already greater than appropriate to provide good patient care, it is my impression that the emphasis on cost-effectiveness will no doubt become stronger.

The future will contain information, data, graphs, figures, statistics, charts, measurements, and new content and presentation formats. Sophisticated electronic systems will collect, analyze and produce electronic images converted into paper for those nurses who still use paper. These systems will provide nurses with costs per bed, per day, per adjusted day, per case mix, per visit, per hour, per minute, per nurse and revenues per all groups and populations of patients.

The most important skills that nurses will need in the future are assessment skills. Nurses must recognize what they should ask for, what they should read, and what they should retain. They will need to ask the important questions. A cartoon I saw recently stated "I may not have all the answers, but at least I am beginning to ask the right questions." For the nurse of the future the world will be filled with answers. Because nurse time is scarce and valued, nurses need to know what questions to ask about resource use.

Christine Tassone Kovner, PhD, RN, FAAN, is an Associate Professor in the Division of Nursing, School of Education, Health, Nursing and Arts Professions, New York University, and a Research Associate at New York University Medical Center. She was the co-principal investigator of the evaluation of the New Jersey Nursing Incentives Reimbursement Awards, which provided $18 million in funding to 37 hospitals to implement innovations in the delivery of nursing care. She is the author of numerous articles and chapters on nursing resource use and costs, and the co-author, with Steven Finkler, of *Financial Management for Nurse Managers and Executives* (1993). She has served on two committees for the New York State Department of Health: the Health Personnel Utilization and Productivity Committee and the Hospital Information Systems Workgroup.

to have in decision making, but nurses will consciously consider cost as one element. Nurses are motivated by multiple forces, including client care quality and nursing convenience. Reducing costs and capturing reimbursement is a part of a healthcare organization's goals that nurses are encouraged to incorporate into their practice.

What cost decisions do nurses control? What can nurses do to reduce costs? The following are suggestions to promote cost control:

- Do the job efficiently. The more efficiently the nursing care delivery is organized and run, and the greater the contribution of individuals to the care provided, the less costly that care is going to be.
- Time is money. For example, simple scheduling errors can increase the length of stay. The time element is especially crucial in care coordination activities.
- Help motivate clients to recover in order to improve their health status and reduce dependency costs.
- Use supplies carefully. Know the costs of those supplies. For example, posting a per-unit cost list by item for the cost of an alcohol swab or a roll of tape helps to keep employees aware of the costs of the supplies they are using. Knowing those costs will facilitate better substitution decisions (Striegel, 1986). For example, Chagares and Jackson (1987) compared price and performance of six pressure-relieving devices, and Smith and Amen (1989) compared the costs of IV drug delivery systems. Their results indicated alternatives for potential substitution decisions.

For a client with poor skin integrity, perhaps the most expensive tape should be used because it has to stick and be waterproof. However, in a routine situation, can a lower-cost item be substituted adequately? Nurses cannot contribute to cost reduction unless they know the per item cost of the supplies they use and then use this information to evaluate substitutions. What is noticed immediately is that over time it becomes costly if a topper sponge or sterile pad is used to wipe up spills, a sterile pack is opened just to get one instrument, or pre-printed chart forms are used as scratch pads.

Nurses need to participate in organization-wide cost containment and take credit for the cost savings generated by nursing. There needs to be a formal, documented way in which decisions made by nurses and the cost savings that result are made visible and rewarded. Knowing the healthcare organization's charges and what treatments and procedures cost clients gives nursing information with which to advocate for clients. Nurses need nursing cost data for analysis and evaluation.

There are areas of nursing practice where nurses can begin to identify inefficient or redundant activities and utilize decision making abilities. Serving on product committees gives nurses an opportunity to advocate for products that save *nursing* time and to put pressure on vendors for adaptations to the technology that decreases *nursing* time. This will assist nurses to work intelligently and efficiently while still enjoying the work of nursing.

In terms of costs and cost awareness, there is a general finding across the literature that "nursing costs," the actual cost of delivering nursing care, are about 20 to 30 percent of hospital costs per DRG, depending on the geographic location (Kirby & Wiczai, 1985; McCloskey, 1989). Therefore, nursing is a reasonably priced service that generates revenue by contributing to the delivery of client care services. Nurses need to contribute to cost control, but this must be balanced by professional decision making. In terms of professional decision making, nurses need to learn to spend money when it is appropriate and avoid being petty or stingy. Nurses also need to learn to save money when it does not need to be spent (McCloskey, 1988). That is part of professional decision making.

Ethical and Legal Issues

Budgeting and financial management involve intensive decision making about the allocation of scarce resources. Conflicts and ethical dilemmas easily can and do arise in the balancing of competing needs and wants. For example, the institution is advantaged if labor budgets are tightly restricted. However, clients may incur greater wait times or diminished direct care time if nurses and other care providers are not readily available. Further, nurses experience greater stress when workloads rise and clients' care needs are difficult to meet in the time available.

Money, personnel, space, and time are scarce resources in organizations and become the focal point for power, politics, and conflict (see Chapters 20, 21, and 30). Ethical and moral problems occur as values clash. Ethical obligations of fidelity can be interpreted as promise-keeping, an obligation to act in good faith, fulfilling agreements, maintaining relationships, and upholding trust and confidence. In law or business the parallel ideas are contracts, trust, or fiduciary relationships (Beauchamp & Childress, 1994). Ethical dilemmas arise over conflicts of loyalty or conflicts of interest.

Professional fidelity or loyalty means upholding the clients' interests as a priority over the professional's self-interest or others' interests in any conflict. Divided loyalties arise from the organizational and financial structures of healthcare. For example, issuing orders, assignment of duties, or allegiance to other providers, employing agencies, funding sources, corporate structures, or governmental agencies may compel an ethical choice. It is unclear what a healthcare provider or institution "owes" a client beyond reasonable or "due care." Because of the structure of healthcare delivery and nursing's traditions, nurses report pervasive moral conflicts among obligations related to fidelity. This means nurses may face choices among obligations to clients, physicians, and employing institutions (Beauchamp & Childress, 1994). Some examples arise over disclosure of information, physicians' orders, respect of clients' wishes, aggressiveness of treatment, impact of teaching and research functions in care delivery, and conflicts of interest with payor restrictions.

The ethical value of stewardship relates to the obligation to oversee and use expertise to decide about the appropriate allocation of resources. Stewardship means that nurses will need to make frequent choices among competing values of client needs balanced with organizational financial survival (Reiser, 1994). The overall effects of nurses' decisions related to budgeting and cost containment impact on clients and organizations. Managed care systems reward restricted or non-intervention and frugality by using economic incentives for clinical decisions. Thus providers and organizations may acquire economic gain by rationing care to clients. Other incentives such as job security may conflict with obligations to clients as financial management decisions are made (Beauchamp & Childress, 1994).

Chart 9.3 illustrates a type of legal and ethical dilemma that may result from the changing structure of healthcare financing. The scenario described in the chart is simplified and, in reality, would probably be much more complex. The purpose of this example is to show the ethical and legal complexities which may be faced by nurses and other healthcare providers as they decide when and when not to provide specific interventions for a client. The example given could impact on the financial solvency of the NICU within the larger institution. It is possible, if not likely, that there may be financial

---

CHART 9.3 ❧ ETHICAL FACTORS CREATED BY HEALTHCARE FINANCING RESTRUCTURING

Scenario—An attending physician in the neonatal intensive care unit (NICU) of a major research hospital has determined that a premature infant (21 weeks gestation) is of questionable viability. Because of underdeveloped lungs and other complications, the physician is considering issuing an order to not provide basic life support, including feeding, to the newborn. Before finalizing the order, the physician consults with the NICU nurse in charge of the infant.

Fee-for-Service
Additional efforts to attempt maintenance of the newborn on life support functions while allowing the lungs an opportunity to develop sufficiently to sustain life will be. . . .
Reimbursed by the newborn's parents, insurance company, Title XIX, etc.

Managed Care
Additional efforts to attempt maintenance of the newborn on life support functions while allowing the lungs an opportunity to develop sufficiently to sustain life will be. . . .
Without additional reimbursement

sanctions against the department and/or healthcare providers who work there, if the department overspends its budget because of deciding in such situations to provide the additional services to the client when there is not any reimbursement that can be achieved.

Organizational loyalty may constrain moral principles and create a tension between nurses' ethic of caring and profit-orientation in corporations (Corley & Raines, 1993). Nurses resolve ethical dilemmas by bending rules, responsible subversion, creating meaning from difficult situations, denial, burnout, quitting, remaining silent, choosing self-interest or organization-interest above the client's interest, or facilitating values clarification (Corley & Raines, 1993). Nurse managers have identified three aspects of an ethical practice environment as autonomy, trust, and communication. Nurse manager characteristics, institutional supports, and organizational values are necessary to create autonomy, trust, and communication orientations that promote ethical professional practice (Corley & Raines, 1993).

Employment arrangements create legal as well as ethical rights and obligations. Financial and budgeting implications arise from legal obligations. Malpractice and negligence place both nurse and employer at financial risk. Both the nurse and the employer can be held liable under the doctrine of respondeat superior, where the employer is named a defendant in a malpractice claim because they are responsible for the acts of their employees. Under the doctrine of corporate negligence, healthcare organizations have a responsibility to monitor or supervise all personnel, including the quality of care, and to investigate physicians' credentials (Aiken, 1994).

While there are clear organizational liabilities for employment issues, less clear are the legal risks related to deployment issues. Unsafe staffing numbers leading to inadequate care remains a major nursing management ethical dilemma (Corley & Raines, 1993). The requirement of the law is that the nurse's actions are reasonable under the circumstances. Reasonable in relationship to short staffing is a matter of judgment. Client safety, accepted professional standards and guidelines, and the language of organizational policies and procedures are major considerations. Budgeting and financial management are managerial decisions fraught with both ethical and legal ramifications.

CURRENT ISSUES AND TRENDS

Costing Out Nursing Services

Costing out nursing services was defined as the determination of the costs of the services provided by nurses. The current application is to identify the cost of nursing for a specific client in a specific diagnosis related group (DRG) category within a hospital setting (McCloskey, 1989). By identifying the specific costs related to the delivery of nursing care to each client, the client can be billed for nursing care based on the actual amount of services received. As a result, nursing would be in a much better position to autonomously monitor, justify, and control the costs of nursing care within a cost-conscious environment (Eckhart, 1993). Scherubel (1994) offered a warning, however. If nurses use costing out nursing care services to decrease costs, nursing budget requests may be reduced through decreased resource allocation to nursing departments. Thus it is important to capture incentives in return for cost control efforts.

There have been a couple of reviews of the literature related to costing out nursing services (Eckhart, 1993; McCloskey, Gardner, & Johnson, 1987). Although a variety of variables were examined, such as length of stay, nursing care costs, direct care costs, and DRG reimbursements, most common was the extrapolation of nursing costs from a specific acuity system. There is a lack of standardization of definitions and elements used to compute direct and indirect nursing care costs (Eckhart, 1993). This lack of standardization impedes comparisons across settings and sites.

The present healthcare system reimburses mostly for medical services aimed at curing diseases. To revise reimbursement to cover nursing services,

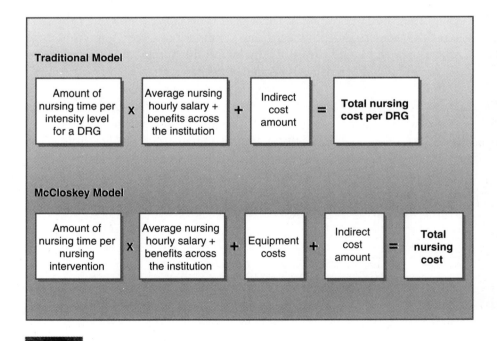

Figure 9.2
Two models of costing out nursing services. (Adapted with permission from McCloskey, J. C. [1989]. Implications of costing out nursing services for reimbursement. *Nursing Management,* *20*[1], 44-49, pp. 46-47.)

nursing costs need to be determined. The usual model identified uses the amount of nursing time per intensity level (for a DRG) multiplied by the average nursing hourly salary and benefits, and added to an indirect cost amount to calculate a total nursing cost per DRG. The result is the nursing cost per DRG or intensity level. Nursing intensity usually is represented by a patient classification measure as a proxy. A serious flaw in this model is the inability to identify what nursing activities are delivered to clients. Patient classification or acuity systems tend to measure average or projected care needs, not actual needs and actual services delivered.

McCloskey (1989) proposed an alternative model to yield nursing cost per nursing intervention or diagnosis. In this model the amount of nursing time per nursing intervention is multiplied by the average nursing hourly salary and benefits and added to equipment costs, to equal direct costs. Direct costs plus indirect costs equal the total nursing cost. As nursing interventions replace intensity in the calculation, the actual nursing care delivered to clients is being measured more accurately. Standardization of nursing interventions will contribute to the ability to compare nursing costs (McCloskey, 1989) (see Fig. 9.2).

RESEARCH NOTE

Source: Bostrom, J. (1994). Impact of physician practice on nursing care. *Nursing Economic$*, *12*(5), 250-255, 286.

Purpose

The purpose of this study was to determine the amount of variation in nursing care hours within a DRG which is attributable to either severity of illness or variation in physician practice style. Nursing time was measured and related to individual physician practice. The setting was one 600 bed tertiary care hospital. From client discharges over a 5 year period, subjects' data were extracted for 11 DRG categories. The sample was 1,964 subjects and 93 physicians. Data were collected on hours of direct nursing care, severity of illness, patient age, DRG, physician code number, total required nursing care hours, and length of stay.

Discussion

The client subjects were analyzed for a demographic profile and length of stay and total required nursing care hours averages. Nursing care hours varied among DRG categories. General linear modeling and ANOVA procedures were used to analyze variables related to physicians. Severity of illness accounted for 17% to 49% of the explained variance; physician practice preferences explained 6% to 38% of the variance; and both physician and severity of illness accounted for 34% to 62% of explained variance in the total hours of care.

Application to Practice

The data add weight to previous studies showing a great variation in hours of required nursing care per DRG category. Understanding the causes of the variation in nursing resources contributes to better resource management, cost control for clients, and financial management by nurses. Client diagnosis and severity of illness account for a substantial portion of length of stay variance. Thus the classification of clients by diagnosis and severity may be useful in predicting resource use, planning care, and allocating costs for reimbursement. Severity of illness does not capture what is needed or overtreatment, only what was done for the client. However, severity of illness does capture to some extent physician practice. The impact of variation in physician practice style has a direct impact on nursing practice and nursing costs. Both nurse staffing and hospital reimbursement are tied to inpatient census and patient diagnosis. In this study, a client's nursing care requirements were driven in large part by diagnosis, severity of illness, and individual physician's practice preferences. This raises issues of the efficient use of nursing care as a scarce and costly component of health care.

SUMMARY

* A budget is a plan designed to control the allocation of resources. It becomes a financial timetable.
* The three types of budgets are cash, capital, and expense budgets.
* The budgetary process is a financial planning and control system.
* Traditional, zero-based, or performance budgeting are typical budgetary processes.
* The budget process follows four stages and is displayed on multiple forms.
* A volume and a cost measure form the basic measurement elements.
* Nurses are concerned with nursing costs, which have been invisible due to not being identified, standardized, and analyzed.
* Focusing on direct, indirect, and supply costs helps to begin to identify the costs of the services provided by nurses.

Study Questions

1. How does budgeting relate to financial planning, control, and management in healthcare?
2. Do nurses raise healthcare costs or lower them?
3. How would a nurse manager manage a revenue budget?
4. How can nursing institute costing out of nursing services for reimbursement? Should this be done?
5. What leadership roles and activities are important in budgeting and financial management?
6. What activities of budgeting and financial management are appropriate at the staff nurse level?

7. How can staff nurses best acquire knowledge and skills in budgeting and financial management?
8. How are budgeting and financial management like balancing a personal checkbook?

Critical Thinking Exercise

Sheryl Little, RN, nurse manager, has a headache. She has been working on budget forms for weeks. The deadline for submission of budget requests for next year is next week. The healthcare facility has been on a cost-containment program for over a year. Sheryl has delayed the purchase of some major equipment and the maintenance costs have been increasing. Today she was working on the staffing worksheet when several staff nurses stopped in to complain that they were consistently working short-staffed. The morning mail had brought a letter of complaint about the timeliness of staff response and the results from a recent client satisfaction survey which Sheryl was afraid to read.

1. *Does Nurse Little have a problem?*

2. *What is the problem(s)?*

3. *How should Nurse Little handle the situation?*

4. *What should Nurse Little do first?*

5. *What creative strategies might be best suited to the situation?*

6. *What would motivate others to assist in this situation?*

7. *What financial management strategies might work?*

REFERENCES

Aiken, T. (1994). *Legal, ethical, and political issues in nursing.* Philadelphia: F. A. Davis.

Beauchamp, T., & Childress, J. (1994). *Principles of biomedical ethics* (4th ed.). New York: Oxford University Press.

Chagares, R., & Jackson, B. (1987). Sitting easy: How six pressure-relieving devices stack up. *American Journal of Nursing, 87*(2), 191-193.

Corley, M., & Raines, D. (1993). An ethical practice environment as a caring environment. *Nursing Administration Quarterly, 17*(2), 68-74.

DeBoer, L. (1990). Organizations as financial systems. In J. Dienemann (Ed.), *Nursing administration: Strategic perspectives and application* (pp. 263-289). Norwalk, CT: Appleton & Lange.

Eckhart, J. (1993). Costing out nursing services: Examining the research. *Nursing Economic$, 11*(2), 91-98.

Finkler, S. (1991). Performance budgeting. *Nursing Economic$, 9*(6), 401-408.

Finkler, S., & Kovner, C. (1993). *Financial management for nurse managers and executives.* Philadelphia: Saunders.

Gardner, D. (1992). The CNS as a cost manager. *Clinical Nurse Specialist, 6*(2), 112-116.

Goldsmith, S. (1981). Financial management of health care organizations. In S. Goldsmith. *Health care management: A contemporary perspective* (pp. 157-175). Rockville, MD: Aspen.

Griffith, H., & Fonteyn, M. (1989). Let's set the payment record straight. *American Journal of Nursing, 89*(8), 1051-1058.

Griffith, H., Thomas, N., & Griffith, L. (1991). MDs bill for these routine nursing tasks. *American Journal of Nursing, 91*(1), 22-27.

Huber, D., Delaney, C., Crossley, J., Mehmert, P., & Ellerbe, S. (1992). A nursing management minimum data set: Significance and development. *Journal of Nursing Administration, 22*(7/8), 35-40.

Johnson, M. (1989). Perspectives on costing nursing. *Nursing Administration Quarterly, 14*(1), 65-71.

Johnson, M., & Carpenter, C. (1990). Financial management for nursing executives. In E. Simendinger, T. Moore, & M. Kramer (Eds.), *The successful nurse executive: A guide for every nurse manager* (pp. 91-106). Ann Arbor, MI: Health Administration Press.

Jones, K. (1993). The ins and outs of financial management: An introduction. *Seminars for Nurse Managers, 1*(1), 4.

Jones, K. (1994). Direct and indirect costs. *Seminars for Nurse Managers, 2*(1), 4-5.

Kirby, K., & Wiczai, L. (1985). Budgeting for variable staffing. *Nursing Economic$, 3*(3), 160-166.

McCloskey, J. C. (1988). Personal communication.

McCloskey, J. C. (1989). Implications of costing out nursing services for reimbursement. *Nursing Management, 20*(1), 44-49.

McCloskey, J., Gardner, D., & Johnson, M. (1987). Costing out nursing services: An annotated bibliography. *Nursing Economic$, 5*(5), 245-253.

Ott, B., Griffith, H., & Towers, J. (1989). Who gets the money? *American Journal of Nursing, 89*(2), 186,188.

Reiser, S. (1994). The ethical life of health care organizations. *Hastings Center Report, 24*(6), 28-35.

Scherubel, J. (1994). Costing out nursing services: Is it happening? In J. McCloskey & H. Grace (Eds.), *Current issues in nursing* (4th ed.) (pp. 483-489). St. Louis: Mosby.

Smeltzer, C., & Hyland, J. (1989). A working plan to understand and control financial pressures. *Nursing Economic$, 7*(4), 208-214.

Smith, R. (1988). The nursing organization budget: Basic principles and concepts. In J. Kirsch (Ed.), *The middle manager & the nursing organization: Human resources fiscal resources* (pp. 129-139). Norwalk, CT: Appleton & Lange.

Smith, C., & Amen, R. (1989). Comparing the costs of IV drug delivery systems. *American Journal of Nursing, 89*(4), 500-501.

Smith, H., Mahon, S., & Piland, N. (1993). Nursing department strategy, planning, and performance in rural hospitals. *Journal of Nursing Administration, 23*(4), 23-34.

Striegel, E. (1986). Cost effective use of supplies in the NICU. *Neonatal Network, 4*(6), 46-48.

PART IV

Organizational Design and Governance in Nursing

Organizational Culture and Environment

Chapter Objectives

∾

explain the importance of organizational culture

∾

define culture and climate

∾

define and describe organizational culture

∾

distinguish among the elements of a culture

∾

explain three levels of culture

∾

compare five critical cultural elements of an organization

∾

define and differentiate implicit and explicit culture

∾

analyze the importance of culture for
leadership and management in nursing

∾

exercise critical thinking to conceptualize and analyze
possible solutions to a practical experience incident

*a*s a nurse it is easy to simply assume that all there is to consider is the narrow perspective of one's own job. On many levels, both personally and professionally, examining an organization's culture and function will improve nurses' effectiveness by providing a perspective about the interpersonal and political forces that operate in any work environment. Learning about organizational culture may further broaden personal management philosophy, style, and success.

FRAMEWORKS FOR ORGANIZATIONAL STRUCTURE

To understand the organizations in which nurses work, nurses can consider that there are different viewpoints or perceptions about how the institution operates. Different viewpoints can be used for thinking about and analyzing organizations. Four different viewpoints have been identified: the structural, human resource, political, and symbolic views. These frameworks focus on one aspect or slice of organizational structure and function.

The structural point of view examines the structure of an organization and its roles and relationships (see Chapter 12 for more information on structural views). The human resource perspective focuses on the integration of individuals with the organization. The political point of view focuses on the importance of the distribution of scarce resources. Power, influence, conflict, bargaining, and coalitions are key concepts in the political perspective. The symbolic point of view focuses on the aspects of organizational behavior that are not analyzed rationally and on the meanings attached to events. Symbols are important for managing chaos and confusion (see Table 10.1).

Table 10.1

Ways of Viewing Organizations

VIEW	PERSPECTIVE	EXAMPLES
Structural	Focuses on formal roles, relationships, and organizational structure	Drawing a formal organizational chart. Listing the officially constituted committees. Rigidly following the reporting structure ("chain of command").
Human resource	Focuses on tailoring the organization to fit the people	Allowing more democratic decision style within a unit of the organization to take advantage of the team style of the workers.
Political	Focuses on organizations as distributing scarce resources	Two departments struggling over use of personnel necessary to both. Two health care provider organizations competing to gain access to the same population.
Symbolic	Focuses on the meaning of events via symbols	Viewing the firing of a seemingly competent employee with a unique personal style as a mandate for conformity. Viewing a merit raise as an entitlement.

Data from Bolman and Deal (1984) and del Bueno and Freund (1986).

The political and symbolic perspectives have been identified as being useful under conditions in which resources are scarce or declining, where there is rapid change, or where uncertainty is high (Bolman & Deal, 1984; del Bueno & Freund, 1986). These conditions are present today in the healthcare industry. Part of a nurse's effectiveness at leadership and management, then, can be derived from assessing and understanding the political and symbolic environment. In analyzing the political and symbolic environment, the nurse's attention is drawn to a careful examination of the organizational culture and environment.

If one is to effectively function in an organization, a good grasp of its characteristic environment and mode of operation is essential. Veninga (1982) noted the importance of understanding an organization before being able to competently manage it. The first step in understanding an organization that employs nurses is to critically analyze the nurse, the job, and the setting in which nursing is practiced.

Think about past experiences as an employee. What kind of experiences were they? What was the nature of any good or bad experiences (e.g., the characteristics of a boss or lousy pay)? Have you had a good job that you hated to leave? And if so, why? Nurses' jobs are influenced by the organizations in which they work. Thus an examination of the organizations that employ nurses is important for nursing.

We think of nurses as being employed by hospitals. There is some evidence that the setting of care is changing and will become community-based. The actual employment settings for nurses may be shifting as well. How much this will shift and into what configuration it will shift is uncertain. For example, there is a trend toward more nurses directing the delivery of a service through creative employment mechanisms such as entrepreneurial ventures, independent practices, owning small businesses, community nursing centers, contracting for services, or working for medical suppliers or as computer consultants. Some predict that under a health care reform process, eventually 70% of nursing jobs will be outside of the acute care inpatient hospital setting. Regardless of the setting in which nursing is practiced, every organization has a history, set of traditions, social structure, values, rituals, and rules (Veninga, 1982). Nurses can list these aspects of an organization and do an organizational analysis of each aspect (see Chart 10.1). For example, do you know the organization's history? What are the enduring traditions? What rituals occur? Culture gives meaning to the distinct way of life in an organization and has a powerful effect on behavior through its influence on decision making (del Bueno & Freund, 1986).

CHART 10.1
∾ CHECKLIST OF CULTURAL COMPONENTS IN ORGANIZATIONS

- History
- Set of traditions
- Social structure
- Values
- Rituals
- Rules

Data from Veninga (1982).

RESEARCH NOTE

Source: Dutcher, L., & Adams, C. (1994). Work environment perceptions of staff nurses and aides in home health agencies. *Journal of Nursing Administration, 24*(10), 24-30.

Purpose

The purpose of this study was to compare staff nurses' perceptions of the work environment to home health aides' (HHAs) perceptions in three home health agencies in one Western state. A convenience sample was used in a descriptive comparative study of 70 RNs and 35 HHAs. An information questionnaire and the Work Environment Scale (WES) were given to subjects. The WES measures three key dimensions of relationships, personal growth, and system maintenance or change. There are ten subscales among the three dimensions.

Discussion

To determine the differences between RNs and HHAs on each of the ten subscales, a multivariate analysis of variance was computed. There were significant role and agency effects. Staff nurses perceived significantly greater levels of involvement, peer cohesion, and work pressure. Control and clarity were significantly higher for HHAs. There were similarities between the job categories on the other subscales. Staff nurses seemed happy with their work environment; HHAs were less happy. Nurses and HHAs perceived equal levels of autonomy. HHAs perceived greater role clarity and greater organizational control than did RNs.

Application to Practice

In the relationship dimension, nurse care managers can use data about HHAs perceived levels of job satisfaction to structure retention strategies. Nurse leaders and managers can foster peer cohesion in the HHA group. In the personal growth dimension, nurse care managers can examine the work of HHAs and look for opportunities to restructure to enhance personal growth and overall productivity. In the systems maintenance/control dimension, nurse leaders and managers can assess the levels of perceived role clarity and explore strategies to build in what RNs need. Creating an innovative work environment is one strategy advocated for improvement of work environments and healthcare systems.

DEFINITIONS

Culture is related to shared values and beliefs and has been described as a "normative glue." It is the sensation perceived about the interpersonal milieu or environment. *Organizational culture* is defined as the shared beliefs, values, and assumptions that exist within an organization (see Chart 10.2). Some authors note a difference between organizational culture and climate. Culture is seen as shared beliefs and values. *Climate* is defined as the perceptions that individuals have of various aspects of the environment in an organization. Thus climate can be characterized as the personality of a setting or environment. The ten components of climate in Moos' Work Environment Scale are: involvement, peer cohesion, supervisor support, autonomy, task orientation, work pressure, clarity, control, innovation, and physical comfort (Flarey, 1991; Moos, 1987).

CHART 10.2
⌒ DEFINITION

Organizational Culture
the shared beliefs, values, and assumptions that exist within an organization.

Veninga (1982) defined organizational culture as the cumulative banking of knowledge, experience, meanings, beliefs, values, attitudes, power, and wealth that is acquired by an organization. Taken together, these variables constitute a cultural mosaic and communal heritage. What this means for nurses is that culture is a complex phenomenon. Like understanding health and illness in a human being, organizational culture is composed of a variety of components that interact. It is subjective and perceptual, making culture more difficult to understand.

Organizational culture has been described as the combination of the symbols, language, assumptions, and behaviors in which an organization's norms and values are manifest. Organizational culture also has been defined as the pattern of basic assumptions and shared meanings developed by a group to survive their tasks (Schein, 1985), a set of solutions devised by a group to solve common problems (Van Maanen & Barley, 1985), and the way things are done around here (Deal & Kennedy, 1982). Every organization has cultural norms and values; modern healthcare organizations are complex blends of social realities and cultures that shape human interactions. At the core of an organizational culture are basic patterns that have worked in the past and are transmitted to new members as the correct way to perceive, think, feel, and act (del Bueno & Vincent, 1986). Culture is learned by making the connection between behaviors and consequences (Sovie, 1993).

Culture can be characterized in four ways: its broadness, subtlety, power, and pattern. These terms are used in describing a culture for purposes of comparison. Culture is a form of internal group control and is based on beliefs about group survival. Thus culture is distinct from external managerial control via organizational charts, policies, and procedures (Coeling & Simms, 1993; Denison, 1990). What this means is that culture is rooted in the group and within the human interpersonal dynamics that occur as a natural result of people in groups. The leader, as a member of a group, may be able to shape and influence the culture if the group accepts this influence. Culture is not generally under management dictate. Managerial control is more obvious in the structural domain, with its focus on organizational structure and rules. However, management control and structure will have an impact on culture through rewards and sanctions available to group members and on the leader's strategies for facilitating a positive culture and climate.

BACKGROUND

Organizational culture is characterized by complexity and multiple interacting components. It is an important component of nurses' work in organizations. Organizational culture is one influence on nurses as individuals and their fit with an organization that employs them. There are four functions that an organizational culture serves.

1. It gives a sense of identity to the members
2. It promotes a sense of commitment to a larger entity
3. It enhances the stability of the social system
4. It helps to make sense of behavior (Smircich, 1983)

Nurses may want to create or modify the work culture and climate. This may be done to better accommodate individuals or professional groups. It may be done as a strategy to enhance the creativity and innovation-readiness of nurses. Creating or modifying the organizational culture may impact on productivity satisfaction and retention outcomes. In order to create or modify organizational culture, nurses need to be aware of the basic elements that make up a culture.

The elements comprising culture include stories, myths, rituals, ceremonies, and metaphors and analogies. Each can be identified and examined for meaning to the group:

- *Stories* may describe conflicts or the traditions and heroes of the organization's history.
- *Myths* are narratives of events that are passed on to inspire belief and establish what is acceptable.
- *Rituals* are honored customs that serve to communicate social relationships and belonging. Rituals serve to socialize, stabilize what works, reduce ambiguity, and convey messages about underlying values.
- *Ceremonies* are attended events, such as retirement parties or company picnics, that serve to benefit both the group and the individual.
- *Metaphors and analogies* explain in "as if" terms situations that are confusing or unexplainable. Complex issues are compressed into simple images. Behavior and attitudes are influenced by these symbols. For example, sports metaphors use concepts such as "the team," "coaches and captains," "stars," and "cheerleaders" (Bolman & Deal, 1984; del Bueno & Freund, 1986; del Bueno & Vincent, 1986).

After nurses examine and analyze the elements of the culture in an organization, they then can assess the manifestations of the culture by level.

Three levels of culture have been identified by Schein (1985):

1. *The visible level:* This includes physical space and social environment. An example of the visible level of a culture might be the luxuriousness of the surroundings. What is visible to clients? What is visible to staff? What image is projected at first encounter with the organization? Who has a close parking space?
2. *The values:* This includes elements of what ought to be. For example, nurses value high quality care and caring. Whose values predominate? How are cost, quality, and access balanced? Are customers important?
3. *The basic underlying assumptions:* This includes the actual guides to behavior that are deeply held and not open to challenge or debate. An

example is the slogan "profit is everything." In some organizations it is assumed that doctors generate profits, whereas nurses generate costs. What assumptions, if challenged, will result in peer pressure or sanctions?

After examining the culture generally and comparing the levels of culture, the nurse can then examine the culture as it is within the specific organization. There are five critical cultural elements in any organization (Veninga, 1982):

1. *The mission statements* outline the organization's philosophy, goals, and objectives.
2. *The formal structure* outlines the hierarchical responsibilities of departments and individuals.
3. *The informal structure* includes networks of relationships.
4. *The political structure* includes the overlay of power within the organization.
5. *The financial structure* includes the fiscal resources to support the organization's activities.

The cultural elements can be viewed as being like an internal road map. Each element is important for understanding how an organization functions. Therefore, the nurse can systematically examine each element in turn. The elements guide the nurse to important areas to assess (see Fig. 10.1).

Within every organization there exists both an explicit culture and an implicit culture. Explicit means written out; implicit means not so formalized.

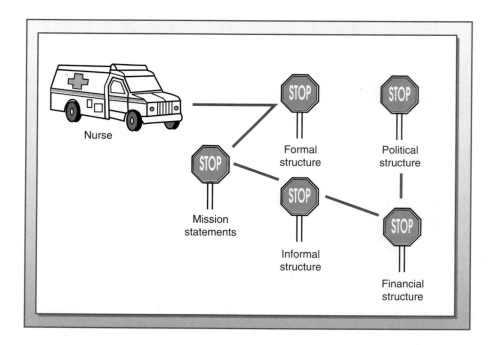

Figure 10.1
Critical cultural elements (Data from Veninga [1982].)

An *explicit culture* is one that is formally written and can be seen in policies, rules, expectations, and ways of doing things that are made known and written down. Some organizations have their cultures well-defined. Norms and values are obvious and pervasive throughout the organization. For example, employees can describe the most important goals and behaviors expected of any employee. Further, there may be posters or cards printed with "guiding principles." Other organizations leave their culture to drift and evolve. Those are the organizations with more implicit cultures.

Implicit culture refers to cultural knowledge that is not verbally communicated. It is shared knowledge that people usually do not discuss (Veninga, 1982). Norms may be subtle and difficult to discern (del Bueno & Vincent, 1986). Rituals, values, traditions, and informal understandings are all a part of the implicit culture. One example of implicit culture is informal work rules. For example, on one hospital unit all of the nurses change into scrub clothes prior to their shift. The implicit work group pattern is that all of the on-coming shift nurses will be changed into scrub clothes and ready for report at least by the stroke of their shift change time. The nurses do not come in late. Report lasts about ten minutes. Then the on-coming shift nurses immediately begin to assess their clients and start their work. At the end of their shift, the on-coming shift is expected to be there, be dressed, and be ready to take report at the stroke of shift change so that the off-going nurses are able to leave. No one tells you this custom. It is not written in a policy statement. However, a violation of the norm will be immediately sanctioned by the peer group. As the violator is confronted with unhappy colleagues, it becomes apparent that this is what the group expectations are.

In contrast, on another work unit, the nurses wander in five or ten minutes late. Then they sit in the break room and socialize. Report will get rolling maybe 15 or 20 minutes into the shift change. The on-coming crew never emerges before a full hour from the time that their shift was supposed to start. As a result, the off-going nurses have to cover the floor past the time that they are actually supposed to go home. Both are very clear cultures to the work group members. The norms are implicit. These patterns reflect the way that the units actually run, and what the people seem to be comfortable with doing. An individual either accommodates to the culture or moves on because of the pressure felt from peers. These are examples of cultural norms related to time use and the rewards or sanctions tied to compliance with group norms.

An organizational culture checklist might be used for a closer examination of the culture as it is manifested in an organization. The checklist could contain the following elements (del Bueno & Freund, 1986):

Image: how does the organization wish to be perceived? Public relations activities and external physical symbols are used to create an image.

- *Deportment:* how do people dress and interact with each other? Dress codes, social stratification, and codes of conduct are used to shape deportment.
- *Status symbols and reward systems:* what is used as a status symbol or reward? Titles and special privileges are frequently used for status and reward.
- *Subcultures:* are there any subcultures that are tolerated and, if so, for what purpose?
- *Environment and ambiance:* how attractive and comfortable is the environment? Attention to colors, music, dining arrangements, and space and furniture are used to promote ambiance.
- *Communication:* what are the permissible modes and channels? Control of information flow and type is used to regulate communication.
- *Meetings:* what practices are established for meetings? Seating, time limits, and group processing procedures are used to regulate meetings.
- *Rites, rituals, and ceremonies:* what are they? Presence or absence serves to communicate social relationships.
- *Sacred cows:* what is revered and protected? Heroes, myths, and taboo subjects are clues to sacred cows

This organizational checklist may be used as a guide to describe and understand an organization's culture (del Bueno & Freund, 1986) (see Table 10.2).

Table 10.2

Organizational Culture Checklist

OBSERVABLE ASPECTS OF CULTURE	EXAMPLES
Image	How professionally dressed are the nurses?
Deportment	What is the level of courtesy shown to clients' family?
Status symbols	Compare the nurses' parking and lounges to physicians' and administrators'.
Subcultures	Will nurses from the same cultural background tend to form friendships with each other more easily?
Environment and ambiance	One hospital has bright hallways and modern abstract paintings on the walls. Another has hallways hung with oil portraits of previous administrators and famous physicians.
Communication	How does the CEO communicate to staff nurses?
Meetings	Count the number and frequency of committees and meetings. Who participates?
Rites, rituals, and ceremonies	How are holidays celebrated? Is longevity recognized?
Sacred cows	Name one hero/heroine and one taboo subject.

Data from del Bueno and Freund (1986).

Organizational culture has been measured for research purposes by the Organizational Culture Inventory (OCI), which measures behavioral norms and expectations associated with shared values and beliefs (Cooke & Lafferty, 1987; Thomas, Ward, Chorba, & Kumiega, 1990). Coeling (1989; Coeling & Simms, 1993) has used her Nursing Unit Cultural Assessment Tool to describe the immediate work group culture in nursing practice. Both are quantitative measures of organizational culture. Culture also has been measured using the variable of climate. The Organizational Climate Audit (OCA) is one such measure (Hart & Moore, 1989).

Organizational climate focuses on employee perceptions of the work environment. Employee perceptions are measured to provide information that helps leaders and managers understand how staff view the environment. This understanding enables leaders and managers to better provide mechanisms that lead to a positive work climate. Work environments have an influence on moods, behaviors, and overall sense of health and well-being in employees (Dutcher & Adams, 1994). Moos's Work Environment Scale (WES) (Moos, 1987) has been used to measure ten elements of the three climate dimensions of relationships, personal growth, and system maintenance/change. The WES has been used to investigate a variety of nursing samples and to compare staff nurses to aides in home health agencies (Dutcher & Adams, 1994). The Work Characteristic Instrument (Simms, Erbin-Roesemann, Darga, & Coeling, 1990) has been used with home healthcare registered nurses to measure work excitement and enthusiasm and commitment to the profession (Baldwin & Price, 1994). Thus there are reliable and valid measures of organizational climate and culture that have been tested in nursing practice.

RESEARCH NOTE

Source: Baldwin, D., & Price, S. (1994). Work excitement: The energizer for home healthcare nursing. *Journal of Nursing Administration*, *24*(9), 37-42.

Purpose

The purpose of this study was to explore home health nurses' perceptions of work and to investigate the relationship between work excitement and nurses' practice settings. A questionnaire that contained 50 items relating to demographics and various aspects of work were administered to 167 RNs who worked in six urban and three rural home health agencies in the southeastern U.S. The instrument asked about interest in work, exciting aspects of work, most exciting work setting, time consuming activities, meaningful and exhausting parts of work, what is a good day, suggested new technologies, and work-related travel.

Discussion

The greatest number of respondents (37%) were very excited about their work on a six-point Likert-type scale. When the sample was split into high

(42%) and low/moderate (58%) categories, the responses were roughly equal. Salaried nurses, less tenured nurses, and rural home care nurses were more excited about their work. The most exciting aspects of work were job flexibility, ability to make a difference for clients, working with people, and being viewed as an important part of the healthcare team. The most meaningful accomplishment is contributing to improved client care. A good day is one in which the nurse achieves a feeling of accomplishment.

Application to Practice

Growth and development and a variety of experiences were positively related to work excitement. Positive aspects of home health nursing were client contact, autonomy, and recognition. These positive aspects can be used to promote nursing recruitment and retention in this setting. They can become motivators and satisfiers to be nurtured and fostered by nurses and leaders and managers. Points of frustration, such as paperwork, can be counteracted by a culture that minimizes frustration and maximizes the exciting aspects of nursing.

LEADERSHIP AND MANAGEMENT IMPLICATIONS

Personal and professional success begins with the knowledge of how to recognize cultural variables. Each nurse will make decisions about whether or not to comply with the cultural norms and values. There may be more or less severe consequences to violating cultural norms and values. For example, colleagues may become irritated, or the violator may be ostracized from the group.

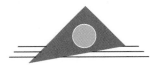 *Leadership & Management Behaviors*

LEADERSHIP BEHAVIORS	MANAGEMENT BEHAVIORS	OVERLAP AREAS
• envisions a dynamic culture	• manages the structure to positively impact on culture	• models constructive interpersonal relations
• inspires a creative climate	• models constructive interpersonal relationships	• influences the group to work together
• models constructive interpersonal relationships	• acts with equity and justice	
• enables followers to be productive	• maintains rituals and ceremonies	
• influences others to work together	• influences employees to work together	
• creates shared values		
• develops stories, rituals, and metaphors		

When first encountering a healthcare organization, absorb a sense of the informal or implicit culture. Look around. Use observation and sensing. Investigate questions like, Is there art work on the walls? If so, who paid for that art work? Is there elaborate landscaping? What is the aesthetic sense? What do the conference rooms look like? What does the nurses' lounge look like, if there is one? Do the nurses have any place to put their coats and purses? Get a sense of how the structure is used, how welcoming the atmosphere is. Are visitors greeted and acknowledged upon entering this organization? Do they have to struggle to get the attention of a receptionist? How do the employees behave? Do people run up and down the halls or walk slowly? Each organization will give a different sense about their culture. Within each organization, each work group similarly will have a sense of culture as manifested by cohesiveness or non-cohesiveness, warmth or coldness, business-like hurriedness or casual non-hurriedness.

Analysis of organizational culture is one element impinging on leadership and relevant to organizational innovation and change. Organizational culture has been seen as important for work redesign, empowerment of nursing staff, and organizational transformation (Coeling & Simms, 1993; McDaniel & Stumpf, 1993).

CURRENT ISSUES AND TRENDS

Nurses' work is influenced by the organization's culture. It is thought that strong cultures either motivate coordinated action and performance or serve as a strong barrier to change. Examples such as mergers and acquisitions, reorganizations, and downsizing highlight the importance of understanding and managing organizational culture (Wilkins, 1983). Leadership at all levels means having a sense of the reality of the setting. This is necessary for functioning within the subjective and expressive domains of the environment that are more emotional than rational. Organizations with strong cultures maintain them by managing human resources: who is hired, how they are developed, and how they are rewarded. Understanding and correctly interpreting the culture enhances success if the nurse is able to fit behavior and management strategies to comply with cultural norms and values (del Bueno & Freund, 1986). Nurses may be expected to reinforce cultural norms, as in the nurses' ethic of providing care to all clients regardless of culture, sexuality, or having a communicable disease such as AIDS.

Nurses may be involved in the leadership and management of organizational change. Organizational culture becomes an important element to manage. The nurse leader may need to help the group learn and accept new values, norms, and assumptions, or match a new program to a prior culture. Many organizations attempting to merge face long periods of unrest until the foundation of a new

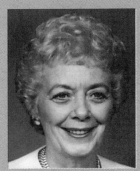

Margaret D. Sovie

Margaret Sovie Envisions
Shifting from Illness Care to Wellness Care

Efforts to reduce healthcare costs through managed care and a capitated environment are forcing a paradigm shift from an illness-oriented care system to a system in which health and health promotion are valued. It matters not that the driving force behind this paradigm shift is preservation of the per member per month capitation dollar. The result is the shift is occurring and healthcare rather than illness care is finally being valued.

Nurses are experts in healthcare and health promotion, and the opportunities for new and expanded roles in these areas will dominate the market. Hospitals will continue to change in size and character with only the most acutely ill being admitted. Alternative care settings including subacute and convalescent care, ambulatory care, home care, long term care and organized community care services will be increasingly in the forefront. These are areas where nurses have expertise and much to offer. Nursing has always been committed to health and wellness and assisting individuals to maximize their health potential and their recovery abilities as well as helping individuals and families cope with chronic illness, disability, and death.

Leadership in this revolution is critical. Leaders must be committed to building learning organizations and creating a culture in which every person is valued and feels valued. A sense of shared ownership will be instrumental to the success of the enterprise since everyone must be committed to working together to create new and better ways of delivering healthcare services. Leaders will strive to create an environment in which every practitioner and staff member is encouraged and empowered to use their individual and collective expertise and creative energies to deliver the most effective and efficient healthcare services possible. The patient and family will be treated as partners in the healthcare enterprise and active members of the healthcare team.

Promoting health, preventing illness and exquisite caring in a culturally sensitive manner will be the new norms. Patient/family satisfaction, provider/staff satisfaction, and clinical outcomes will be routinely measured and reported to the purchasers and consumers of health care services. The value of nursing, including advanced practice nursing, will be obvious, recognized and remunerated. Nurses working together with others, including the consumers and purchasers of care, will make it happen.

Margaret D. Sovie, PhD, RN, FAAN, is Associate Deputy Executive Director and Chief Nursing Officer, Hospital of the University of Pennsylvania, and the Jane Delano Professor of Nursing Administration and Associate Dean for Nursing Practice at the University of Pennsylvania School of Nursing, as well as a Senior Fellow at the Leonard Davis Institute of Health Economics. Dr. Sovie has published and spoken on a wide variety of subjects related to nursing leadership and administration, including patient outcomes, the cost of nursing care, and organizational culture. She was one of the co-authors of the landmark study of "magnet hospitals," which looked at how certain hospitals attracted and retained professional nurses of superior quality.

culture can be forged. Which norms and values will be retained, which let go (del Bueno & Vincent, 1986)? Because values and norms are basic and provide comfort, changing or merging cultures is very difficult for nurses to deal with.

Cultural management is a leadership issue. What the leader stands for and communicates to others is considered important if the objective is to stir human consciousness, interpret and enhance meanings, identify key cultural strands, and link members to the organization. Developing and nurturing norms about what to believe and how to behave represent a response to the needs of individuals and groups for stability, order, and meaning (Sergiovanni, 1984). Sovie (1993) noted that a culture helps determine the success of an organization and that a major responsibility of each hospital's leadership is to create and maintain a culture that will enable the organization to execute its mission effectively and cope successfully with a changing environment.

Values drive the way resources are distributed. They contribute to a general attitude and sense about the quality of working life. They reflect the organization's core goals. Clues can be gleaned from organizational documents such as philosophy statements and meeting minutes. Caring values of the organization are reflected in the way the organization treats its staff. Organizational values may or may not be similar to professional values. The leader's role is to bridge these with individuals' values.

Building a culture is based on a framework of support (see Fig. 10.2). Values support the mission and the related vision, which support strategies and action plans. The key platform is shared values. A nurse who wants to build a culture would (1) start wherever the group currently is at and build from there, (2) use appropriate communication skills and personal contact to establish open discussion, (3) identify shared values and mission so the group knows where it is going, (4) determine strategies, and (5) take planned action. For example, trust, risk-taking, and positive self-esteem may be values identified to promote innovation. Decision making at the grass roots level may be an action strategy (Kerfoot, 1991).

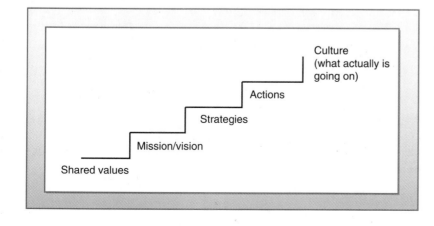

Figure 10.2
Framework of support for building a culture.

Within the environment of work there are real human variables like job satisfaction, commitment, and turnover that affect nurses and relate to how the product of nursing is delivered. Of the four different conceptual frameworks taken to understand organizations and how they function, the human resource viewpoint focuses on the interface of the work environment with the human employees such as nurses in a work unit. The human resource point of view focuses on the importance of the people who work in the organization. Their needs and feelings are seen as significant for organizational effectiveness. The concept of the fit of the organization to its people is emphasized.

Cultural elements have been viewed as intervening variables in models of turnover and retention. In the Hinshaw, Smeltzer, & Atwood (1987) path model, group cohesiveness, defined as how integrated a nursing staff member felt as a part of the organization and collegial environment, was an important aspect of job satisfaction and the prediction of retention. The three other aspects were job stress, control over nursing practice, and autonomy. It is thought that when there is a lack of shared values and a lack of a sense of cohesion and direction, turnover is likely to increase. Positive culture has been found to be related to productivity, retention, high morale among providers, and decreased mortality among acute care clients (Shortell et al., 1991; Thomas et al., 1990).

Some healthcare organizational practices expose a philosophy that nurses are interchangeable cogs, using the industrial model metaphor or analogy of machinery: that one part can be interchanged for another part. For example, an institution that floats a nurse from one unit to another, especially if it is to an area outside the same practice specialty, is assuming that the nurse is interchangeable with any other nurse. Specialization in both medicine and nursing has progressed to the point where the specialties vary significantly, and it may not be safe to "pull" or "float" without specific cross-training. Functioning in organizations and as service workers means that nurses need to know the system. Nurses are advised to know the power structure, network with each other, and build a support system to alleviate some aspects of the organization that may create job dissatisfaction.

Culture and climate are elements of the work of nursing. They are symbolic and political. They are related to nurses' successful functioning in organizations. They can be studied, measured, and analyzed. Cultures and climates can be improved or may degenerate. Nurses can have an influence on the outcome.

SUMMARY

- Understanding organizational culture is important for successful functioning.

- ✷ Culture gives meaning to behavior and influences decision making.
- ✷ Culture is shared values and beliefs.
- ✷ There are levels of culture.
- ✷ Cultures are both explicit and implicit.
- ✷ Cultures have elements that can be identified and measured.
- ✷ Culture management is a leadership issue.
- ✷ Cultures can and should be built by nurse leaders.
- ✷ Culture elements can influence nursing turnover and retention.

Study Questions

1. What is the relationship between an organization and its values?
2. To what extent does an organization's culture determine job satisfaction?
3. How can you assess an organization's culture?
4. How long does it take to really perceive the culture?
5. Is caring the central value for nursing?
6. What are the effects of leadership on culture?
7. Does organizational culture reflect an individual's perception of the organization, or is it a relatively enduring characteristic?
8. How can you build a culture?
9. What is the best kind of organizational culture for nursing?
10. What values are important in an entrepreneurial nursing environment?
11. What nursing values create dilemmas?

Critical Thinking Exercise

Nurse Nancy Coggeshall has been employed by Loving Care Home Health Agency less than a year. She was excited to get this job after graduation with her BSN. She holds a strong commitment to quality client care. Most of the other nursing staff hold long tenure with the agency. They also state a belief in quality client care. Nurse Coggeshall has proposed the introduction of laptop computers and cellular phones as an efficiency and effectiveness measure. She has arranged for product demonstrations at the staff meeting coming up in two days. Now Nurse Coggeshall's Nursing Director is expressing vague doubts about this "new technology." Nurse Coggeshall notices that the Director does not have a computer on her desk.

1. What is the problem?

2. Whose problem is it?

3. What should Nurse Coggeshall do next?

4. What cultural elements are operative in this situation?

5. What cultural analysis could be done?

6. Has Nurse Coggeshall violated any cultural norms?

7. How can Nurse Coggeshall be successful in her proposal?

REFERENCES

Baldwin, D., & Price, S. (1994). Work excitement: The energizer for home healthcare nursing. *Journal of Nursing Administration, 24*(9), 37-42.

Bolman, L., & Deal, T. (1984). *Modern approaches to understanding and managing organizations.* San Francisco: Jossey-Bass.

Cody, B. (1990). Shaping the future through a philosophy of nursing. *Journal of Nursing Administration, 20*(10), 16-22.

Coeling, H. (1989). *Nursing unit cultural assessment tool: NUCAT-1.* Kent, Ohio: Harriet Coeling.

Coeling, H., & Simms, L. (1993). Facilitating innovation at the nursing unit level through cultural assessment, part 1: How to keep management ideas from falling on deaf ears. *Journal of Nursing Administration, 23*(4), 46-53.

Cooke, R., & Lafferty, J. (1987). *Level V: Organizational culture inventory.* Plymouth, MI: Human Synergistics.

Deal, T., & Kennedy, A. (1982). *Corporate culture.* Reading, MA: Addison Wesley.

del Bueno, D., & Freund, C. (1986). *Power and politics in nursing: A casebook.* Owings Mills, MD: National Health Publishing.

del Bueno, D., & Vincent, P. (1986). Organizational culture: How important is it? *Journal of Nursing Administration, 16*(10), 15-20.

Denison, D. (1990). *Corporate culture and organizational effectiveness.* New York: John Wiley & Sons.

Dutcher, L., & Adams, C. (1994). Work environment perceptions of staff nurses and aides in home health agencies. *Journal of Nursing Administration, 24*(10), 24-30.

Flarey, D. (1991). The social climate scale: A tool for organizational change and development. *Journal of Nursing Administration, 21*(4), 37-44.

Hart, S., & Moore, M. (1989). The relationship among organizational climate variables and nurse stability in critical care units. *Journal of Professional Nursing, 5*(3), 124-131.

Hinshaw, A., Smeltzer, C., & Atwood, J. (1987). Innovative retention strategies for nursing staff. *Journal of Nursing Administration, 17*(6), 8-16.

Kerfoot, K. (1991). Personal communication.

McDaniel, C., & Stumpf, L. (1993). The organizational culture: Implications for nursing service. *Journal of Nursing Administration, 23*(4), 54-60.

Moos, R. (1987). *The social climate scales: A user's guide.* Palo Alto, CA: Consulting Psychologists Press.

Schein, E. (1985). *Organizational culture and leadership.* San Francisco: Jossey-Bass.

Sergiovanni, T. (1984). Cultural and competing perspectives in administrative theory and practice. In T. Sergiovanni & J. Corbally (Eds.), *Leadership and organizational culture: New perspectives on administrative theory and practice* (pp. 1-11). Chicago: University of Illinois Press.

Shortell, S., Rousseau, D., Gillies, R., Devers, K., & Simons, T. (1991). Organizational assessment in intensive care units (ICUs): Construction, development, reliability, and validity of the ICU nurse-physician questionnaire. *Medical Care, 29*(8), 709-726.

Simms, L., Erbin-Roesemann, M., Darga, A., & Coeling, H. (1990). Breaking the burnout barrier: Resurrecting work excitement in nursing. *Nursing Economic$, 8*(3), 177-187.

Smircich, L. (1983). Concepts of culture and organizational analysis. *Administrative Science Quarterly, 28*(3), 339-358.

Sovie, M. (1993). Hospital culture-why create one? *Nursing Economic$, 11*(2), 69-75, 90.

Thomas, C., Ward, M., Chorba, C., & Kumiega, A. (1990). Measuring and interpreting organizational culture. *Journal of Nursing Administration, 20*(6), 17-24.

Van Maanen, J., & Barley, S. (1985). Cultural organization: Fragments of a theory. In P. Frost, L. Moore, M. Louis, C. Lundberg, & J. Martin (Eds.), *Organizational culture* (pp. 31-53). Beverly Hills, CA: Sage.

Veninga, R. (1982). *The human side of health administration: A guide for hospital, nursing, and public health administrators.* Englewood Cliffs, NJ: Prentice-Hall.

Wilkins, A. (1983). The culture audit: A tool for understanding organizations. *Organizational Dynamics, 12*(autumn), 24-38.

Organizations, Mission Statements, Policies, and Procedures

Chapter Objectives

∞

define and describe an organization

∞

explain the product of nursing

∞

compare the two dimensions of a social system

∞

explain the three main parts of a mission statement

∞

distinguish among philosophy, purpose, and objectives statements

∞

analyze policies and procedures

∞

relate organizational philosophy to nursing practice

∞

exercise critical thinking to conceptualize and analyze
possible solutions to a practical experience incident

*t*he provision and management of nursing care to clients usually is embedded within an organization. Thus understanding organizations and how they function is important to nurses who are employed by organizations. This is because there are practical aspects to the managerial structure imposed by an organization. An organizational structure can be both efficient and effective. It is thought that operationalized documents like mission statements give a thoughtful direction for planning and directing functions of the management process (Trexler, 1987).

Within an organization there is an established framework for management. For each organization there is a characteristic collective of power and authority that is vested in the managerial hierarchy. This legitimated authority, given by position, is used with the management process, management skills, and whatever resources are available to meet the organization's goals. Together, the elements of management plus the resources available combine to form the basic framework for the management and functioning of an organization. Organizations have a mission. That mission is to produce a product or service. This will be expressed in mission statements and carried through into policies and procedures.

DEFINITIONS

 n *organization* is a group of people with specific responsibilities acting together for the achievement of a specific purpose determined by the organization (see Chart 11.1). An organization usually is thought of as an institution like a hospital or manufacturing company. All organizations have a purpose, structure, and some collection of people (see Fig. 11.1). The actual character or nature of any organization is highly variable, depending upon the purpose, structure, and collection of people that form the organization.

BACKGROUND

Business management theory has contributed ideas about how to organize a business so that it makes money and runs efficiently. Theories based on busi-

CHART 11.1
DEFINITION

An Organization
a group of people with specific responsibilities acting together for the achievement of a specific purpose determined by the organization.

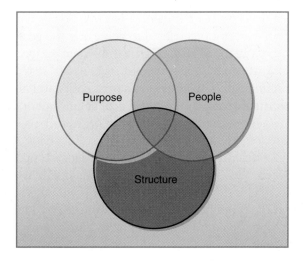

Figure 11.1
Components of an organization.

ness firms do not always apply directly to nursing because nursing is a service industry. Drucker (1973), a prominent business management theorist, said that service institutions are more complex than either businesses or governmental agencies. In a service industry such as nursing, the two key aspects of effectiveness are quality and cost control. Further, service agencies like hospitals rely on professional staff to accomplish their mission. Thus the relationship of professionals to their employing institutions affects organizational effectiveness in healthcare. Nurses primarily work in groups, thus making work group functioning and the interactions among people important for effectiveness and mission accomplishment in nursing.

As a service industry, healthcare has a product. What is the product of healthcare? What is the product of nursing? Are they the same? Health may be the ultimate outcome to be achieved. Do nurses deliver health as a product? Quality care is one ideal product of healthcare. Kramer and Schmalenberg (1988) said that the product of a hospital is a quality, accessible, cost-effective service called client care, and in hospitals 90% of client care is delivered by nurses. If the product is "quality care," then there needs to be valid and reliable measurement to assure that "quality care" is delivered and received. More recently, the idea has arisen that the product of nursing is not a service composed of tasks, but rather a business with a product of enhanced client outcomes and contained costs (Zander, 1992). This idea takes Drucker's conceptualization and merges ideas about a service industry with ideas about traditional for-profit business.

Organizations are designed to produce goal accomplishment and can be understood as social systems. The Getzels and Guba model (Getzels, 1958) indicated that there are two dimensions to a social system. One part is the environment of the organization. An institution has certain role expectations, a culture, ethos, and values. If an organization has certain goals, for example, quality client care and cost containment, then individuals have a role in the system with certain expectations related to achieving the goals.

The other part of the social system is the individual person, who has a personality and certain needs. For example, the needs may be for power, achievement, or affiliation. The individual's personality and needs disposition will interact with the institution's need for goal achievement. Somewhere in that dynamic interaction, the behavior seen in organizations is manifested as a result. Sometimes organizations appear to be in total chaos; sometimes they run smoothly and efficiently. The manifest result depends upon the dynamic interaction between the organization on the one hand with its need to achieve goals, and the individual with their own personality and unique drives and desires on the other hand (Getzels, 1958) (see Fig. 11.2). Thus nurses can examine their personal and group "fit" with any organization as one criterion for effectiveness.

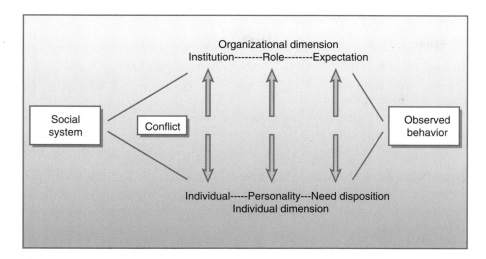

Figure 11.2
Social system and behavior.
(Data from Getzels [1958].)

For nurses as professional employees, the question is, who do you serve? Do you serve the needs of the organization as a business with pressures for efficiency, mass production, and cost containment, or do you serve the needs of the client who may want teaching and counseling time, rehabilitation time, home care planning coordination, and individualized but time consuming care? There is an underlying dynamic tension between bureaucratic and professional values identified as a problem for nurses called "reality shock" (Kramer, 1974). This parallels the organizational-individual tensions that arise in social systems. The behavior of any nurse in a healthcare organization can be seen as a dynamic interaction and outcome of the nurse interacting with the specific social system in which the nursing care delivery is embedded.

When a nurse accepts a position in a healthcare agency, that nurse makes a commitment to the goals and philosophy of the nursing service department within that organization. Likewise, when one assumes a managerial position in an organization, that same commitment is made, as well as a commitment to subscribe to the philosophy of management of that organization. Although an individual may or may not personally believe in or subscribe to the organization's philosophy, taking a position in an organization implies an agreement to accommodate to the organization's philosophy while at work. Therefore, an examination of organizational mission statements such as the philosophy, goals, and objectives statements promotes a greater understanding of the specific institution and may promote more effective organizational participation by nurses. To begin to learn how the organization runs, examine the philosophy, structure, and policies. The functional aspects of organizations include the culture, philosophy, purposes, objectives, policies, and procedures related to the work environment. They are key aspects of managerial planning.

Organizational Mission Statements

Veninga (1982) identified the mission statement as one of the critical culture elements in any institution. The mission statement explicitly outlines the organization's philosophy, values, goals, and priorities. There are three main parts to a mission statement:

- *philosophy:* the philosophy states the values and beliefs.
- *purpose:* the purpose states the reason for existence.
- *objectives:* the objectives state specific and measurable outcomes desired.

Some believe that the mission statements are the standard against which performance is to be judged. Following these statements into actual practice is a way to ensure that an organization delivers to the clients what was promised (Martin & Hughes, 1993).

Philosophy Statements

The written statements of philosophy, purpose, and objectives are found in an administrative manual. The administrative manual is a companion to the disaster, safety, isolation, policy, and procedure manuals. It forms a ready reference to the mission statement documents.

A *statement of philosophy* is defined as an explanation of the systems of beliefs that determine how a mission or a purpose is to be achieved (see Chart 11.2). An organization's philosophy states the beliefs, concepts, and principles of an organization. It serves as a guide for and an explanation of actions (Poteet & Hill, 1988). The philosophy is abstract: it describes a vision and gives direction to achieving the purpose. It often begins with "We believe that. . . ." For example, the system of beliefs, or philosophy, might be stated as follows: we believe that everyone has a right to the highest quality client care; we believe that we have an obligation to render quality client care at a cost-effective price; or we believe that any person who walks through the door should get care regardless of their ability to pay.

The philosophy has implications for a nurse's practice role. If an organization's stated mission includes client care, teaching, and research, then all employees will be expected to be involved in all three aspects of the mission. Part of the nurse's job will be to teach students and be involved in research. The nursing service philosophy should be congruent with the organization's philosophy. The three vital components that form the core of a nursing service philosophy are the client, the nurse, and nursing practice (Poteet & Hill, 1988).

The organization's philosophy is important to assess as it relates to one's personal philosophy. For example, a potential employee on a job search might compare his or her own philosophy, both of nursing practice and of management, to the philosophy of the organization with which she or he might secure employment. Is there a match? For example, hospitals that are owned by reli-

CHART 11.2
∾ DEFINITION

Philosophy
an explanation of the systems of beliefs that determine how a mission or a purpose is to be achieved.

gious organizations may prefer to hire people of their own religious faith. If you are not of that religious faith, or if you have a prejudice or a lack of knowledge about that religious faith, it is advisable to assess your fit with that particular organization. If there is some part of the philosophy that is personally distasteful, it can have implications for functioning within the practice environment. For example, there may be a specific religious tradition still pervasive within the organizational culture, even though the stated philosophy may say that they provide care to people of all faiths. That may bother you. One example occurs when an organization that is owned and run by a religious group opens each administrative meeting with a prayer. Another example occurs when a nurse believes in providing the total scope of public health services to clients, but the organization is run by for-profit principles that dictate only the provision of services that make a profit. Taking a job in an organization suggests a silent agreement to cooperate with their particular values while at work.

RESEARCH NOTE

Source: Wolf, G., Boland, S., & Aukerman, M. (1994). A transformational model for the practice of professional nursing: Part 1, the model. *Journal of Nursing Administration, 24*(4), 51-57.

Purpose

The purpose of this article is to present and explain the Transformational Model for the Practice of Professional Nursing, which was developed in response to the healthcare system's imperative to reduce healthcare costs while improving quality and access. The authors identify four values and assumptions within nursing that need to be reassessed and shifted in a transformation. Then a phenomenological study of 500 nurses from one tertiary care teaching hospital was done to determine the critical factors necessary to support professional practice. Then nursing exemplars (clinical stories) were elicited from staff nurses to identify expert clinical nursing practices.

Discussion

The results of the phenomenological study were used to form the core components of the professional practice model. The model was presented and discussed. The four core components are professional practice, process, primary outcome, and secondary outcome. The professional practice component contains four elements at the heart of the model: transformational leadership, care delivery systems, professional growth, and collaborative practice. Concepts that support each of the four elements at the heart of the first (professional practice) component of the model were identified.

Application to Practice

Philosophy and values form important underpinnings of two of the four elements that compose the professional practice component of this model: transformational leadership and collaborative practice. Of the seven concepts of transformational leadership, empowerment, vision, decentralization, participative management, and organizational culture emphasize philosophy and values. Of the four concepts supporting collaborative practice, unit norms and professional shared governance use philosophy and values as a basis. This model can be applied in practice. It can serve as a conceptual framework for a nursing department's philosophy statement. It can drive the philosophy, purpose, and vision for a nursing department or organization. It could be used in planning and unit management.

Purpose Statements

The statement of purpose describes the reason for being, or why the healthcare organization is operating. *Purpose* is defined as the service or services to be provided and for which an organization or unit exists (Trexler, 1987) (see Chart 11.3). Each institution exists for a specific purpose or mission and to fulfill a specific social function. For a healthcare organization, of course, this means healthcare services, for example, client care, teaching, and research. Trexler (1987) reviewed mission statement documents and found that the purpose of carrying out physicians' legal orders·was not acknowledged in nursing departments' purpose statements. This may mean that the purpose was not clearly and realistically defined.

For a nursing department's purpose, constraints include the organization's purpose, the state nurse practice act and other legal parameters, the context of the local community, and directives of regulating agencies. The purpose statement should be short, concise, and clear. The purpose of the nursing department should mesh with the purpose of the institution.

Objectives

Objectives are written, behaviorally-specific statements of desired outcomes. *Objectives* are defined as the identified outcomes directing activity toward achieving the purpose of the organization or unit (Trexler, 1987) (see Chart 11.4). Organizations use written, behaviorally specific objectives so that each employee knows what it is that the organization is trying to achieve. Objectives are the fundamental strategy of an institution (Drucker, 1973). The objectives of each work unit are used for establishing priorities, strategies, plans, work assignments, and the allocation of resources (Drucker, 1973; Trexler, 1987). Objectives need to be specific, realistic, attainable, challenging, fit with the organization's goals, and emphasize the work of greatest importance. Chart 11.5 displays examples of how philosophy, purpose, and objectives may be stated.

Policies and Procedures

Policies and procedures are two functional elements of an organization that are extensions of the mission statements. Policies and procedures both are

---

CHART 11.3
〜 DEFINITION

Purpose
the service or services to be provided and for which an organization or unit exists.

Data from Trexler (1987).

CHART 11.4
〜 DEFINITION

Objectives
the identified outcomes directing activity toward achieving the purpose of the organization or unit.

Data from Trexler (1987).

written rules that are derived from the mission statement and together determine the nursing systems of the work unit and the department of nursing. The purpose of policies and procedures is to provide some order and stability so that the unit works as a coordinated group and functions coordinatively within the larger structure of nursing and the institution. Organizations need to integrate the behaviors of the employees to avoid random chaos and maintain some order, function, and structure.

These plans are often referred to as standard operating policies and procedures. They guide the personnel in decision making. A *policy* is a guideline that has been formalized (see Chart 11.6). It directs the action for thinking about and solving recurring problems related to the objectives of the organization.

There will be specific times when it is not clear who is supposed to do something, under what circumstances, or what should be done about unusual circumstances. For example, often there are controversies about the dress code because of disagreements about the definition of what is "appropriate." This occurs, for example, when the dress code says, "Nurses will come to work dressed in appropriate attire."

Policies direct decision making and serve as guides to increase the likelihood of consistency in decisions and actions. Policies should be written, understandable, and general in nature to cover all employees. If written, they should be readily available in the same form to all employees. Policies should be reviewed in orientation, because they indicate the organization's intentions for goal achievement.

After institutional approval, policies should be placed in a manual, indexed, classified, and noted in the table of contents. Policies so organized are easily replaceable with revised ones, because policies need to be revised in light of new environmental circumstances. Policy formulation in any organization is an ongoing core process. Hospitals will have a standing committee for the review of policies as a part of the organizational structure. Policies establish broad limits on and provide direction to decision making yet permit some initiative and individuality.

Policies can be implied, or unwritten, if they are essentially established by patterns of decisions that have been made. In this case, the informal policies represent an interpretation of observed behavior. For example, the organization may expect caring treatment for all clients. This expectation may not be written as a policy of the organization. But by the decisions and disciplinary actions that occur, an employee can infer that there is a policy that will be enforced even though it is not written. However, the vast majority of policies are and should be written. Informal and unwritten policies are less desirable because they can lead to systematic bias or unfairness in their application and enforcement (see Chart 11.7).

There are some general areas in nursing that require policy formulation. These are areas in which there is confusion about the locus of responsibility

CHART 11.5
↪ MISSION STATEMENT EXAMPLES

Philosophy
We believe that nursing services are organized to optimally manage client care and produce improvement in clients' outcomes with cost-effective use of resources.

Purpose
The purpose of the institution is to provide compassionate care to the sick and injured of all religions and races.

Objectives
To decrease nursing turnover by 10%.

CHART 11.6
↪ DEFINITION

Policy
a guideline that has been formalized.

CHART 11.7
↪ POLICIES

- Serve as guides
- Help coordinate plans
- Control performance
- Increase consistency of action
- Should be written
- Usually are general in nature
- Refer to all employees

and where lack of guidance might result in the neglect, malpractice, or malperformance of an act necessary to the client's welfare. In those areas in which it is important that all people adhere to the same pattern of decision making given a certain circumstance, it is important to have a policy so that the policy can be used as a guideline. Also, areas pertaining to the protection of clients' or families' rights should have policies written. Areas involving matters of personnel management and welfare, such as vacation leave policy should have written policies. The lack of a uniform policy would be considered unfair. Many conflicts arise related to the scheduling of vacations: how many people can be off at any one point in time, how long in advance must a vacation request be put in, or how is the priority for granting requests to be determined (e.g., seniority or by the first person to put a request in). The policy is the guideline for determining specific decisions.

Procedures

CHART 11.8
∾ DEFINITION

Procedure
a description of how to carry out an activity.

Procedures are detailed directions for action that provide step-by-step directions and methods for common situations. *Procedures* are descriptions of how to carry out an activity (see Chart 11.8). They are usually written in sufficient detail to provide the information required by all persons engaging in the activity. What this means is that procedures should include a statement of purpose and who is to perform the activity. Procedures should include the steps necessary and the list of supplies and equipment that are needed. A procedure is a more specific guide to action than is a policy statement. Procedures usually are departmental or divisionally specific, so they will vary across an institution. They may be very detailed as to how to perform a specific procedure on a specific unit. They help to achieve regularity. They are a ready reference for all personnel (see Chart 11.9).

CHART 11.9
∾ PROCEDURES

- Provide step-by-step methods
- Are written in detail
- Provide guidelines for commonly occurring events
- Provide a ready reference
- Guide performance of an activity
- Should include:
  – statement of purpose
  – who performs activity
  – steps in procedure
  – list of supplies and equipment needed

The similarities and the differences between policies and procedures are that both are a means for accomplishing goals and objectives. Both are necessary for the smooth functioning of any work group or organization. The difference is that a policy is a more general guideline for decision making about actions, whereas a procedure gives directions for actions. For example, in a hospital there may be a policy about what to do if a client leaves against medical advice. The policy will most likely be a little bit different for a psychiatric unit than it would be in a general hospital. There should be a policy written as a guide for the decisions needed in recurrent and anticipated situations. For example, there may be a policy about assisting with an abortion or whether abortions are performed. A policy is a more general guide for decision making; a procedure is more like a cookbook recipe or a how-to guide giving specific directions about how to perform a certain act or function. There are legal implications to the application of policies and procedures. For example, the nurse may be held liable for failing to follow written policies and procedures. Thus it is important for nurses to be informed about policies and procedures governing practice in an institution.

LEADERSHIP AND MANAGEMENT IMPLICATIONS

Change and competition in healthcare create circumstances that may drive the need to revise an organization's or a department of nursing's philosophy. The philosophy should be a dynamic and vital values statement. Graham et al (1987) described how to implement a new or changed philosophy. They used a marketing-based perspective to transform a traditional philosophy statement into a positioning statement. Rather than merely survive, they articulated a vision and provided a framework for planning to thrive in times of change. This implies that a philosophy *may* be different from the vision in an organization. Graham et al (p. 15) set a goal of having a philosophy statement that was "unique, concise, measurable, and easy to remember." In order to accomplish this through group work, a marketing strategy called positioning was used as a basis for discussion and communication. A positioning statement about four areas of excellence was developed and integrated into all aspects of the organizational documents and nursing care processes.

Clearly the philosophy needs to be reviewed periodically and may need to be completely revised if major changes occur. This is especially true in the case

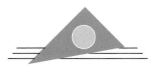 *Leadership & Management Behaviors*

LEADERSHIP BEHAVIORS	**MANAGEMENT BEHAVIORS**	**OVERLAP AREAS**
• inspires a vision that is reflected in a philosophy	• ensures that the nursing department philosophy is meshed with the organization's philosophy	• develops a philosophy, purpose and objectives
• enables followers to accomplish the purpose		• develops policies and procedures
• motivates followers to achieve objectives	• measures outcomes	
• influences the group to creatively develop the philosophy	• reviews and revises policies and procedures	
• provides personal consideration	• directs subordinates to achieve objectives	
• guides the development of policies and procedures	• monitors purpose and objectives	
	• implements the "philosophy in action"	

of a merger (Appenzeller, 1993). Normally the philosophy guides actions. However, in times of rapid change, the philosophy may require revision to reflect current practices.

Periodic review is necessary to keep a philosophy consonant with what is or should be occurring in the work environment. With a rapid pace of change, it may be easy to overlook the philosophy and mission statements. If the philosophy needs to be revised, who does this? Commitment to a philosophy of nursing is fostered by input from all members and group participation in its formulation. In one facility this process included task force selection, preparation of the task force, review of strategies to develop a philosophy, details of the process used, and presentation of the resulting document (Cody, 1990).

Brown-Stewart (1987) discussed "thinly disguised contempt," or the translation of managerial decisions into the work environment. The reality of effectiveness in a managerial role is that managers can have a tremendous impact on the work environment by virtue of their basic personality, problem solving and decision making strategies, and managerial and leadership style. When the organization's environment promotes contempt, it may impact on the availability of competent nurses. Specifically, through the strategic construction of a philosophy and culture, leaders and managers affect the morale and job satisfaction of the nurses.

Behaviors that reflect a lack of concern for people and a contempt for employees create barriers to developing excellence in organizations. Brown-Stewart (1987) listed four ways in which contempt for people is demonstrated: telling clients what they want instead of responding to the client's perceived needs, casting aspersions on or depersonalizing clients, lack of habitual courtesy, and contempt for employees. The concept of "thinly disguised contempt" is closely related to the idea of a "philosophy in action." While there are written mission statements, the implementation of these documents comes through people, especially in managerial decision making and resource allocation. Some examples of contempt behaviors are (Brown-Stewart, 1987) a consumptive as opposed to investment attitude toward employees; lack of orientation; ambiguity of mission, values, and job requirements; parking areas; physicians treated preferentially, ignoring the client's family; lack of attention to client's comfort; amount and type of nursing staff on duty; failure to communicate; and insensitivity when creating an inconvenience. Thus the leadership and management style becomes important at the interface of culture and philosophy with any individual nurse in a work environment.

One result of organizational philosophies and cultures that create barriers to quality nursing practice is that nurses manifest a sense of job dissatisfaction, feelings of frustration or powerlessness, a feeling of not being a part of the decision making process, and a feeling that supervisors are not empathetic. Since nurses as professionals work primarily as employees, tension in the relationship with the work environment results in a concern about job satisfaction, commitment, and turnover. There is an extensive literature on job satisfaction in nursing. The research on social integration, for example, indicates that nurses feel happy and more satisfied if they have a cohesive work group. Thus the philosophy and mission statements may need to be examined to see if they support work group cohesion. For example, leaders and managers can operationalize a philosophy that promotes positive resolution of conflict in work groups. Resources can be allocated to work group functioning. Philosophy statements can speak directly to valuing a positive work climate.

It is important to look at the factors in the environment that might impede the functioning of nursing and that therefore make nurses job dissatisfied, unhappy, or perhaps at risk for a high degree of turnover. Nurses feel strongly about needing job autonomy and having control over their practice. They feel they need autonomy in order to adequately meet legal requirements and clients' care needs. Generally nurses want improvements in pay, image, and working conditions (Minnick, Roberts, Curran, & Ginzberg, 1989) (see Fig. 11.3). In these three areas nurses are most concerned that there be substantial changes. The working conditions issues relate to shift work and rotation, floating, the number of weekends, job security, workload, the amount of recognition for the actual work done and the level of legal liability carried, as well as a sense of autonomy. If nurses are vested with the responsibility to carry out complex client care, then they feel the urgency to be free from interference as they make basic decisions about the care of clients that are necessary to be able to effect outcomes.

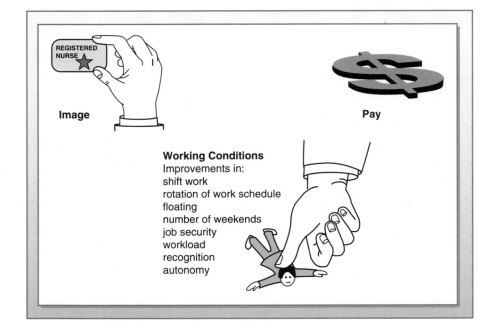

Image

Pay

Working Conditions
Improvements in:
shift work
rotation of work schedule
floating
number of weekends
job security
workload
recognition
autonomy

Figure 11.3
What nurses want. (Data from Minnick, Roberts, Curran, and Ginzberg [1989].)

McCloskey (1991) suggested that nurse leaders and managers can create and maintain an environment that facilitates the practice of the professional nurse. Leadership is required to bring out a good environment. She suggested that three elements form the basis for the creation of a positive professional work environment: fun, hope, and trouble. Nurses can use fun, hope, and trouble to support each other, stimulate creativity, and successfully work together.

Nurses are a key and critical component of the functioning of a healthcare organization. In today's environment, clients come to a hospital for nursing care. As care delivery shifts toward home and community settings, clients still seek nursing care because of needing the assessment, education, and evaluation skills of nurses. Thus, keeping a happy, stable, and satisfied nursing work force is an organizational pressure for hospitals and other healthcare organizations delivering nursing services.

The Concept of Caring

Caring is one fundamental philosophical principle of nursing. It has been described as the essence of nursing, and the visibility of caring as an important nursing concept is growing (Pepin, 1992). Caring has been defined as meaning that persons, events, projects, and things matter to an individual (Benner & Wrubel, 1988). Caring in nursing is seen as related to attention and concern for the client; responsibility for the client; and regard, fondness, or attachment to the client (Gaut, 1983). Swanson (1991, p. 162) offered the following definition of caring: "a nurturing way of relating to a valued other toward whom one feels a personal sense of commitment and responsibility." The five categories or processes of caring are (Swanson, 1991) knowing, being with, doing for, enabling, and maintaining belief.

As the basis or essence of nursing practice, caring can be seen to be a crucial component of nursing department and unit philosophy statements. It then should be explicit in the written philosophy and obvious in the "philosophy in action." Perhaps, however, not all organizations value caring. If caring is valued by an organization, then this will be reflected in decisions, resource allocations, types of power used, handling conflict, recognition of nurses as professionals, and strategies chosen to motivate nurses. Thus the philosophy of the institution provides a glimpse at the concept of caring and its intersection with leadership and management. If it is a cherished value, then the concept of caring will be incorporated into leadership styles. For example, does caring about the employees come through in the day-to-day work situation? Caring can be manifested in resource decisions about personnel, equipment, and supplies. How do organizations respond to a nursing shortage? What strategies are used when there is a need to reduce the size of the workforce? Nurses can examine the written philosophy and the obvious decision patterns to see if caring is valued and promoted in the organization.

CURRENT ISSUES AND TRENDS

In times of change, organizational philosophies, policies, and values may undergo change. What would happen if nurses were the supervisors of physicians: if physicians were employees and the nurses actually managed the work flow? There are places where nurses have admitting privileges and physicians do not. Across the country alternative systems of care delivery are being tested, and some of those systems are focused on nurse-managed centers. In some places, physicians are salaried employees of the healthcare organization. There is a persuasive argument that nurses are more cost-effective providers of primary care. In an era of fiscal constraint, there is an opportunity for nurses to redefine and reposition their roles within the healthcare delivery system. Healthcare reform processes are driving reconfigurations of care delivery systems. Mission statements and philosophies may need to change in response.

Positive job motivation is an important element in the functioning of human service organizations. It could be assumed that job satisfaction should follow from an environment in which each person's expertise is acknowledged and respected, and nurses go home at the end of their shift feeling good about their work. Thus the influence of philosophy on organizational culture and values may be more visible if it is practiced as well as being written.

One example of how hospitals have been examined in terms of effectiveness is in their recruitment and retention record as analyzed in the Magnet Hospital Study of McClure et al (1982). They discovered that managers, the work culture, and the work environment made a difference in nurse recruitment and retention. Three common elements emerged in terms of successful organizations that nurses like and stay at (Mallison, 1982):

- *management commitment to nursing and nurses:* there has to be evidence that the management of the organization is committed to nursing and nurses.
- *strong nursing leadership:* the goal is to find strong nurse leaders with good academic and experiential backgrounds, good problem solving skills, and facilitative interpersonal styles.
- *competitive salaries and benefits:* being paid well and having good benefits is an important attractor and retainer.

This work has been updated by Kramer (1990) and Kramer and Schmalenberg (1988a, 1988b), who did a comparative analysis of a nationally representative subset of the original 41 magnet hospitals (N = 16). The hospitals were visited and studied. Magnet hospitals evidenced a valuing of quality of care and excellence. Caring and quality values were pervasive and deliberately promoted. Further, caring about the nurses was exhibited. Emphasis on quality built up the hospital's reputation in the community. The hospital environments supported autonomy and innovation, risk taking, and decreased bureaucratic rules. Thus they created conditions conducive to excellence, positive work environment, and decreased nurse shortage.

SUMMARY

- An organization is a group acting to achieve a goal.
- The two dimensions of a social system are the environment and the individual.
- Behavior in organizations is a function of the dynamic interaction of these two dimensions.
- Service industries, like nursing and healthcare, emphasize quality and cost control.
- The three main parts of a mission statement are the philosophy, purpose, and objectives statements.
- Policies and procedures are two functional elements of an organization that flow from the mission statements and help to guide decision making and performance.
- Organizational philosophies impact on nursing practice through elements related to culture, job satisfaction, and turnover.
- Philosophies may need to be revised as circumstances change.

Study Questions

1. How do previous employee experiences color perception and attitude? Why do these perceptions linger?
2. Do nurses profess loyalty to the organization/job or to the profession/work of nursing? Can an individual have both?
3. How do you use the change process to implement a new philosophy in a pre-established work group?
4. What is the "philosophy in action"? Cite some examples. Describe why this makes a difference.
5. What problems are solved by having policies and procedures?
6. What decisions can nurses make without a written policy?

Critical Thinking Exercise

Nurse Nathan Lyzotte believes in order and efficiency. He is known for his ability to complete his nursing care tasks in record time, chart, and complete a shift's work before the oncoming shift arrives. His motto is organize, organize, organize. He views most nurses as disorganized and inefficient. Recently he has approached his nurse manager to discuss some frustrations he has encountered in practice. For example, he disagrees with the extension of visiting hours into the late evening. Some patients want to take their medicines from home. He is feeling irritated at telephone and call light interruptions, especially about the cold coffee and lack of diverse menu selections.

1. *Is there a problem?*

2. *What is the problem?*

3. *Whose problem is it?*

4. *What should the nurse manager do?*

5. *What interactions should have occurred prior to this point?*

6. *Whose philosophy is in operation in this situation?*

7. *Is there a clash of philosophies?*

8. *If so, how should they be resolved?*

REFERENCES

Appenzeller, L. (1993). Merging nursing departments: An experience. *Journal of Nursing Administration, 23*(12), 55-60.

Benner, P., & Wrubel, J. (1988). Caring comes first. *American Journal of Nursing, 88*(8), 1072-1075.

Brown-Stewart, P. (1987). Thinly disguised contempt: A barrier to excellence. *Journal of Nursing Administration, 17*(4), 14-18.

Drucker, P. (1973). *Management: Tasks, responsibilities, practices.* New York: Harper & Row.

Gaut, D. (1983). Development of a theoretically adequate description of caring. *Western Journal of Nursing Research, 5,* 313-324.

Getzels, J. (1958). Administration as a social process. In A. Halpin (Ed.), *Administrative theory in education* (pp. 150-165). Chicago: University of Chicago Press.

Graham, P., Constantini, S., Balik, B., Bedore, B., Hooke, M., Papin, D., Quamme, M., & Rivard, R. (1987). Operationalizing a nursing philosophy. *Journal of Nursing Administration, 17*(3), 14-18.

Kramer, M. (1974). *Reality shock: Why nurses leave nursing.* St. Louis: C.V. Mosby Company.

Kramer, M. (1990). The magnet hospitals: Excellence revisited. *Journal of Nursing Administration, 20*(9), 35-44.

Kramer, M., & Schmalenberg, C. (1988a). Magnet hospitals: Institutions of excellence: Part 1. *Journal of Nursing Administration, 18*(1), 13-24.

Kramer, M., & Schmalenberg, C. (1988b). Magnet hospitals: Institutions of excellence: Part 2. *Journal of Nursing Administration, 18*(2), 11-19.

Mallison, M. (1989). Hospitals that succeed with nurses. *American Journal of Nursing, 89*(3), 313.

Martin, L., & Hughes, S. (1993). Using the mission statement to craft a least-restraint policy. *Nursing Management (long-term care edition), 24*(3), 65-66.

McCloskey, J. (1991). Creating an environment for success with fun, hope, and trouble. *Journal of Nursing Administration, 21*(4), 5-6.

McClure, M., Poulin, M., Sovie, M., & Wandelt, M. (1983). *Magnet hospitals: Attraction and retention of professional nurses.* Kansas City, MO: American Nurses Association.

Minnick, A., Roberts, M., Curran, C., & Ginzberg, E. (1989). What do nurses want? Priorities for action. *Nursing Outlook, 37,* 214-218.

Pepin, J. (1992). Family caring and caring in nursing. *Image, 24*(2), 127-131.

Poteet, G., & Hill, A. (1988). Identifying the components of a nursing service philosophy. *Journal of Nursing Administration, 18*(10), 29-33.

Swanson, K. (1991). Empirical development of a middle range theory of caring. *Nursing Research, 40*(3), 161-166.

Trexler, B. (1987). Nursing department purpose, philosophy, and objectives: Their use and effectiveness. *Journal of Nursing Administration, 17*(3), 8-12.

Veninga, R. (1982). *The human side of health administration: A guide for hospital, nursing, and public health administrators.* Englewood Cliffs, NJ: Prentice-Hall.

Zander, K. (1992). Nursing care delivery methods and quality. *Series on Nursing Administration, 3,* 86-104.

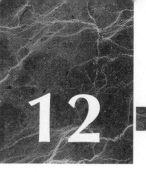

12

Organizational Structure: Concepts

Chapter Objectives

∽

explain what an administrative structure organizes

∽

define and describe organizational structure

∽

describe four classic foundations of organizational theory

∽

distinguish among four major influences on structure

∽

compare coordinating mechanisms

∽

analyze authority, responsibility, and accountability

∽

compare centralization/decentralization

∽

analyze current trends in restructuring

∽

exercise critical thinking to conceptualize and analyze
possible solutions to a practical experience incident

*a*n organization exists for the purpose of achieving some goal or a set of
goals. For example, in healthcare the obvious goals might be the reduction of cost, increased efficiency, and higher quality of care. The general goal of
nursing might be defined as the delivery of a service that is caring, high quality,
and cost-effective. Yet whether this goal is realized or not may depend heavily

on the decisions made by people in an organization. The structure of an organization is one important variable affecting nursing practice. Exploring organizations means examining their structures as well as their patterns of functioning.

How nurses' roles intermix with the structure of the organization influences the accomplishment of organizational goals. An organizational structure configures the work, power, and control elements within an institution. The core elements of organizational theory address these work, power, and control variables. Power, authority, and control relate to the way people are motivated to accomplish the work tasks. Power and how power is used are interrelated with work structuring, as well as being associated with how organizations are structured, how to control and motivate people to accomplish tasks, and how to maintain a sense of order and goal accomplishment.

One of the four ways of viewing organizations, identified in Chapter 10, is the structural perspective. The structural point of view focuses on the importance of the structure of an organization, with its formal roles and relationships. The concept of the fit of the structure to the environment and technology is emphasized in this viewpoint (Bolman & Deal, 1984; del Bueno & Freund, 1986).

DEFINITIONS

CHART 12.1
∾ DEFINITION

Structure of an Organization
the sum total of the ways its labor is divided into distinct tasks and then the way coordination is achieved among these tasks.

The *structure of an organization* is defined as the sum total of the ways its labor is divided into distinct tasks and then coordination is achieved among these tasks (see Chart 12.1). Structure is a by-product of two fundamental and opposing needs of every organized human activity: to divide the labor into the specific tasks to be performed and to coordinate these tasks to accomplish the activity or goal. The elements of structure should be selected to achieve internal consistency and consistency with the external environment. Factors of size, age, technical systems used, and environment in which the organization functions are important in considering the structural design of an organization (Mintzberg, 1983). In general, organizational structure refers to the mechanisms developed to balance specialization of work roles with a sufficient amount of coordination in order to accomplish tasks and goals (Mark, 1989) (see Fig. 12.1).

A structure in an organization is built as a way to accomplish goals. People either work within an organization or as a solo individual. Most nurses work within an organizational structure and as employees of an organization. This structure gives the system some kind of order, distinction, and framework. The purpose of structure is to control variations in behavior among individuals, avoid chaos, direct the flow of information, determine the positions, and provide some orderliness to the flow of work.

Structure is the established pattern of relationships among the component parts of the organization. The structure is comprised of both the formal orga-

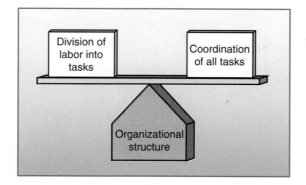

Figure 12.1
Organizational structure.

nization and the informal organization. The formal organization is the structure that can be seen on an organizational chart. It is the planned structure. It is a deliberate attempt to lay out a patterned relationship among the parts within the system. The formal structure is the result of explicit decision making. The informal structure is more often thought of as the "grapevine," or the network of informal social relationships outside the formal structure.

One way to view structure is to think of it as a gating mechanism or interface. Structure, then, is the linkage or network between the outer environment and the organization as a system. It is a binding element. It provides for internal integration. It is like a glue that helps the parts of an organization adhere together so that they can work toward their goals. In healthcare organizations, structure is an interface between the clients and the staff (see Fig. 12.2).

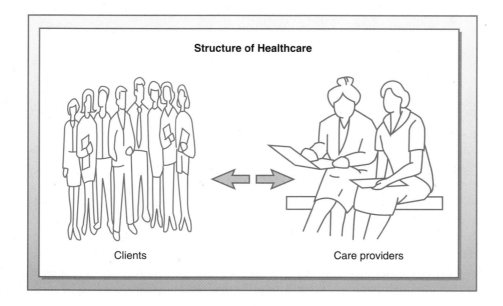

Figure 12.2
Structure as an interface.

RESEARCH NOTE

Source: Strasen, L. (1994). Reengineering hospitals using the "function follows form" model. *Journal of Nursing Administration, 24*(12), 59-63.

Purpose

The purpose of this article is to describe the development and outcomes of a "function follows form" model for consultants to use to assist hospitals to reengineer their operations. Organizational reengineering is a hot topic. The favored model uses a "form follows function" process, where tasks and activities are assessed, evaluated, and redesigned to reduce inefficiencies, costs, and poor quality of service. New functions and roles then determine the structure (form) of the organization.

Discussion

Kubler-Ross's loss model from the death and dying literature was used to understand and work with employees' predictable reactions to a major organizational change in structure and roles. After observing that "form follows function" was not the most effective way to reengineer the work of professionals because of issues related to professional role socialization, it was decided to use a reversal of form/function. A "function follows form" model resulted. This model shortens the reengineering time frame, focuses on cross-training and streamlining documentation, moves employees through the loss process, and documents financial outcomes. The outcomes in three facilities that used this approach were reported.

Application to Practice

This "function follows form" model requires strong and visible leaders. A high level of interpersonal and conceptual skills are required. The process can be threatening in so far as changes in the structure of the organization force nurses and nurse managers to change the way they function at work. Some do not want to make a transition. The author documents costs savings recouped through implementation of the new model. The model also incorporates humanistic elements of employee assistance with coping with loss triggered by changing the organizational structure. Thus the "function follows form" model may be better suited to nursing practice.

BACKGROUND

In organizational theory, the concept of management is associated with structure. Structure includes the elements of division of labor, hierarchy of authority, rules and regulations that govern behavior, span of control, and lines of communication. It is thought that by using the classic foundations of organizational theory—division of labor, span of control, scalar process, and line and staff—any human undertaking can be managed and organized.

Division of labor is one of the classic elements of management (see Chart 12.2). Because managers cannot complete the work by themselves, the job is broken up into pieces and assigned as responsibilities to others. In nursing this is described as *delegation. Span of control,* the number of subordinates any one manager can manage, is limited. In nursing this would be the number of staff nurses and non-nurse nursing personnel reporting to a nurse manager (Pabst, 1993). The *scalar process* is the creation of levels in an organization, or the direct line of command from top to bottom. In nursing, a hierarchical bureaucracy creates layers of positions with differing amounts of power attached to them. *Line and staff* are concepts that refer to the ordering of positions according to mission centrality. Line positions are in the direct line of hierarchical authority that is arrayed from top to bottom in an organization. Line positions are central to producing the product of the organization. Staff positions are outside of the direct hierarchical authority chain. Staff positions provide expertise and knowledge to assist the line positions in meeting the organization's goals. The whole purpose of an organization and the management structure behind it is to convey the vision of the top person all the way down to the bottom, thereby accomplishing work through others.

Influences on Structure

There are four major influences on structure: technology, the social environment, size, and the repetitiveness of the tasks (Mintzberg, 1983). Structures can be highly influenced by the nature of the technology. For example, within nursing and the healthcare system, technology such as computerization, all of the equipment in ICUs, the vast array of monitors and pumps, and technological devices that are used to deliver nursing care can and do affect the type of structure that might be effective for nursing.

Like the nature of the technology, the character of the social environment will impact on a specific organization and most likely require some changes in the structure. For example, today U.S. healthcare is affected by trends in which consumers are active and concerned. Further, social change in the larger environment creates financial, psychological, and care delivery implications and drives change. Also, generational demographics and age cohorts like the "baby boomers" influence both national financial and political structures as well as healthcare delivery.

The size of the organization and how repetitive the work tasks are further influence structure. There is a different type of structure that works in manufacturing firms such as automobile assembly plants, as compared to the work of nurses in healthcare. In general, larger organizations are slower to make decisions and more complex to manage. This is partially a function of the greater number of interpersonal interactions that occur.

Organizations generally appear to show evidence of a life cycle or growth and development changes that occur in spurts and are associated with changes in

---

CHART 12.2
❧ DEFINITIONS

Division of Labor
the work is broken up into pieces or tasks, then assigned.

Span of Control
the number of workers supervised by a manager.

Scalar Process
the creation of levels of authority in a hierarchy.

Line and Staff
the array of positions into direct producers and support positions.

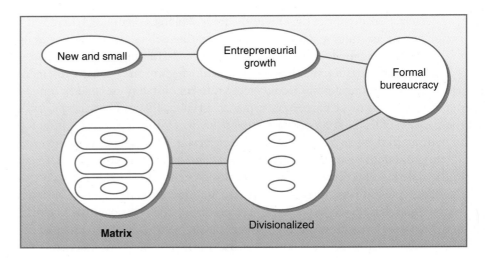

Figure 12.3
Organizational life cycle.
(Data from Mintzberg
[1983].)

structure. New organizations start out small, with an organic and nonelaborated structure. As they begin to grow, they shift to an entrepreneurial stage with a powerful chief executive and coordination by direct supervision. Further growth brings a more formalized structure and the eventual shift to a bureaucratic structure and coordination by standardization. As still further growth and aging occur, organizations may split into divisionalized structures that overlay the functional bureaucratic structure. Finally, a matrix structure may develop to rise above the divisionalization and partially create a regression back toward a more organic structural form (see Fig. 12.3). A number of forces influence this process, for example, complexity, technical sophistication, stability, competition, hostile environments, and external control (Mintzberg, 1983).

Types of Structures

The elements of structural design and the situational factors faced by organizations cluster into configurations. There are five basic types of structural design: (1) the simple structure, (2) machine bureaucracy, (3) professional bureaucracy, (4) divisionalized form, and (5) adhocracy (Mintzberg, 1983). These will be explored further in Chapter 13.

In designing organizational structures, the division of labor occurs largely in relationship to the job to be done and the technical system available. Coordination of tasks and jobs is more complex, involving both control and communication. Coordination is the element of "glue" holding organizations together. There are five basic coordinating mechanisms or ways in which organizations coordinate their work: mutual adjustment, direct supervision, standardization of work processes, standardization of work outputs, and standardization of workers' skills (Mintzberg, 1983).

- *Mutual adjustment* coordinates work through simple informal communication. In nursing, mutual adjustment occurs when one nurse consults another nurse about practice issues such as how to interpret a policy.
- *Direct supervision* coordinates work through the use of a supervisor taking responsibility for the instruction and monitoring of the work of others. In nursing, direct supervision occurs when a nurse supervises the work of unlicensed assistive personnel.
- *Standardization of work processes* coordinates work through specifying or programming content before the work is undertaken. In nursing, standardization of work processes occurs when nurses use standardized critical paths or plans of care.
- *Standardization of work outputs* coordinates work through the specification, before the work is undertaken, of the results, product, or performance desired/expected. In nursing, standardization of work outputs occurs when care is specified as outcome objectives.
- *Standardization of worker skills* coordinates work by specifying the kind of training or education required to perform the work. It is a more indirect way to control or coordinate work. In nursing, the standardization of worker skills occurs for Advanced Practice Nurses when a Master's degree is required or certification is mandated.

It is thought that as work becomes more complex, the means of coordination shifts from mutual adjustment to direct supervision, and then to standardization, preferably of work processes, otherwise of outputs or skills. In highly complex environments, coordination may revert back to mutual adjustment (Mintzberg, 1983).

Essentially, there is no one right way to structure; there is no one ideal structure. This means that there is no one absolute answer to the question, what is the best way to structure? Structure depends upon a number of variables and their combinations, such as the environment and the nature of the work to be done (Mark, 1989). There are different structural types. When faced with a situation of low organizational effectiveness, one strategy is to examine the structure and determine if that structure has to change to better fit the situation or a changed environment.

Positions, Authority, Responsibility, and Accountability

Structure establishes patterns of authority and collegiality. The pattern results in roles that are played in an organization. For example, there are top level managers, middle managers, and workers in a pyramidal pattern typical of a bureaucracy. This means that the structure takes the shape of a pyramid. Bureaucracies tend to assume a pyramidal shape. In a bureaucracy, there is a controlling or policy making body at the top of the structure, usually called a

Board. The primary function of a Board is to control fiscal resources and make policy. A Chief Executive Officer (CEO) manages the organization and reports to the Board. Then there are successively larger layers of managers in the middle. At the bottom is a broad base of workers who implement the work tasks. For nursing, it is important to identify the Board of Trustees or Directors and determine what duties they fulfill. Generally these are overall organizational policy making decisions and fiscal oversight. Through such policy decisions, nursing practice will be impacted. Nurses need to know and influence the top executive officers with their insights into issues of access, quality, and costs. The first-line nursing manager's role is to be an interface or linking pin between the executive level and the individual nurses. At this level, policies and decisions move into actual implementation.

Within organizational structures there are identified positions with attached titles. A *position* is defined as a collection of tasks that are configured together for performance, usually by one individual (see Chart 12.3). For example, nurse manager, assistant nurse manager, and staff nurse are organizational positions, each with a job description. Each job on the organizational chart is a certain position that carries a predetermined degree of authority, accountability, and responsibility.

Authority is defined as the right to act or to command the actions of others (see Chart 12.3). It includes the power to issue instructions for others to follow. Authority is granted by a boss to a subordinate. It is based on position and flows down the hierarchical organizational chain. Because of being in a position in an organization, each job contains a certain amount of authority to command the actions of others. It then is the responsibility of the occupant of the position to utilize the authority granted (Callahan & Wall, 1987; Scanlan & Keys, 1979). Authority involves power and its use (Manthey, 1989).

Schmieding (1992) differentiated between organizational authority and professional authority. Organizational authority for nurses is the responsibility to fulfill the professional role with the specific job or management position. Professional authority is the right to practice professional nursing. This distinction sometimes is associated with line or position power and staff or expertise power.

Responsibility is defined as the allocation and acceptance of a task. Thus responsibility is an obligation for oneself and for the completion of tasks. It means that there is a certain amount of obligation for the self in each position, as well as for subordinates. Responsibility is the obligation to take on and accomplish work. It denotes an obligation to secure the desired results. It also is assigned or delegated by a boss to a subordinate and thus flows down the organizational chain. Responsibility must be accepted by each person who fulfills a position. The power to command is meaningless unless the subordinate accepts the obligations of the assignment or acts to accept the responsibility to complete the assigned task (Callahan & Wall, 1987; Scanlan & Keys, 1979). Re-

CHART 12.3
∾ DEFINITIONS

Position
a collection of tasks that are configured together for performance, usually by one individual.

Authority
the right to act or command the actions of others.

Responsibility
allocation and acceptance of a task.

Accountability
the liability for task performance.

sponsibility means the ability to respond and refers to both the allocation and acceptance of responsibility for a task or function (Manthey, 1989).

Accountability denotes liability and is defined as the liability for task performance. It is created by the assignment of responsibility and the grant of authority. It means that the subordinate is answerable and liable to the superior for the quality and quantity of the assigned task. Accountability flows upward from the subordinate to the boss (Callahan & Wall, 1987; Scanlan & Keys, 1979). It is the concept of "the buck stops here." Accountability is a retrospective analysis of what occurred in order to determine if what occurred was appropriate in the situation (Manthey, 1989).

Each nurse is accountable, answerable, or liable for their own actions, the completion of the assigned task, and their acts of delegation. Each nurse is accountable to the boss and clients. Accountability is the one element that cannot be delegated. If the responsibility is great, so is the accountability. Upon taking a job, the nurse accepts the authority and the responsibility for the position. For example, as a staff nurse, the nurse accepts the authority to perform client care within the scope of the practice of a staff nurse in that organization and accepts the responsibility for completing that assigned task.

It is important that organizations match the authority to the responsibility. Nurses may be responsible for accomplishing the work but not be given the corresponding authority to carry out the job. For example, nurses carry legal liability for the quality and safety of care delivery to clients. However, if staff mix and numbers available are decided based on financial pressures without nursing input or recourse, nurses may be liable for care, yet be without sufficient caregivers to carry out the care needs. While there is some room for argument about what is "adequate numbers" of staff, clearly there is a point where clients' safety is in jeopardy because no nurse is physically available. Nurses may face similar dilemmas with any resource constraint, such as available equipment. Suggestions for avoiding the mismatch of authority to responsibility include clear and explicit communication. This may need to be coupled with negotiation strategies. One useful technique is responsibility charting: a structured process for documenting and visualizing how each member will participate in a set of decisions (Gilmore & Peter, 1987).

Accountability relates to legal aspects and parameters of the practice of a registered nurse. As a part of the role, the professional nurse is assumed to be a manager and supervisor because there are ancillary workers whom the nurse delegates to and supervises. Leadership and management skills thus become a useful supplement to clinical psychomotor skills. Further, RNs are obligated to understand the reality of practice within the parameters of the legal definition of nursing practice. Some resources include The Code for Nurses, state laws and administrative rules, and literature from state nurses' associations about RNs' supervisory and managerial accountability.

Centralization/Decentralization of Power

Organizational structuring overlaps with the concept of power. The question is how is power flowing around the organization? Power can be centralized or decentralized. Centralized/decentralized refers to the structure and the way that power is dispersed throughout the organization (see Chart 12.4).

Centralized means that the power to make decisions is concentrated at the top of the organization and flows down. The person at the top has power by position and uses the power to make decisions. There are advantages to centralized organizations, although nurses do not like them very well. When the organization is facing a serious threat, like an imminent fiscal crisis, a centralized structure works the best because there is not time for participative deliberation or to make consultative decisions. The leader has to make decisions and face the threat.

Decentralized means that power filters down toward the bottom level. At the individual worker level, people may be empowered: given the authority, responsibility, and autonomy to make decisions about the work and the work processes. With decentralization, decision making is diffused down to the lower organizational levels. Decentralized means that the power is delegated down, but that power delegation may or may not be to the lowest levels. The power actually may settle in reality at the middle level and not "trickle down."

Decentralized structures work the best when organizations are trying to improve quality and cut down costs as a long-term strategy because the people at the worker level know the work and can provide input about what works best, if given the skills and ability to make decisions. If empowered to make decisions and do the work the way they know will work the best for the client, the whole organization may become more cost efficient. The result is a higher quality product, in this case client care.

LEADERSHIP AND MANAGEMENT IMPLICATIONS

Leadership in nursing can occur in any group. Management, however, is a process and function specifically more associated with organizations. Both leaders and managers need in-depth knowledge of the organizations in which they function. Taking the structural perspective, an organization and its structure can be analyzed. Leaders and managers can influence the structure in which goals are accomplished. In nursing, determining the structure is a planning and organizing aspect of the management process. As the environment changes, the manager may need to re-think the structure and decide if a change needs to be made to better match the structure to the work group and its changing environment.

Structure is a managerial decision. For nurses, the results of decision making about structure have a direct impact on the work of nursing by setting pa-

---

CHART 12.4
∾ DEFINITIONS

Centralization
power to make decisions concentrated at the top of the organization.

Decentralization
power to make decisions filtered down toward the individual worker.

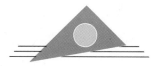

Leadership & Management Behaviors

LEADERSHIP BEHAVIORS	**MANAGEMENT BEHAVIORS**	**OVERLAP AREAS**
• develops a vision of a structure to further group goals	• develops an organizational chart	• develops the structure
• models the acceptance and use of decentralized power	• plans for restructuring to match environmental conditions	• influences people to work within a structure
• inspires the group to restructure when necessary	• decides on line and staff positions	
• influences the design of the structure	• delegates tasks	
• enables followers to function within a structure	• provides authority to match responsibility	
	• monitors accountability	
	• influences the implementation of the structure	

rameters on physical work space, amount and type of equipment and support services, workload demands, and limits on autonomy. Job structure is one of the organizational factors influencing nursing's work and work excitement (Simms, Erbin-Roesemann, Darga, & Coeling, 1990).

Structure becomes a central focus for managerial strategies when the environment is turbulent. It is thought that modern healthcare cannot be delivered efficiently and effectively using classic hierarchical bureaucratic organizations. Frustration is caused by trying to force contemporary outcomes such as collaborative interdisciplinary teams for cost containment from organizational designs and structures geared toward different purposes. Thus the structure has to change or be restructured or reengineered.

Because of the turbulent environment in healthcare and the rapid change of advancing technology and environmental conditions in society, decentralized structures are considered to be the structures that are going to work the best for nursing. The reason is because the flattened structure and a minimum of layers gives nurses job-related decision authority (Manthey, 1989). Decision autonomy has been equated with professionalism and job satisfaction, although some research indicates that nurses vary in their preferences for decision making autonomy (Dwyer, Schwartz, & Fox, 1992). Nurses need to be developed toward the knowledge and expertise level of mature workers, so that they are well prepared for client care decision authority.

Leaders and managers also will be involved in revising or changing organizational structures. Restructuring means revising or modifying the structure to reshape it or switch to another structural type. Restructuring efforts typically have been geared toward fixing existing operational processes. Tasks are examined and reconfigured. Reengineering is considered to be a more radical process of re-thinking the operational processes. In order to begin anew, the processes are analyzed from the point of view of what is needed by the customer and to achieve greater cost containment, quality, service, and speed. Thus reengineering is called a radical redesign of business processes (Hammer & Champy, 1993; Moss, Eagen, & Russell, 1994). Curtin (1994) differentiated job redesign from restructuring and reengineering. Job redesign focuses on who does what tasks. Flexibility, cross-training, and productivity become key ideas. Restructuring focuses on the architecture of an organization. Lean, decentralized, self-governing organizations that empower first line caregivers are preferred structures to evolve and emerge. Reengineering focuses on renovating the processes used to accomplish goals. User friendly processes, efficiency, and economy become key ideas.

Curtin (1994) developed a differentiation between what works and what does not work for nursing and clients. What works are restructuring to nurse case management, reengineering to implement critical paths, physician-nurse collaboration, cross-training, and moving services to the community. What does not work are poor communication, diminished morale, low staffing, high mix of assistive personnel to supervise, and replacing RNs with less prepared substitutes. Nurses will need to educate themselves about these structures and process changes and analyze how organizational structures facilitate or impede nursing care delivery. Leaders and managers will need to make strategic decisions about structures and what works for nursing.

CURRENT ISSUES AND TRENDS

Part of the current swirl of changes in hospitals and healthcare organizations includes changing organizational structures to decentralize, drawing new organizational charts, and instituting collaborative teams to reform bureaucracies and create a structure within an organization to utilize workers of multiple skill levels. The idea is that flattened, decentralized, highly empowered-at-the-bottom structures will make a difference in terms of effectiveness. Related terms and concepts are case management, use of nurse extenders, professional practice models, contractual models and alternative structures, shared governance, product line management, and total quality management (see Chapters 13 to 16). What these "new" management ideas really are implying is restructuring in some manner or form.

Beyond restructuring and reengineering is a current trend in healthcare to integrate different types of organizations across the continuum of care. The idea is for clients to move along the health-illness continuum across settings and sites of care delivery without fragmentation of service delivery. This means coordinating care, a role ideally suited to nurses. From the client's perspective, a continuum of care exists but has not been seamless. Care is not viewed as a total experience or managed as an ongoing process instead of as an episode needing medical intervention. In fragmented parts, care becomes costly, uncoordinated, and fraught with duplicated effort. Frustrations arise from the effects of fragmentation (Lumsdon, 1994).

Consumer and payor frustration with rising cost burdens in healthcare began to drive managed care initiatives. Managed care initiatives began to drive care coordination and a re-examination and transformation of the organizational structures in healthcare delivery. New structures emerged. Parts of the healthcare delivery system began to align into integrated systems as the reimbursement incentives began to change from "patient days" to "covered lives." In this process, traditional organizational structures that were vertical and hierarchical began to give way to new structures that were horizontal and organized around processes rather than tasks (Moss, Eagen, & Russell, 1994).

The challenges for nursing in the restructured, reengineered, new organizational structures are many and extensive. Organizational cultures may facilitate or impede nursing's work and the need for nurses to change as the environment changes. For example, the organizational culture may or may not support a seamless continuum of care. Nurses will need to learn new behaviors and new strategies for working across an organization that owns different types of care agencies. The most proactive stance for nursing is to seize the opportunities inherent in nurses' natural care coordination role, reconfigure organizational structures to match care delivery needs and the environment, and advocate for those elements of "what works" for nursing and for clients.

RESEARCH NOTE

Source: Moss, M., Eagen, M., & Russell, M. (1994). Service integration in the reform era. *Nursing Economic$, 12*(5), 256-260, 286.

Purpose

The purpose of this article was to discuss the redesign of care delivery processes, or reengineering, in one southern United States hospital's perioperative services. Healthcare reform efforts initially were predicated on "fixing up" restructuring efforts. Now actions are focused on restructuring via reengineering and drastic reshaping of organizational structures. Change is painful. Major transformations of organizational cultures are required in order to change systems and manage in new ways.

Discussion

After major steps were taken to reduce costs in one perioperative service, further cost reductions were again requested. As traditional cost cutting measures were exhausted, reengineering of the perioperative services was needed. Phase 1 began with an analysis. The core process was identified. Three departments merged into one integrated team. The change required a meshing of skill mix, quality control, and materials management. Many different strategies of collaboration were employed. The redesign was labeled "integration," and it resulted in a new multidepartmental team that operated like a company called Perioperative Services.

Application to Practice

Risk taking is basic to reorganization. Change creates a sense of loss. Leaders and managers can promote acceptance by reshaping perceptions, positive and open communication, and intensive education of staff. Policies of shared leadership and empowerment promote involvement in decision making and commitment. Change, while seen as painful, also can be exhilarating and an opportunity to grow.

SUMMARY

- Organizational structure is built to accomplish goals.
- Structure organizes work, power, and control elements.
- Structure is a binding and integrating element, an interface.
- Structure creates order by establishing a framework and pattern of relationships.
- Division of labor, span of control, scalar processes, and line and staff are the classic management structure elements.
- Technology, environment, size, and task repetitiveness influence structure.
- The simple structure, machine bureaucracy, professional bureaucracy, divisionalized form, and adhocracy are the five types of structural designs.
- There is no one right way to structure.
- Organizational positions carry authority, accountability, and responsibility.
- Power can be structurally centralized or decentralized.
- Healthcare is undergoing a turbulent era of restructuring and reengineering.

Study Questions

1. What purposes for nursing does the structure of an organization serve?
2. What elements of organizational structure are found in nursing organizations?
3. What elements are most important for nursing practice?
4. How are the structures of community agencies the same as or different from hospitals?
5. What coordinating mechanisms are used in nursing and healthcare organizations?

6. How effective are the coordinating mechanisms used by nursing?
7. How have authority, responsibility, and accountability been used in nursing practice? What feelings do they create?
8. Is power in nursing centralized or decentralized?

Critical Thinking Exercise

Kory Danielson is an Emergency Department staff RN. One day a 66-year-old indigent male patient is brought in complaining of crushing chest pain. Nurse Danielson assesses the patient on arrival and documents his assessment on the standard forms. The physician diagnoses gastroenteritis and tells Nurse Danielson to send the patient home. Nurse Danielson is very uncomfortable with the physician's medical diagnosis and discharge decision without further testing. He tries to decide if he should tell the physician he disagrees, report his concern to his nurse manager, or just chart his disagreement.

1. Is there a problem?

2. What is the problem?

3. What should Nurse Danielson have done?

4. What was Nurse Danielson's authority, responsibility, and accountability?

5. What interaction(s) should have occurred between Nurse Danielson and the physician?

6. What other interactions should Nurse Danielson initiate?

7. What elements of organizational structure could be helpful in this situation? Which could be barriers?

8. Is Nurse Danielson in administrative or legal jeopardy?

REFERENCES

Bolman, L., & Deal, T. (1984). *Modern approaches to understanding and managing organizations*. San Francisco: Jossey-Bass.

Callahan, C., & Wall, L. (1987). Participative management: A contingency approach. *Journal of Nursing Administration*, 17(9), 9-15.

Curtin, L. (1994). Restructuring: What works and what does not! *Nursing Management*, 25(10), 7-8.

del Bueno, D., & Freund, C. (1986). *Power and politics in nursing: A casebook*. Owings Mills, MD: National Health Publishing.

Dwyer, D., Schwartz, R., & Fox, M. (1992). Decision-making autonomy in nursing. *Journal of Nursing Administration*, 22(2), 17-23.

Gilmore, T., & Peter, M. (1987). Managing complexity in health care settings. *Journal of Nursing Administration*, 17(1), 11-18.

Hammer, M., & Champy, J. (1993). *Reengineering the corporation: A manifesto for business revolution*. New York: HarperCollins.

Lumsdon, K. (1994). Crash course: Piecing together the continuum of care. *Hospitals & Health Networks, 68*(22), 26-28.

Manthey, M. (1989). Control over practice: Who owns it? *Nursing Management, 20*(7), 14-16.

Mark, B. (1989). Structural contingency theory. In B. Henry, C. Arndt, M. Di Vincenti, & A. Marriner-Tomey (Eds.), *Dimensions of Nursing Administration: Theory, research, education, practice* (pp. 175-182). Boston: Blackwell.

Mintzberg, H. (1983). *Structure in fives: Designing effective organizations*. Englewood Cliffs, NJ: Prentice-Hall.

Moss, M., Eagen, M., & Russell, M. (1994). Service integration in the reform era. *Nursing Economic$, 12*(5), 256-260, 286.

Pabst, M. (1993). Span of control on nursing inpatient units. *Nursing Economic$, 11*(2), 87-90.

Scanlan, B., & Keys, J.B. (1979). *Management and organizational behavior*. New York: John Wiley & Sons.

Schmieding, N. (1992). The complexity of an authority role. *Nursing Management, 23*(1), 57-58.

Simms, L., Erbin-Roesemann, M., Darga, A., & Coeling, H. (1990). Breaking the burnout barrier: Resurrecting work excitement in nursing. *Nursing Economic$, 8*(3), 177-187.

Organizational Structure: Types

Chapter Objectives

ↂ

explain the three common types of organizational structures
found in healthcare organizations

ↂ

define and differentiate among bureaucracy, matrix, and adhocracy

ↂ

explain and compare the five basic parts of an organization

ↂ

define five basic organizational types

ↂ

compare the five basic organizational types

ↂ

analyze organizational types best suited to nursing

ↂ

define and analyze an organizational chart

ↂ

exercise critical thinking to conceptualize and analyze
possible solutions to a practical experience incident

*h*ealthcare is a service industry segment of the U. S. economy that had been largely outside of the private business sector. Business and manufacturing firms in the private sector have been the template for most business management theory. Because of this, and because healthcare systems appear to have some characteristics which differentiate them from the private sector, it is necessary to analyze the private sector template for adjustments which are indicated before use in the healthcare domain. Healthcare delivery systems, as a subset of all organizations, traditionally have utilized one of three basic types of administrative

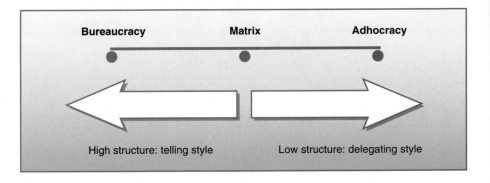

Figure 13.1
Continuum of
organizational structures.

organizational structure: bureaucracy, matrix, or adhocracy. These three types of structures can be thought of as fitting across a continuum from a telling-oriented organization, the classical bureaucracy, on one end; to the other end of a highly delegating organization that uses sophisticated specialists, called an adhocracy (see Fig. 13.1). Thus an organization's administrative structure can be assessed, analyzed, and identified. For example, in the U. S. most hospitals adopted a classic hierarchical bureaucratic form. Some, faced with the need to better utilize and reward highly trained professional staff, evolved a matrix structure. Some physicians' office practices, however, used an adhocracy to structure their work. As healthcare reform drives restructuring and reengineering efforts, administrative organizational structures will need to change.

DEFINITIONS

Administrative organizational structures are formal structures adopted and used by organizations to organize and direct the flow of work and activity and to define the relationships among the parts of an organization (Mintzberg, 1983). There are three basic types:

A *bureaucracy* is defined as an administrative organizational structure that is pyramidal, hierarchical, and centralized.

A *matrix* is defined as an administrative organizational structure that is a complex combination or an interweaving of a bureaucratic structure with an adhocracy or project team component.

An *adhocracy* is defined as an administrative organizational structure that is flat, decentralized, and uses ad hoc committees or project teams to produce the work of the organization.

BACKGROUND

Hierarchical Bureaucratic Structures

The first basic type of organizational structure is the *classic hierarchical bureaucracy* (see Fig. 13.2). The ancient Roman army under Julius Caesar and

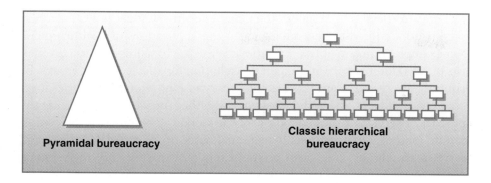

Pyramidal bureaucracy

Classic hierarchical bureaucracy

Figure 13.2
Pyramidal and hierarchical structures.

the Roman Catholic Church became the examples for studying what structure works for large sized and geographically dispersed endeavors (Townsend, 1970). This template evolved into one structural form, known as a classic hierarchical bureaucracy. Large governmental agencies often assume the bureaucratic form, which has both positive and negative aspects to it. The bureaucratic structural form, predominant in hospitals and many healthcare organizations in the U.S., is described as being pyramidal.

Pyramidal means shaped like a pyramid with a wide base and narrow apex (see Fig. 13.2). Bureaucracies are called pyramidal because, when diagrammed, the structure actually is shaped like a pyramid with a wide base of workers and a narrow apex of decision makers. This model is designed to include a hierarchy of power and authority, arrayed from high to low, among the various organizational positions.

A *line and staff bureaucracy* is a variation of the pyramidal bureaucratic form, which emerges when there is a need for technical experts (see Fig. 13.3). The experts are designated as *staff*. They are resource experts who provide expertise to the people who do the main work of the organization. Some exam-

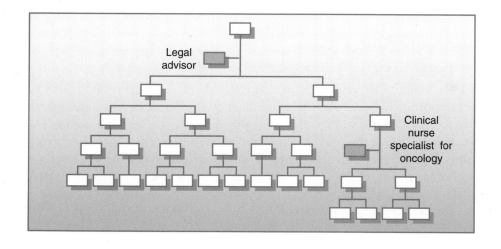

Legal advisor

Clinical nurse specialist for oncology

Figure 13.3
Line and staff bureaucracy.

ples are attorneys as legal staff to the Chief Executive Officer (CEO) of a hospital, who are hired to give advice about the applications of healthcare law. An example in nursing of staff positions is the use of Clinical Nurse Specialists (CNSs) for inservice and expert consultation for selected client groups. By contrast, *line* workers are those employees whose positions are in the direct chain of command line and are assigned as either the workers producing the product or service or the supervisors of the workers who produce the organization's output. Line positions have formal authority to make decisions; staff serve in an advisory role. Staff positions rely on expertise and interpersonal power bases.

Mintzberg (1983) called the people who perform the basic work of producing the product or rendering the service in an organization the *operators* who form the *operating core*. The *middle line* is the hierarchy of authority between the *operating core* and the *strategic apex* of top decision makers who have overall responsibility for the organization. He differentiated among two types of staff: the *technostructure* and the *support staff*. The technostructure includes analysts who design, plan, change, or train people to do the work. For example, scheduling, inservice education, fiscal management, and quality assurance/improvement personnel form part of the technostructure in healthcare. The support staff include units that exist to support the organization outside of its operating work flow. For example, payroll, billing, security, janitorial, and cafeteria services are support functions in healthcare. The operating core, middle line, strategic apex, technostructure, and support staff form the five basic parts of an organization.

Note that *line* and *staff* are terms used to describe workers' functions (see Chart 13.1). However, the titles given to positions may not correspond to their functions. Thus the designation of a line or staff position is not made based on the title used, but rather on the function the position performs in the organization. For example, "staff nurses" in a hospital function in a line position because they work directly to produce the product, in this case client care.

Matrix Structures

The second major way of organizing is to use a *matrix* structure (see Fig. 13.4). A matrix structure is more complicated and may seem confusing. Organizations may try to adapt to a turbulent environment by first moving to a matrix structure as a way to solve some problems of operating. It is used in environments where the work itself is complex. Essentially, this is a hybrid structure of bureaucracy plus another form of structure, called adhocracy, overlaid and combined together. Thus a matrix really is two structures in one, making it the most complex structure. It is the combination of the two co-existing structures that makes it a matrix form (Allcorn, 1990; Mintzberg, 1983).

CHART 13.1
～ LINE AND STAFF FUNCTIONS

Line Positions
- Responsible for achievement of organizational objectives
- Indicate lines of authority and accountability

Staff Positions
- To support line positions
- Advisory in nature
- Have no direct authority; use expertise and knowledge

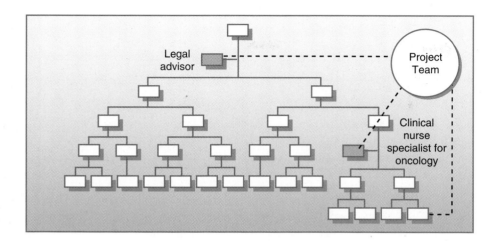

Figure 13.4
Matrix structure within an organization.

In a matrix structure, the line manager and a project manager function in a collaborative arrangement. Included in this structure are the elements of the classic hierarchical bureaucracy: a boss, intermediate bosses, and workers. For example, in nursing there would be a Chief Nurse Executive, nurse managers, and staff nurses in a line of authority to accomplish client care. In a matrix structure, some of the nurses' time is allocated to project or committee work. Nursing care is delivered in a teamwork setting or within a collaborative model. This means that the individual worker essentially may have two bosses. The nurse manager is the superior for the line job, which is taking care of clients; the committee chair is the superior when working on a project within the matrix overlay (Wright Jr., 1984).

A matrix organization is identified and characterized by management responsibilities that are shared between the line manager and the project manager, including the sharing of staff and sharing the evaluation of their work (see Chart 13.2). In this type of combined structure, a staff nurse's performance appraisal may have input from multiple sources, based on differing work assignments in the organization. There occurs collaborative behavior and an increased need for communication and coordination.

In hospitals, especially in larger facilities, the matrix structure is characterized by liaison roles, task forces, standing committees, and a dual authority structure. As a result the communication becomes more horizontal than vertical. In a classical bureaucracy, the communication would occur down and up the chain of authority. In a matrix structure, the communication occurs in a more horizontal fashion as staff talk with peers in other departments across the organization because of collaborating on projects.

Matrix structures use connecting links within the organization or across the integrated parts of a large and complex integrated network (see Fig. 13.5).

CHART 13.2
⌒ PROFILE OF A MATRIX ORGANIZATION

Where management responsibilities are shared between the line manager and the project manager, and where both managers share staff and evaluative responsibilities for staff.

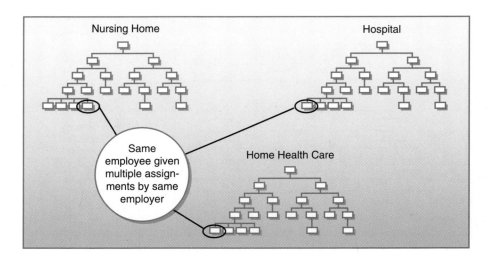

Figure 13.5
Matrix structure in an
integrated network.

There are certain liaison roles. For example, in a hospital there may be a nurse liaison to purchasing, radiology, and quality improvement committees. Matrix organizations are characterized by teamwork, multidisciplinary specialists, and problem-centered, problem-oriented teams. The major disadvantage of a matrix structure is that it requires sophisticated management skills. Further, success is based on having well educated workers who can handle a complex communication and authority web. For nurses, this would mean an advanced level of interpersonal relationship skills and group and teamwork skills. Matrices require people at the individual worker level who have expertise in some area, and who are able to function within a dual authority structure (Allcorn, 1990).

One example of a matrix arrangement in hospitals is cardiopulmonary resuscitation (CPR) teams. In a CPR or code team, members from various departments such as respiratory therapy (RT), intensive care unit (ICU) nursing, and the cardiopulmonary electrocardiogram (EKG) unit respond to and run a code. This team forms a matrix group, with their own structure and procedures, who are evaluated as a group. A renal dialysis or oncology nurse expert might likewise move across the structure to do referrals. Another example might occur when a psychiatric nurse consultant moves across departments to evaluate a client who has a psychiatric as well as a physical disorder.

Adhocracy Structure

On a continuum of highly structured to loosely structured, the third basic form of organizational structure is a loosely structured project organization called an adhocracy (see Fig. 13.6). The word *adhocracy* comes from the term ad hoc committee. This is an organizational structure that reflects the use of teams of specialists who are organized to complete specific jobs (Fuszard, 1983;

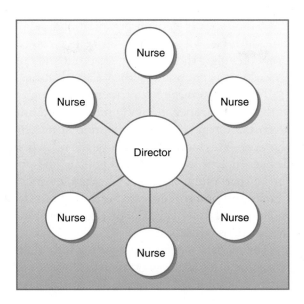

Figure 13.6
Adhocracy.

Mintzberg, 1983). This structure is not yet seen often in nursing; it primarily is used with highly specialized professional group practices, such as those in accounting, engineering, architecture, or space exploration. In an adhocracy the whole organization is made up of project teams. The project work comes in to the organization, and the expertise of the various members is utilized according to specialty and needed expertise. Examples are a research grant team or a National Aeronautics and Space Administration (NASA) project to put a spaceship on the moon or to launch a spy satellite. However, some entrepreneurial nursing businesses or community nursing centers are organized as adhocracies.

In leadership theory, if the situation contains workers who have job readiness, or both the willingness and knowledge to do the job, then the leader simply delegates to them. An organizational structure that allows delegation of the work is an adhocracy. There is one main coordinator who oversees the financial resources and the job flow, usually called a Director. The work then is delegated out to the member specialists, who are formed into collaborative teams that form and reform in response to the work and the expertise needed.

Five Basic Organizational Types

As noted in Chapter 12, the elements that come together to highly influence administrative structural design (e.g. size, age, and technology) and the situational factors faced by organizations in general (e.g. social environment, amount of change) tend to cluster into groupings. Examining how these clusters tend to occur over all types of organizations, Mintzberg (1983) grouped

CHART 13.3
↪ ORGANIZATIONAL
ADMINISTRATIVE
STRUCTURES

- Simple structure
- Machine bureau-
  cracy
- Professional bureau-
  cracy
- Divisionalized form
- Adhocracy

Data from Mintzberg (1983).

the basic types of general organizational administrative structures into five categories (see Chart 13.3). These five categories look broadly at organizations, including those that are for-profit and not-for-profit, manufacturing and service producers, and healthcare and non-healthcare institutions.

The *simple structure* is a structure in which there is a wide span of control at the strategic apex, no staff units, and a minimal or absent middle line. It is a centralized and organic structure that uses direct supervision to coordinate the work. This form is not elaborated and avoids many of the formal structural devices such as well-developed policies and procedures. The strategic apex is the key part of the structure. The simple structure is best suited to new, small, simple, and non-sophisticated organizations. It often is seen in small and entrepreneurial firms. For example, nurses opening their own new small business might choose this form.

The *machine bureaucracy* type has fully elaborated administrative and support structures, large operating units, and a tall hierarchy of authority. Coordination is achieved by standardizing work processes. The key part was called the "technostructure" by Mintzberg (1983). This means people who function in staff roles such as control analysts, accountants, quality control, inservice education, and recruiters. Machine bureaucracies are characterized by highly specialized, routine operating tasks, formalized procedures in the operating core, proliferation of rules and regulations, formalized communication, large sized units at the operating level, relatively centralized power and decision making, and an elaborate administrative structure with a sharp distinction between line and staff. It is a structure obsessed with control and found in environments that are simple and stable. Mass production firms are examples of the best known machine bureaucracies. In healthcare, U. S. acute care hospitals historically evolved into classic machine bureaucracies.

The *professional bureaucracy* type is common in universities, hospital medical staffs, school systems, accounting firms, and social work agencies where the organization relies on the skills and knowledge of the operating professionals to produce standard products and services. They are flat structures with thin middle lines, a tiny technostructure, and fully elaborated support staff. They are highly decentralized and use the standardization of worker skills to coordinate the work. The key part is the operating core, with professionals who seek to control their own work and collective control over the administrative decisions that affect them. Medical staff structures and physician practices within acute care hospitals traditionally adopted this form.

The *divisionalized form* of structure is one in which a set of quasi-autonomous units are coupled together by an integrated central administrative structure. The units are called divisions; the central administration is called headquarters. The key part of the organization is the middle line. The standardization of outputs is used as the primary coordinating mechanism. The divisionalized form works best with machine bureaucracies in a for-profit field with market diversity. This structure does not seem to work very well outside of the private sector, although some hospitals have experimented with "product line management" and spinning off for-profit divisions. This structural form may be used more in the future as healthcare organizations merge and integrate healthcare functions beyond the traditional acute care services.

The *adhocracy* is the structural form most conducive to promoting sophisticated innovation in organizations. An adhocracy is a highly organic structure with all the parts mingled together in one large mass in the middle. There is little formalization of behavior and high job specialization based on formal training. The tendency is to group specialists into units for housekeeping purposes but to form the work around small project teams that involve various mixtures of line managers, staff, and operating managers. The key part of the organization is the support staff together with the operating core. Person-to-person mutual adjustment is the prime method of coordinating the work. Top managers handle battles ensuing over strategic choices, disturbances in the fluid structure, monitoring of the various projects, and relating to or liaisoning with the external environment. Multidisciplinary teams of experts such as in think-tanks, consulting firms, creative and advertising agencies, engineering firms, and NASA are examples of adhocracy-type organizations (Mintzberg, 1983). In healthcare some examples occur in hospice organizations, community health, nursing centers or nurse-run clinics, and multispecialty group practices. This structural form may be used more in the future by nurse practitioners in private practice.

Mintzberg (1983) included the simple structure to reflect small and emerging businesses. The machine bureaucracy most closely resembles the classic hierarchical bureaucracy. The professional bureaucracy and the divisionalized form were seen as distinct by Mintzberg (1983) but can be similar to matrix structures. The adhocracy form may emerge as more important in nursing practice in the future, as the healthcare field restructures.

The Organizational Chart

Organizations contain both a *formal structure* and an *informal structure*. The informal structure is simply the network or pattern of social relationships and friendship circles that are outside the formal structure. The informal structure is an interconnected web of relationships that operate in and around the formally designated lines of communication. The informal structure does not appear on the formal organizational chart.

The formal structure can be identified on an organizational chart. An *organizational chart* is a visual display of what the organization says is their formal structure. The extent to which the organizational chart reflects the reality of decision making, resource allocation, and actual communication patterns may

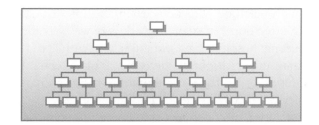

Figure 13.7
Vertical structure.

vary (del Bueno, 1987). The organizational chart can be found in the administrative manuals along with the mission statement, philosophy, purpose, and objectives documents.

The organizational chart identifies the formal channels of communication. It is a schematic drawing of the various positions and the formal relationships between and among the positions and, by extension, the people who are a part of the organization. Organizational charts display the administrative structure in vertical and horizontal dimensions. When applying for a job, one of the pieces of information to ask for is the organizational chart. This document can help to give an idea about how the organization is structured, or at least how decision makers think it is structured, as one part of assessing the organization and any individual's place within it.

A *vertical structure* goes from top to bottom and includes multiple layers (see Fig. 13.7). Vertical structures are referred to as tall organizational charts. Tall organizational charts are elongated structures and are found in large bureaucratic institutions. They typify chain of command, unity of command, and span of control. A tall vertical structure that goes from top to bottom implies a bureaucracy.

In contrast, a *horizontal or flat structure* has few administrative layers between management and employee (see Fig. 13.8). Flat organizational charts reflect a decentralized approach to structuring the organization. Decentralization means flattening out the organizational chart, making it more horizontal, and diminishing the layers between management and employee. It is an attempt to permit the employees to organize their work to obtain more efficient and effective results.

Organizational charts help with administrative control, policy making and planning, and evaluating the organization in terms of strengths and weak-

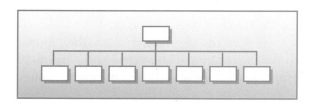

Figure 13.8
Horizontal structure.

nesses. They are used to help orient personnel because they show relationships and thus make it clear as to how people are to interact within the formal organization. They display positions and position titles. For example, an organizational chart of a matrix structure may show dotted lines for the project relationships. Dotted lines mean that there is a relationship to the position or the group that would form for a project (see Figs. 13.4 and 13.5).

LEADERSHIP AND MANAGEMENT IMPLICATIONS

It appears that organizational structures coalesce into one of several basic types. The organizational structure is a management decision but may be the result of needing to alleviate pressures or solve certain problems of management. For example, as the size of an organization grows, employees need to be able to interact and communicate in an orderly fashion. On the other hand, a small organization may need the creativity and flexibility of a loose structure. As the environment changes, managers may be forced to restructure to survive and thrive. Theory about organizational structures provides a knowledge base with which to have a greater awareness of options. The research may indicate which types are more effective under which conditions. The leader and manager is challenged to assess and use organizational structure and restructuring efforts to ease frictions where the structure, the environment, and the needs of the workers create sparks or serious threats to organizational effectiveness.

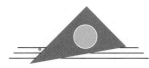 *Leadership & Management Behaviors*

LEADERSHIP BEHAVIORS	MANAGEMENT BEHAVIORS	OVERLAP AREAS
• envisions an ideal or desired structure	• plans the structure	• plans and develops the structure
• inspires restructuring decisions	• organizes needed positions	• makes decisions about the administrative structure
• enables the group to use structure to further the group's goals	• decides on number and types of positions and related duties	
• generates an empowering environment within the administrative structure	• implements structural design	
	• implements restructuring designs	
	• evaluates structure for effectiveness	
	• monitors stresses and strains created by structure	

Restructuring the ICU Leadership Team

When I arrived to work as Director of Critical Care at a large tertiary care referral center, one of the major complaints I heard from intensive care unit (ICU) nursing staff was they "never saw" their nurse manager. "She is always away in meetings" and "never available" within the unit and "can no longer relate" to our nursing practice issues. I realized this was a major issue facing nurses at the bedside since the unit clinical leadership figure was frequently unavailable within an environment where major changes were occurring.

Over the years, nurse managers have been gradually pulled away from the clinical arena to address critical fiscal and operational issues related to patient care. As a result, clinical leadership has assumed a secondary role at a time when practice issues are of primary importance. Because of the complexity and rapidly changing healthcare environment, a review and possible revision of the role of the nurse manager position was undertaken.

A small task force of individuals was charged with assessing the nursing leadership structure in the area and developing a plan for change. Three ICU's were involved; a 12 bed medical, an 8 bed neuro and an 18 bed surgical ICU. The original leadership structure for the area was organized in a traditional hierarchical fashion (see Fig. 13A). More specifically, the nurse manager was responsible for providing both clinical and operational direction for each unit. Understandably, as cost containment issues soared, clinical leadership diminished, resulting in the concerns voiced by the staff.

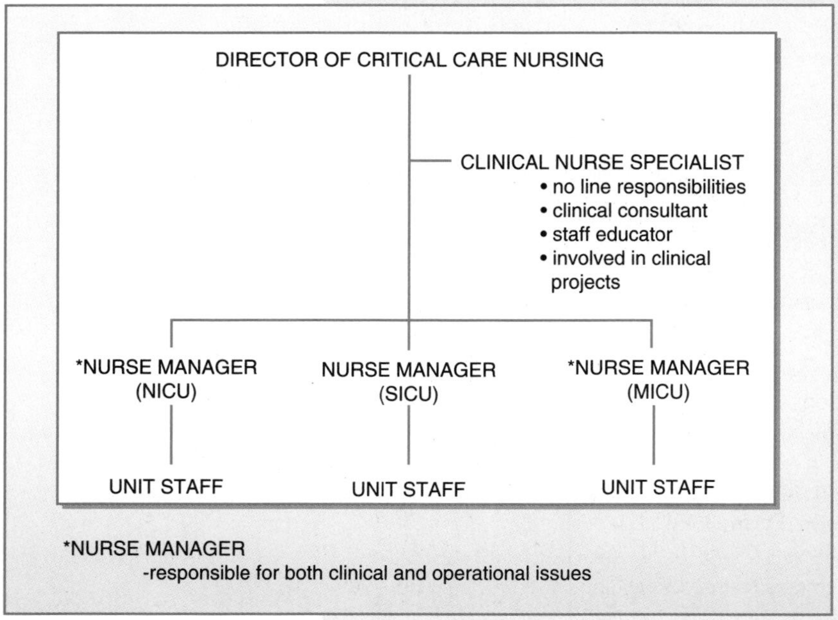

DIRECTOR OF CRITICAL CARE NURSING

CLINICAL NURSE SPECIALIST
- no line responsibilities
- clinical consultant
- staff educator
- involved in clinical projects

*NURSE MANAGER (NICU) **NURSE MANAGER (SICU)** ***NURSE MANAGER (MICU)**

UNIT STAFF   **UNIT STAFF**   **UNIT STAFF**

*NURSE MANAGER
-responsible for both clinical and operational issues

Figure 13A

After much discussion, a new structure evolved with a goal to provide strong clinical leadership and presence within the units while maintaining fiscal accountability. Instead of having three nurse managers and one clinical nurse specialist to cover the area, the positions were changed to include one operations nurse manager and three clinical nurse specialists (see Fig. 13B). A matrix alignment of the positions facilitated a collaborative approach to leadership and equally emphasized both the clinical and operational components of the original nurse manager's role.

The operations nurse manager role was designed to assume responsibility and accountability for various operational areas such as budget, staffing, scheduling, payroll and more. The clinical nurse specialist role was outlined to assume clinical responsibility for each unit which involved establishing an appropriate care delivery system, clinical evaluation and professional development of staff, and establishment of practice standards. Both the operational manager and clinical nurse specialist would have line responsibility related to the role's particular function. For example, if an employee had attendance questions or problems, the operations nurse manager would address those issues. If an employee had clinical ideas or problems, the clinical nurse specialist would assist in ensuring their resolution.

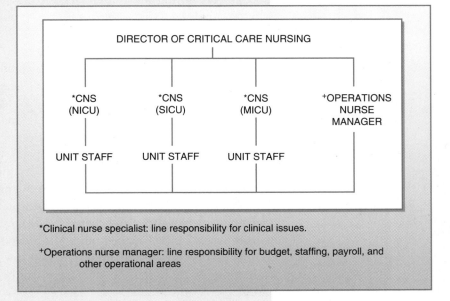

Figure 13B

The new structure has now been in place for over a year and both positive and negative aspects have surfaced. Since many situations cross over clinical and operational boundaries, effective communication and collaboration patterns between the clinical nurse specialist and operations manager are now considered essential. Individuals in the roles who have strong communication and management skills have adapted well. Individuals who required a high degree of environmental structure in the workplace have struggled at times with the new design. The nursing staff have adjusted well in relating to "two bosses." As turnover occurs, we realize that constant education is required to facilitate a clear understanding of the structure. The original goal of providing a strong, visible clinical leader within the unit while maintaining fiscal accountability has been achieved. The new challenge will be to adapt the structure as the healthcare environment and practice arenas continue to change.

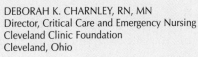
DEBORAH K. CHARNLEY, RN, MN
Director, Critical Care and Emergency Nursing
Cleveland Clinic Foundation
Cleveland, Ohio

The traditional hospital was not designed to respond to the needs of clients. The challenge today is for hospitals to restructure and reorganize to insure effective outcomes for clients. The four major initiatives are downsizing management, decentralizing the support services, centralizing supply distribution, and organizing labor around technology. These initiatives are opposite to what hospitals used to do: decentralizing supplies and centralizing support services (Strasen, 1991).

Leaders and managers may face power and control barriers as systems reconfigure, network, and become more integrated. As interdependent and interconnected facilities integrate, they will need to develop structures to support and coordinate across departments and boundaries. Mergers and associations create turmoil. The leader and manager needs to begin by creating a shared vision. Through differentiation of functions and specific clinical areas plus integration of organizational parts, the nurse designs an organizational structure that may affect the performance of the entire organization. Structure and system integration is a developmental process (Stichler, 1994).

It has been thought that decentralized structures work best for nursing service delivery. However, Mintzberg (1983) noted that in times of adversity or threat to an organization, centralization of decision making is needed. Further, as organizations grow large, there is a pull toward bureaucratization and centralization. Nurse leaders and managers will be challenged to analyze organizational structure as healthcare reform initiatives trigger changes.

A fundamental challenge will occur as to how to integrate and structure nursing within new configurations such as "hospitals without walls." The nurse's role may expand and broaden as the key coordinator across care settings. New structures may be necessary for nursing practice. Vision and strategic planning are key activities. Where restructuring occurs, an analysis of what works for nursing practice may need to be done independently of what works for the healthcare organization.

Flannery & Williams (1990) described seven patterns predicted to combine to reconfigure hospital structures in the near future. Creating a simpler and more responsive organization, these trends are flattened organizations, more fluid structures, outcomes (not functions) orientation, redefined staff functions by managers who are better developed and held accountable, reduced staff costs, more subcontracting of services, and a refocus on the core business. The result will be a streamlined structure, and a fundamental change in jobs and positions. Perhaps management will be done primarily by pulling together a "swat team."

Certainly structures in healthcare organizations are changing. Just as pyramidal shapes gave way to internal matrix structures, internal matrix structures are giving way to flat organizations linked via networks of integrated healthcare organizations. Smaller organizations of providers are configuring as adhocracies (see Fig. 13.9). Work design, defined as changing the actual struc-

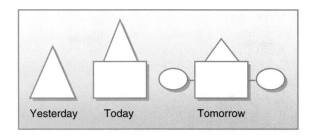

Figure 13.9
Changing shape of healthcare organizations.

ture of jobs people perform by measuring the workload and fitting people into jobs, is one area of high activity in nursing. This is the opposite of fitting jobs to people (Tonges, 1992). Reengineering, defined as the fundamental re-thinking and radical redesign of business processes to achieve dramatic improvements in critical measures of performance, also is a popular term (Hammer & Champy, 1993). Nursing service delivery is directly affected by these processes. The nursing leadership and management challenge is to use the best ideas and make them work for nursing. In describing the Transformational Model for Professional Nursing Practice, the authors noted this challenge and offered a "road map" for nursing through major organizational transformation (Wolf, Boland, & Aukerman, 1994).

CURRENT ISSUES AND TRENDS

Regardless of the final form that government-initiated healthcare reform takes, changes are occurring throughout the nation in the healthcare delivery system. As the largest health professions occupation, nurses are directly affected by the shape and form of healthcare reform. Layoffs, downsizing, substitution of assistants for RNs, and restructuring have affected nursing. Leadership and management challenges arose as nursing struggled to decide upon a structure to deliver high quality, low cost nursing service.

Case management and patient-centered care ideas have taken hold. However, they present structural questions such as, what is the best structure to reach these desired outcomes? Other changes in the financial structure of healthcare, such as reimbursement for "covered lives" instead of "patient days" and competition on price and quality, have triggered restructuring. As the nursing shortage abated, the focus shifted from what structure is best suited to attracting and retaining nurses to what structure will help the organization survive under capitated reimbursement. Immediate solutions were implemented to reduce the size of the nursing staff and to substitute assistants in order to ease financial pressures. However, history indicates that these actions set the stage for another nursing shortage.

Reduction-in-force (RIF) and decreasing the nursing staff skill mix to 50% or less RNs are short-term measures. They bring about other issues such as costs of supervision, appropriate care modality, nurse satisfaction, and how to restructure. Nurse leaders and managers will be challenged to analyze the theoretical structuring issues, match them to a specific organization, and manage to lead the nursing staff toward personal adaptation to growth and change.

RESEARCH NOTE

Source: Pabst, M. (1993). Span of control on nursing inpatient units. *Nursing Economic$*, *11*(2), 87-90.

Purpose

The purpose of this research was to explore and describe the managerial span of control on inpatient units of two Midwestern tertiary care centers. Manager-to-worker ratios were computed and displayed. Managerial spans of control were displayed. Nursing hours per patient day (NHPPD), unit size, and percent of RN staff were computed to facilitate a financial analysis.

Discussion

Hospital 1 had 22 units analyzed. Manager-to-staff ratios ranged from approximately 1:12 to 1:63. Hospital 2 had 13 units and managerial spans of control that ranged from approximately 1:11 to 1:41. The ideal or optimal span of control is not certain. There were large variations among the units in managerial span of control in both hospitals. The amount of variation raised issues related to finances, characteristics of the workers, job preparation, different patient characteristics, unit size, percent occupancy, and nursing care delivery model.

Application to Practice

Clearly there are financial impacts to the span of control for each manager. Knowledge of the ratio of salary resources spent on managerial positions is important for making decisions and may create potential savings if the span is changed. However, other variables may contribute to the span of control. For example, skill mix, experience level of staff, and duties of the charge nurse may contribute to feasibility issues that prevent decentralization and efforts to increase span of control. Other issues are stability of work, complexity of work, degree of coordination required, geographic proximity, similarity of jobs, amount of direction of workers needed, and amount of planning of work needed. Nurse managers often directly supervise more employees than heads of other departments. Financial savings may be captured by instituting parity in span of control across units and departments.

SUMMARY

- The classic hierarchical bureaucratic structure is one of the major forms of structure found in healthcare.

- A line and staff bureaucracy is one modification of a bureaucratic structure.
- The second major form of structure is a matrix: the combined, complex, or overlaid structure.
- The third form, an adhocracy, is at the other end of the continuum away from bureaucracy and toward a delegating structure.
- Organizations may try to adapt to a turbulent environment by first moving to a matrix structure as a way to solve some problems.
- The operating core, middle line, strategic apex, technostructure, and support staff form the five basic parts of an organization.
- The five broad, general types of organizational design are simple structure, machine bureaucracy, professional bureaucracy, divisionalized form, and adhocracy.
- Organizational charts show the formal structure; they may look horizontal or vertical in shape.

Study Questions

1. Discuss the different types of organizational structures. Which best suit the practice of nursing?
2. What factors need to be assessed prior to changing the organizational structure?
3. Why are organizations resistant to changing their structure?
4. How do nurses foster or hinder restructuring?
5. How do complex organizations adapt to their environment?
6. What changes are needed in nursing organizations? Why?
7. How are healthcare structures changing under healthcare reform? Why?

Critical Thinking Exercise

Renewed Hope Medical Center had been a 300 bed community hospital until healthcare reform swept the state a year ago. The hospital downsized, laying off 20% of the nurses. Nurse extenders were hired. The hospital bought the local public health nursing agency and privatized it. The hospital formed an alliance with a for-profit healthcare chain and its network of healthcare facilities. Renewed Hope is expanding its long-term care and hospice services. Now the nursing department is being told to provide staff for the new services without hiring any new RNs. The Director of Nursing has decided to restructure the Department of Nursing.

1. *Is there a problem(s)? What would this be?*

2. *What structure was most likely in place prior to the reform changes?*

3. *What should the Director do for restructuring?*

4. *What options are there to restructure?*

5. *How could this be done?*

6. *What new structure would work best for nursing?*

7. *What problems and decisions face the staff nurses?*

8. *What implementation challenges face the Director?*

REFERENCES

Allcorn, S. (1990). Using matrix organization to manage health care delivery organizations. *Hospital & Health Service Administration, 35*(4), 575-590.

del Bueno, D. (1987). What's in a name—or shape? *Journal of Nursing Administration, 17*(7/8), 31-34.

Flannery, T., & Williams, J. (1990). The shape of things to come: Part 1. *Healthcare Forum Journal, 33*(3), 14-20.

Fuszard, B. (1983). "Adhocracy" in health care institutions? *Journal of Nursing Administration, 13*(1), 14-19.

Hammer, M., & Champy, J. (1993). *Reengineering the corporation: A manifesto for business revolution.* New York: HarperCollins.

Mintzberg, H. (1983). *Structure in fives: Designing effective organizations.* Englewood Cliffs, NJ: Prentice-Hall.

Stichler, J. (1994). System development and integration in healthcare. *Journal of Nursing Administration, 24*(10), 48-53.

Strasen, L. (1991). Redesigning hospitals around patients and technology. *Nursing Economic$, 9*(4), 233-238.

Tonges, M. (1992). Work designs: Sociotechnical systems for patient care delivery. *Nursing Management, 23*(1), 27-32.

Townsend, R. (1970). *Up the organization: How to stop the corporation from stifling people and strangling profits.* Greenwich, CT: Fawcett.

Wolf, G., Boland, S., & Aukerman, M. (1994). A transformational model for the practice of professional nursing. *Journal of Nursing Administration, 24*(5), 38-46.

Wright Jr., N. (1984). The dynamics of matrix management. *Manage, 36*(4), 29-32.

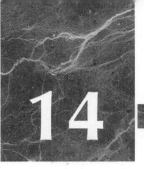

14

Decentralization and Shared Governance

Chapter Objectives

❧

define and differentiate centralization and decentralization

❧

explain the continuum of control over a decision

❧

distinguish vertical from horizontal decentralization

❧

define and describe shared governance

❧

analyze how shared governance models are constructed

❧

compare shared governance models

❧

analyze problems related to the implementation of shared governance

❧

explain recent trends in reorganization

❧

exercise critical thinking to conceptualize and analyze
possible solutions to a practical experience incident

*t*he power to make decisions is a key structural and functional issue for organizations. The way in which power over the decisions to be made in an organization is distributed is frequently described in terms of centralization or decentralization. These terms relate to the degree to which power is differentially distributed within an organization (Price & Mueller, 1986). Who makes decisions is important to the functioning of professionals who are employed in organizations. Both professional and job autonomy are at stake in the location of decision power in nursing practice. Nurses need to be able to make the necessary decisions about care management that allow them to affect outcomes for clients.

DEFINITIONS

entralization is the concentration of power to make decisions at a single point, usually at the top of the organization (see Chart 14.1). In a centralized organization, power flows vertically from the top down the line to the bottom of the organizational structure.

Decentralization is the dispersal of decision making power to many points in the organization (see Chapter 12). It is a characteristic of an organization in which employees at lower levels have the authority to make certain decisions and participate in the general process of organizational decision making (Hage & Aiken, 1967). Participation in decision making occurs when employees or subordinate groups consult and are involved in making decisions that affect them and their work (Likert, 1960; McGregor, 1960; Melcher, 1976).

In considering the exercise of power over decision making (see Chapter 7), it is helpful to recall the series of steps that are followed in making a decision. The steps are (Mintzberg, 1983):

1. Collect information.
2. Process information into advice.
3. Make the choice.
4. Authorize the implementation.
5. Execute what is done.

If there is power over any one step in the process, then some power is exerted over the whole process. Power is maximized if there is control over all the steps. If there is control over the input information, then there is control over what variables will be considered in relation to the decision (Mintzberg, 1983; Paterson, 1969) (see Fig. 14.1). If the decision process occurs in a number of steps, then there is a continuum of control over the decision process and a potential dispersion of the power to make decisions (Mintzberg, 1983; Paterson, 1969). Some examples of the types of decisions made in nursing organizations are strategic priorities, budget and resource allocation, work standards, outcomes, work processes such as staffing and making assignments, care modality, and implementing clinical care.

Mintzberg (1983) noted that there are three different ways that the term decentralization is used:

1. To refer to the distribution of formal power down the chain of line authority. This is called *vertical* decentralization.

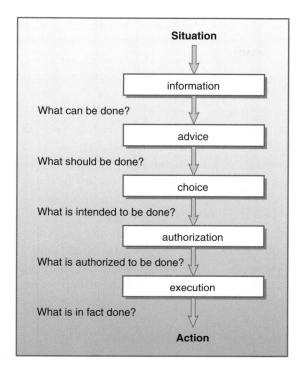

Situation

↓

information

What can be done?

↓

advice

What should be done?

↓

choice

What is intended to be done?

↓

authorization

What is authorized to be done?

↓

execution

What is in fact done?

↓

Action

Figure 14.1
Continuum of control over the decision process. (Adapted with permission from Mintzberg, H. (1983). *Structure in fives: Designing effective organizations.* Englewood Cliffs, NJ: Prentice-Hall, p. 100.)

2. To refer to decisional power flowing outside the line structure, for example, to support staff or analysts. The extent to which nonmanagers have power over decision processes is called *horizontal* decentralization (see Chart 14.2).

3. To refer to the physical distribution of services. This does not relate to power, but rather to the concentration versus dispersal over the location of services such as central pharmacy and pharmacy substations.

The two meanings of the term decentralization that are important for the design of organizational administrative structures are vertical and horizontal decentralization. The third meaning relates to the idea of a structure as a physical location, building, or space arrangement. Mintzberg (1983) visually depicted five combinations of vertical and horizontal decentralization as overlaid onto the five basic parts of the organization (see Chapter 13).

CHART 14.2
⤺ DEFINITIONS

Vertical Decentralization
power distributed down the line of authority.

Horizontal Decentralization
power distributed outside the line structure to nonmanager.

Data from Mintzberg (1983).

BACKGROUND: DECENTRALIZATION

Centralization/decentralization is a classic topic in the design of administrative structures for organizations. It is a central strategy for resolving tensions between the division of labor and the need to coordinate. Centralizing is the tightest way to coordinate decision making and control power. However, under conditions such as complexity and information overload, decentralizing allows the people at the bottom of the hierarchy who have the necessary knowledge to make the necessary decisions. Advantages include a faster response time and greater innovation, creativity, and motivation (Mintzberg, 1983).

It is important to view centralization and decentralization as a matter of degrees. Mintzberg (1983) viewed this as two ends of a continuum, as opposed to these two terms having absolute meanings. Thus an organization is not "decentralized," but rather more (or less) decentralized. Decentralization is most specifically aimed at decision step 3—making the choice—by involving the operating core workers in more of the entire decision process. Clearly, the operating core workers are involved in the implementing and executing steps no matter who makes the choice.

Among the obstacles to decentralization in nursing is the fact that knowledge and skill levels vary among the several types of basic nursing preparation. Further, strong hierarchical systems in the past have not given individual nurses autonomy with authority and accountability. Overcoming barriers may occur by defining what nursing's service is, making explicit how this service benefits clients, and standardizing nursing's skills, service, and the products provided to clients (Porter-O'Grady, 1987).

There are reasons to decentralize. Complexity may prohibit one decision maker from having or being able to process all of the needed information for success. Decentralization frees up the organization to be flexible and respond more rapidly to local or environmental conditions. It may be a stimulus for motivation and innovation (Hess, 1994; Mintzberg, 1983).

Decentralized nursing has been defined as a style of organization, communication, and decision making that fosters autonomy, accountability and authority at the individual nurse level (Althaus, Hardyck, Pierce, & Rodgers, 1981). Effective and continuing communication is necessary for its success because communication flows in all directions. Usual methods of decision making must be changed as administrators share power and staff nurses learn to handle the extra workload of being involved and accountable.

RESEARCH NOTE

Source: Cassard, S., Weisman, C., Gordon, D., & Wong, R. (1994). The impact of unit-based self-management by nurses on patient incomes. *Health Services Research*, 29(4), 415-433.

Purpose

The purpose of this research was to compare patients discharged from a self-managed nursing unit to those from traditionally managed units as to their post-discharge outcomes. The article examines whether the management strategy of unit-based professional practice model affects the quality of patient care in one large Eastern teaching hospital. Four self-managed units were matched to four traditional units, and primary data were collected from all discharged patients over a three month period. There were 165 enrolled patients from the self-managed units and 163 from the traditional units. The outcome variables measured were perceived health status, perceived functional status, postdischarge needs for care and unmet needs, postdischarge unplanned healthcare visits, and 31-day rehospitalizations.

Discussion

The two groups of patients varied significantly as to age, gender, and distribution of medical diagnosis category. The groups varied significantly as to severity of medical illness. On outcome variables, the two groups varied significantly as to need for care and unmet needs for care, with the results unfavorable to the self-managed units group. However, patient sociodemographic characteristics emerged as an explanation for the difference.

Application to Practice

The analyses in total demonstrated no significant effect, positive or negative, in patient postdischarge outcomes due to unit-based self management or traditional nursing practice models. Previous research has indicated a positive effect of unit-based self management on nurses' job satisfaction and retention. With self-management contributing to improving the quality of nurses' work life and having no detrimental effects on patient postdischarge outcomes, self-management structures might be expected to be positive for nursing service departments to implement.

DEFINITION: SHARED GOVERNANCE

Shared governance is defined as one form of a professional practice model that includes an accountability-based governance system for professional workers (see Chart 14.3). It is an organizational structure and process that legitimizes nurses' control over practice and extends their influence to administrative decision areas previously controlled by management. Shared governance means some type of shared decision making by nursing staff and management (Maas & Specht, 1994). Authority is vested in specified processes, formal committee structures, and board-adopted bylaws (Hess, 1994; Porter-O'Grady, 1987). The organizational structure of shared governance is constructed from the center of the workplace outward. The core of the structure is the practicing nurse. The next levels are the four major nursing service components of practice, quality, education, and peer process/governance. The outer levels are the nursing management and healthcare organization levels that coordinate, integrate, and facilitate the core operating system (Porter-O'Grady, 1987).

CHART 14.3
↪ DEFINITION

Shared Governance
a professional practice model that includes an accountability-based governance system for professional workers.

BACKGROUND: SHARED GOVERNANCE

The first wave of hospital restructuring in the 1980s employed the concepts of decentralization and shared governance. The idea was to empower staff nurses by involving them in client care decision making (Jones, Stasiowski, Simons, Boyd, & Lucas, 1993). Shared governance was conceived to be a radical departure from the traditional hospital management structure in which nurses had limited governance, little authority, and low control within the organization (Hess, 1994). Shared governance was adopted as a strategy for involving staff nurses in decision making and for fostering professional nursing practice by empowering nurses with the ability to make decisions affecting their clients and their practice. Evaluation data supported claims that implementing shared governance improved staff nurse perceptions of job and practice environment satisfaction (Jones et al., 1993). This issue of staff nurse job satisfaction was especially important during the most recent round of nursing shortage, turnover, and recruitment challenges that were acute in the late 1980s.

Searching for solutions, reorganization to decentralization and shared governance became popular. Hess (1994) noted that although nursing shared governance was first introduced in the late 1970s, over half of the 145 articles published about it appeared after 1988. Two problems related to the implementation of shared governance arose: (1) professional vs. bureaucratic control tensions and (2) true change vs. cosmetic imitation of change.

Bureaucratic characteristics may impede professional practice. For example, strong hierarchies, clear authority structures, rigid approval mechanisms, and extensive policies and procedures constrain peer-based, lateral, and collegial dialogue and governance. Working relationships, attitudes, and conditions faced by nurses have been characterized as narrow, autocratic, sexist, controlling, and devaluing. The result is a real need to change the structure at the practice level and directly influence the work of nursing in a manner that assures a professional practice environment (Porter-O'Grady, 1987). Sharing governance comes from the need to accommodate two systems of authority: organizational authority vested in positions and professional authority to meet society's needs. Professional employees face the danger that societal needs entrusted to the profession will be subordinated to the needs of the organization (Maas & Specht, 1994).

At issue is whether reorganization and decentralization are real or cosmetic. At the heart of the issue is the fact that nurses, even in shared governance or professional practice models, are still employees of the hospital or healthcare organization. Professional models and shared governance imply a peer status or the separateness of having outside self-management or contractual status. Independence may be an illusion when applied to governance shared among organizational members. When governance is restricted to the level of the nursing unit, staff autonomy and participative decision making may increase without affecting the overall organizational structure (Hess, 1994). Nursing shared governance does not exist unless the authority and accountability for decisions defining and regulating nursing practice and those

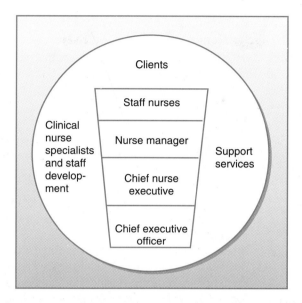

Figure 14.2
Decentralized nursing
structure.

shared with management are solidified with actual decision making structures and processes (Maas & Specht, 1994). This primacy of clients and direct care providers, truly reflecting a decentralized structure, should be evident in resource allocation decisions, the structure, and the organizational chart. One example is displayed in Figure 14.2. If this structure were truly in operation, resources would be concentrated at the staff nurse level. For example, staff nurses would receive the travel money allocations as first priority. There is some evidence that professional governance for staff RNs is not being fully implemented (Havens, 1994).

In participative decision making, employees are expected to participate in decisions. The same is true for decentralization and shared governance. However, the number, type, degree, areas, and authority to implement the decisions may vary substantially. There may be different approaches to clinical decisions as opposed to administrative decisions.

Nurse autonomy is the key concept related to shared governance. The dimensions of nurse autonomy include peer determination and control of functions and processes. Control is exercised by defining the (Maas & Specht, 1990):

- scope of practice
- standards of practice
- nursing care delivery system
- knowledge specialization
- knowledge and resource development priorities
- self or peer evaluation component.

Collegial nursing governance procedures and decentralization of the nursing hierarchy are integral to nurse autonomy via control of the nursing care delivery system. Also critical to these systems are peer evaluations as a feedback and control mechanism.

RESEARCH NOTE

Source: DeBaca, V., Jones, K., & Tornabeni, J. (1993). A cost-benefit analysis of shared governance. *Journal of Nursing Administration, 23*(7/8), 50-57.

Purpose

The purpose of this article was to conduct a cost-benefit analysis to evaluate the fiscal impact of the implementation of shared governance in one Western hospital. The direct costs of implementation and ongoing maintenance of the shared governance model were compared to cost savings that the organization realized as a result of shared governance and the resulting elimination of managerial positions as the organization flattened out. For the first three years following the implementation of shared governance, no other major projects or restructuring occurred.

Discussion

Restructuring involved redesign of caregiver roles, decentralization of ancillary services, and bedside computers. Direct costs were for staff hours in planning and implementation meetings. Expenses were for consultant fees, education, and newsletters. Cost savings were in registry and travel nurse usage, decreased turnover costs, and management position reductions. The net savings, due to shared governance, over a five year period was estimated to be (conservatively) 11.5% of a calculated $5,837,126.

Application to Practice

It is possible to calculate the financial aspects of a change to shared governance. A cost-benefit analysis can be conducted to aid in decision making. In this article, cost savings exceeded cost outlays over a five year period. Thus the financial investment was recovered and exceeded. Further, non-monetary or intangible benefits have been documented with shared governance models. These relate to improvement in nurses' working conditions and greater nurse job satisfaction which may lead to lower absenteeism and turnover. Reducing turnover and dissatisfaction was associated with less need for expensive registry and travel nurse staffing supplementation.

Models

The models implemented under the term shared governance vary as to the degree of nurse participation in decision making, from minimal or informal participation to true sharing of authority and accountability. Part of the tension relates to whether or not nurses who are not managers can decide about resource allocation (Maas & Specht, 1994).

Porter-O'Grady (1987) described three operating models of professional governance approaches: the councilar, congressional, and administrative models. The *councilar model* uses council formats for structuring staff and managing governance. The *congressional model* uses a president and elected cabinet of officers, similar to our representative system of government. The *administrative model* separates clinical and administrative tracks and divides authority between the two. Representation may be evenly divided or weighted. One example of the administrative model as implemented in a long-term care setting used two structures of nurse autonomy and nurse accountability to build a governance model based on a specialized body of knowledge and the commitment to serve clients (Maas, 1989).

Some examples of what a changed organizational structure would look like were depicted by Porter-O'Grady (1987). These examples are of new organizational structures and ways that people are trying to reconfigure the organizational structure of nursing to fit the changing environment:

- *Shared governance* model: In this model it is difficult to identify the one person at the top. Shared governance implies that all of the nurses are involved in determining nursing practice, the related quality improvement, assessing educational needs, and maintaining positive peer relationships so that there is high morale and minimal disruptive conflict. There is an executive leadership group at the core for central guidance. It means that clients are at the top of the organization, the staff is the next highest priority, and then comes management (see Fig. 14.2).
- A *councilar* model: This model uses a number of committees called councils, usually elected, with defined authority and functions. Practice, quality improvement, education, and management are the primary councils (see Fig. 14.3).
- A *congressional* format: This structure patterns itself after our constitutionally empowered representative system of government. Officers and a cabinet are elected from the staff. They oversee the operation of the service. Power and control governance mechanisms are defined between the nurse executive and the cabinet (see Fig. 14.4).
- An *administrative shared governance* model: This structure has a number of committees or forums. Management forums and clinical forums are the method for people to communicate and share ideas. Rather than going through a chain of command from nurse to nurse manager, to Director of Nursing, to Chief Executive Officer (CEO), there is a series of forums within the structure based on peer interrelationships. This is where the policies are made, procedures are determined, and the various particulars of the actual work decision making occurs (see Fig. 14.5).

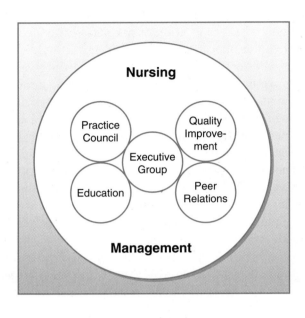

Figure 14.3
Councilar model. (Reprinted from *Nursing Economic$,* 1987, Volume 5, Number 6, pp. 281-286. Reprinted with permission of the publisher, Jannetti Publications, Inc., East Holly Avenue Box 56, Pitman, NJ 08071-0056; Phone [609] 256-2300; FAX [609] 589-7463.)

Figure 14.4
Congressional format. (Reprinted from *Nursing Economic$,* 1987, Volume 5, Number 6, pp. 281-286. Reprinted with permission of the publisher, Jannetti Publications, Inc., East Holly Avenue Box 56, Pitman, NJ 08071-0056; Phone [609] 256-2300; FAX [609] 589-7463.)

Decentralization and shared governance are strategies for shifting the responsibility and authority for both policy and day-to-day decision making from upper level management down to the unit level. An atmosphere that fosters nurse autonomy, control over work environment, mutual trust, and respect is essential. Problem solving is done at the unit and department of nursing levels, but starts as a grass-roots effort. The organizational structure can be streamlined to reduce the positions allocated to administration, thereby gen-

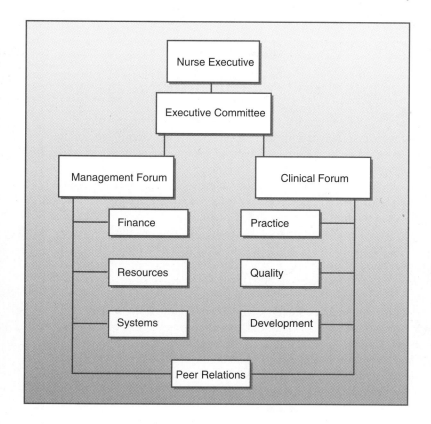

Figure 14.5
Administrative shared governance.
(Reprinted from *Nursing Economic$*,
1987, Volume 5, Number 6, pp. 281-
286. Reprinted with permission of the
publisher, Jannetti Publications, Inc., East
Holly Avenue Box 56, Pitman, NJ 08071-
0056; Phone [609] 256-2300; FAX [609]
589-7463.)

erating cost savings. However, movement to this type of structure requires professional development of staff nurses in decision making, team building, group dynamics, leadership, and budgeting (Jacoby & Terpstra, 1990). Leaders and managers need to nurture staff participation, empowerment, and effective communication patterns (Davis, 1992).

A shared governance organizational design has become widespread in U.S. hospitals (Porter-O'Grady, 1994). This design appears to be effective for empowering nurses as professional employees and represents values of interdependence and accountability (DeBaca, Jones, & Tornabeni, 1993; Porter-O'Grady, 1994). Shared governance is instituted for a variety of reasons. Some seek greater efficiency, quality, and cost containment, such as by decreasing the overtime budget (Leftridge & Lydford, 1993). The general effort in decentralizing and moving to a shared governance model is to empower nurses and foster their autonomy, leading to enhanced job satisfaction, positive perceptions of the job environment, and lowered anticipated turnover (Jones, et al., 1993). A side agenda is the growth and development benefits that accrue as nurses mature and improve their self-image in the process of adopting adult, collaborative, and active decision making roles more on par

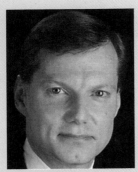

Tim Porter-O'Grady

Tim Porter-O'Grady Envisions Decentralization and Shared Governance

Shared governance for nursing has formed the foundation for organizational change for nursing for the past fifteen years. In one form or another the principles of shared governance have been explored and systems models created in a large number of nursing systems around the world. Shared governance is an accountability based organizational structure that creates a framework for partnership, equity, accountability and ownership through every component of the nursing organization. Through the use of service based or unit based councils or teams and systems wide councils or forums, a formal structure unfolds, requiring inclusion and investment of nurses in critical decision making affecting practice and patient care.

Shared governance, however, is a system's model and is therefore invitational to all partners in the delivery of care of services. If it stops at the doors of the nursing discipline, it essentially fails to make the necessary linkage to advance the delivery of patient care and build true integration around the patient or client. Next steps in creating a whole systems shared governance framework mean ultimately joining the structure with the system and the inclusion of other disciplines and service providers in a partnership for health care. An interdisciplinary, collegial approach to providing health service is essential if a true health script is to be written between providers and patients.

Organizing the health system around the point of care and building the relationships necessary to sustain it is a cornerstone of the whole systems approach to shared governance. Building the integrated clinical team, strengthening the organization's support structures, and linking with the board and community all form the underpinnings of an effective integrated health system. Shared governance structures create the fluid parameters that sustain the partnership between the providers of care and establish a format for their building together a service system that operates effectively along the continuum of care.

In the new social paradigm for work, relationships form the foundations for the organization. The integration of roles rather than the definition of jobs becomes the foundation for successful service structures. Patient care is based on healthy relationships. It is therefore appropriate that models which delineate relationships predominate in the future designs of health care systems. Shared governance is increasingly a viable structure for both creating and sustaining patient based and integrated approaches to providing health care services.

Tim Porter-O'Grady, EdD, PhD, RN, CS, CNAA, FAAN, is Senior Partner, Tim Porter-O'Grady Associates, Inc., Senior Consultant, Affiliated Dynamics, Inc., and Assistant Professor, Emory University, Atlanta, Georgia. Porter-O'Grady is an international consultant and advisor. He helps create the relationships, structures, and behaviors that reflect the principles of shared governance in a wide variety of health care settings throughout the world. He is the author of several books, including *Implementing Shared Governance: Creating a Professional Organization* (1992), and *The Nurse Manager's Problem Solver* (1994).

with other professional care providers in healthcare organizations (Porter-O'Grady, 1994).

However, decentralization and shared governance innovations can be major changes for nursing organizations. This new structure sets up an expectation of staff nurse participation and acceptance of personal responsibility. It has not been uniformly accepted or successful (Hess, 1994). Staff nurses may exhibit resistance due to a reticence to assume accountability and lose a traditional target for blame (Jacoby & Terpstra, 1990). Further, not all organizational change efforts balance the principles of centralization and decentralization through analysis of what can feasibly be decentralized, to what level, and in what way. Not all jobs and functions can be decentralized (Dirschel, 1994).

Thus nurses need to analyze and evaluate decentralization and shared governance for their fit to the organization and level and degree of implementation. Another level of analysis may be necessary as healthcare reform and revised payment mechanisms drive changes in the structure and delivery of care. As integrated networks form into new "organizations," lateral and relational designs are emerging to support community-based healthcare delivery. These organizations are challenged to create delivery structures that ensure seamless delivery of care. Clinical accountability will need to emerge from multidisciplinary and multi-site care environments. Shared governance, with its emphasis on responsibility and accountability, can form the basis for an integrated services structure. This is what Porter-O'Grady (1994) calls whole systems shared governance. With experience in hospital decentralization and shared governance, nurses are better prepared to function in integrated care networks.

LEADERSHIP AND MANAGEMENT IMPLICATIONS

A major leadership function is to provide vision during times of turbulent change. A major management function is to determine the structure of the department. The lessons of the last nurse shortage pointed out nurses' disenchantment with organizations that obstruct nurse autonomy and professional practice. Reorganization to achieve self-governance in organizations was thought to be a way to improve work performance, satisfaction, and quality of nursing care (Maas, 1989). Thus restructuring could be used as a leadership strategy to increase nurses' motivation. However, to enable professional nursing shared governance, management styles and roles have to change. The leader's role shifts from leading, organizing, and controlling to activities of integrating, facilitating, and coordinating (Jacoby & Terpstra, 1990). The manager's role becomes more concentrated on coaching, teaching, collaborating, consulting, and creating the environment with structures and resources to share decision making (Maas & Specht, 1994). Not all managers are prepared to do this and not all nurses are ready to assume reconfigured roles.

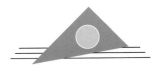

Leadership & Management Behaviors

LEADERSHIP BEHAVIORS	**MANAGEMENT BEHAVIORS**	**OVERLAP AREAS**
• integrates work effort	• coaches individual employees	• communicates
• facilitates communication	• teaches others how to handle conflict	• coordinates activity
• coordinates plans and actions	• collaborates with staff	• enables participation in decision making
• envisions an empowered decision making environment	• consults across units	
• enables participation	• creates a participative governance environment	
• liaisons with group members and outside the group	• communicates widely	
	• coordinates work activities	

Balancing the needs of the nursing staff with the organization's strategic needs is a nurse manager's challenge. Structure is a choice-based decision. Careful and deliberate alterations of organizational structure provide one mechanism for leading and managing with newer care models in a resource constrained environment. It is not always clear as to what works for nursing. Innovative governance models are likely to develop and evolve as nursing grows within a reformed healthcare delivery system. Clearly the structure of healthcare needs to change. Visionary leadership will help nurses find a way that best suits clients and their care needs. Decentralizing in a way that allows nurses to function to their fullest capabilities across a seamless continuum of care is a more cost-effective care management structure.

RESEARCH NOTE

Source: Anderson, R., & McDaniel, Jr., R. (1992). The implication of environmental turbulence for nursing-unit design in effective nursing homes. *Nursing Economic$*, *10*(2), 117-125.

Purpose

The purpose of this study was to examine the relationship of environmental turbulence to nursing unit organizational design in effective nursing homes. Some studies indicated that the degree of professionalization of the work force, decentralization, and participation depended on environmental turbulence. The professional nature of the organization and the cost constrained nature of the industry were two characteristics of nursing organizations thought to be related to the relationship of organizational structure to the environment. Information processing and decision making formed the theoretical framework for an exploratory study of 14 nursing homes in Texas. Environmental turbulence and decentralization were measured.

Discussion

Perceived environmental turbulence varied across facilities. There were generally low levels of decentralization and participation. At the organizational unit of analysis, decentralization was significantly correlated with environmental turbulence. There was greater decentralization with higher perceived environmental turbulence. When stratified by caregiver category, there was a statistically significant correlation between RN participation in decision making and environmental turbulence.

Application to Practice

The study was exploratory and used a small sample size of only effective nursing homes in one region. However, nurse managers who perceived higher environmental turbulence reported greater use of decentralization and greater participation of RNs in decision making. Apparently, they are compelled to more creatively and effectively utilize RNs. Healthcare organizations have heterogeneous core workers. Uncertainty and cost constraints should be matched to efforts to decentralize decision making, professionalize the workforce, and increase participation of RNs.

CURRENT ISSUES AND TRENDS

Shared governance in nursing is a recent innovation. The concept has been linked to ideas about decentralization and participation, both of which vary across time and vary by degree within specific situations. Staff nurses may be allowed to only make limited decisions, or not be involved at all in certain areas such as resource allocation. Authority may not be given or may be taken back. There are few generalizable evaluations of the effects of shared governance beyond specific sites (Hess, 1994).

As the innovation of shared governance diffused via consultants, publications, conferences, networking, and nursing education, the external pressures of cost and quality began to affect hospitals and healthcare organizations. As the national environment began to change to anticipate healthcare reform, reimbursement and financial management ideas focused on reducing costs by lowering the skill mix percentage of RNs and substituting nurse extenders.

Reorganization became reengineering. Work redesign promised to retool worksites for more effective and efficient outcomes (Porter-O'Grady, 1993). For nursing this meant looking at the delivery and organization of nursing care in a changing framework. Traditional frameworks were no longer seen as adequate to meet the needs for lower costs, higher consumer satisfaction, and pressures of the marketplace for quality and price (Porter-O'Grady, 1990). According to Hammer and Champy (1993), reengineering in healthcare is a radical redesign of the critical systems and processes used in delivering client care in order to achieve dramatic improvements in organizational performance measures such as cost, quality, service, and speed within a short time (Bergman, 1994).

The trends triggered by anticipation of healthcare reform also include an emphasis on the community, mergers, multihospital systems, consolidations, and uncertainty about payment mechanisms. Nurse practitioners are being promoted as primary care providers and substitutes for physicians. Case management and managed care are popular concepts in acute care service delivery.

Shared governance may go through an evolutionary change or simply fade under the pressure of greater organizational threat and change. For example, at one site, shared governance has moved from a traditional representational committee model to an interactive planning model using unit boards with multidisciplinary membership (Minnen, Berger, Ames, Dubree, Baker, & Spinella, 1993). In other places, client care delivery system redesigns are being called organizational transformations to outcome models for patient-focused care. These redesigns redefine tasks, work processes, jobs, roles, services, and systems. A series of transitions restructures roles:

- decentralizing to the point of service
- empowering staff decision making on the units
- multitasking and decreased task specialization
- development of new work processes and systems to support the delivery of client care
- creating new skill mixes and staffing templates (Cummings & O'Malley, 1993).

Porter-O'Grady (1990) has advocated the restructuring of nursing services to decentralize into smaller units of activity at a basic level of common function, such as a client need or nursing diagnosis classification. At the same time, the organization needs to integrate and establish centralized control in order to maintain control over services and functions. He views this not as a contradiction, but as the complementary process of differentiation. This is a way of organizing work processes and activities to provide needed and responsive services to clients. Porter-O'Grady (1990) called this the creation of a custom shop. One outcome goal is to provide an environment that leads the consumer to see the unique differences offered by the service and understand the difference it made. Service is knowing what you do, cost is knowing what it costs, and quality is delivering what you promised. A whole new approach to structure may be needed to reflect the changes and new views on the outcomes of nursing services.

SUMMARY

- Decision power is a key element of organizational structure.
- Centralization is the degree of decision power concentrated at the top.

❧ Decentralization is the degree of decision power dispersion to lower levels.

❧ Vertical decentralization is distribution of power down the line of authority.

❧ Horizontal decentralization is the flow of power outside the line of authority.

❧ Centralization/decentralization occur along a continuum, as a matter of degree.

❧ Shared governance is one form of a professional practice model and is a governance system designed to involve staff nurses in decision making.

❧ Shared governance implementation is affected by professional/bureaucratic conflicts and depth/degree of true change that occurs.

❧ Councilar, congressional, and administrative are the three identified operating models of professional shared governance.

❧ Leadership is needed to balance the staff's needs for governance and the organization's needs for lowered risk and higher control.

❧ Reorganization and restructuring are currently popular but evolving concepts.

Study Questions

1. What is the relationship between decentralization and shared governance?
2. How are shared governance and structure related?
3. What conditions in the facility in which you are a student or employee would facilitate shared governance?
4. Are decentralization and shared governance characteristic of current hospital nursing organizations? Current community health and long-term care organizations?
5. Does changing to a shared governance model change nurses' roles? If so, how?
6. What is the governance structure of the nursing organization you are most familiar with?
7. What questions should be asked to determine how decentralized an organization is in reality?

Critical Thinking Exercise

The RNs who work on the Mother-Baby Unit at High Care Hospital are frustrated with being floated to other units in times of low census. Morale is deteriorating. They perceive that they send out more staff to other units than they receive when busy. At the last unit meeting, the staff demanded that the nurse manager minimize their floating. The nurse manager announced an option: self-staffing. This would minimize floating, but the nurses would be accountable to cover their own unit at all times. This might mean on-call systems or mandatory overtime, which had never been used in the past. The nurse manager wanted the staff's decision in one month.

1. *What is the problem?*

2. *Whose problem is it?*

3. *What should the staff do first? Do next?*

4. *What organizational structure would be helpful?*

5. *What else should the nurse manager do?*

6. *What decision making strategy or process might be helpful?*

7. *Should the staff adopt a shared governance model? Which one?*

REFERENCES

Althaus, J., Hardyck, N., Pierce, P., & Rodgers, M. (1981). *Nursing decentralization: The El Camino experience.* Wakefield, MA: Nursing Resources.

Bergman, R. (1994). Reengineering health care. *Hospitals & Health Networks, 68*(3), 28-36.

Cummings, S., & O'Malley, J. (1993). Designing an outcome model for patient-focused care. *Seminars for Nurse Managers, 1*(1), 16-21.

Davis, P. (1992). Unit-based shared governance: Nurturing the vision. *Journal of Nursing Administration, 22*(12), 46-50.

DeBaca, V., Jones, K., & Tornabeni, J. (1993). A cost-benefit analysis of shared governance. *Journal of Nursing Administration, 23*(7/8), 50-57.

Dirschel, K. (1994). Decentralization or centralization: Striking a balance. *Nursing Management, 25*(9), 49-51.

Hage, J., & Aiken, M. (1967). Relationship of centralization to other structural properties. *Administrative Science Quarterly, 12*(6), 72-91.

Hammer, M., & Champy, J. (1993). *Reengineering the corporation: A manifesto for business revolution.* New York: HarperCollins.

Havens, D. (1994). Is governance being shared? *Journal of Nursing Administration, 24*(6), 59-64.

Hess, Jr., R. (1994). Shared governance: Innovation or imitation? *Nursing Economic$, 12*(1), 28-34.

Jacoby, J., & Terpstra, M. (1990). Collaborative governance: Model for professional autonomy. *Nursing Management, 21*(2), 42-44.

Jones, C., Stasiowski, S., Simons, B., Boyd, N., & Lucas, M. (1993). Shared governance and the nursing practice environment. *Nursing Economic$, 11*(4), 208-214.

Leftridge, D., & Lydford, C. (1993). Decentralizing an overtime budget. *Nursing Management, 24*(8), 52-53.

Likert, R. (1960). *New patterns of management.* New York: McGraw-Hill.

Maas, M. (1989). Professional practice for the extended care environment: Learning from one model and its implementation. *Journal of Professional Nursing, 5*(2), 66-76.

Maas, M., & Specht, J. (1990). Nursing professionalization and self-governance: A model from long-term care. In G. Mayer, M. Madden, & E. Lawrenz (Eds.), *Patient care delivery models* (pp. 151-168). Rockville, MD: Aspen.

Maas, M., & Specht, J. (1994). Shared governance in nursing: What is shared, who governs, and who benefits? In J. McCloskey & H. Grace (Eds.), *Current issues in nursing* (4th ed.) (pp. 398-406). St. Louis: Mosby.

McGregor, D. (1960). *The human side of enterprise.* New York: McGraw-Hill.

Melcher, A. (1976). *Structure and process of organizations: A systems approach.* Englewood Cliffs, NJ: Prentice-Hall.

Minnen, T., Berger, E., Ames, A., Dubree, M., Baker, W., & Spinella, J. (1993). Sustaining work redesign innovations through shared governance. *Journal of Nursing Administration, 23*(7/8), 35-40.

Mintzberg, H. (1983). *Structure in fives: Designing effective organizations.* Englewood Cliffs, NJ: Prentice-Hall.

Paterson, T. (1969). *Management theory.* London: Business Publications.

Porter-O'Grady, T. (1987). Shared governance and new organizational models. *Nursing Economic$, 5*(6), 281-286.

Porter-O'Grady, T. (1990). *Reorganization of nursing practice: Creating the corporate venture.* Rockville, MD: Aspen.

Porter-O'Grady, T. (1993). Work redesign: Fact, fiction, and foible. *Seminars for Nurse Managers, 1*(1), 8-15.

Porter-O'Grady, T. (1994). Whole systems shared governance: Creating the seamless organization. *Nursing Economic$, 12*(4), 187-195.

Price, J., & Mueller, C. (1986). *Handbook of organizational measurement.* Marshfield, MA: Pitman.

Delegation

Chapter Objectives

❧

define and describe delegation

❧

define supervision

❧

explain characteristics of true delegation

❧

analyze the relationships among delegation, authority,
responsibility, and accountability

❧

identify four principles of delegation

❧

explain four steps in the process of delegating

❧

explain delegation pitfalls

❧

analyze legal and regulatory aspects of delegation and supervision

❧

analyze the use of nurse extenders and delegation to
unlicensed assistive personnel (UAPs)

❧

exercise critical thinking to conceptualize and analyze
possible solutions to a practical experience incident

*d*elegating is a fundamental aspect of every leader's and manager's job.
The effective assignment of work to others is essential in every type of
group and organization. Further, effective delegation skills are important for

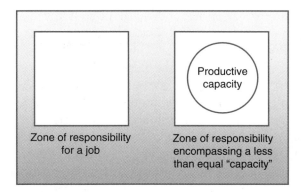

Zone of responsibility
for a job

Zone of responsibility
encompassing a less
than equal "capacity"

Productive
capacity

Figure 15.1
Zones of responsibility.

managers whose function is to get work done through the labor of others (Poteet, 1989). For most nursing jobs the zone of responsibility exceeds one person's capacity to produce (see Fig. 15.1). What this means is that most nursing jobs encompass responsibility beyond one individual's ability to get all the work done by themselves. This is especially true for the care coordination aspects of nursing care management. Thus nurses need to delegate parts of nursing care delivery to others.

Delegation is becoming a more urgent issue in nursing practice. Changing staff mix and job restructuring are national trends in hospitals. With healthcare reform movements, new roles for nurses have emerged, and care tasks are being redistributed and delegated within a multidisciplinary team (del Bueno, 1993). Throughout the history of nursing, nurses have delegated to personnel in the healthcare environment, whether this was to a student, LPN/LVN, corpsman, nursing assistant, or some other form of nurse extender. The most recent cycle of the nurse shortage created a pressing need for either nurses or substitutes for nurses. Subsequent cost concerns under healthcare reform initiatives brought downsizing and substitution of assistive personnel for RNs. One result of this shortage was a discussion about what tasks are appropriate to nursing, which of these tasks are appropriate to be delegated, and what level of personnel is appropriate for which tasks.

DEFINITIONS

Delegation essentially is getting things done through other people. It involves transferring a task or procedure to someone else. It is a leadership and management strategy designed to maximize time management. The American Nurses Association has defined *delegation* as the transfer of responsibility for the performance of an activity from one individual to another while retaining accountability for the outcome (American Nurses Association, 1993; Dietz, 1994). Delegation in nursing has been defined as transferring to a competent individual the authority to perform a selected nursing task in a selected situation (National Council of State Boards of Nursing [NCSBN], 1990). It relies on trust. The goal of delegation is workload distribution.

The *delegator* is the nurse or manager making the delegation (see Chart 15.1). The *delegate* is the assistant or staff person receiving the delegated task or procedure. *Supervision* in nursing is defined as a qualified nurse providing guidance for the accomplishment of a nursing task or activity, with initial direction and periodic inspection of the actual accomplishment of the task or activity (NCSBN, 1990). Supervision is the active process of directing, guiding, and influencing the outcome of a person's performance of an activity. Supervision can be categorized as on-site or off-site (American Nurses Association, 1993).

What delegation is not: (1) the indiscriminate assignment of work to others is dumping work, not delegating, (2) giving orders is directing the flow of work and is not the same as delegating, and (3) abdicating control or responsibility is not delegation.

True delegation is real to the participants: the manager intentionally creates tension by really letting the participants go on their own, but only after instilling in them the highest standards of performance and adherence to a shared vision. The participants then function within the standards set by the manager (Peters, 1987). True delegation implies that the subordinate is given the authority to do the job, can make independent decisions, and has the responsibility for seeing that the job is done well. Effective delegation requires that subordinates have the authority to accompany their responsibility.

However, ultimate responsibility and accountability rests with the manager because, in the end, the manager is accountable to his or her own superiors for fulfilling the responsibility to get the job done right and on time. Thus true delegation means giving up some of the authority and holding onto the ultimate responsibility and accountability. Delegation benefits managers and organizations by gaining freedom, time, and greater efficiency from its effective implementation.

Nursing activities include all tasks and activities, both mental and physical, necessary to care for clients and produce nursing and health outcomes. Nursing activities involve tasks and direct client contact, as well as the full scope of the nursing process. It is inappropriate to delegate the core activities of the nursing process and those that require specialized knowledge and judgment. *Nonnursing tasks* are those tasks necessary to support client care. These typically are tasks related to housekeeping and clerical duties, not usually involving direct client care (American Association of Critical Care Nurses [AACN], 1991).

BACKGROUND

The NCSBN issued a concept paper on delegation in 1990. According to the NCSBN (1990) the acceptable use of the authority to delegate is based

---

CHART 15.1
∽ DEFINITIONS

Delegation
the transfer of responsibility for the performance of an activity from one individual to another while retaining accountability for the outcome.

Delegator
the manager making the delegation.

Delegate
the staff person receiving the delegated task.

Supervision
providing guidance for the accomplishment of a task or activity, with initial direction and periodic inspection of the actual accomplishment of the task or activity.

Data from American Nurses Association (1993) and from NCSBN (1990).

upon a determination of the task to be accomplished. Delegation also involves an assessment of each person's competency as an essential part of the delegation activity. The questions to ask are, what is the task to be delegated, how complex or simple is it, and how much intensive decision making is needed to do this task? Factors to be considered include the task, the staff available, and the client's needs; the potential delegate's competency, and the level of supervision available (see Chart 15.2). The delegation dilemma relates to how to select, based on the client's needs, the best caregiver from among the available staff. The six principles related to delegation are (Hansten, 1991):

1. Know yourself and your team members well.
2. Assess strengths, weaknesses, job descriptions, the situation, and the skills of yourself and the team members.
3. Understand the state practice act, practice limitations, and job descriptions.
4. Know the job requirements.
   a. Assess the assignment.
   b. Diagnose the situation.
   c. Plan appropriate strategies.
5. Keep communication clear, complete, and constant.
   a. Communicate expectations.
   b. Validate understanding.
   c. Provide ongoing communication.
6. Evaluate.
   a. Review what happened.
   b. Measure the results.

What is the competency of the staff available for delegation? The job title of nursing assistant does not mean that a nurse automatically can delegate to any assistant certain tasks. Assignments must fall within the person's scope of practice. The delegate must understand the assignment and be competent (Barter & Furmidge, 1994).

The nurse's delegation responsibility includes (1) assessing the competency of the person and (2) assessing how much supervision time is available. The nurse's two main legal responsibilities when making work assignments are to appropriately delegate duties and adequately supervise afterward (Barter & Furmidge, 1994). Both factors may vary depending on the situation and the employee's job maturity. The amount of time needed to supervise after delegation and the needed proximity of the supervisor affect the nurse's workload.

From the perspective of the delegate, if delegated to, it is important to understand the parameters around the delegation: how is the task to be done, when is it to be done, where is it to be done, and by whom? How much actual or potential authority is being transferred in this delegation? Delegation means being given a responsibility, but the amount and type of authority actually being transferred along with the responsibility is important for task per-

CHART 15.2
∽ DELEGATION CHECKLIST

- How is the task to be done?
- When is the task to be done?
- Where is the task to be done?
- By whom is the task to be done?
- What is the responsibility and authority for decision making (approves, is responsible, is consulted, is informed)?

CHART 15.3 ◆ DELEGATION TRACKING FORM

Date _____

Task Outcome _____

Task Steps _____

Task Location _____

Delegator _____

Delegate _____

Time Frame _____

Decision Responsibility/Authority _____

Next Communication _____

Other_____

---

formance. A device such as a written tracking form can be used as a communication and planning aid to make the process clearer (Gilmore & Peter, 1987). (See Chart 15.3.)

RESEARCH NOTE

Source: Jung, F. (1991). Teaching registered nurses how to supervise nursing assistants. *Journal of Nursing Administration*, 21(4), 32-36.

Purpose

The purpose of this article was to describe the evaluation of a program to improve the direction and supervision of nursing assistants (NAs) developed at one eastern hospital. It was identified that NAs were not being used effectively. Most RNs who had to direct NAs had little background in the supervision of NAs. Consequently, NAs had large amounts of nonproductive time. A pilot project was instituted on one 40 bed medical-surgical unit as part of an evaluation of alternative care delivery models. RNs were taught how to supervise NA staff and redistribute the workload. Subsequently, a four hour educational program was developed for other areas. Then changes were made in RN and NA job descriptions, performance evaluations, and staff workload distribution.

Discussion

The RN teaching program was divided into two 2-hour sessions. In the first session, roles and responsibilities of staff were reviewed by category. Principles and guidelines for effective staff supervision and utilization were presented. Application of the knowledge was made afterward, on the home unit. Four weeks later the second session used small unit groups and focused on the implementation of the workload distribution program. Role playing was used to critically think through specific difficult supervision situations of NA malingering, poor quality of work, avoiding assignments, tardiness, and blatant refusal of work assignment. After six months, significant improvement in NA utilization was observed.

Application to Practice

The author discusses some of the barriers encountered in a workload redistribution program. The NA's role in patient care was not clearly identified nor valued. Clearly, a move toward greater implementation of NAs is underway in healthcare. Yet many RNs and nurse managers much prefer all-RN staffs. Thus there is a clash of philosophies. Lack of cooperation and support for a program makes it difficult to implement. A clear delineation of how NAs are to be used in direct care is needed if the RNs' time is to be refocused. RNs benefit from educational programs that provide the knowledge, skills, and tools to delegate and supervise effectively.

Process of Delegation

The benefits of delegating are many and important. Delegation encourages the initiative of subordinates and creates room for them to grow. It frees management for other priorities, including planning, organizing, directing, and controlling the organization itself. Viewed abstractly, delegating appears to be a fairly straightforward and simple process. Four basic steps involved in the process of delegating are:

1. Select a capable person.
2. Explain the task and outcomes to occur.
3. Give the necessary authority and means for doing the job.
4. Arrange to keep in contact and give feedback.

The process is to give a directive, set a time frame, and have periodic reviewing from the beginning of the task or project through the end of the task or project. In most cases, it is very wise for the manager and the subordinate to agree upon the job, its essentials, and the objectives and then to arrange for continuing series of feedback sessions in which the subordinate reports on progress. One way to make certain that both manager and subordinate understand what the objectives are and reach them effectively is to follow up a verbal directive with written instructions so that each person can refer to them at some later point. Set a specific time frame in which the entire task or project is going to be completed. Establish specific review dates throughout the entire time frame, so that no one is surprised at any point as to what is expected of them or as to what is expected as an outcome (Delegating, 1981; Poteet, 1989). Nelson (1994) provided a list of delegation preparations for delegators that can be used as a checklist of activities for delegation (see Chart 15.4). In making a decision to delegate nursing activities, the following five factors can be assessed (AACN, 1991):

- the potential for harm
- the complexity of the nursing activity

CHART 15.4
∾ DELEGATOR'S CHECKLIST

- Develop a good attitude.
- Decide what to delegate.
- Select the right person.
- Communicate responsibilities.
- Grant authority.
- Provide support.
- Monitor the delegation.
- Evaluate.

Data from Nelson (1994).

- the required problem solving and innovation
- the predictability of the outcome
- the extent of client interaction.

The process of delegation incorporates the right task delegated to the right person and with the right communication and the right feedback. The most crucial legal issue remains nursing judgment. The nurse must ask questions and give direction. The success of the delegation process relies on an ability to communicate with clear direction and motivational appeal (Hansten & Washburn, 1992a, b, c, d).

Although it is in everyone's best interest to delegate, the process may be undermined from within. Many managers find it hard to let go of control psychologically. The central aspect of delegation is trust. When called upon to delegate something important, individuals may suddenly discover that for some reason they do not trust subordinates quite as much as they thought they did. How can work be delegated to people if they are not trusted? On the other hand, how can they earn our trust if we do not delegate to them? This is a real dilemma, facing both manager and subordinate. The absence of trust by the manager arouses in the subordinates one of the most powerful of all feelings: fear. Yet in delegation there is for the manager a loss of control that also can arouse fear (Delegating, 1981).

Further, there is an emotional reality that surrounds delegation. Delegation inevitably involves risk. On the one hand, managers may fear that something a subordinate initiates will damage their reputation. In nursing this translates into the fear of harming a patient or incurring a lawsuit. On the other hand, subordinates' successes may be as threatening as their failures. This occurs naturally as a fear that a subordinate might surpass the manager in ability or prestige.

In nursing, conventional wisdom and anecdotal experiences indicate how difficult it is for nurses to delegate effectively. For some this is an ability issue. The ethic of primary care was that the RN was responsible for providing most of the direct client care. Therefore, nurses became used to providing care themselves and may not have learned how to delegate. For others, it is a willingness or motivation issue. Interdependency creates some practical difficulties. Staff nurses do not have the legitimacy of position to support delegation decisions that line managers have. Thus nurses may find that they need to direct and supervise others, yet they have no power over the rewards and punishments that motivate cooperation. This issue is especially acute in highly unionized environments. Other issues of trust and control, the need for approval and affiliation, beliefs in equality and democracy, and a desire to avoid confrontation all create sticky or threatening relationship difficulties that may sabotage delegation (del Bueno, 1993).

However, organizations must run on delegation. Therefore, managers who will not delegate cause difficulties and confusion. Despite reluctance, time pressures eventually may force even the hesitant the manager to delegate.

RESEARCH NOTE

Source: Jung, F., Pearcey, L., & Phillips, J. (1994). Evaluation of a program to improve nursing assistant use. *Journal of Nursing Administration, 24*(3), 42-47.

Purpose

The purpose of this research was to evaluate a workload redistribution program that focused on delegating patient care activities by RNs to NAs. This article is an update and extension of the Jung (1991) article that introduced the teaching program for RNs on delegation and supervision. In the current article, the program was evaluated for effects on outcomes of nurses' job satisfaction, quality of nursing care, workload, ability to supervise NAs, and coordination of care. Quality and workload data were trended quarterly for nine months before implementation and 12 months after implementation. Transformational nursing leadership was the conceptual framework used. The program was described in Jung (1991). A questionnaire was administered to 98 RNs. Both pre-and post-implementation measures were designed to assess job satisfaction, quality of care, workload, and care coordination.

Discussion

The workload redistribution program increased the amount of work delegated by RNs to NAs. Patient satisfaction, nurse job satisfaction, and quality of care were maintained or slightly improved. NAs were more available and productive. Workload for RNs improved. However, RNs continued to report a significant level of discomfort with supervising NAs, even after the teaching program. The need for follow-up was indicated.

Application to Practice

Overall, the workload redistribution project was a major change in RN role: from solo practitioners to delegators and supervisors of NAs. Findings indicated that RN workload was decreased while holding steady quality of care and patient satisfaction. NA productivity was increased following an RN teaching program. However, discomfort lingered and indicated either a need for follow-up activities with RNs or a genuine systems problem with NA utilization. This article highlights the use and value of capturing systematic evaluative data when implementing a major innovative change in nursing practice.

Delegation Pitfalls

When delegating work to someone, strong feelings and reactions occur, including the manager's desire to hold on (see Chart 15.5). In effect, the man-

CHART 15.5
∾ DELEGATION RELUCTANCE

- Getting trapped in the "I can do it better myself" fallacy
- Lack of ability to direct
- Lack of confidence in subordinates
- Lack of confidence in self
- An aversion to taking a risk
- Need to feel indispensable and difficulty letting go
- Fear of losing authority or personal satisfaction

Data from Delegating (1981) and from Poteet (1989).

ager takes some of the delegation back by reclaiming some of the delegated authority or responsibility. Nothing is more demoralizing for subordinates than to discover that the manager has undercut their authority. Managers who are novice, insecure, or needing to feel indispensable are most likely to resist delegation or to renege on it later. Their motto is, "If you want a job done right, you have to do it yourself." The reasons why delegators are reluctant to delegate include feeling that they need to do it themselves, lack of ability to do the directing, lack of confidence in the subordinates, a temperamental aversion to delegation, fear of losing authority or personal job satisfaction, and having difficulty with letting go (Delegating, 1981; Poteet, 1989).

Some subordinates attempt to avoid a delegation by fostering a myth that the delegators are so indispensable that they therefore need to do the work themselves. The illusion of the manager's indispensability may be actively fostered by a subordinate. Sometimes this belief is genuine, but it may be a reason for the subordinate to avoid being delegated to and, therefore, avoid accepting personal responsibility. The issue may be the reluctance of subordinates to accept responsibility. The subordinate may simply be responding to the manager's unique personality. Perhaps the employee does not feel like taking on the responsibility, so it is easier to ask someone else to make all the decisions rather than to take the initiative and the risks personally. Subordinates may fear criticism of mistakes or may simply feel that they already have more work than they can handle. They may not have confidence in their own abilities (Delegating, 1981). Sometimes it is a matter of reminding them that they do have the necessary skills and abilities, especially if they would push themselves a little bit. The supervisor may feel that the subordinates do have the job maturity, knowledge, and ability to handle the task, but the subordinates may feel that positive incentives are not present. From the employee's perspective, why take on something extra or put in more effort if the perception is that they are not going to be positively rewarded? (See Chart 15.6.)

Managers sometimes reestablish their claim on authority by hovering after a job has been delegated. But hovering, or "breathing down somebody's neck," usually conveys a feeling of distrust, not the helpful concern it is masked with. The manager's actions may lead to the feeling that maybe the lack of trust is justified. Thus hovering often causes the very mistakes it was intended to prevent and undermines the subordinate's self-esteem (Delegating, 1981).

To help nurses work through the reluctance to delegate, Hansten and Washburn (1992a) posed six scenarios with accompanying multiple choice foils to help nurses examine their delegation style. For example, one statement asks nurses to identify what they would do if they were uncertain about a nursing assistant's skill at giving an enema. Another statement asks nurses to identify what they would do if they were a nurse assigned to 10 patients on a medical-surgical floor with only one assistant. Testing with this simple exercise gives an indication of predisposition to overcome obstacles to delegation such

CHART 15.6
∾ Why
Subordinates
Avoid
Responsibilities

- Fits with manager's personality
- Easier to ask the boss than to decide how to deal with a problem
- Fear of criticism for mistakes
- Lack necessary information and resources to do a good job
- Subordinates may already have more work than they can do
- Lack of self-confidence
- Positive incentives may be inadequate

Data from Delegating (1981).

as feeling you can do it better yourself, thinking it takes too much time to teach, not trusting others, or preferring to work alone.

Legal Aspects of Delegation and Supervision

There are legal regulations that pertain to the role of the nurse and the nurse's supervision of others in the delivery of client care. That occurs because nursing is defined in state laws that require a license to practice nursing. Nurses at all levels may be unclear about the legal accountability in a delegation situation. For example, a nurse preceptor might ask: "What is my responsibility if I take on a student and that student creates an error or is negligent?" A staff nurse may be uncertain about the legal parameters of delegating to a nursing assistant who may have had only two weeks of training or a short orientation to client care. It has been reported that the trend for hospitals is to provide less than 20 hours of classroom orientation and less than 40 hours of on-the-job training to newly hired unlicensed assistive personnel (Barter & Furmidge, 1994; Barter, McLaughlin & Thomas, 1994). For what kinds of things will a nurse be sued? This has been described as the age-old fear that the nurse's license is on the line (Herrick, Hansten, O'Neil, Hayes & Washburn, 1994).

Delegation is considered to be part of the nurse's role. Nurses will be delegating and participating in being delegated to. When the nurse delegates, the nurse assumes responsibility for supervision, whether physically present or not. Each nurse is accountable to practice according to state law. The nurse delegator is accountable to assess the situation and for the decision to delegate. Thus the nurse delegator is accountable for the acts of delegation and may incur liability if found negligent in the process of delegating and supervising. The person delegated to is accountable for accepting the delegation and for their own actions in carrying out the delegated tasks (see Table 15.1).

Table 15.1

Who Has Accountability

DELEGATOR	DELEGATE
Own acts	Own acts
Acts of delegation	Accepting the delegation
Acts of supervision	Appropriate notification and reporting
Assessment of the situation	Accomplishing the task
Follow-up	
Intervention	
Corrective action	

If a delegating nurse makes an acceptable delegation to a competent delegate and an error occurs, then the delegate is accountable for his or her actions in its performance, and the delegator is accountable for supervision, follow-up, intervention, and corrective action. Assessment, evaluation, and nursing judgment should not be delegated; tasks and procedures may be delegated. While others may suggest which acts to delegate, the individual nurse ultimately decides the appropriateness of delegation in a specific situation (NCSBN, 1990).

The Nurse Practice Act and the related laws that govern nursing practice in each state, along with the accompanying administrative rules and regulations, are the main legal regulations. Each state's legislature has set up a Board of Nursing, whose function is to interpret and enforce the law. When they interpret the law, the formal interpretations become administrative rules that have the force of law. Obviously, then, state nurse practice acts and their official interpretations constitute a body of rules, codified within the legal regulatory system, that govern nursing practice and provide direction about delegation and supervision. The professional nursing association, the American Nurses Association, and each state's nurses association are the bodies that speak for the profession of nursing to define and guide the professional practice of nursing.

The American Nurses Association's Code for Nurses is the source to use for ethical dilemmas. It gives guidance in terms of ethical accountability for nurses' actions and for those they supervise in the scope of practice. These are the basic sources to use as guides about incompetent, unethical, or illegal practice on the part of anyone concerned with the client's care. The nurse has an obligation to act under such circumstances.

In one state the nurses association developed a pamphlet that discussed the nurse's supervisory obligations and accompanying regulations. Called "Supervision by Professional Nurses" (Iowa Nurses' Association, 1984), it noted that the Nurse Practice Act in the state defined accountability as being obligated to answer for one's acts, including the act of supervision. The registered nurse is expected to recognize and understand the legal implications of accountability by knowing what accountability is and what it means in terms of nursing practice. Accountability includes acts of supervision, among other things. In a legal sense supervision means personally observing a function or activity, providing leadership in the process of nursing care, delegating functions or activities while retaining the accountability, and evaluating or determining that nursing care being provided is adequate and delivered appropriately. While this document is dated, the definitions and principles of the law related to supervision have not changed.

The state administrative code also identifies nursing behavior that constitutes illegal conduct. This includes delegating nursing functions to others contrary to statute or state rules. Such nursing behavior is subject to discipline. The state regulatory body can utilize any measure of discipline across the continuum, including revoking a license. In a legal sense, negligence or malpractice consists of failure of a professional person to act in accordance with the prevalent professional standards or failure to foresee possibilities and consequences that a professional person, having the necessary skill and training to act professionally, should foresee. The nurse must perform at a level that exceeds or equals that of a reasonably prudent registered professional nurse. Generally, practice issues are tested in courts of law. In this process, expert witnesses are used to interpret the standard of a reasonably prudent professional registered nurse.

The nurse has an obligation or duty to act in the event of a breakdown in client care wherever in the chain that breakdown occurs. This means that the nurse is never permitted under law to passively observe substandard care. The most common situation is of a fellow nurse or other healthcare provider demonstrably or clearly failing to provide the appropriate care to clients. Substandard care also may come about because a healthcare agency is failing to exercise its corporate duty in providing quality care. Under both of these circumstances, the nurse must act and cannot hide behind the fact that "the doctor knows best" or that "the administration does not listen to nurses."

The next issue is what to do in these situations. The nurse begins with an assessment of how much client safety is being compromised. If there is clear actual or potential harm, the nurse must act directly. If the situation is ambiguous, such as an ethical issue, then the nurse must take some action appropriate to the circumstance. For example, this may be reported to the immediate superior, or there may be a refusal to participate if that is appropriate.

Some situations are less complex and more clear as to the appropriate actions to take. For example, when an ICU nurse walks away from the bedside of a patient who is comatose with an intracranial pressure screw in place and leaves the siderails down, patient safety is clearly compromised and action must be taken. If an overdose level of a chemotherapy drug is ordered, action must be taken. However, many situations fall into a "gray area." For example, providers use a variety of practice patterns. Situations are complex and multidimensional. Ethical values may be at odds. One provider might not have complete information about an observed situation. For example, behaviors interpreted as due to substance abuse can be manifested because of physical or psychological organic illness.

Legal and ethical issues surround the tensions and trade-offs between quality and cost. For example, it is not clear as to what constitutes an "unsafe" level of nurse staffing. Nurses face uncomfortable situations when deciding between labor budget pressures and staffing for clients' care needs. At what point does the nurse take action to report "unsafe" staffing levels? What action strategies are effective? How does the nurse who calls the fire department to report serious overcrowding of patients into hallways reconcile the duty to protect client safety with accusations of insubordination and potential job termination?

There is a whole continuum of circumstances in clinical practice that challenge the duty and obligation to act and not passively observe substandard care. What is substandard care and what is a reasonable standard are professional judgments. Novices must learn ways of handling situations both for themselves and within the context of an organization so as to not get fired or be at risk for a lawsuit.

One example occurs when a colleague is either known or suspected to be suffering from a chemical dependency. When that person comes onto the work area clearly in an altered level of awareness state and not capable of providing safe care to clients, the nurse must act in order to protect clients' safety. See Chapter 5 for further discussion.

Another example can occur when questioning a physician's order or treatment regimen. For example, the physician involved in the care of the client prescribes a medication that seems unusual, wrong, or inappropriate. Perhaps the concern is about the effects of the medical regimen, such as when a client has not been attended to and is decompensating. The nurse is faced with a decision about how to act. Analysis of the situation may lead to the conclusion that there are a variety of ways in which physicians may treat any condition. Or action may be necessary to report the situation and obtain remediation.

In ambiguous circumstances or situations in which a choice must be made between competing ethical values, the actions to be taken must be carefully weighed and considered. Clearly, client safety and the obligation to do no harm is a fundamental starting point. The nurse then can analyze the situation and decide upon a strategy. A framework for ethical analysis can be chosen to help clarify values and ethical choices (see Chapter 7). A legal analysis can be done to assess whether the elements of a malpractice claim appear to be in evidence: duty, breach of duty, proximate cause, and damages (see Chapter 5). Other assessments can be done by consulting organizational policies and standards, the state's Nurse Practice Act and administrative rulings from the Board of Nursing, nursing's Code of Ethics and standards of practice, and standards and guidelines of specialty organizations. A clear legal duty to act is more urgent than is a question of ethics. Through reasoned investigation and analysis of the situation, the nurse decides to act immediately, investigate further, document, report, or analyze the situation for future decision making. The standards of "reasonable," "prudent," and "good faith" form the foundations for legal and ethical decision making strategies.

LEADERSHIP AND MANAGEMENT IMPLICATIONS

Delegation is related to leadership effectiveness and the use of leadership styles. For example, the nurse manager would use the leadership style of selling and supervise the task accomplishment more closely with novices or in

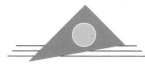

Leadership & Management Behaviors

LEADERSHIP BEHAVIORS

- enables followers to learn delegation and supervision skills
- creates a positive work climate and teamwork
- matches leadership style to readiness of followers and situation
- is visible and available
- communicates clearly
- uses interpersonal relationship facilitation to aid group functioning
- delegates
- facilitates delegation and acceptance of responsibility

MANAGEMENT BEHAVIORS

- coaches subordinates to improve task maturity
- performs careful assessments of abilities
- makes assignments to match skills and abilities
- monitors performance through supervision
- documents
- evaluates task accomplishment
- disciplines employees
- communicates clearly
- delegates

OVERLAP AREAS

- facilitates delegation and acceptance of responsibility
- communicates clearly
- delegates

• •

complex situations (see Chapter 4 for Hersey & Blanchard's leadership style theory). Following leadership principles, this is similar to matching the leadership style to the readiness of the followers. It appears that leaders and managers may adopt one of two problem solving styles: adaptation or innovation. Adaptors generate ideas to solve problems. Innovators detach the problem, critically think about it, and search for a solution. Individuals tend to remain in an organizational environment that has a problem solving style that matches their personal inclination (Adams, 1993). The same may be true for styles of delegation. Individuals may adopt unique styles, and these styles may be a "fit" or a mismatch.

Leader behaviors for delegation and supervision include being around, being available, and helping the subordinate through the task actions and decisions. Coaching actions are employed. Nursing practice in community health or home healthcare settings may include supervision off-site. Careful assessment, regular visits, and complete documentation are used when delegating (Barter & Furmidge, 1994).

The manager should never attempt to delegate three aspects of managerial work (see Chart 15.7). One is personal accountability. Technically, personal accountability literally cannot be delegated, but some people try. The manager is accountable for his or her personal acts and the quality and quan-

CHART 15.7
∾ WHAT NOT TO DELEGATE

- Personal accountability
- Discipline of employees
- Recognition and praise

tity of his or her supervision. For example, within the clinical setting of nursing practice, the nurse manager of a particular area has the accountability for the quality of the client care. This is always retained and cannot be delegated.

Second, the discipline of employees should be accomplished by the manager. Direct managerial intervention maintains a climate within the work group, communicates a message, and shows discharge of duty. If there is an area in which the client care is not bringing about quality results, or if there is some problem in regard to the delivery of client care, the manager needs to be directly active in the remediation of the problem.

The third area relates to morale problems. Morale, and its associated aspects of motivation and job satisfaction, should be addressed directly as a function of leadership. Leadership style and the interpersonal and communication skills of the leader have a strong influence on the subordinates' morale. Recognition and praise do not lend themselves to delegation.

When nurses practice as employees, they act for the employer and work within a setting where the employer may control the work of the nurse and nurse's role enactment. Nurses must manage and coordinate their responsibility to the employer for employment activities with their responsibility to the Board of Nursing for nursing practice. Issues arise over the amount of allocation of resources, the locus of decision making over allocation of resources, the level of supervision required in the nursing role, and the nurse's autonomy to determine nursing work and working conditions. The employer is primarily responsible for the allocation of resources. While it may be uncomfortable to work in an unfamiliar setting, it may be unsafe to work in a new setting without adequate orientation, education, and supervision. Further, the nurse ultimately decides and is accountable for appropriate and safe delegation, even when faced with employer pressure and staffing problems (NCSNB, 1990).

CURRENT ISSUES AND TRENDS

The Use of Nurse Extenders

Delegation and supervision are intertwined with issues surrounding the use of nurse extenders and unlicensed assistive personnel (UAPs). In the past, a nurse extender meant a nursing assistant or a corpsman. A nurse extender was an ancillary person trained to perform some basic client care tasks who may have been given a client assignment. Today, there are many names for and types of nurse extenders, and they can be classified by clinical and nonclinical job duties (Gardner, 1991). The basic distinction is whether or not the nurse extender does direct client care. Nurse extenders range from licensed practical and vocational nurses (LPNs and LVNs) to UAPs, who have no formal healthcare education or training. Alterations in the skill mix percentage of RNs to UAPs have been moving toward an increase in UAPs and a decrease in RNs. Nurses argue that inadequate staffing ratios can create a potentially dangerous circumstance for client care and safety. In California, nurses lobbied to legislate minimum nurse-patient ratios in acute care hospitals (Sherer, 1993).

The Tri Council for Nursing (1990) has stated that it is extremely important that assistants be used in a way that assures appropriate delegation and assignment of nursing functions as well as adequate supervision of those to whom nursing activities are delegated. The Joint Commission on Accreditation of Healthcare Organizations (JCAHO) requires sufficient RNs to ensure safe care. Without national standards for RN to client ratios, facilities usually set a number ratio (e.g., 1:8 or 1:12) that stresses speed and increases the chance for distractions to cause errors (Davis, 1993). However, hospitals say that they must trim costs, that ratios have little to do with clients' needs, and that this is a turf issue about RN job security (Anders, 1994; Sherer, 1993).

Decisions about the use of nurse extenders focus on what tasks there are to do and which ones belong only to the registered nurse. For example, what tasks can registered nurses do with extenders to help them out? What tasks could be delegated completely to non-licensed or minimally trained personnel? Some guidelines include routine care needs, predictable outcomes, and nonthreatening illness states (see Chart 15.8). The nursing profession is challenged to find ways to balance the tension between professional judgment about care needs and organizations' fiscal pressures.

Hiring UAPs increases an organization's responsibility for screening, orientation, and training. The direct care RNs assume a major responsibility for supplementing minimally trained UAPs and for supervising their delegated tasks (Barter & Furmidge, 1994). Joel (1994) recommended that nursing's bottom line remain "what is best for the client." Thus staffing patterns and methods of care delivery should be scrutinized in terms of client outcomes.

A reasonable first decision rule is to be able to delegate the care of clients whose care requirements are routine and standard. Once it is assessed that the person to be delegated to has the minimal competencies, then if the outcomes of care are relatively predictable, delegation is probably fairly safe. If the client's reaction to illness and hospitalization is not threatening to his or her mental health or sense of self, it probably is relatively safe to assume that that is the kind of care that can be delegated to a UAP.

Delegation is part of the RN's role that occurs as a part of a job within the context of a care delivery system. The skill mix and care modality structure to best fit care delivery needs varies over time and in specific settings and sites. Learning when and how to delegate is a key skill for developing effective leaders and managers and for maintaining quality of care under conditions of rising client acuity, fiscal pressures, and shorter lengths of hospital stays (Hansten, 1991).

CHART 15.8
∿ DELEGATION TO UAPS

Patients whose
- care requirements are routine and standardized
- outcomes are predictable
- reaction to illness and hospitalization is not threatening to their mental health.

Changing the Skill Mix

Our University Hospital was undergoing reorganization and redesign of our patient care delivery system. As a manager, I was faced with altering the skill mix of staff in an intensive care unit and an acute transplant/general surgery unit. The staff in both areas had worked with nurses aides (NAs) in limited numbers. The traditional role of the NA was to aide in comfort and safety, assist with activities of daily living and hygiene, accompany patients during off unit transport, stocking and supplying carts and bedsides. In addition, the acute unit NA would measure blood pressure, pulse, temperature, and respiratory rate on a routine basis.

The ICU skill mix changed from 90% RN:10% NA to 70% RN:30% unlicensed assistive personnel (UAP). The acute unit skill mix changed from 70% RN:30% NA to 60% RN:40% UAP. The changing skill mix drove the need to upgrade and expand the skills and size of the NA group per unit. This necessitated role expansion, a change in job title, the development of the unlicensed assistive personnel (UAP) role description, a skills checklist, and training programs.

Registered nurse, respiratory therapy, and physical therapy staff participated in developing a comprehensive list of the things it would be helpful and safe to have the UAP trained to perform. After consulting resources from the state Board of Nursing and other literature, the UAP role description and skills checklists were developed. These skills included simple dressing changes, catheterizations, airway care in a stable tracheostomy patient, ECG performance, setting up oxygen therapy and sterile procedures, measuring and recording vital signs and intake and output, emptying drainage bags, assisting with meals, assisting with progressive mobility by getting ICU patients in and out of bed, ambulating patients, performing range of motion exercises, responding to patient requests, etc. The department of continuing education designed and conducted the training for the UAPs. Training was provided in a skills lab setting.

In addition to UAP training, it was clear we would need to offer education and ongoing support to the nursing staff. Adjusting to the implementation of the UAP role was a stressor. The RN staff questioned their liability in working with UAPs. Not only would they need to learn about the UAP role description and performance expectations, they would need to learn methods of supervision, delegation, and risk management related to this newly expanded role. Registered nurses were also responsible for the orientation and skill verification of the UAP group.

We chose to implement this program slowly. We began with the skills training of the existing NA group and delegation and supervision for the RN staff. Our selection criteria for UAP applicants focused on individuals with a nurses aide certification (CNA), emergency medical skills and patient care experience, or other healthcare background.

RN delegation has also occurred slowly. Staff have viewed their responsibility for the development and implementation of UAP seriously. A level of trust and confidence in the skills of the individual UAP is necessary before the RN will delegate comfortably. There have been some interpersonal conflicts between UAP and RN staff along the way. Most have centered on issues of delegation and the approach of the RN toward the UAP. The UAP training was amended to include a session on communication and conflict management. This has proven beneficial to all parties.

DONNA W. MARKEY, MSN, RN
Patient Care Services Manager
Transplant and Surgical Subspecialties
University of Virginia Health Sciences
    Center
Charlottesville, Virginia

RESEARCH NOTE

Source: Barter, M., McLaughlin, F., & Thomas, S. (1994). Use of unlicensed assistive personnel by hospitals. *Nursing Economic$, 12*(2), 82-87.

Purpose

The purpose of this research was to investigate the restructuring of nursing care services in acute care hospitals by the addition of unlicensed assistive personnel (UAPs). Another purpose was to evaluate how much data are being collected on the utilization of UAPs, their costs for orientation and training, and their effect on nurse job satisfaction, patient and physician satisfaction. A cross-sectional descriptive survey design was used to elicit data from 102 California hospitals. The survey instrument asked 23 questions about the use of UAPs.

Discussion

Hospitals were dispersed among rural, suburban, and urban areas. Most had more than 200 beds and 64% were not-for-profit. Team nursing was used in 75%, with primary nursing being used in 26% of hospitals. Only eight hospitals did not employ UAPs. A variety of supervision models was used, raising issues of consistency in evaluation and quality control. Only 20% required a high school diploma for UAPs. Classroom instruction for new UAP hires totaled less than 20 hours for 59% and less than 40 hours for 88% of hospitals. Little data were reported for orientation costs or cost-effectiveness of UAP use. Exit interviews, dialogue during staff meetings, discharge questionnaires, and performance evaluations were the methods used (if any) to capture job, physician, and patient satisfaction with UAP use.

Application to Practice

The absence of collected evaluative data on the use of UAPs was a striking outcome of this study. Most hospitals did *not* have a standardized hiring requirement, more than token training and orientation, procedures to measure UAPs' cost effectiveness, consistent RN supervision, or measures of nurse job satisfaction, physician satisfaction, or patient satisfaction. Clearly the use of UAPs is becoming widespread in hospitals. However, evaluative measures and data need to be implemented before restructuring occurs. Evaluative data are used for improvement of organizational effectiveness. Without this, restructuring efforts may be misguided or unsafe.

SUMMARY

- Delegation is essential in every organization.
- Delegation is the transfer of responsibility and authority to perform a task while retaining accountability.
- Supervision is guiding and influencing the outcome of a person's performance.

- True delegation is giving authority and responsibility while keeping ultimate accountability.
- Delegation involves an assessment of competency.
- The delegation process is to select a capable person, explain the task and outcomes, give authority and means to do the task, and keep in contact.
- Managers may be reluctant to delegate or subordinates may resist delegation when strong feelings and reactions occur.
- Delegation and supervision are part of the nurse's role.
- Laws and regulations influence delegation and supervision in nursing.
- The nurse must balance obligations to an employer with obligations to the state laws governing practice.
- The nurse ultimately must decide about appropriate and safe delegation.
- Delegation is related to leadership effectiveness.
- Delegation and supervision are issues surrounding the use of UAPs.

Study Questions

1. What does your nurse practice act say about delegation and supervision?
2. Should a nursing student delegate work?
3. How extensively is delegating to non-RN personnel used in the work settings you have experienced?
4. How comfortable do you feel with delegation?
5. How do you delegate to assist others to further develop?
6. What criteria can be used to assess workers' competency?
7. Do these criteria differ for RNs and UAPs? For nursing students?
8. What routine activities can RNs delegate to others?
9. When you delegate your work, what do *you* do?
10. What is a safe or minimum nurse to client ratio? Does this differ across care settings?
11. What is a nurse really responsible for when she or he is responsible for care coordination and delivery?

Critical Thinking Exercise

It's been a bad day on the floor. There have been five new admissions and several crises as patients decompensated. The patients' families are complaining about the food and the cleanliness of the rooms. Charge Nurse Danielle Nau has a headache. Three of the seven evening shift personnel have called in sick. She cannot get them replaced, and the decision has been to float in one RN and two aides from another unit. She just found out that the RN coming to cover for the shift has no experience in the specialty area. Nurse Nau knows that her staff hate floats, and the floats hate to come to her unit. In the past, her strongest RN, who is assigned to the oncoming shift, has stated a preference for Nurse Nau to stay and cover sick calls instead of covering with floats. However, Nurse Nau had promised her daughter that she would make it to her 5 pm dance recital.

1. What is the problem?

2. Who "owns" the problem?

3. What should Nurse Nau do in the situation?

4. What leadership and management styles are best suited to the situation?

5. What delegation issues are brewing?

6. What legal liability issues are operative?

7. How should Nurse Nau handle the strong RN?

REFERENCES

AACN. (1991). *Delegation of nursing and non-nursing activities in critical care: A framework for decision making.* Laguna Niguel, CA: American Association of Critical Care Nurses (AACN).

Adams, C. (1993). The impact of problem-solving styles of nurse executives and executive officers on tenure. *Journal of Nursing Administration, 23*(12), 38-43.

American Nurses Association. (1993). *Position statement on registered nurse utilization of unlicensed assistive personnel.* Washington, DC: American Nurses Association.

Anders, G. (1994, January 20). Nurses decry cost-cutting plan that uses aides to do more jobs. *The Wall Street Journal,* p. B1.

Barter, M., & Furmidge, M. (1994). Unlicensed assistive personnel: Issues relating to delegation and supervision. *Journal of Nursing Administration, 24*(4), 36-40.

Barter, M., McLaughlin, F., & Thomas, S. (1994). Use of unlicensed assistive personnel by hospitals. *Nursing Economic$, 12*(2), 82-87.

Davis, N. (1994). Concentrating on interruptions. *American Journal of Nursing, 94*(3), 14.

del Bueno, D. (1993). Delegation and the dilemma of the democratic ideal. *Journal of Nursing Administration, 23*(3), 20-25.

Delegating (1981). [Videotape]. Del Mar, CA: McGraw-Hill.

Dietz, E. (1994). Should nurses use assistants? In J. McCloskey & H. Grace (Eds.), *Current issues in nursing* (4th ed.) (pp. 212-219). St. Louis: Mosby.

Gardner, D. (1991). Issues related to the use of nurse extenders. *Journal of Nursing Administration, 21*(10), 40-45.

Gilmore, T., & Peter, M. (1987). Managing complexity in health care settings. *Journal of Nursing Administration, 17*(1), 11-17.

Hansten, R. (1991). Delegation: Learning when and how to let go. *Nursing 91, 21*(2), 126-133.

Hansten, R., & Washburn, M. (1992a). Delegation: How to deliver care through others. *American Journal of Nursing, 92*(3), 87-90.

Hansten, R., & Washburn, M. (1992b). How to plan what to delegate. *American Journal of Nursing, 92*(4), 71-72.

Hansten, R., & Washburn, M. (1992c). Tips for delegating to the right person. *American Journal of Nursing, 92*(6), 64-65.

Hansten, R., & Washburn, M. (1992d). What do you say when you delegate work to others? *American Journal of Nursing, 92*(7), 48, 50.

Herrick, K., Hansten, R., O'Neil, L., Hayes, P., & Washburn, M. (1994). My license is not on the line: The art of delegation. *Nursing Management, 25*(2), 48-50.

Iowa Nurses' Association. (1984). *Iowa Nurses' Association Resource Directory: Supervision by professional nurses*. Des Moines, IA: Iowa Nurses' Association.

Joel, L. (1994). Restructuring: Under what conditions? *American Journal of Nursing, 94*(3), 7.

National Council of State Boards of Nursing (NCSBN). (1990). *Concept paper on delegation*. Chicago: National Council of State Boards of Nursing.

Nelson, R. (1994). *Empowering employees through delegation*. Burr Ridge, IL: Richard D. Irwin.

Peters, T. (1987, March 8). Delegation is never simple; a manager's most nettlesome problem. *The Cedar Rapids Gazette*, p. 3E.

Poteet, G. (1989). Nursing administrators and delegation. *Nursing Administration Quarterly, 13*(3), 23-32.

Sherer, J. (1993). Nurses call for regulations on hospital staffing ratios. *Hospitals & Health Networks, 67*(14), 56.

Tri Council for Nursing (1990). *Statement on assistive personnel to the registered nurse*. Washington, DC: American Association of Colleges of Nursing.

16

Nursing Care
Delivery Systems

Chapter Objectives

ᐧᐧᐧᐧ

define and describe nursing care delivery systems

ᐧᐧᐧᐧ

compare and contrast six common nursing care modalities

ᐧᐧᐧᐧ

analyze the advantages and disadvantages of each care delivery system

ᐧᐧᐧᐧ

explain trends shaping the development and use
of care delivery systems in the U.S.

ᐧᐧᐧᐧ

exercise critical thinking to conceptualize and analyze
possible solutions to a practical experience incident

*O*ne specific way in which organizations use the concept of delegation in nursing is in the determination of the nursing care modality, or system of nursing care delivery, that is established for the work unit. Structure is a deliberate decision. The conscious decisions made to use a specific structure in any organization are based on the work to be done, the staff mix of people, and the environmental circumstances that the organization faces. Structures that organize nursing practice may inhibit or facilitate the work of nurses (Neidlinger & Miller, 1990).

Nurses deliver and coordinate client care. Nurse managers design nursing systems for the provision of client care and the betterment of the organization. The care modality has a direct relationship to the allocation of control over decisions about client care. It is the means through which nurse managers delegate effectively and thereby free up and manage time as a scarce resource. Manthey (1989) said that the type of care delivery system or care modality determines whether professional practice exists among the nursing staff on a particular unit because delivery systems define control over nursing decision making. This means that autonomy over practice decisions largely is determined by the care modality and the resultant nurse decision making latitude. The type of care delivery system used has implications for job satisfaction, the character of professional practice, and the amount of authority that is actually transferred to the staff.

DEFINITION

A nursing *care modality,* or the method or *system of nursing care delivery,* is defined as a method of organizing and delivering nursing care (see Chart 16.1). The client care assignment system is one aspect of the care modality. The system of nursing care delivery is the manner in which the nursing care is organized and delivered to meet the needs of the clients. It is how the work is delegated. Utilizing human resource decisions such as staffing and skill mix, the care modality forms a framework for the deployment of nursing staff and their assignment to client care. Manthey (1990) identified the basic elements of nursing care delivery systems as clinical decision making, work allocation, communication, and management (see Chart 16.2).

The practice model can be thought of as a link between the problems presented by client populations, the purposes of professional occupations, and the purposes of healthcare organizations. For any practice model, the degree of integration of the nursing care given to a client, the degree of continuity in assignment of nursing personnel caring for a client, and the type of coordination used to plan and organize the client's care need to be consistent with general client characteristics, available nursing resources, and the organizational support available to nursing (Mark, 1992).

CHART 16.1
∾ DEFINITION

Care Modality
a method of organizing and delivering nursing care.

CHART 16.2
∾ ELEMENTS OF NURSING CARE DELIVERY

The four fundamental elements of any nursing care delivery system are:
• Clinical decision making
• Work allocation
• Communication
• Management

Data from Manthey (1990).

RESEARCH NOTE

Source: Lengacher, C., Kent, K., Mabe, P., Heinemann, D., Van Cott, M., & Bowling, C. (1994). Effects of the partners in care practice model on nursing outcomes. *Nursing Economic$, 12*(6), 300-308.

Purpose

The purpose of this research was to evaluate the effects of a nursing practice model on outcomes of nurse job satisfaction, autonomy, and retention/turnover. The nursing practice model was tested with an experimental pretest/posttest design on two randomly selected nursing units of one 518-bed medical center. The nurses were a convenience sample from the two units. Total patient care was delivered on both units. The intervention of the Partners in Patient Care (PIPC) Nursing Practice Model was implemented on the experimental unit.

Discussion

The PIPC model used the four components of staff participation in decision making, partner in patient care extenders, change education classes, and delegation process classes for RNs. Data were gathered baseline and after implementation on retention/turnover, nursing staff satisfaction, and autonomy. Six months after implementation, there were significant differences on interaction, task requirements, and autonomy. There were no significant differences on retention/turnover rates at six months after implementation. Thus the practice model had an effect on some elements of job satisfaction and on autonomy.

Application to Practice

The strength of this study is in the experimental design used and in the baseline and post-implementation measures of effect. It is important to test and evaluate the effects of a new care delivery model. Job satisfaction and autonomy perceptions were improved with the new model, without any deleterious consequences to important outcome variables like retention and turnover.

BACKGROUND

Organizations exert a strong influence over nursing care delivery. Nursing care delivery can be seen as the dynamic balance between routine resource management and the structure, process, and content of practice. One outcome is that the system for distribution of nursing personnel must assure that staff of the right skill mix and numbers are promptly deployed so that clients are cared for in an appropriate and timely manner. There are four strategic decisions to make: a philosophy of resource utilization, a choice of delivery system, common and individual practice expectations, and a development of the role of the registered nurse (Manthey, 1991). These four strategic decisions may be made at different levels in any organization. If made only by the chief nurse executive, shared governance and decentralization do not exist.

Six Major Types of Delivery Systems

Historians mark the emergence of modern nursing from Nightingale's work in the Crimea. She instituted reforms centering on hygiene, cleanliness, and nutrition. She also was the first nurse educator, researcher and administrator. The Nightingale model was transported to the U.S., and nursing practice evolved from there over the course of the 20th century (Kalisch & Kalisch, 1978).

There have been six major types of nursing care modalities in the history of American nursing: private duty, functional, team, primary, case management, and current evolving types (Lee, 1993). Of these six, four care modalities were associated with hospital nursing practice: functional, team, primary, and case management. Private duty, later called case or case management, was the original way nursing care was delivered; it later became the foundation for public health nursing and community service delivery.

Private duty nursing, sometimes called case nursing, is the oldest care modality in the United States. Private duty nursing is the nursing care modality of one nurse caring for one client (see Chart 16.3). It is the modality where complete and total care is provided by one nurse, but the nurse only carries one client assignment. Originally when the nurse went into the home, the nurse did the cooking, cleaning, bathing of wounds, and the organizing of the household functions, basically functioning as a home manager. In American nursing practice, private duty was the original way that graduate nurses found employment, although some had administrative positions in hospitals, and some worked in public health (Reverby, 1987). A form of hospital case nursing evolved between 1900 and the 1930s when the Depression hit. Most families were too poor to afford private duty nurses, thus nurses were without jobs. Hospitals began to employ graduate nurses.

Reverby (1987) noted that during the Depression years a great transformation from private duty to hospital staffing took place in nursing. As the graduate nurses who had been doing private duty came into the hospital, they wanted the type of care modality that they had been used to transferred into the hospital setting. Private duty, the idea that one nurse does the total care of one client, was transplanted into hospital settings for as long as nurses were paid as "specials" by clients. When nurses became employees of hospitals, the kind of client care that private duty allowed was not possible to give in hospital staff nursing. The organization of work in hospitals was task, not client, focused (Reverby, 1987).

The advantage of private duty nursing was that the nurse's focus was entirely on one client's needs. This fostered closeness in the nurse-client relationship and increased RN and client satisfaction with care delivery. The disadvantage was that private duty is a very costly modality because of low efficiency. Further, job security was tenuous and irregular (Lee, 1993; Reverby, 1987). Nurses had little job mobility and were relatively isolated from colleagues.

There were two main variations to the basic pattern of private duty nursing that developed: group nursing and total patient care. Group nursing was an early alternative model that combined private duty concepts with hospital staff nursing. Total patient care was a hospital care modality characterized by eight hour shift accountability.

Group nursing was a care modality proposed in the 1930s by Janet Geister, the ANA's Executive Director. The plan was to reorganize private duty from individual to group practice, both inside and outside of the hospital. Thus the registry of private duty nurses would be transformed into a group practice and linked to a community's public health nursing service. Facing political pressure,

---

CHART 16.3
⤳ DEFINITIONS

Private Duty
one nurse to one client.

Group Nursing
private duty nurses in group practice.

Total Patient Care
one-shift responsibility for a client.

Data from Glandon, Colbert, and Thomasma (1989), Hegyvary (1977), and Reverby (1987).

the plan died. Hospitals also experimented with a group nursing care modality, described as being halfway between a "special," or private duty arrangement, and graduate nurse hospital staff nursing. Under this plan, clients were grouped together in a special unit where several clients shared a private nurse. Thus three nurses could do eight hour shifts for two clients instead of four nurses on 12 hour shifts. The hospital paid the nurses' wages but charged the clients directly as a surcharge on the hospital bill. The advantages included shorter hours for nurses, order and regularity in hospital staffing, steady employment for nurses, slightly cheaper rates for clients, and responsibility for the total care of several clients for the nurse. Nurses obtained the autonomy and care delivery method of private duty without its isolation and uncertainty. The nurse was a member of the hospital's staff, yet her time was specifically allocated only to a set number of clients who paid for this service directly. However, economic and political pressures for more efficiency, productivity, and service cut off the adoption of this system in hospitals (Reverby, 1987).

Total patient care has been defined as a case method for organizing nursing care where nurses are responsible for total care of a client but only for the hours in which that specific nurse is present (Glandon, Colbert, & Thomasma, 1989; Hegyvary, 1977). The distinguishing feature of total client care is the shift-only (usually eight hours) accountability for care. Some examples occur in intensive care units, hospice care, and home health care. The term has come to mean the assignment of each client to a nurse who plans and delivers care during a work shift (McCloskey, Blegen, & Gardner, 1991). With this connotation, the term total patient care has become confused with team or primary nursing care delivery systems.

Functional nursing is a care modality that utilizes the division of labor according to specific tasks and technical aspects of the job (see Chart 16.4). It has been defined as assignment by functions or tasks such as passing medicine, giving baths, or taking vital signs (McCloskey, Blegen, & Gardner, 1991). Under functional nursing, the nurse identifies the tasks to be done for a shift. The work is divided up and assigned to personnel, who focus on completing the assigned task. Functional nursing can be efficient for taking care of the tasks related to handling a large number of patients.

Functional nursing was the norm in U.S. hospitals from the late 1800s through the end of World War II. Factors such as increases in client acuity, greater complexity of care delivery, and expansion of the number of paying clients increased demand for hospital nursing services. As hospitals searched for ways to get more efficiency and service yet control labor costs, the functional division of tasks was instituted to get the work done. Cyclical shortages of nursing labor, exacerbated during times of war, accelerated staffing shortages and the demands of work. This organization of work, combined with frequent understaffing, forced nurses to be task oriented rather than client ori-

CHART 16.4
∾ DEFINITION

Functional Nursing
assignment by functions or tasks.

ented. It was a major reason why the graduate nurses hated staff nursing as compared to private duty (Reverby, 1987).

In the early 1900s, business and industry concepts of "scientific management" emphasized efficiency. The efficiency was gained by breaking down a work process into its component task steps and then analyzing and timing the steps, establishing standards, and determining the best way to perform each task. Thus managerial control over the planning and execution of work could be established. Assembly lines in factories were one result. Functional nursing was developed out of this concern for task analysis and proper division of the nursing workload. Under this modality, there might be a "temperature nurse," "medication nurse," "right-side nurse," and "left-side nurse" (Kalisch & Kalisch, 1978; Reverby, 1987). Functional nursing was less oriented to client care and more oriented to task accomplishment. There was little confusion about roles and duties. When applied to nursing, it was efficient and cheap, but nurses and clients hated it. Client satisfaction dropped under this kind of care delivery system. Clients felt they could not identify who was their nurse caretaker.

Team nursing is a care modality that uses a group of people led by a knowledgeable nurse (see Chart 16.5). Team nursing is a delivery approach that provides care to a group of clients by coordinating RNs, LPNs, and aides under the supervision of one nurse, called the team leader (Glandon, Colbert, & Thomasma, 1989; Hegyvary, 1977). Team nursing has been defined as the assignment of a group of clients to a small group of workers under the direction of a team leader. Each team member would provide most of the care to their assigned patients, although some tasks such as medications may be assigned separately (McCloskey, Blegen, & Gardner, 1991).

Team nursing is designed to make use of each member's capabilities to meet the nursing needs of their group of clients. It is a delegation of care to a designated team of staff members. The staff members have various levels of expertise, but they are formed into a team. The nurse leader takes into account the level of expertise, and then divides up the assignments accordingly so that a group of patients who are assigned to a team of caregivers have their needs met appropriately. Team nursing developed in the early 1950s in response to a shortage of RNs and in reaction to the dissatisfaction with functional nursing.

The advantages of team nursing are that each member's particular capabilities can be used to the maximum. This modality supports group productivity and the growth of team members. Communication is vital. A sense of contribution via the team can be fostered. However, it takes a skilled RN to be a team leader. Further, an RN team member may not be functioning up to her or his full potential because of being assigned an ancillary role. This creates some underutilization of the RN personnel.

CHART 16.5
∾ DEFINITIONS

Team Nursing
care to a group of clients by a mixed-staff team.

Modular Nursing
construction of geographic modules to facilitate team nursing.

One variation of team nursing that developed was *modular nursing*. Modular nursing is predicated on facilities and actual structural and spatial changes to enable hospital nurses to stay near the bedside. Modules based on client acuity are clustered into larger districts based on geography. Nurses are stationed near their clients, and a wider range of responsibility is delegated to them. Open design and convenient access architecture provides for geographic decentralization of care delivery and enhanced communication (Magargal, 1987). Modular nursing is a spatial arrangement resulting in a care delivery system with philosophy of care implications. The development of an innovative new care delivery system needs to echo themes set forth in the philosophy of care (Guild, Ledwin, Sanford, & Winter, 1994). The essential features of modular nursing are (Anderson & Hughes, 1993):

- a module consists of a group of nurses and a group of clients
- clients are grouped by geography
- nurse/client assignment is standardized
- modular care planning rounds occur regularly
- a unit-based modular committee is established

In one facility, decentralizing nursing activity to three modular substations for a 50-bed unit allowed for a reduction in RN skill mix from 63 to 46% (Abts, Hofer, & Leafgreen, 1994). In general, functional nursing was a precursor of team nursing. Both models emphasized efficiency and care delivery with limited RNs, but team nursing corrected some deficiencies in care fragmentation and regimentation.

Primary nursing began in the 1970s as a way to overcome the discontent with functional and team nursing's emphasis on tasks and discrete functions that focused nurses' attention off holistic care of the client. This matched a societal trend toward accountability and nursing's rising level of professionalism. Primary nursing is an approach in which a nurse has responsibility and accountability for the continuous guidance of specific clients from hospital admission through discharge. Thus the primary nurse provides for the total nursing process for the client during a period of hospitalization (Glandon, Colbert, & Thomasma, 1989; Hegyvary, 1977). Primary nursing has been defined as the assignment in a hospital of each patient to a primary nurse who plans, delivers, and monitors care under a 24-hour responsibility from admission to discharge (McCloskey, Blegen, & Gardner, 1991) (see Chart 16.6). The hallmark of the primary nursing concept is the 24-hour accountability aspect; autonomy, authority, and accountability in the primary nurse's role are basic to primary nursing. When the nurse is not actually taking care of clients, an associate delivers the care. However, the primary nurse makes the care and treatment coordination decisions, supervising the entire stay, 24 hours per day, for the length of the hospital stay. This increases continuity of care and con-

CHART 16.6
∽ DEFINITION

Primary Nursing
24-hour accountability by a nurse for specific clients from hospital admission through discharge.

Data from Glandon, Colbert, and Thomasma (1989), Hegyvary (1977), and McCloskey, Blegen, and Gardner (1991).

sistency in assignments. Primary nursing does not mean that the primary nurse takes care of clients 24 hours a day, as the 24-hour accountability is for the supervision and delegation of client care. Primary nursing has been called the first formal professional model in hospital nursing (Zander, 1992).

The advantages of primary nursing include a focus on the client's needs, greater nurse autonomy, and greater continuity of care. Primary nursing came to be associated with all-RN staffing, but has moved away from that position. Problems in the implementation of primary nursing include the wide variation in its operationalization and implementation. The result has been confusion and lack of a structure to enable primary nurse autonomy. Total accountability may create burnout, and a poorly prepared RN may feel threatened by primary nursing.

Research conducted to compare team nursing to primary nursing care modalities has found higher quality of nursing care, higher levels of nurse satisfaction, increased continuity of care, improved nurse retention, and positive patient outcomes with primary nursing. Levels of patient satisfaction were equal, and cost comparisons were inconclusive between the two modalities (Gardner, 1991; Lang and Clinton, 1984; Lee, 1993).

Private duty was a precursor of primary nursing (Poulin, 1985). Both care delivery models emphasized the closeness of the nurse-client relationship, but primary nursing was more cost-effective. Primary nursing was a care modality that evolved in reaction to the desire of RNs to return to active caregiving over supervision of ancillary workers in the team nursing care modality. Primary nursing promoted greater RN professional authority, accountability, autonomy, and continuity of care. Initially, an all-RN staff was thought to be needed. Compatible support systems were needed for a primary nursing care modality to be effective. Primary nursing is highly sensitive to human resource distribution, skill mix, staff competency levels, and client care needs. However, as budget constraints, shortened lengths of stay, increased patient severity, and pressures for cost containment hit hospitals in the late 1980s and early 1990s, it was difficult to maintain primary nursing care modalities (Cohen & Cesta, 1993).

RESEARCH NOTE

Source: Allred, C., Michel, Y., Arford, P., Carter, V., Veitch, J., Dring, R., Beason, S., Hiott, B., & Finch, N. (1994). Environmental uncertainty: Implications for practice model redesign. *Nursing Economic$*, *12*(6), 318-326.

Purpose

The purpose of this research was to explore and describe the practice environment of selected nursing units in order to understand the relationship of the environment and the design of the practice model. The literature suggests that the environment exerts an effect on the performance of a practice model by means of uncertain or unanticipated events occurring with frequency. This study was conducted at one 517 bed Southeastern medical center using a stratified random sample of RNs. A questionnaire elicited data on subject demographics, environmental factors, the environmental state, and uncertainty.

Discussion

Nursing units were classified and analyzed according to type. There were three distinct nursing environments that varied on knowledge complexity, change and unpredictability of environmental factors, on a scale of high-medium-low. As the environment increased in complexity, changeability, and unpredictability, nurses perceived increasing levels of environmental uncertainty. Important information about the changing environment and its impact and options were perceived to be lacking by nurses.

Application to Practice

Nurses interact with the environment and divide and coordinate work to facilitate the interaction. Compatibility between the care delivery model and the environment may facilitate efficient and effective care outcomes. This study offered an approach to measuring and examining nursing practice environments which may be useful in the design and redesign of care delivery systems.

Case management, as a general term, has been defined as a system of health assessment, planning, service procurement, service delivery, service coordination, and monitoring through which the multiple service needs of clients are met (American Nurses Association Task Force on Case Management in Nursing, 1988; Zander, 1990) (see Chart 16.7). Case management today is an attempt to reconfigure the delivery of hospital care away from previous care modalities. It has been used for years by public health and community health nurses, where case management and care coordination have been the care delivery modality employed (Mikulencak, 1993). In these settings, case management has been client needs centered, rather than shift or unit centered and centered on the system. Case management can occur in the hospital only, extend across the healthcare continuum, or be linked to a population focus (Lee, 1993; Lyon, 1993).

Case management is defined as a system of client care delivery that focuses on the achievement of client outcomes within effective and appropriate time frames and resources. It is a system of health services delivery, coordination, and monitoring through which multiple service needs of clients are met. It is focused on an entire episode of illness, crossing all settings in which the client receives care. New services across the continuum of healthcare are incorporated as needed. Care is directed by a case manager, ideally a nurse. Case management incorporates the ideas of managed care and critical paths (Fuszard, 1988).

CHART 16.7
❧ DEFINITIONS

Case Management
a system of health services delivery, coordination, and monitoring used to meet multiple service needs across the continuum of health care.

Managed Care
managing care to achieve fiscal restraint and client outcomes.

Critical Path
written tracking system for health outcomes.

Data from Fuszard (1988).

Patient-Centered Care

Several nursing care delivery systems have been in place at our 553-bed, academic, public, and tertiary medical center. The choice of nursing care delivery systems has undergone constant change and has also evolved through the years. The majority of our patient care areas utilize primary and modular nursing. However, we have also utilized team and functional nursing in several services over the years. In the 90s, our nursing organization is continuing to explore effective nursing care delivery systems and has embraced the evolution of another care delivery modality—patient-centered care.

What is Patient-Centered Care?

Patient-centered care is a new care delivery system based on the principles of primary nursing and case management. Whereas primary nursing works in isolation of other team members, and case management coordinates care across a continuum, patient-centered care addresses existing structures, systems, roles/reporting relationships, and the work of each stakeholder group and encourages a patient focus. Patient-centered care is a new organizational paradigm reflecting the need to put the patient at the center of all of our redesign and restructuring efforts.

This model encourages feedback from all stakeholders as well as our customers—the patients. In this model, an interdisciplinary team may utilize any of the existing modalities of care, but the work is redesigned around the patient.

Operationalizing Patient-Centered Care

In our facility, patient-centered care was operationalized through the development of an interdisciplinary design team comprised of nurses, physicians, respiratory, laboratory, dietary, administration, patients, occupational and physical therapy (OT/PT), housekeeping, and admitting representatives. This team was responsible for reengineering unit operations for a 36-bed medical ward. Formal and informal meetings, focus groups, etc., were held with each role group to identify the "ideal" picture/outcome (vision) that they wanted to achieve with patient-centered care. The outcomes were categorized into quality patient care, quality work life, and organizational effectiveness.

Incorporating the patient's perspective into the design of the unit was accomplished through analysis of initial baseline information from patient surveys, patient focus groups, and informal meetings. The unit operations were assessed for efficiency related to admission/discharge/transfers, admitting practices, communication patterns, staffing mix, staff competency, and patient mix. Structures were analyzed related to information retrieval, reporting relationships, existing care modality, governance, policies/procedures, etc.

The roles of each stakeholder group were addressed by each discipline. The design team initiated a "walk through of the patient's continuum of care," and analyzed what each role group was doing for the patient. A greater understanding of teamwork stemmed from this preliminary work and these concepts were applied in the development of the continuum of care. Additionally, critical paths were developed for the high volume, high risk, problem-prone patients to promote quality, efficient, and cost effective care. Reporting relationships and the resultant work of the disciplines were discussed and roles were expanded to meet the needs of the patients. Following are examples of role expansion that are presently being implemented: nursing attendants were cross trained to pass dietary trays and perform other job duties; OT/PT worked with the nursing staff to cross train them in physical therapy techniques; nurses were cross trained to phlebotomize patients;

and patients were given guidelines indicating their role in this new unit.

Numerous components were involved with the implementation of this patient-centered care environment. To promote a patient centered approach to unit operations, we first needed to communicate the mission, vision, and values of the organization to the staff. Interviews were necessary to ascertain that new and existing staff have congruence with the mission, vision, and values of the organization. To promote professional competence, we developed extensive competence and cross training learning opportunities. We created a design team to explore and develop the framework for reengineering and effective utilization of resources, exploring which care provider should and could do the work. Patient and staff mix was established. Our teams explored care modalities and the principles of case management as a framework for promoting continuity and collaboration across disciplines and departments.

We continue to develop systems that support the health care providers and promote communication. We are presently marketing the program to other units, encouraging the various disciplines to promote patient-centered care and sharing the successes with patients, visitors, and existing staff. We continuously monitor and evaluate our progress toward goal achievement and patient and staff satisfaction.

Conclusion

Care delivery systems continue to evolve. Whether we are using primary, team, or functional nursing, it is important that we continually assess the effectiveness and quality of our care delivery system. Creating a new design for the delivery of patient care takes time, initiative, involvement, support, and innovation. Through careful planning, implementation, and evaluation, this process can be achieved. Consistency of information, the development of staff, and the involvement of all stakeholders are all essential to the success of such a program.

PAULA SILER, RN, MS
Director, Professional Practice Affairs
Harbor–University of California Los Angeles
    Medical Center
Torrance, California

CATHY LOPEZ HOUSTON, RN, MBA
Analyst, Department of Nursing
Harbor–University of California Los Angeles
    Medical Center
Torrance, California

Special recognition to Thresia Nayagam, RN, MBA, Associate Director of Nursing; Elisa Sanchez, BS, Administrative Assistant; Amy Lentz, RN, BA, Nurse Manager; and Divina Apolinario, RN, BSN, Clinical Nurse Educator, Harbor–University of California Los Angeles Medical Center, Torrance, California.

Managed care is unit-based care that is organized to achieve specific client outcomes, given fiscal and other resource constraints. Resources appropriate in amount and sequence to a specific case type and individual client are managed for length of stay, critical events and timing, and anticipated outcomes. A *critical path* is a written plan that identifies key, critical, or predictable incidents that must occur at set times to achieve client outcomes within an appropriate length of stay in a hospital setting. The critical path is a tracking system for health outcomes, complications, activity, and teaching/learning (Fuszard, 1988).

In the face of strongly economic external forces, acute care hospitals turned to case management. Nursing did not desire to return to team nursing care delivery and the associated issues of care fragmentation and the use of nurse extenders. Instead, nurses advocated the use of professional practice care delivery models. Case management was seen as a way to incorporate and build on the strengths of earlier care modalities yet provide a professional practice model. Zander (1985) has described case management as second generation primary nursing. (See Chapter 17 for further discussion.)

Current evolving or "new" types of care modalities can be identified in the literature. In general these new types are mixed models, some form of second generation primary nursing, or professional practice models that emphasize outcomes management, collaboration, the use of a variety of caregivers with variable competency and preparation, and integrated practice (Bard, Jimenez, & Tornack, 1994; Jones-Schenk & Hartley, 1993; Lengacher et al., 1993; Parkman & Loveridge, 1994; Wolf, Boland, & Aukerman, 1994; Zander, 1985) (see Chart 16.8). The terms case management and managed care are joined with concepts of accountability, cost containment, effectiveness, seamless continuum of care, integration, multidisciplinary collaboration, new roles, alteration in skill mix, and new assignment systems. All seek to reconfigure nursing's work within resource constraints, care needs, and current ideas about professional nursing practice. Some models have focused on the need for integration, when the healthcare system begins to relate to other systems in the environment in a mutually cooperative way (Newman, 1990). Others still tinker with the existing modes of care delivery, seeking to develop a hybrid that incorporates the best features of all (Hyams-Franklin, Rowe-Gilliespie, Harper, & Johnson, 1993).

Fundamentally, a nursing care delivery system is the way clients' needs are matched to nursing resources. Through some complex relationships, the nursing care delivery system influences the quality of nursing care provided and its cost. There are a number of nursing care modalities that have been developed; there is some evidence of evolutionary changes and repeating cycles (Barnum, 1990). Over time, nursing care delivery methods were changed and adapted to better fit external forces and the balance of the needs of clients and the needs of employing organizations. With the changes came variations in assignment systems, skill mix, and the role of the nurse. Nursing care delivery has become more complex, and nurses have evolved professional practice models. Future trends point to greater integration and multidisciplinary team collaboration models for service delivery as healthcare reform drives changes in the organizations within the healthcare industry.

LEADERSHIP AND MANAGEMENT IMPLICATIONS

During the last round of a nurse shortage and into the early 1990s, salaries for registered nurses substantially increased. As RNs cost more, nurses were pressured to demonstrate better utilization of their skills and abilities. Changes in the model of care delivery began to occur in hospitals. Hospitals examined their traditional reliance on RNs via the percentage of RNs in the staff mix, the role of the organization and structure of nursing care delivery, and the size of nursing units on their labor costs. The role of the organization of nursing care delivery

CHART 16.8
〜 DEFINITION

Evolving/New Types mixed models emphasizing outcomes management and integrated professional practice.

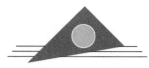 *Leadership & Management Behaviors*

LEADERSHIP BEHAVIORS	MANAGEMENT BEHAVIORS	OVERLAP AREAS
• envisions an effective and professional care delivery system	• plans a care delivery modality	• develops a care modality
• enables professionals to deliver quality and cost-effective care	• organizes staff for client care assignments	• communicates
• communicates about delivery of care issues	• communicates clearly	• delegates
• influences shared decision making about care modalities	• delegates assignments	
• balances tensions from competing stakeholders	• monitors resource utilization	
• delegates	• evaluates the effectiveness of care delivery	
	• makes care delivery system adjustments as needed	
	• implements care delivery system changes	

in labor costs and efficient, cost-effective use of nursing resources can be addressed by examining whether the method of organizing nursing service delivery influences nursing labor costs and affects quality. Analyzing 392 hospital medical/surgical nursing units from the Medicus System Corporation's National Comparative Data Base, wide variations in nursing cost per day by delivery model were found. Total client care and primary care units were the most costly, provided more care by RNs, were smaller in size, and had clients with higher average acuity. Team nursing units had the lowest cost per day, lowest average acuity, and largest average size (Glandon, Colbert, & Thomasma, 1989). This means that nurses need to be concerned about whether their care, embedded within the context of a larger organization, is both quality and cost effective. This ensures a greater degree of client satisfaction and organizational survival.

The nurse leader and manager has a key role to play in the development and selection of a care delivery model. Under true shared governance, staff nurses play this key role. Although there appears to be no one right model of care, nurses will be involved in the planning for care delivery, tinkering with improvements in the current model, exploring new models developed by others, and/or attempting to develop their own new model of care delivery. The leadership and management challenge is to balance risk taking and adoption of innovations with the pragmatic necessity to be systematic, evaluative, and realistic. Consistency with operating systems and resources available is a key driving component for evaluating a care delivery model (Armstrong & Stetler, 1991). The key components of practice that need to be considered in the construction of a nursing care delivery model are the make-up of staff, the assignment system, the care based on MD orders and physical care, the comprehensiveness of nursing intervention, end-of-shift reporting, decision making about care, accountability of nurses, communication, and cost-effectiveness (Armstrong & Stetler, 1991; Kron & Gray, 1987). Nurses' autonomy and job satisfaction is affected by the work environment and the structure of the care modality used. Leadership is needed to strike a balance between nurses' needs and preferences and those of clients, physicians, and organizations.

CURRENT ISSUES AND TRENDS

Influential Trends

A number of social, technological, environmental, economic, and political trends have shaped and influenced the type of nursing care delivery systems in use in U.S. hospitals. From 1900 to 1950 the following trends were influential (Lee, 1993):
- the status of women and expectations of altruism
- the apprenticeship model of nursing education
- advances in healthcare scientific knowledge
- transfer of equipment-based technologies from physicians to nurses
- task analysis and division of labor
- hospital control of nursing education
- patient location by disease diagnosis
- cyclic nurse shortages precipitated by epidemics, war, and the peak of the efficiency movement in nursing care delivery
- the Great Depression
- the strike as a negotiation strategy
- passage of state registration laws
- upgrading of nursing education standards
- unsatisfactory working conditions in hospitals and inadequate salaries for nurses

Since 1950, general trends that were influential included (Lee, 1993):
- changes in demographics, social mores, and lifestyle patterns
- advances in professional self-regulation and nursing knowledge
- changes in the role of the nurse and in nursing education
- changes in the focus of healthcare delivery from episodic acute care to a continuum of healthcare services, including prevention, ambulatory care, and chronic illness care

- new communication and computing technology
- new drugs and medical devices
- a revival of nurse extenders
- swings in the organization of hospital nursing care delivery from functional (before the 1950s) to team (early 1950s) to primary nursing (1970s) to case management (late 1980s) and client-focused care (1990s)
- participatory management and shared governance
- inadequate working conditions, salary compression, and poorly administered institutions
- reform of healthcare financing and the rise of competition in healthcare
- cost containment pressures
- restructuring and reengineering
- cycles of nurse staffing shortages
- increasing hospital patient acuities, underutilization of professional nursing, and lack of system supports for nursing
- political activism, advocacy, legislation, and regulation
- rise of consumer concern about cost, quality, and access
- healthcare reform movement and legislation
- hospital and healthcare service
- mergers and integration
- emerging role of advanced practice nurses
- the rise of nursing centers and nurse-run clinics
- shift in emphasis to community health care

Both recurring themes and new evolutionary issues can be seen in a review of trends affecting care delivery systems. Clearly, forces and pressures outside of professional nursing work to influence nursing care modalities. Nurses are urged to follow the clients, come to grips with the business aspects of healthcare, and remain vigilant in analyzing emerging economic and nursing staffing/skill mix trends (Lee, 1993).

It is not known which form is the best care modality for each setting in which nursing is practiced. Although there is some knowledge about the advantages and disadvantages of different modality types, we are not certain which setting is most appropriate for which care modality, where each is most cost effective, or which one is going to produce a higher quality of care delivery.

Restructuring today means looking at new care modalities as they relate to a cost-quality balance. The question is how can nursing service delivery be organized better, and what is the best way to restructure, reconfigure, or change the work environment so that both nurses and clients are more satisfied and care delivery is less costly. In the restructuring process, the desired outcome is that the client care be delivered more efficiently, the people be more satisfied, and the costs be minimized.

RESEARCH NOTE

Source: Guild, S., Ledwin, R., Sanford, D., & Winter, T. (1994). Development of an innovative nursing care delivery system. *Journal of Nursing Administration, 24*(3), 23-29.

Purpose

The purpose of this article is to discuss the development of a care delivery system for one Northeastern hospital's obstetric nursing service. As the environment changed to shortened length of stay, single room maternity care as a standard, managed care, demand for tertiary services, and emphasis on the consumer, an evaluation of facilities and care delivery systems was done by a task force who developed recommendations for a new system. The task force initially brainstormed a vision of the ideal system of care delivery. An outline/mapping wheel visual displayed the multiple elements of a care delivery system that were deemed important to effectiveness.

Discussion

The essential elements were patient/family-centered philosophy, efficient and effective physical layout, comprehensive staff education, a blend of nursing care models, effective use of staff, cost-effective use of resources, comprehensive patient education, collaboration/continuity of care, high RN satisfaction/retention, efficient flow of patients, effective marketing, and a streamlined documentation/communication system. Important themes were philosophy of care, continuity, comprehensiveness, collaboration, effectiveness, and efficiency. The task force went through a process of being selected, getting organized, developing a work plan, reviewing the literature, surveying other hospitals, doing internal interviews, collating data, developing recommendations, and writing a report. The result was a new care delivery system that was a blend of case management, primary nursing, and mother-baby nursing models.

Application to Practice

New delivery systems are a key part of the changes occurring in healthcare. Nurses can play a central role in constructing the architecture of new care delivery systems. A systematic process using work teams, organization, creativity, and commitment can produce a high quality result that is acceptable to users. Success was considered to be largely the result of the process used.

SUMMARY

- Organizations use delegation in the process of establishing the nursing care delivery system.
- The care modality influences whether professional practice exists.
- A nursing care modality is a method of organizing and delivering nursing care.

- The six types of nursing care modalities are private duty, functional, team, primary, case management, and evolving types.
- The four major care modalities used in hospitals are functional, team, primary, and case management.
- Private duty is one RN to one client.
- Functional nursing is assignment to tasks.
- Team nursing is the care of a group of clients by a skill-mixed team.
- Primary nursing is 24-hour accountability by an RN for specific clients over a hospital stay.
- Case management is the coordination and monitoring of services across the continuum of health care.
- Evolving care modalities focus on effectiveness, resource management, and professional practice.
- Social, technological, environmental, economic, and political trends have shaped and influenced nursing care delivery systems.

Study Questions

1. Who has the authority to establish the nursing care delivery modality for the institution?
2. How do nurses decide on which nursing care delivery system to use?
3. Why are nursing care delivery systems being revised and restructured?
4. What issues arise when the care delivery system is changed?
5. What common themes emerge among the newest care delivery systems being developed? How do they compare to older modalities?
6. What care delivery system best fits a merger of hospital and community agencies, or are multiple care modalities needed?

Critical Thinking Exercise

Nurse Ryan Danielson worked in an adult ICU for five years. He then pursued a master's degree and became certified as a nurse practitioner. As he finished his certification, he found the local nursing employment situation turbulent. Area hospitals had been downsizing by laying off nurses. Nurse Danielson did a needs assessment of unmet nursing care needs and wrote a business plan for opening a nurse-owned and nurse-run neighborhood clinic. He found financial backing and opened the clinic. In two months he was overwhelmed with clients. Nurse Danielson immediately hired 50 new staff in addition to the 25 already in place. In doing so, Nurse Danielson decided to redesign the nursing care delivery model used at the clinic.

1. *What is the problem?*

2. *Why is it a problem?*

3. *What should Nurse Danielson do first?*

4. *What leadership and management styles might be effective in the situation?*

5. *What decision procedure might be effective?*

6. *What care delivery model would be most suited to this situation?*

7. *How should the redesign take place?*

REFERENCES

Abts, D., Hofer, M., & Leafgreen, P. (1994). Redefining care delivery: A modular system. *Nursing Management, 25*(2), 40-46.

American Nurses Association Task Force on Case Management in Nursing. (1988). *Nursing case management.* (Publication No. NS-32). Kansas City, MO: American Nurses Association.

Anderson, C., & Hughes, E. (1993). Implementing modular nursing in a long-term care facility. *Journal of Nursing Administration, 23*(6), 29-35.

Armstrong, D., & Stetler, C. (1991). Strategic considerations in developing a delivery model. *Nursing Economic$, 9*(2), 112-115.

Bard, J., Jimenez, F., & Tornack, R. (1994). An outcome-focused, community-based health support program. *Journal of Nursing Administration, 24*(3), 48-54.

Barnum, B. (1990). Cycles of nursing. *Nursing & Health Care, 11*(8), 395.

Cohen, E., & Cesta, E. (1993). *Nursing case management: From concept to evaluation.* St. Louis: Mosby.

Fuszard, B. (1988). What is case management? *The Facilitator, 4*(1), 3-4.

Gardner, K. (1991). A summary of findings of a five-year comparison study of primary and team nursing. *Nursing Research, 40*(2), 113-117.

Glandon, G., Colbert, K., & Thomasma, M. (1989). Nursing delivery models and RN mix: Cost implications. *Nursing Management, 20*(5), 30-33.

Guild, S., Ledwin, R., Sanford, D., & Winter, T. (1994). Development of an innovative nursing care delivery system. *Journal of Nursing Administration, 24*(3), 23-29.

Hegyvary, S. (1977). Foundations of primary nursing. *Nursing Clinics of North America, 12*(6), 187-196.

Hyams-Franklin, E., Rowe-Gilliespie, P., Harper, A., & Johnson, V. (1993). Primary team nursing: The 90s model. *Nursing Management, 24*(6), 50-52.

Jones-Schenk, J., & Hartley, P. (1993). Organization for communication and integration. *Journal of Nursing Administration, 23*(10), 30-33.

Kalisch, P., & Kalisch, B. (1978). *The advance of American nursing.* Boston: Little, Brown.

Kron, T., & Gray, A. (1987). *The management of patient care: Putting leadership skills to work* (6th ed.). Philadelphia: Saunders.

Lang, N., & Clinton, J. (1984). Assessment of quality of nursing care. *Annual Review of Nursing Research, 2,* 135-163.

Lee, J. (1993). A history of care modalities in nursing. *Series on Nursing Administration, 5,* 20-38.

Lengacher, C., Mabe, P., Bowling, C., Heinemann, D., Kent, K., & Cott, M. (1993). Redesigning nursing practice: The partners in patient care model. *Journal of Nursing Administration, 23*(12), 31-37.

Lyon, J. (1993). Models of nursing care delivery and case management: Clarification of terms. *Nursing Economic$, 11*(3), 163-169.

Magargal, P. (1987). Modular nursing: Nurses rediscover nursing. *Nursing Management, 18*(11), 98-104.

Manthey, M. (1989). Of bandwagons and partnerships. *Nursing Management, 20*(8), 22-23.

Manthey, M. (1990). Definitions and basic elements of a patient care delivery system with an emphasis on primary nursing. In G. Mayer, M. Madden, & E. Lawrenz (Eds.), *Patient care delivery models* (pp. 201-211). Rockville, MD: Aspen.

Manthey, M. (1991). Delivery systems and practice models: A dynamic balance. *Nursing Management, 22*(1), 28-30.

Mark, B. (1992). Characteristics of nursing practice models. *Journal of Nursing Administration, 22*(11), 57-63.

McCloskey, J., Blegen, M., & Gardner, D. (1991). Who helps you with your work? *American Journal of Nursing, 91*(4), 43-46.

Mikulencak, M. (1993). Public health stands as a proven model for future delivery systems. *The American Nurse, 25*(6), 18.

Neidlinger, S., & Miller, M. (1990). Nursing care delivery systems: A nursing administration practice perspective. *Journal of Nursing Administration, 20*(10), 43-49.

Newman, M. (1990). Toward an integrative model of professional practice. *Journal of Professional Nursing, 6*(3), 167-173.

Parkman, C., & Loveridge, C. (1994). From nursing service to professional practice. *Nursing Management, 25*(3), 63-68.

Poulin, M. (1985). Configuration of nursing practice. In American Nurses Association (Ed.), *Issues in professional practice* (pp. 1-14). Kansas City, MO: American Nurses Association.

Reverby, S. (1987). *Ordered to care: The dilemma of American nursing 1850-1945.* Cambridge: Cambridge University Press.

Wolf, G., Boland, S., & Aukerman, M. (1994). A transformational model for the practice of professional nursing: Part 2, implementation of the model. *Journal of Nursing Administration, 24*(5), 38-46.

Zander, K. (1985). Second generation primary nursing: A new agenda. *Journal of Nursing Administration, 15*(3), 18-24.

Zander, K. (1990). Case management: A golden opportunity for whom? In J. McCloskey & H. Grace (Eds.), *Current issues in nursing* (3rd ed.) (pp. 199-204). St. Louis: Mosby.

Zander, K. (1992). Nursing care delivery methods and quality. *Series on Nursing Administration, 3*, 86-104.

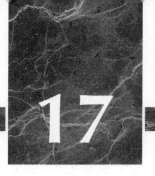

Case Management and Managed Care

Chapter Objectives

∽

define and describe case management

∽

define and describe managed care

∽

differentiate case management and managed care

∽

compare differences in definitions between
hospital-focused and general definitions of case management

∽

analyze the development of case management
as a nursing care modality

∽

explain the main service components in case management models

∽

analyze nursing role changes under case management and managed care

∽

exercise critical thinking to conceptualize and analyze
possible solutions to a practical experience incident

*i*nternal and external pressures on the healthcare delivery system have
been intensifying. A combination of cost, quality, and access demands
have combined to create a complex and volatile environment. Complexity arises from the simultaneous balancing of quality, productivity, and flexibility. Healthcare providers are directed to manage the resources by providing cost-efficient and cost-effective healthcare services and be

accountable for the value of services relative to the costs of those services. Specifically, the pressure on nurses is to balance quality of care with client advocacy. Thus nurses need to demonstrate and document the effect of nursing care on client outcomes and on the efficiency and price competitiveness of provided services. The benefits achieved need to exceed the costs incurred. Further, nurses need to demonstrate that they can provide services more cost-effectively than other providers (Hicks, Stallmeyer, & Coleman, 1992). The mounting pressures on the healthcare delivery system since the mid-1980s provided an impetus for case management as an economically important strategy for hospitals and an opportunity for hope during economic hard times.

DEFINITIONS

Managed Care

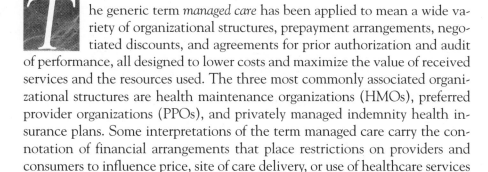

The generic term *managed care* has been applied to mean a wide variety of organizational structures, prepayment arrangements, negotiated discounts, and agreements for prior authorization and audit of performance, all designed to lower costs and maximize the value of received services and the resources used. The three most commonly associated organizational structures are health maintenance organizations (HMOs), preferred provider organizations (PPOs), and privately managed indemnity health insurance plans. Some interpretations of the term managed care carry the connotation of financial arrangements that place restrictions on providers and consumers to influence price, site of care delivery, or use of healthcare services (Hicks, Stallmeyer, & Coleman, 1992). Utilization review and gatekeeper functions are emphasized.

In the nursing literature, *managed care* is defined as a clinical system that organizes and sequences the process of caregiving at the client-provider level (see Chart 17.1). The objective is to better achieve cost and quality outcomes (Zander, 1991). It serves to restructure the tools and systems used in client care. It is based on a process of anticipating and describing care requirements in advance and then comparing actual occurrences to the anticipated path. The emerging definition includes client assessment, care planning, clinical analysis, and quality and cost of care measured and analyzed (Beyers, 1993). Managed care is project management at the provider-client level (Zander, 1992).

Managed care is unit-based care that is organized to achieve specific client outcomes, given fiscal and other resource constraints. Resources appropriate in amount and sequence to a specific case type and individual client are managed for length of stay, critical events and timing, and anticipated outcomes (Fuszard, 1988; Hampton, 1993).

CHART 17.1
‿ DEFINITION

Managed Care
a clinical system that organizes and sequences the process of caregiving at the client-provider level in order to better achieve cost and quality outcomes.

Data from Zander (1991).

RESEARCH NOTE

Source: Weilitz, P., & Potter, P. (1993). A managed care system: Financial and clinical evaluation. *Journal of Nursing Administration, 23*(11), 51-57.

Purpose

The purpose of this program evaluation was to evaluate the impact of care paths on clinical and financial outcomes of resource utilization, length of stay, and client outcomes in one midwestern university medical center. The care paths were central to a managed care system and the improvement of clinical practice outcomes. Multidisciplinary documentation occurs on the care path. A comprehensive clinical and financial evaluation system is integrated with the hospital's total quality management program. Clinical evaluation was based on success in delivering recommended interventions and meeting projected outcomes. Financial evaluation was done by an analysis of key financial indicators such as length of stay, charge per case, cost per case, and payor.

Discussion

Clinical evaluation data were captured on variance reports and examined for trends in practice and resource use. Financial measures were retrieved from the hospital's financial system. Analysis of results demonstrated a decreased length of stay and overall cost savings. Outcomes also included improved communication and greater efficiency. Tools and processes to measure clinical outcomes have been developed to collect admission and post discharge data.

Application to Practice

Care paths are an important alternative strategy for delivering quality care, managing resources, and reducing lengths of stay in hospitals. They can incorporate multidisciplinary care planning, discharge planning, and documentation. This article highlights the incorporation of both clinical and financial impact evaluation strategies as well as the importance of multidisciplinary documentation on the care path. Care paths help ensure a consistent standard of care across settings and caregivers.

CHART 17.2
↩ DEFINITION

Case Management
a system of health assessment, planning, service procurement, service delivery, service coordination, and monitoring through which the multiple service needs of clients are met.

Data from American Nurses Association Task Force on Case Management in Nursing (1988) and from Zander (1990).

Case Management

Case management, as a general term, has been defined as a system of health assessment, planning, service procurement, service delivery, service coordination, and monitoring through which the multiple service needs of clients are met (American Nurses Association Task Force on Case Management in Nursing, 1988; Zander, 1990) (see Chart 17.2) (see Chapter 16 for a discussion of case management as a nursing care modality). Thus the general meaning of case management is any method of linking, managing, or organizing services to meet client needs. Client assessment, service integration, and follow-up are typically included (Zawadski & Eng, 1988). Thus, case management entails the coordination and sequencing of care. It helps to tighten the plan of care and link direct caregivers across facility and service boundaries.

Hospital nursing case management is a system in which the accountability for the care management of clients in a specific diagnosis-related group (DRG) category and over an entire hospitalization are assigned to an RN. The nurse case manager coordinates care across the continuum of services. Hospital nursing case management usually is targeted to high risk populations. While all clients need coordinated care, case management functions best to coordinate healthcare services for high risk populations across community, acute, and long-term care settings (Simpson, 1993). Zander (1988; 1991) defined case management as a matrix model at the clinician-provider level in acute care. Zander's (1994) display of the CareMap® system infrastructure reflects a matrix structure.

Case management today is an attempt to reconfigure the delivery of hospital care away from previous care modalities. It has been used for years by public health and community health nurses where case management and care coordination have been the care delivery modality employed (Mikulencak, 1993). In these settings, case management has been client needs-centered rather than shift or unit-centered. Case management can occur in the hospital only, extend across the healthcare continuum, or be linked to a population focus (Lee, 1993).

Case management is described as a system of client care delivery that focuses on the achievement of client outcomes within effective and appropriate time frames and resources. It is a system of health services delivery, coordination, and monitoring through which multiple service needs of clients are met. Case management is an umbrella program in a healthcare facility for systems management. Case management operates at the intersection of organizational systems and the delivery of clinical care. It is focused on an entire episode of illness, crossing all settings in which the client receives care. New services across the continuum of healthcare are incorporated as needed. Care is directed by a case manager, ideally a nurse. Case management incorporates the ideas of managed care and critical paths (Fuszard, 1988).

A *critical path* is a written plan that identifies key, critical, or predictable incidents that must occur at set times to achieve client outcomes within an appropriate length of stay in a hospital setting. The critical path is a tracking system for health outcomes, complications, activity, and teaching/learning (Fuszard, 1988). Critical paths have been described as protocols of interdisciplinary treatments, based on professional standards of practice and placed in order on a decision tree (Simpson, 1993).

A critical pathway is a document that organizes the sequence of events for an episode of care. Both processes and outcomes are incorporated. Some see critical paths as creating a cookbook approach to care delivery. However, critical paths do organize and sequence the usual path of client care and form a standard of care. Variances are noted and analyzed. The process of developing and using critical paths encourages both critical thinking and accountability. One critical path document reads from left to right. It begins with nursing assessment and ends with client outcomes and teaching needs for each day during an episode of care (Sperry & Birdsall, 1994). Critical paths can be used to educate, prepare and orient, negotiate expectations, and negotiate care roles with clients. Critical paths can and should be individualized to each client. They are major tools of outcomes management and coordination of care delivery.

Case Management vs. Managed Care

What is case management? To healthcare insurers it is viewed as utilization review. Hospitals use it as a care modality for linking various inpatient activities (Lumsdon, 1994). Confusion about case management arises secondary to a confusion in definition of terms, inconsistently used labels, and the variety of applications of the concept. The terms associated with case management include managed care, care management, critical paths, and care coordination. Some terms refer to comprehensive models and others refer to utilization, access, and cost control mechanisms (Capitman, 1988). Specifically, case management and managed care are the two terms most often used interchangeably, creating a lack of clarity.

Managed care is the broader term, viewed as a system that provides the structure and focus for managing the use, cost, quality, and effectiveness of health services. Managed care is the umbrella under which case management may be one cost containment strategy. However, managed care has evolved into meaning a separate hospital professional nursing care delivery model that is unit-based and focused on support for standardized patterns of care and length of hospitalization. Case management differs from managed care in that the focus for delivery of care is based on an entire hospitalization for a targeted DRG group and is not geographically confined to the patient's unit. It implies consistency of coordinator or provider across healthcare settings. Both managed care and case management employ critical paths, case management care plans, and variance analysis. Case management can be a hospital-based within-the-walls or a community-based beyond-the-walls program (Cohen & Cesta, 1993). Managed care organizes the sequence of work; case management is the method that appoints accountability for work outcomes (Zander, 1991). Managed care is targeted to 100% of clients; case management may be targeted to 10% to 20% of clients who are at high risk.

RESEARCH NOTE

Source: Sperry, S., & Birdsall, C. (1994). Outcomes of a pneumonia critical path. *Nursing Economic$, 12*(6), 332-339, 345.

Purpose

The purpose of this research was to identify the relationships among length of stay, hospital charges, care listed on a critical path, and quality of documentation in randomly selected charts of patients with pneumonia at one 300-bed community teaching hospital in the Northeast. First, 35 charts from 1991 were reviewed. A case management project had been instituted after that and included the development of a critical path for simple pneumonia, DRG 89. The 1991 results were compared to 38 charts from 1992, post critical paths. Data were collected on patient demographics, length of stay, hospital charges, modalities of care, and documentation.

Discussion

There were not statistically significant differences between the two sets of charts on patient population demographics. The overall major findings showed a decrease in length of stay, an average decrease in hospital charges per admission, and improved quality of multidisciplinary documentation after implementation of the pneumonia critical path. After the chart review, the critical path was revised to make compliance with documentation easier. Clearly, the implementation of a critical path had a positive effect on outcomes of care management.

Application to Practice

Case management programs are implemented for a variety of reasons. The management of outcomes is a key feature. Critical paths are used to establish a standard of care within the framework of a reimbursed length of stay. Comparative and descriptive research data can be generated by analysis of critical path outcomes. These data can identify practice and systems issues and problems. Critical paths give a framework for decision making and variance management. Therefore, they assist with the quality of decisions and the quality of executed actions.

BACKGROUND

In nursing, case management historically has been the care modality associated with public health and community health nursing. Thus it was operational in settings outside of hospitals and operated without the umbrella of managed care. In these settings, case management focused on accountability of process and outcomes of care delivery. Traditional case management principles were operational in several nursing care modalities. Private duty, sometimes called the case method, was the assignment of one nurse to one client. Later forms like total patient care involved the assignment of one nurse to a case load of clients to provide complete care. The role of care giving was more primary than the role of care coordination. Case management also was used in social service agencies, community mental health services, rehabilitation settings, and long-term care. Since 1985, case management has been adopted by acute care hospitals as a "new" care modality and applied to their specific care setting.

In acute care settings, case management focuses on and restructures the way clinical work is organized and processed. Adopting case management highlights the need for better clinical and financial information systems, clarification of standards, incentive programs, and improved integration of operations. Case management incorporates an interdisciplinary aspect that contributes to care integration and successful care management. Case management is reported to be effective for targeting specific client populations for improved quality, increasing coordination and continuity of care, improving care effectiveness, and enhancing an institution's competitiveness for managed care contracts (Zander, 1990).

Clearly, various configurations have evolved for the delivery of nursing care. There is a parallel between nursing care modalities and major economic, social, demographic, and political trends. Current forces include the rise of consumerism, imposed economic constraints, technological advances, and changing social values and expectations (Cohen & Cesta, 1993).

Private duty was a precursor of primary nursing (Poulin, 1985). Both care delivery models emphasized the closeness of the nurse-client relationship, but primary nursing was more cost-effective. Functional nursing was a precursor of team nursing. Both models emphasized efficiency and care delivery with limited RNs, but team nursing corrected some deficiencies in care fragmentation and regimentation (see Chapter 16 for more discussion).

Primary nursing was a care modality that evolved in reaction to the desire of RNs to return to active caregiving over supervision of ancillary workers in the team nursing care modality. Primary nursing promoted greater RN professional authority, accountability, autonomy, and continuity of care. Initially, an all-RN staff was thought to be needed. Compatible support systems were needed for a primary nursing care modality to be effective. Primary nursing is highly sensitive to human resource distribution, skill mix, staff competency levels, and client care needs. However, as budget constraints, shortened lengths of stay, increased patient severity, and pressures for cost containment hit hospitals in the late 1980s and early 1990s, it was difficult to maintain primary nursing care modalities (Cohen & Cesta, 1993).

In the face of strongly economic external forces, acute care hospitals began to restructure and reengineer care delivery systems. To balance professional care provider needs with fiscal constraints, many hospitals turned to case management. Nurses did not desire to return to team nursing care delivery and the associated issues of care fragmentation and the use of nurse extenders. Instead, many nurses advocated the use of professional practice care delivery models. Case management was seen as a way to incorporate and build on the strengths of earlier care modalities yet provide a professional practice model. Zander (1985) has described case management as second generation primary nursing model.

A variety of case management models have arisen; some are nursing models, others are nonnursing models. The core elements center around a case manager who coordinates and monitors the care given to clients by multiple services in an attempt to decrease service fragmentation and improve the quality of care (Rheaume, Frisch, Smith, & Kennedy, 1994). Weil & Karls (1985) identified eight main service components common to all case management models. (See Chart 17.3.)

Case Management Implementation

In case management, the nurse may or may not be the direct care provider. For example, public health nurses often provide direct care. On the other hand, nurse case managers who work for insurance companies are not the direct care providers. The four basic principles that guide nursing case management are:

- the coordination and integration of a continuum of holistic care
- the promotion and preservation of health through periods of transition and risk
- the conservation and allocation of scarce resources
- the provision of follow-up care that tracks and guides service delivery over the long term and across episodes and settings

Thus the nurse case manager remains in a relationship with clients over time and across boundaries. The nursing concept of discharge is replaced by accompaniment, as the nurse follows the client, acting to connect and coordinate a broad continuum of sites and services (Hinitz-Satterfield, Miller, & Hagan, 1993). Nurses "accompany" clients in a cognitive and communication sense. Only in certain models will nurses literally provide care across the continuum.

Coordination and continuity are the keys to managing care over the healthcare continuum and across organizational boundaries. Thus care must be managed carefully within each area or unit and between healthcare areas. Case management focuses on provider continuity; managed care focuses on the continuity of the plan. Both must be integrated into the care delivery system using a systems perspective (Falk & Bower, 1994).

The unit or area is the most basic locus to begin the coordination of care. In nursing, the care delivery system functions to coordinate care at the unit level. Coordination and continuity can be shift-based or unit-based. If the existing care delivery system does not accomplish goals of coordinating care, then a unit- based role with accountability for coordinating care across time will need to be developed (Falk & Bower, 1994).

Development of Case Management Programs

Case management programs are developed using a number of situation-specific elements. Two initial assessments are helpful: assessment of the organization and assessment of client populations. The organizational assessment focuses on identification of resources while the client population assessment

---

CHART 17.3
～ SERVICE COMPONENTS OF MANAGEMENT MODELS

- Client identification and outreach
- Individual assessment and diagnosis
- Service planning and resource identification
- Linking clients to needed services
- Service implementation and coordination
- Monitoring service delivery
- Advocacy
- Evaluation

Data from Weil and Karls (1985).

CHART 17.4 ∽ CASE MANAGEMENT ASSESSMENT QUESTIONS

Organizational Assessment
- What clinical and support services are needed?
- When in the client experience are services most appropriately provided?
- How should services be provided?
- Where are services best delivered?
- Who are the most appropriate providers?
- Where and by whom are services best managed?

Client Assessment
- What are the major client populations served by the organizations, by volume, diagnosis, cost, payor mix, and high intensity/resource use outliers?
- What is the service path followed by client populations, by entry point, internal flow, discharge, and recidivism?
- What groups of clients fall into high-risk categories, by volume?
- What clients are at risk for less than desired outcomes, by morbidity, mortality, infection rates, falls, and clinical outcomes?

---

focuses on how care is experienced by clients and the characteristics of client populations served by the organizations. (See Chart 17.4 for related assessment questions.) If case management is used for specific client populations, then priority would go to clients who:

- have a high recidivism or frequent emergency department encounters
- have unpredictable needs for care
- have significant complications, comorbidities, or variances in usual care patterns
- fall into high-risk profiles
- are high cost (Falk & Bower, 1994)

The general process for the development of a case management program can be synthesized as follows:

1. Assess the organization and the client population served. This assessment provides a baseline for implementation.
2. Identify high-volume or high-risk case types. This assessment will indicate priority areas for care coordination.
3. Determine the usual client care problems, issues, or difficulties related to the high-volume or high-risk case types. Determine desired goals.
4. Form an interdisciplinary care team of the interrelated care providers who will be involved with the case types.
5. Develop and design a critical pathway for each selected case type. The path should outline and specify measurable clinical outcomes, key professional care processes, and exact corresponding timelines as based on practice patterns, professional standards of care, and length of stay parameters. The input and involvement of the client and each provider

group, in relation to achieving client outcomes, should be clearly specified. The pathway would mark the occurrence of routine treatments, tests, consults, client activities, medications, diet, educational interventions, and discharge planning. Variance from the path triggers analysis and intervention.

6. Develop a pilot program or trial site.
7. Evaluate the pilot program and consider system-wide implementation. Review the pilot program's articulation with the existing mode of nursing care delivery.

RESEARCH NOTE

Source: Goodwin, D. (1994). Nursing case management activities: How they differ between employment settings. *Journal of Nursing Administration, 24*(2), 29-34.

Purpose

The purpose of this research was to describe the differences in case management activities across various employment settings in nursing. A descriptive survey of two groups of nurse case managers from one western area: from home health agencies (N = 23) and from case management companies, insurance companies, or HMOs (N = 9) was conducted. Data were collected from the Competency Behaviors of Case Managers Inventory (CBCMI), which was modified to ask the frequency with which case management activities were performed by the respondents.

Discussion

Responses to the CBCMI were grouped according to assessment, planning, implementation, and evaluation components of the nursing case management process. Results were compared between the two groups. There was a higher frequency of response by the home health case managers to activities of assessment, planning, and implementation. The case manager group indicated 100% involvement in evaluation activities; this was responded to by 83% of the home health nurses. Regulatory mandates may drive the activities of the home health nurses, whereas the case management group may be balancing care provided with the benefits plan. Case management nurses were not the direct care providers.

Application to Practice

The CBCMI was a useful tool to identify case management activities. The majority of all activities on this instrument were reported as performed by both groups, although with some variation in frequency. Thus there may be some potential for duplication of service between the two groups. This study highlights the focus of case management services: some are provided to the client as customer while others are provided to the agency or insurer as customer. Further research is needed in fully defining the appropriate activities of case management.

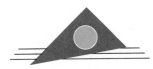

Leadership & Management Behaviors

LEADERSHIP BEHAVIORS	MANAGEMENT BEHAVIORS	OVERLAP AREAS
• enables nurses to coordinate care	• develops critical paths	• integrates clinical nursing practice
• creates a vision of high quality and cost effective care delivery	• tracks variances	• communicates
	• integrates clinical nursing practice	• evaluates care delivery
• communicates care management concepts	• communicates care management needs	
• integrates clinical nursing practice	• organizes nursing care delivery	
• evaluates care delivery systems	• directs others in coordinating care	
• influences policy and organizational systems	• evaluates care coordination	
• inspires a multidisciplinary team	• influences employees to implement managed care	

LEADERSHIP AND MANAGEMENT IMPLICATIONS

All nursing roles contain a component of management. McClure (1991) has noted that nurses have two roles: caregiver and care coordinator. Nurses in management positions in an organizational hierarchy are organization managers. Management of client care by nurses makes them clinical managers. The emphasis on managed care in integrated health systems requires a new type of clinical nursing practice system with an emphasis on practice management and empowerment of nurses (Beyers, 1993).

Future effectiveness is thought to be based on decisions about what types of organizational structures and nursing care delivery systems best enable nurse-managed client care and best support nurses in practice. One related question is, how much management does a nurse require? One assessment is the extent to which a nurse provides client care or manages the care of clients. Case management is one specific approach to redesigning care delivery for client care improvement. This may mean that some traditional management practices and habits will need to change or be discarded. As new ideas and methods about how to design nursing services emerge, they will need to be evaluated for fit and appropriateness to nursing's care delivery needs (Beyers, 1993).

Mark (1992) advocated an approach to determining the organization of practice that begins with clients at the core of care delivery systems. Then the goals, roles, and activities valued by nursing staff, medical staff, critical support services, and other stakeholders can be explored. A new practice model and structure can then be created to be consistent with client characteristics, nursing resources, and available organizational support. Various practice models incorporate dimensions of:

- the degree of integration of nursing care given to a client
- the degree of continuity of assignment of nurses to clients
- the type of coordination used to plan and organize care

As nursing care delivery systems evolve, the configuration of these dimensions will need to be addressed and evaluated. Nurse leaders can examine the state of healthcare management in their organizations and develop strategies to implement coordination of care models to best meet client, organizational, societal, and professional priorities (Kelly, 1992). Given the interdisciplinary nature of case management, model development and success may require a "buy in" by other healthcare disciplines and other organizational stakeholders.

CURRENT ISSUES AND TRENDS

Managed care has been described as an outstanding trend currently growing and projected to increase in the future healthcare environment. The critical need to control costs while providing quality healthcare underlies the importance of the managed care trend (Beyers, 1993). Case management as a professional practice model is under development in hospital settings. It is promoted as a means to address the issues of allocation of resources, effectiveness of care, cost containment, and accountability. It has the potential to increase nurse satisfaction and autonomy (Zander, 1990).

In the shift of nursing care delivery systems toward case management, the balance between nurses' roles may shift. Some of the primary caregiving component may be exchanged for care coordination roles. This is the movement away from service provision and into service coordination as the central component of nurses' practice. The expansion of coordination roles may influence the character and nature of nurse-client relationships (Rheaume et al., 1994).

Continued pressure for cost-effective healthcare may push buyers into managed care arrangements. Managed care organizations use case management as one strategy to control costs. The nurse case manager is pivotal to overseeing critical paths and facilitating interventions and coordination activities. There is opportunity in the strategic economic importance of the case management process. However, it must be remembered that the common thread weaving through various forms of managed care is the placing of constraints through the use of rewards, penalties, and mandates on both consumers and providers to modify their production/consumption of healthcare services (Hicks, Stallmeyer, & Coleman, 1992). If managed care becomes a system in which the provider receives a set dollar amount for any delivery of service, then new challenges and role changes will arise. Many former assumptions about what we think is appropriate and many former activities and roles will be challenged and re-thought. This will take leadership, creativity, innovation, and risk-taking.

SUMMARY

- Cost, quality and access pressures in healthcare have provided an impetus for case management and managed care.
- Managed care is a clinical system that organizes and sequences caregiving by providers.
- Case management is a system of health assessment and service coordination.
- A critical path is a written plan that identifies key incidents needed to achieve client outcomes.
- Managed care is a broader term than case management.
- Case management is a nursing care modality historically associated with community health nursing but now adapted to hospitals.
- There are a variety of case management models.
- In developing case management programs, both the organization and client populations should be assessed.
- One of nursing's two main roles is care coordinator.
- Organizational structures and nursing care delivery systems need to mesh to support nurses and clients.
- Managed care may be the wave of the future.

Study Questions

1. What are the goals of case management?
2. What are the goals of managed care? How do they compare to those of case management?
3. What are the outcomes anticipated by case management? By managed care?
4. How is case management affecting the role of the nurse?
5. Who should be the case manager?
6. Does the Public Health model apply to hospital settings? Why or why not?
7. Do all clients need case management?

Critical Thinking Exercise

Nurse Lisa Lucky has been working as a case manager for a large HMO. Recently she was assigned a group of cases to manage that all were clients with AIDS. Nurse Lucky knows that care for AIDS clients was poorly coordinated in the past. Further, the corporate philosophy of the HMO discourages the authorization of expensive services or treatments. In fact, Nurse Lucky's supervisor said, "Our goal here is to hold down costs" when Nurse Lucky was given the assignment. Nurse Lucky anticipates a real challenge.

1. What is the problem?

2. Whose problem is it?

3. What should Nurse Lucky do?

4. What approach to care coordination should Nurse Lucky take?

5. What other resources might Nurse Lucky enlist?

6. How can Nurse Lucky develop an interdisciplinary approach?

REFERENCES

American Nurses Association Task Force on Case Management in Nursing. (1988). *Nursing Case Management* (Publication No. NS-32). Kansas City, MO: American Nurses Association.

Beyers, M. (1993). Managing nursing: Emerging roles in the current health care environment. *Series on Nursing Administration, 5,* 3-19.

Capitman, J. (1988). Case management for long-term and acute medical care. *Health Care Financing Review, Annual supplement,* 53-55.

Cohen, E., & Cesta, E. (1993). *Nursing case management: From concept to evaluation.* St. Louis: Mosby.

Falk, C., & Bower, K. (1994). Managing care across department, organization, and setting boundaries. *Series on Nursing Administration, 6,* 161-176.

Fuszard, B. (1988). What is case management? *The Facilitator, 4*(1), 3-4.

Hampton, D. (1993). Implementing a managed care framework through care maps. *Journal of Nursing Administration, 23*(5), 21-27.

Hicks, L., Stallmeyer, J., & Coleman, J. (1992). Nursing challenges in managed care. *Nursing Economic$, 10*(4), 265-276.

Hinitz-Satterfield, P., Miller, E., & Hagan, E. (1993). Managed care and new roles for nursing: Utilization and case management in a health maintenance organization. *Series on Nursing Administration, 5,* 83-99.

Kelly, K. (1992). Managing care: A search for role clarity. *Journal of Nursing Administration, 22*(3), 9-10.

Lee, J. (1993). A history of care modalities in nursing. *Series on Nursing Administration, 5,* 20-38.

Lumsdon, K. (1994). Beyond four walls. *Hospitals & Health Networks, 68*(5), 44-45.

Mark, B. (1992). Characteristics of nursing practice models. *Journal of Nursing Administration, 22*(11), 57-63.

McClure, M. (1991). Introduction. In I. E. Goertzen (Ed.), *Differentiating nursing practice: Into the twenty-first century* (pp. 1-11). Kansas City, MO: American Academy of Nursing.

Mikulencak, M. (1993). Public health stands as a proven model for future delivery systems. *The American Nurse, 25*(6), 18.

Poulin, M. (1985). Configuration of nursing practice. In American Nurses Association (Ed.), *Issues in professional practice* (pp. 1-14). Kansas City, MO: American Nurses Association.

Rheaume, A., Frisch, S., Smith, A., & Kennedy, C. (1994). Case management and nursing practice. *Journal of Nursing Administration, 24*(3), 30-36.

Simpson, R. (1993). Case-managed care in tomorrow's information network. *Nursing Management, 24*(7), 14-16.

Sperry, S., & Birdsall, C. (1994). Outcomes of a pneumonia critical path. *Nursing Economic$, 12*(6), 332-339, 345.

Weil, M., & Karls, J. (1985). *Case management in human service practice*. San Francisco: Jossey-Bass.

Zander, K. (1985). Second generation primary nursing: A new agenda. *Journal of Nursing Administration, 15*(3), 18-24.

Zander, K. (1988). Nursing case management: The strategic management of cost and quality outcomes. *Journal of Nursing Administration, 18*(5), 23-30.

Zander, K. (1990). Case management: A golden opportunity for whom? In J. McCloskey & H. Grace (Eds.), *Current issues in nursing* (3rd ed.) (pp. 199-204). St. Louis: Mosby.

Zander, K. (1991). Case management in acute care: Making the connections. *The Case Manager, 2*(1), 39-43.

Zander, K. (1992). Nursing care delivery methods and quality. *Series on Nursing Administration, 3*, 86-104.

Zander, K. (1994). Nurses and case management: To control or collaborate? In J. McCloskey & H. Grace (Eds.), *Current issues in nursing* (4th ed.) (pp. 254-260). St. Louis: Mosby.

Zawadski, R., & Eng, C. (1988). Case management in capitated long-term care. *Health Care Financing Review, Annual supplement*, 75-81.

PART V

Managing Professionals and Their Practice

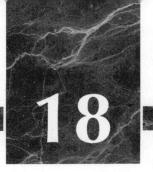

Communication

Chapter Objectives

☙

define and describe communication

☙

differentiate verbal and nonverbal communication

☙

explain four ways communication is distinguished

☙

explain five steps of information exchange

☙

compare communication net studies

☙

analyze elements of personal communication effectiveness

☙

relate feedback and criticism to communication

☙

relate appearance and behavior to forms of communication

☙

discuss aspects of professional communication effectiveness

☙

analyze organizational communication

☙

describe the relationship between communication and leadership

☙

compare organizational communication assessment areas

☙

analyze current issues in work-related communication in nursing

❧

explain managing multicultural diversity in nursing

❧

exercise critical thinking to conceptualize and analyze
possible solutions to a practical experience incident

*C*ommunication is the lubricant of organizations. Communication is a vital aspect of both leadership and management. Human beings communicate naturally and frequently. In nursing practice, communication is focused on both client care management and organizational outcomes.

As nurses work within organizations to deliver nursing care, they need to be able to work together to reach common goals. Communication can facilitate positive working relationships or can contribute to stress, lack of recognition, and feelings of alienation. Organizations face the challenge of creating communication pathways that lead to professional, productive, and comfortable work environments. Faulty communications take a toll on self-esteem and a sense of work-related well-being (Cornell, 1993).

DEFINITIONS

ommunication is the art of being able to structure and transmit a message in a way that another can easily understand and/or accept. *Organizational communication* is defined as the degree to which information is transmitted among the members and parts of an organization (see Chart 18.1). Information can be transmitted through a variety of verbal, written, electronic, and oral communication modes. Some examples are fliers, memos, letters, faxes, e-mail, formal discussions, committees, informal networking, newsletters, videos, bulletin boards, and telephone calls. When defined as information exchange, the two dimensions of accuracy and openness are relevant to communication (Price & Mueller, 1986). Communication encompasses both verbal and nonverbal information transmission. *Verbal communication* is both written and spoken (oral). *Nonverbal communication* is unspoken and is composed of affective or expressive behaviors. Verbal communication effectiveness depends on vocabulary, language, phrases, sentence structure, sentence clarity, rate of speech, diction, tone, rhythm, and volume. Nonverbal behavior includes elements of gestures, facial expression, eye contact, body language, and positioning (Hersey & Blanchard, 1993). Communication can be thought of as a continuum from nonverbal forms such as art, music, and body language, to general verbal expression, to precise special purpose languages such as computer language and mathematical applications (Henry & LeClair, 1987).

CHART 18.1
↪ DEFINITIONS

Organizational Communication
the degree to which information is transmitted among the members and parts of an organization.

Verbal Communication
communication through the use of words, either spoken or in writing.

Nonverbal Communication
communication which does not use words but rather affective or expressive behaviors.

Communication can be characterized by four distinctions: formal/informal, vertical/horizontal, personal/impersonal, and instrumental/expressive. These distinctions are defined as (Price & Mueller, 1986):

- *formal:* officially transmitted information, supported by organizational sanctions
- *informal:* unofficial information exchange
- *vertical:* transmission of information in superior-subordinate relationships
- *horizontal:* transmission of information among peers
- *personal:* information transmitted in situations where mutual influence may occur
- *impersonal:* information exchange without mutual influence
- *instrumental:* transmittal of information necessary to do the job
- *expressive:* the residual category of nonjob information transmittal

Thus, in the complex situations of organizational environments, information of a variety of types will be communication in a variety of ways. Nurses need to analyze all aspects of communication at work.

BACKGROUND

Communication and relating are linked to each other in that effective communication enhances interpersonal relations, and positive interpersonal relations promote effective communication. Communication models described in the literature include the sender-receiver, human needs, and transactional analysis models (Grant, 1994).

The sender-receiver model describes communication as messages or signals passed between the sender and the receiver. A single communication can be broken down into five steps of information exchange (Gerrard, Boniface, & Love, 1980; Grant, 1994):

- *message formation:* the message develops in the sender's mind
- *message encoding:* the decision by the sender as to verbal and nonverbal components
- *message transmission:* the spoken, written, and/or nonverbal information is expressed
- *message reception:* the receiver receives the information
- *message decoding:* the receiver interprets the message

Communication can be viewed as a pathway between two people. Communication occurs in a variety of interactive patterns (Cornell, 1993) (see Fig. 18.1). What this means is that the equality of exchange may be balanced or skewed. Sometimes people only desire to express themselves or depart information and do not engage in listening to the other or in reciprocity of communication exchange. When both people take turns, the conversation can be productive and show fewer signs of faulty communication.

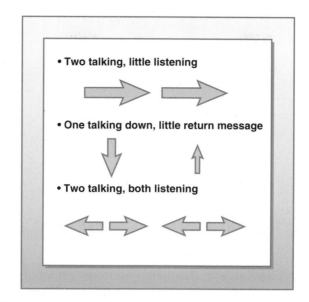

Figure 18.1
Interactive communication patterns. (Data from Cornell [1993].)

Perception and interpretation form filters for messages and create a potential for communication breakdown. Both sender and receiver have separate perceptual filters. On both ends, then, what was meant and what was understood may vary.

Problems can occur at any point and result in miscommunication. Successful communication is promoted by utilizing simplicity, clarity, appropriate timing, relevance, adaptation to circumstances, and credibility. On the other hand, successful communication is hindered by actions that distract, cut off communication, insert unhelpful advice, remove the other person's decision making power, or negate the importance of the other person or his or her message. Specific behaviors of offering inappropriate reassurance, rejecting the other, agreeing uncritically, stereotyping, belittling, or being egocentric tend to harm or hinder communication (Grant, 1994).

Communication also has been conceptualized within the framework of interpersonal skills or transactional analysis models. These models emphasize therapeutic communication techniques of active listening, attending, questioning, paraphrasing, reflecting feelings, assertion, challenging, confrontation, and interviewing skills (Thies & Williams-Burgess, 1992).

Communication in Groups

Group communication is even more complex because of the exponential way interactions duplicate as the number of active participants increases. This makes effective communication a greater challenge. In order to better comprehend what makes group communication effective, communication net studies have been done. Communication net studies have been conducted by social

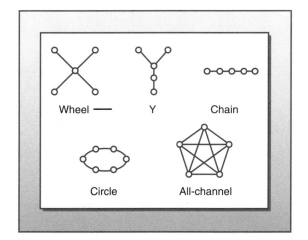

Figure 18.2
Communication networks.
(Data from Mintzberg
[1979].)

psychologists and communication researchers. In these experiments a few subjects are put into networks with selectively restricted channels of communication, given simple games or tasks, and then observed for patterns of interaction. The five commonly used networks are the wheel, the Y, the chain, the circle, and all-channel (see Fig. 18.2). The wheel, Y, and chain restrict communication the most and tend to be centralizing and hierarchical; the wheel network passes all communication through one person. The all-channel form has no communication restrictions. The circle and the all-channel networks tend to be more democratic configurations. The circle is the least efficient network (Mintzberg, 1979). In a hierarchical network, all members have to pass messages through one person. Sometimes a circle is formed and communication only allowed to either side. In a democratic network, all members can communicate freely. Hierarchical networks organize more quickly, make fewer errors, and have less satisfied members at the periphery. Democratic networks often develop hierarchies by themselves (Mintzberg, 1979; 1983).

In organizations, a parallel finding is that centralized organizations are more efficient in certain circumstances. Horizontally decentralized organizations seem better for morale but tend to become unstable and revert to a more centralized structure to complete tasks. This is especially true for organizations that do simple, repetitive, and unskilled tasks. Complex and knowledge-based work by professional workers tends to pull the organization toward decentralization (Mintzberg, 1979; 1983). There seems to be a pattern of relationships among group communication networks, effective communication, and the structure of an organization.

Personal Communication Effectiveness

Structuring a message for effectiveness is an important concept to consider. The sender has a choice of channels, whether it is by dress, nonverbal behavior, or a written or oral communication. To plan for personal effectiveness, decide on what message is desired and how it can be structured so that the message will be received positively and will engender the response preferred. Effectively communicating takes into consideration decisions about how to communicate, including aspects such as message structure, delivery style, and mode of communication.

Effectiveness in communication is related to timing and the choice of channel. For example, people respond to personal contact or appeal. It is much more difficult to say no to someone who comes personally to ask for participation, as opposed to a memo of request. It is more difficult to say no on the phone to someone who is a colleague than it is to rip a memo up and throw it in the wastebasket.

Consider the choice of words used in structuring a message. When using oral communication, select the words with care to structure the presentation for maximum impact. There are certain red flags, or emotionally charged words, that people respond to. Most of the emotion-laden words are superlatives, but there are certain words that are emotionally charged triggers. An example is racist or sexist language. Even though the sender thinks it to be normal conversation, any hint of discrimination or exclusion may raise sensitivities. Orators and preachers deliberately include inflammatory words as a motivation and persuasion technique. Because people will respond to the inflammatory words and not listen critically to the message, it may be necessary to deliberately delete certain words. If a person has an emotional response to the choice of words, then the message may be obscured or completely lost.

It is so easy to overlook the basic necessity of checking whether a message was understood. This is especially true for nursing, a field prone to jargon. Whether nurses are teaching clients or delegating work, it is tempting to assume that instructions given are clear. This is not always the case, as one group of nurses found out. They constructed 34 acontextual sentences using common nursing jargon such as vitals, NPO, ambulate, void, stool, flatus, and analgesic. They asked 101 adult patients to define the general meaning of each term. Correct responses ranged from 16% for flatus to 98% for OR, stethoscope, and bloodwork. If communication is key to understanding, then care must be taken to avoid misperceptions in translation (Cochrane et al., 1992).

RESEARCH NOTE

Source: Libbus, M., & Bowman, K. (1994). Sexual harassment of female registered nurses in hospitals. *Journal of Nursing Administration, 24*(6), 26-31.

Purpose

The purpose of this research was to explore and describe the extent to which practicing RNs in one state reported being subjected to sexual harassment in a hospital. A random sample of 78 female RNs employed for at least six months as staff nurses on a patient care unit were surveyed. Respondents were asked to report sexual harassment from any source and to describe the type of behavior and nurse response.

Discussion

Sexual harassment in the hospital work setting was reported by 56 nurses. Some form of sexual harassment by male co-workers, including physicians, was reported by 46 respondents reporting sexual harassment experiences. Clients were identified as the perpetrator by 30 nurses. Twenty-eight nurses responded to the harassment they experienced by choosing to ignore it. Only eight of the nurses reported confronting the perpetrator. Respondents described feelings of anger, embarrassment, and disgust in response to incidents of sexual harassment.

Application to Practice

It appears that nurses are frequent targets for sexual harassment. This behavior originates from a variety of sources and comes in a variety of forms. Little research has been done to identify the extent and form of sexual harassment in nursing. Perhaps ignoring the behavior is counterproductive. Sexual harassment contributes to lowered levels of self-esteem, work performance, and productivity. Nurse leaders and managers need to develop detection, assessment, and intervention strategies to identify, eliminate, and constructively manage incidents of sexual harassment.

Feedback and Criticism

Feedback is a basic and essential communication principle. It is tied into the concept of delegation: after choosing what to delegate (the right task), matching the task to the delegate's competence (the right person), and making an effective assignment (the right communication), then sharing the evaluation (the right feedback) closes the loop by providing closure and future motivation. Giving effective feedback provides a sense of recognition for task accomplishment. What is said and how the message is communicated affects the results of an interaction and the working relationships. Clear, timely, tactful communication with shared input and perceptions promotes effectiveness (Hansten & Washburn, 1992).

Part of feedback is learning to be able to give constructive criticism. Criticism is not inherently negative. It takes time and exposure to giving and receiving positive criticism to be able to take the ideas and use them to improve. Nurses may be targets for criticism for the following reasons (Deering, 1993):

- being on the front lines
- being the focus for displaced criticism when others are upset with the system

- working with people who have health problems
- working in high-stress environments requiring frequent critical decisions

The most natural human response is to become defensive. Defensive reactions may prompt defensive counterreactions. A heated argument, not a civil discussion, ensues. The opportunity to see a problem more clearly evaporates. The three communication techniques recommended to respond effectively to criticism are: ask for more information, agree with the critic, and use listening skills to guide the critic toward the real problem source (Deering, 1993).

There are group situations in which feedback, brainstorming, or open discussion is asked for. One of the essential characteristics of followership is to be able to dissent. However, when that dissent is formed as a personal attack or as the defamation of a person, it is not appropriate. Personal attacks merely tear down another person. Constructive criticism is not focused on blame or on a person's characteristics; it is focused on an analysis of the problem. Problem solving is a way of practicing positive communication. The appropriate communication approach when there is a problem with the system or the process is to use a critiquing: balancing the positives and negatives and pointing out problems and solution options.

Giving criticism may be avoided because it tends to provoke defensiveness and arguments. However, conflict may erupt if the skills of positive criticism are not employed to defuse frustrations. The first consideration is when and whether to criticize. The key is to take charge of the situation without losing control of emotions and alienating others. After choosing an appropriate time and place to deliver criticism, communication techniques such as phrasing the criticism in terms of outcomes desired and avoiding blanket statements are helpful. Criticism may have its basis in perception, not reality (Deering, 1993).

Appearance and Behavior

Communication behavior includes both the content of the communication and the expression or communication style. Research has shown that 55% of audience interpretations for speaker messages are determined by the speaker's nonverbal communication, such as facial expression and body language; 38% by the speaker's vocal quality, including tone, pitch, volume and variation; and 7% by the literal words. Overall, audiences remember concepts and emotional expression more than the content (Yepsen, 1988). Further there appear to be gender-based differences in communication behavior. For example, the communication of females may fulfill a socioemotional or expressive function; the communication of males may fulfill a task or instrumental function (Bales, 1950; Kennedy, Camden, & Timmerman, 1990).

Psychologists have analyzed job interviews and found that they consist of two parts. The first part is what is called the 30-second hurdle, because research has shown that most employers make up their minds about job applicants in the first 30 seconds. This 30-second decision is based on the halo effect. As psychologists use the term halo, it means the effects of the person's first impression. The halo effect radiates out from all directions and can be positive or negative. Unfortunately, first impressions are not always good impressions. It is this initial effect or impression that is extremely difficult, if not impossible, to overcome. What content can be expressed in 30 seconds to make a critical difference? Therefore, it is not the content of the message that forms the initial impression, it is the packaging. Facial expression, clothing, body posture, and hair form a total image. Appearance and behavior create a dramatic communication. The total picture, both verbal and nonverbal, can and does effectively communicate a message. If you mess up on this first impression part, the chances of getting the job are slim no matter how brilliantly the second part, the actual interview, is handled (Brothers, 1986). It may be tempting to ignore the impact of appearance and behavior. However, it appears to be a natural human response and one that nurses need to recognize and use for effectiveness.

Professional Communication Effectiveness

The importance of positive communication may be neglected in nursing. For example, how often are compliments and positive feedback given to others? Are nurses able to express their needs? Does verbal abuse exist and create a climate of intimidation where nurses feel they should not ask questions at all? What kind of environment is nursing practiced in, and what kind of person is each nurse in that environment?

Communication includes both verbal and nonverbal modalities, put together so that a message is communicated in a package. One application in nursing relates to image. The problem of image in nursing includes the portrayal of nurses in the media and dissention about uniforms and dress codes.

Nurses have identified their portrayal in the media as a concern related to stereotyping, lack of professionalism, and low esteem (Aber & Hawkins, 1992). Occupational prestige, both internal and external, was an issue during the most recent nurse shortage (Bream, Bram, Bantle, & Krenz, 1992). This means that it is easier to recruit into an occupation that has a high prestige in society and/or pays a lot of money. This societal view of nursing is called external prestige. Nurses also need to examine internal prestige, which is how nursing values nursing and nurses.

One media strategy evolved into a national advertising campaign. In 1990, the National Advertising Council, along with nursing's Tri-Council, put out a series of ads as a way of helping to alleviate the prevailing nursing shortage of the time. Called the "National Nursing Image Campaign," the theme of this campaign was, "If Caring Were Enough, Anyone Could Be a Nurse." One ad said, "At 10:26 AM Sandy Hardwick brought her 57-year old cardiac patient back to life. What did you accomplish this morning?" Another ad said, "After four years of college, you look for a job. After nursing school, a job's looking for you." The idea was to convey a different image of nursing: that it is an important and essential service with a good job market. At the same time, the Nurses of America published *Media Watch*, a communicative strategy to monitor the media for sexism and negative images of nurses. Their major impact was on the TV program "The Nightingales," which eventually was cancelled.

Who determines what is appropriate nursing attire? An interesting small group activity is to ask a group to come up with their ideal professional uniform. Policy committees may have lively discussions about nursing dress codes. This is because clothing is a form of nonverbal communication that stimulates judgmental responses from others (Kalisch & Kalsich, 1985).

Research has shown that the consumer prefers white uniforms with skirts and a cap as a nurse's uniform, possibly due to the persistence of traditional views and images of nursing (Franzoi, 1988; Kucera & Nieswiadomy, 1991). In one research study a series of photos of a woman in three styles of nursing attire were given to students and consumers to rate (Franzoi, 1988). One pose was the traditional white dress, white hose, white shoes, and white cap. The second was a modern style that consisted of white slacks and shoes with a multicolored, vertically striped blouse and no cap. The third style was scrubs. The study found that most of the people thought that the person in scrubs was a physician. The people identified the woman in the traditional outfit 90% of the time as a nurse. Sixty percent of the people preferred the traditional uniform, 35% the modern uniform, and only 5% preferred the picture of the person in the scrubs. Although nurses think scrubs are practical and comfortable, the public would prefer to see the traditional nurse attire.

The issue is projecting the perception of and communicating an attitude of competence and professionalism. The way nurses dress symbolizes role identity, function, authority, professional image, and confidence in ability and judgment, as well as how nurses feel about themselves (Mangum et al., 1991). It is even possible to find designer uniforms that attempt to blend professional tailoring with the uniform style (Barnum, 1990).

Institutions try to balance the public's perception of a nurse as a female in a white uniform and a cap with the practical reality of nursing practice. Caps are not really functional for nurses, and they are silly for male nurses. In healthcare facilities it is possible to see nursing staff dressed in a way that appears to be casual, soiled, ugly or unattractive, tight fitting, disheveled, or seductive. The leader and manager might be concerned about the image that

Communicating Vision, Mission, and Values

The task of communicating the vision, mission, and values of a 553-bed, academic, public, and tertiary medical center to campus stakeholders was approached utilizing various interdisciplinary campus members, existing structures (committees, teams), and numerous communication strategies. The expected outcomes of our communication strategies require that components of the vision, mission, and values be demonstrated in various forms. The vision, mission, and values must be reflected in staff interactions, recognized through role modeling, identified in printed documents, reflected in performance evaluations, and promoted through implementation of recognition programs.

Communication Methods

Realizing that communication styles differ vastly for individuals and/or groups, various strategies were utilized to reach the critical mass of stakeholders throughout our campus. The implementation strategies were derived through the collaborative efforts of staff from various departments within the campus. Both formal and informal communication strategies were implemented.

Formal Communication

In accomplishing our goals, formal communication methods were utilized in our facility. These methods included several passive techniques such as the display of the mission, vision, and values message in posters, banners, and bulletin boards. Written materials included memos and newsletters. Employee badges were produced with the mission, vision, and values imprinted on the back. Computer network systems relayed the messages to all users upon its initiation. Active communication techniques included focus groups which were developed to promote greater analysis, input, and feedback.

Our use of passive formal communication techniques were advantageous in reaching a large number of individuals and in creating awareness. However, we were unable to measure the direct result of this communication method as input and feedback were minimal. The focus group sessions were much more valuable in terms of problem identification and resolution. Input and feedback were important concerns in the use of focus groups. Although useful in some situations, formal communication methods had the added problem of creating a barrier to communication for the members involved. This barrier included staff discomfort in a formalized environment. This barrier was addressed through the use of informal sessions where input and feedback were less restricted by formality.

Informal Communication

Informal communication methods included brown-bag lunch sessions where interested members spent their lunch breaks with administrators and/or other executive level staff for the purpose of discussing issues within the facility. These sessions were informal, with no agenda, and were designed to address the immediate concerns of members in attendance. The informal atmosphere encouraged members to address their issues without concern for protocol and were successful in attracting the voices of the "every day worker." Other informal communication methods incorporated were one-on-one discussions (versus group discussions). These sessions were extremely helpful in identifying the specific needs of individuals and enabled us to work closely with them in developing more coherent agendas for problem resolution. It was especially critical for us to carefully select the individuals on these one-on-one discussions as assumptions regarding a larger population may be based on the answers of a few individuals.

Results

Whether informal or formal communication techniques were utilized, the dissemination of information utilized top-down, bottom-up, and lateral communications as foundations for our methods. To determine the results of our communication strategies, we acquired qualitative and quantitative data. Anecdotal feedback and some structured evaluations were obtained and utilized. Performance evaluations were also linked with the behavioral objectives of our campaign. Feedback was easily obtained from these evaluations. Communication through experiential learning yielded the best results.

Environmental Issues

In addition to developing and initiating communication methods, we also addressed environmental issues to promote communication and ownership of the mission, vision, and values of our organization. We analyzed our existing work (hiring, orientation practices) and linked them with the objectives of the mission, vision, and values of the organization. We developed learning interventions that applied the concepts of our mission, vision, and values and provided experiential learning for our staff. Additionally, we created developmental opportunities for new leaders to emerge.

Conclusion

This campaign reaffirmed the importance of a comprehensive marketing program when communicating the mission, vision, and values of an organization. To reach the target audience, particularly the broad masses, communication methods must be visible, diverse, and often tailored for specific populations. The collaborative efforts of an interdisciplinary staff and the creation and/or utilization of structures (committees, teams) play a critical role in communication strategies.

PAULA SILER, RN, MS
Director, Professional Practice Affairs
Harbor–University of California Los Angeles
   Medical Center
Torrance, California

CATHY LOPEZ HOUSTON, RN, MBA
Analyst, Department of Nursing
Harbor–University of California Los Angeles
   Medical Center
Torrance, California

the nurses portray and may decide that a certain uniform is required as a part of enhancing the nurses' image.

Further, organizations may feel the need to be responsive to consumer preferences, desiring to use image and professional polish as a competitive edge (Mangum et al., 1991). Marketing and imaging have become a communication imperative as competition increases in healthcare. The choice of clothing is in and of itself an important statement about nurses' professionalism and affects the amount of trust, confidence, and respect from the consumer.

Organizational Communication

Communication in organizations is not a simple sender, receiver, channel concept. Group dynamics and the interaction of multiple people provide complexity and challenges to the communicative process and the influence of perception in organizations. There are political and interpersonal subtleties and complexities to take into account. For example, people inherently have a strong reaction to written memos, especially those tacked up on bulletin boards. In an employee lounge, a general memo posted on the bulletin board may have graffiti written on it, partially because the employees are not able to give feedback to what is perceived as an edict or proclamation. There can be strong negativity to a written memo.

Notice how organizations choose to deliver various messages. Consider an example from an employee's perspective as to how an organization might communicate when a hospital is laying off nurses. In nursing there have been periods where reductions in force (RIFs) were common, as well as periods of nursing shortage. Each institution makes choices if they decide to lay people off. The kinds of controversies include how to choose who will be laid off, how to tell them, what kind of outplacement help is extended to them, the extent of unionization, and other personnel requirements that need to be followed. Conversely, the messages that organizations give when heavily recruiting nurses may reflect either an attitude of valuing professionalism or offering short-term inducements.

The question, then is: In reviewing instances in life and examining other ways to act, what are the options to increase personal and professional effectiveness? Job satisfaction in nursing can be augmented as nurses perceive themselves to be more effective and more in control of their practice environment.

LEADERSHIP AND MANAGEMENT IMPLICATIONS

Communication is a process in which information, perception and understanding are transmitted from person to person. As an integral part of any relationship, communication is important to nurses. Nurse leaders and managers can view communication as a tool to accomplish work and meet goals. The sig-

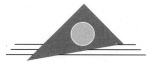 *Leadership & Management Behaviors*

LEADERSHIP BEHAVIORS

- communicates a vision
- structures messages to inspire
- motivates by communication strategies
- projects a professional image
- models positive communication
- influences frequent communication
- coaches followers
- structures symbols and shared meanings

MANAGEMENT BEHAVIORS

- communicates with superiors and subordinates
- structures messages for clarity
- directs the performance of others by communication strategies
- influences organizational goal accomplishment by communicating

OVERLAP AREAS

- communicates with others
- influences others

nificance of communication revolves around its effectiveness and the climate in which communication occurs. Effective communication is enhanced by clear, direct, straightforward, and frequent message transmission. Trust, respect, and empathy are the three ingredients needed to create and foster effective communication. Communication flows throughout any organization in upward, downward, and horizontal directions. Collaboration, conflict, and confrontation are often found in the communication "traffic" in organizations (Lancaster, 1982).

For leaders, communication is a key element of the role. Bennis and Nanus (1985, p. 33) noted that "success requires the capacity to relate a compelling image of a desired state of affairs." Such a compelling image is thought to induce enthusiasm and commitment in others. Thus the leader's role is to communicate a vision. Within organizations, leaders need to be "social architects" (Bennis & Nanus, 1985). This means that leaders will be shaping values and norms in a way that binds and bonds individuals and groups. Communication is key to this effort. Visions are communicated by means of managing meaning and creating understanding, commitment, and ownership of a vision. Leaders use communication as a tool for building trust. Trust is the glue that adheres leaders and followers together.

Communication is a basic and essential skill for leaders and managers. Communicating, along with diagnosing and adapting, is one of the three basic competencies of influencing and leadership (Hersey & Blanchard, 1993). Communication is a critical and important tool for effectiveness, in engaging and motivating people, and in getting the work done through others. As a manager, structuring messages so that people understand them clearly and avoiding emotion-laden triggers enhances communication effectiveness.

Acquiring interpersonal relationship skills, including the ability to communicate, is as essential to a leader's "kit bag" of leadership skills as psychomotor skills are for a nurse. Leadership and management ability is predicated on a facility for communication. In nursing leadership and management, communication is a skill that is essential for effective implementation of the change process. Communication is an intervention that leaders and managers in nursing use in order to accomplish their goals.

Language is used by leaders to give meaning to work. Metaphors and political language are used by leaders to influence and motivate (Henry & LeClair, 1987). Farley (1989) identified six areas of organizational communication that can be assessed for communication problems (see Chart 18.2). Communication problems may be a source of dissatisfaction. Research has indicated that a positive communication atmosphere, positive communication between staff nurses and immediate superiors, and personal feedback on job performance are related to nurse job satisfaction (Pincus, 1986).

A couple of examples from nursing leadership and management are worth considering. In hospital nursing, situations occur where nurses are sent

CHART 18.2
❧ COMMUNICATION ASSESSMENT

- Accessibility of information
- Communication channels
- Clarity of messages
- Span of control
- Flow control/communication load
- The individual communicators

Data from Farley (1989).

Exemplar 18.2

Personal Touches

Communication among approximately 200 employees in the department of Ambulatory Clinic Nursing can occur in many forms. Information regarding clinical issues is conveyed by the usual means—memos, bulletins, and meetings. Personal communication with staff members also receives formal emphasis. Here are two examples:

For the past several years, we have sent birthday cards to the homes of each member of our nursing staff. This simple goodwill measure is intended to communicate that his or her birth date is a special occasion worth recognizing. The overall response from the nursing staff is positive, and recently hired staff are genuinely surprised and pleased to learn of this friendly practice, which is easy to implement, minimal in cost, and an effective way to acknowledge each individual nurse.

Another personal touch is for those who experience the death of immediate family members. On the first month anniversary of that loss, a fresh bouquet of cut flowers is sent to their home—to say that we are thinking of them at this time of change and challenge. We chose the first month date because about that time life has usually returned to a normal routine yet with some changing dynamics. It is an attempt to acknowledge what is often a difficult time in their lives.

Recently one of our nurses lost her mother after two years of treatment for lung cancer. Gloria's role was that of primary caregiver, coordinator, and communicator between her seven adult siblings, the healthcare team, and her mom; she also worked full time. Her mom died in February, and we sent a bouquet of flowers exactly one month later. Gloria sent a note to us that was particularly poignant. She recalled how she and her mom would drive home from clinic appointments through a particularly beautiful area of town. On one of their last trips her mom remarked that she would miss seeing the beautiful flowers bloom this spring—her way of communicating realization and acceptance of her impending death. The one month anniversary date happened to be a particularly beautiful day, and Gloria was reminded as she was driving home that afternoon of her mom's comment about not seeing the flowers bloom in spring. She arrived home to find this bouquet of flowers and wrote of her combined joy and sadness in having her mother's death remembered that particular day—in that particular way.

If ever we doubt whether it is right to reach out and touch our staff, we are reminded that it is important for leaders to remember and recognize nurses as individuals who share the profession of nursing. Our efforts are focused on recognizing the happy and sad times in everyone's life.

E. MARY JOHNSON, RN, BSN, CNA
Director, Ambulatory Clinic Nursing
Cleveland Clinic Foundation
Cleveland, Ohio

(pulling, floating, or farming are the terms used) from the unit they normally work on to another unit. The person who has to deliver the unpleasant news determines whether to call the unit and leave a little note on the assignment sheet or go to the nurse and talk directly. Some might offer to take the nurse to the other unit, introduce them to the charge nurse, and smooth out the transition. How is the message best structured and delivered? There are different ways to be effective in difficult situations.

One leadership moment happens when a nurse must present a proposal to a committee which must be convinced to release the money for a project that is vitally important to the care of clients. Strategic planning is used to figure out what will maximize the message delivery. This may include how to structure the communication, nonverbally as well as verbally, so that a positive impression is created, and the second stage of receiving your message has an opportunity for a full and impartial hearing.

Leaders and managers always communicate two things to others whether they want to or not: they always communicate their attitude and their goals and expectations. Trust or distrust is communicated. Whether it is direct or subtle, the leader communicates a vision and a sense of where they are going and what they expect from their followers.

CURRENT ISSUES AND TRENDS

In the practice of nursing, communication techniques can be applied to the remediation of work-related issues and to the communication of professional messages to each other and to the larger public. Three examples are verbal abuse, physical violence, and the use of work teams.

Verbal abuse is a job issue in nursing. Nurses perceive that they are exposed to verbally abusive situations in excessive amounts (AJN Newscaps, 1993; Braun, Christle, Walker, & Tiwanak, 1991). That creates some conflict for nurses and some stressful situations to deal with. Principles of caring, assertiveness, and communication apply in a verbally abusive situation. In one reported scenario, a physician was repeatedly verbally abusive to nurses. The nurses collectively devised a creative and empowering solution. They decided that what they would do is call a specific "code" when a verbal abuse incident was taking place. They established a code call, similar to a code blue or fire alert, but with another name. The nurses agreed that if this code was called over the public address system, then any nurse who was available would go to the unit where there was a nurse under verbal barrage. They would gather and simply stand there. Imagine what happened: the social pressure of public display and a crowd of witnesses tended to change behavior immediately.

In one hospital the nurses instituted a system of restraints because of the level of drug and alcohol-related violence in the emergency room. This was happening especially on nights, weekends, and holidays. The nurses were feeling personally threatened because there were enough incidents of serious violence. The Nursing Department arranged for training in non-violent restraint. One staff member subsequently formed a specially trained restraint team, and when there was a violence potential, the nurses were told to call the restraint team. The team was composed of four people who had been trained in one of the non-violent Japanese martial arts. With these three or four people, even the most violent patients were restrained very quickly. The team simply walked into the room. They were trained to be very calm. They knew exactly how to restrain the person if motor activity occurred: team members took up positions on each shoulder and hip and applied manual restraint. Frequently, the client calmed down without the team's having to apply restraints. These techniques, based on interpersonal communication and a conveyance of calm competence, did work. Nurses can create a difference in behavior when they structure their messages and when they have confidence that as a group they will be able to handle problems positively and constructively.

The concepts of team and team process are enjoying a resurgence of interest. There may be work teams, self-managed work teams, project teams, and cross-functional teams. Most involve people working in a group together to produce a product or service. Stages of team development have been described as forming, storming, norming, performing, and adjourning; as initial, transition, working, and final; or as awareness, conflict, cooperation, productivity, and separation. Effective teams rely on interpersonal skills and communication. Listening and open communication characterize effective teams (Anderson, 1993). (See Chapter 8 for further discussion of teams.)

Managing Multicultural Diversity

Rapid changes in the ethnic composition of the U.S. population has been cited as one of the major sociodemographic forces taking place in this decade (see Chapter 2). Issues related to multicultural diversity impact the leadership and management of nursing and healthcare. The projections indicate a modest growth in the African-American population and a rapid increase in the Asian and Hispanic ethnic groups. Because there is diversity of opinion within various ethnic groups, based on geographical, economic, political, and age differences, concerning appropriateness of nomenclature, the terminology "people of color" will be used here when referring collectively to African-Americans, Hispanics, Native Americans, Asians, and other ethnic groupings.

Two general challenges to nursing and healthcare from the changing ethnic diversity revolve around the provision of healthcare on the one hand and the provision of jobs on the other. Nursing and healthcare leadership and management must be prepared to face challenges in meeting the healthcare needs and expectations of increasingly diverse populations as reflected in ethnic, cultural, and linguistic components. Challenges also will be faced in healthcare industry employment activities as the people seeking employment in the industry continue to grow in ethnic, cultural, and linguistic diversity (Castiglia, 1994; Poteet & Goodard, 1989).

The demographic profile of the RN population and the nursing student population does not reflect the demographics of the general population (Castiglia, 1994). Increases in the proportion of nurses, nursing faculty, and nursing students who are people of color have been small. However, nursing needs to draw from the societal population base that it serves. This means deliberate strategies to place value on cultural diversity in nursing, to nurture people of color within the profession, and to teach and learn about managing multicultural diversity.

Furuta and Lipson (1994) suggested eight ways to facilitate cultural diversity in the nursing student body: develop an applicant pool of people of color, create orientation and preceptor programs, personalize recruitment, formalize nontraditional admissions criteria, enroll a cohort of students who are people of color, create a culturally sensitive learning environment, mainstream student services, and recruit faculty who are people of color. These strategies make a stronger effort to attract diversity among students in nursing.

There are barriers and difficulties to increasing multicultural diversity in nursing. Diversity is the opposite of homogeneity. In educational institutions, homogeneity makes the task of teaching easier and more efficient. Students from other cultures or who have English as a second language add complexities for the faculty members. However those same students also add a rich accumulation of experiences, values, and beliefs to the benefit of both faculty members and other students and should not be overlooked (Brink, 1994).

Brink (1994, p. 664) has said, "cultural diversity does not happen peacefully, without struggle and strain." Managing multicultural diversity challenges nurse leaders and managers to handle conflict constructively and learn to negotiate new perceptions. For example, cross-cultural educational programs in human resources, education, and nursing departments may be needed as one measure to deal with potential misunderstandings among clients, employees, providers, and employers related to dissimilar perceptions or expectations (Poteet & Goddard, 1989).

Specific approaches to managing diversity in the workforce vary by organization and not infrequently by manager within an organization. Managerial strategies for handling workforce diversity can be divided into three general categories: deny, minimize, and energize.

Those who *deny* the realities of the situation either may resent the growing cultural diversity in their workforce or may welcome it. In either event they feel that this diversity does not impact on the organization or that any impact is negligible. Frequently, this type of manager or organization views his or her way of operating as the only acceptable way. Those who work for this organization or manager will either buy into the "acceptable way" to operate or will move out. The cultural background employees bring to the workplace will not be viewed as capable for contributing to or detracting from the organization's central mission. The most likely outcome of this strategy is that problems will occur (Adler, 1986).

The manager and organizations who use a *minimize* strategy perceive cultural impact as primarily negative for the organization. These minimizers may well try to maintain a culturally homogeneous workforce and, where that is not possible, will attempt to socialize those of different cultural backgrounds into the primary culture of the workplace. The most likely outcome of this common strategy is some problems and few advantages (Adler, 1986).

Some organizations and managers try to *energize* the influence of cultural diversity in their workplace. In these situations the manager views cultural diversity as containing positive and negative elements. The manager attempts to control the negative elements and to increase the positive elements by managing the impacts of that diversity rather than the diversity itself. This view operates on the premise that the whole is greater than the sum of the parts and leads to the development of new operational methods for the organization which transcend the cultures of individual workers. This energizing approach to cultural diversity views the similarities and differences between cultures to be of equal importance. It operates on the premise that there are many equally valuable ways to achieve a desired end and the best way for this specific organization is dependent on the makeup of its workforce. The most likely outcome of this strategy is some problems and many advantages (Adler, 1986).

To entice performance from a workforce characterized by multicultural diversity, Thomas (1990) outlined ten managerial guidelines:
- Clarify your motivation to learn to manage diversity.
- Clarify your vision or image of a diverse workforce.
- Expand your focus to include a dominant heterogeneous culture across many characteristics.
- Audit your corporate culture for current operative assumptions.
- Modify your assumptions to embrace equal opportunity.
- Modify your systems for hiring, promoting, mentoring, and evaluating.
- Modify your models of both managerial behavior and employee behavior.
- Help your people pioneer a change to greater diversity.
- Apply the special consideration test: does this initiative give special consideration to one group, or does it contribute to everyone's success?
- Continue affirmative action in order to achieve a diverse workforce, then move beyond it.

Thomas (1990, p. 112) noted that "managing diversity does not mean controlling or containing diversity." Rather, managing diversity is seen as empowering each unique member of the workforce to attain his or her potential and as encouraging and massaging disparate talents to the end of accomplishing a common goal. It is imperative that the nurse manager audit the organizational culture and then identify a set of values and a common purpose that will "transcend the interests, desires, and preferences of any one group" (Thomas, 1990, p. 116).

When nurses lack knowledge and exposure to people from different cultures, encounters with people different from themselves may be uncomfortable or difficult. Stereotyping is a common occurrence and is a challenge to overcome. However, nursing will need to capture the energy of people with diverse experiences and better reflect and represent the population served. Nurse leaders and managers can recognize multicultural diversity issues and institute strategies to counteract stereotyping and lack of knowledge.

SUMMARY

- Communication is the art of being able to structure and transmit a message in a way that another can easily understand and/or accept.
- Communication is defined as the degree to which information is transmitted among the members and parts of an organization.
- Verbal communication is both written and spoken (oral).
- Nonverbal communication is unspoken but affective or expressive behaviors.
- Communication can be characterized by four distinctions: formal/informal, vertical/horizontal, personal/impersonal, and instrumental/expressive.
- Communication models described in the literature include the sender-receiver, human needs, and transactional analysis models.
- Interpersonal relationships include an element of communication.
- A single communication can be broken down into five steps of information exchange.
- Communication occurs in a variety of interactive patterns.
- Perception and interpretation form filters for messages and create a potential for breakdown.
- Effectiveness in communication is related to timing and the choice of channel.
- Feedback is a basic communication principle tied into the concept of delegation.
- Constructive criticism is focused on an analysis of the problem.
- Appearance and behavior add to the total communication to effectively communicate a message.
- One issue in nursing is how to project and communicate an attitude of competence and professionalism.
- Group dynamics and the interaction of multiple people provide complexity and challenges to the communicative process and the influence of perception in organizations.

- Communicating, along with diagnosing and adapting, is one of the three basic competencies of influencing and leadership.
- There are six areas of organizational communication that can be assessed for communication problems: accessibility of information, communication channels, clarity of messages, span of control, flow control/communication load, and the individual communicators.
- In nursing, communication techniques can be applied to the remediation of work-related issues, for example, verbal abuse, physical violence, and the use of work teams.
- Changes in the ethnic composition of the U.S. population create multicultural diversity management opportunities and challenges.

Study Questions

1. What are the essential components of the communication process?
2. What are the barriers to effective communication in organizations?
3. What problems of communication occur frequently in nursing?
4. Are superior-subordinate communication problems more common than peer-to-peer difficulties?
5. What solutions tend to help communication effectiveness?
6. What is the relationship of communication skill to leadership effectiveness?
7. What is the leader's role in helping others improve written and oral communication?
8. How important is written communication skill in influencing an individual's image?
9. How do you personally communicate, both verbally and nonverbally?
10. How might you choose some other message or some other channel in order to increase personal effectiveness?
11. Do nurses, from the staff nurse to the chief nurse executive, present an image of nursing that you agree or disagree with?
12. What does the ideal nurses' uniform look like? Analyze your response.
13. Why do nurses need to look professional?

Critical Thinking Exercise

Nurse Harry Albert is assigned to the skilled nursing unit of a community hospital and has the responsibility for passing meds to the clients this afternoon. When he arrives at room 605 at approximately 4 PM, he reviews the new admission client's chart and determines that oral morphine is scheduled. However, when Nurse Albert starts to give the morphine to the client, the client's son stops him and asks what medication he is administering. When told, the client's son has a strong negative reaction and tells Nurse Albert that the client just had his morphine an hour and a half ago and that morphine hallucination has been a problem for the client. Nurse Albert rechecks the chart and tells the client's son that there is no record of morphine being administered an hour and a half ago. The son explains that when he brought the client into the hospital there was no doctor's order yet for morphine. The nurse who did the admission left the room so that the family could give the client the morphine dose that was brought from home. The day shift admission nurse has left the hospital for the day and has left no special information for Nurse Albert about the morphine.

1. *What is the problem?*

2. *Whose problem is it?*

3. *What should Nurse Albert do?*

4. *What mode of communication should Nurse Albert use?*

5. *How can Nurse Albert structure a clear message?*

6. *To whom should Nurse Albert communicate first? Then who else needs to be in the communication flow?*

7. *What leadership and management strategies should Nurse Albert use?*

REFERENCES

Aber, C., & Hawkins, J. (1992). Portrayal of nurses in advertisements in medical and nursing journals. *Image, 24*(4), 289-293.

Adler, N. (1986). *International dimensions of organizational behavior*. Boston: Kent Publishing.

AJN Newscaps. (1993). RNs cite physical and verbal abuse. *American Journal of Nursing, 93*(1), 85.

Anderson, L. (1993). Teams: Group process, success, and barriers. *Journal of Nursing Administration, 23*(9), 15-19.

Bales, R. (1950). *Interaction process analysis: A method for the study of small groups*. Reading, MA: Addison-Wesley.

Barnum, B. (1990). Wear your designer clothes on duty: The Diane Von Furstenberg collection. *Nursing & Health Care, 11*(9), 484-485.

Braun, K., Christle, D., Walker, D., & Tiwanak, G. (1991). *Nursing Management, 22*(3), 72-76.

Bream, T., Bram, K., Bantle, A., & Krenz, K. (1992). Beyond the ordinary image of nursing. . . . *Nursing Management, 23*(12), 44-47.

Brink, P. (1994). Cultural diversity in nursing: How much can we tolerate? In J. McCloskey & H. Grace (Eds.), *Current issues in nursing* (4th ed.) (pp. 658-664). St. Louis: Mosby.

Brothers, J. (1986, November 16). How to get the job you want. *Parade*, pp. 4-6.

Castiglia, P. (1994). Increasing the pool of minority students. In J. McCloskey & H. Grace (Eds.), *Current issues in nursing* (4th ed.) (pp. 676-682). St. Louis: Mosby.

Cochrane, D., Oberle, K., Nielson, S., Sloan-Roseneck, J., Anderson, K., & Finlay C. (1992). Do they really understand us? *American Journal of Nursing, 92*(7), 19-20.

Cornell, D. (1993). Say the words: Communication techniques. *Nursing Management, 24*(3), 42-44.

Deering, C. (1993). Giving and taking criticism. *American Journal of Nursing, 93*(12), 56-61.

Farley, M. (1989). Assessing communication in organizations. *Journal of Nursing Administration, 19*(12), 27-31.

Franzoi, S. (1988). A picture of competence. *American Journal of Nursing, 88*(8), 1109-1112.

Furuta, B., & Lipson, J. (1994). Cultural diversity in the student body revisited. In J. McCloskey & H. Grace (Eds.), *Current issues in nursing* (4th ed.) (pp. 665-670). St. Louis: Mosby.

Gerrard, B., Boniface, W., & Love, B. (1980). *Interpersonal skills for health professionals.* Reston, VA: Reston.

Grant, A. (1994). *The professional nurse: Issues and actions.* Springhouse, PA: Springhouse.

Hansten, R., & Washburn, M. (1992). What's your feedback style? *American Journal of Nursing, 92*(12), 56-61.

Henry, B., & LeClair, H. (1987). Language, leadership, and power. *Journal of Nursing Administration, 17*(1), 19-25.

Hersey, P., & Blanchard, K. (1993). *Management of organizational behavior: Utilizing human resources* (6th ed.). Englewood Cliffs, NJ: Prentice-Hall.

Kalisch, B., & Kalisch, P. (1985). Dressing for success. *American Journal of Nursing, 85*(8), 887-893.

Kennedy, C., Camden, C., & Timmerman, G. (1990). Relationships among perceived supervisor communication, nurse morale, and sociocultural variables. *Nursing Administration Quarterly, 14*(4), 38-46.

Kucera, K., & Nieswiadomy, R. (1991). Nursing attire: The public's preference. *Nursing Management, 22*(10), 68-70.

Lancaster, J. (1982). Communication as a tool for change. In J. Lancaster & W. Lancaster (Eds.), *The nurse as a change agent: Concepts for advanced practice nursing* (pp. 109-131). St. Louis: Mosby.

Mangum, S., Garrison, C., Lind, C., Thackeray, R., & Wyatt, M. (1991). Perceptions of nurses' uniforms. *Image, 23*(2), 127-130.

Mintzberg, H. (1979). *The structuring of organizations: A synthesis of the research.* Englewood Cliffs, NJ: Prentice-Hall.

Mintzberg, H. (1983). *Structure in fives: Designing effective organizations.* Englewood Cliffs, NJ: Prentice-Hall.

Pincus, J. (1986). Communication: Key contributor to effectiveness—The research. *Journal of Nursing Administration, 16*(9), 19-25.

Poteet, G., & Goddard, N. (1989). Issues in financial management. In B. Henry, C. Arndt, M. DiVincenti, & A. Marriner-Tomey (Eds.), *Dimensions of nursing administration: Theory, research, education, practice* (pp. 699-709). Boston: Blackwell.

Price, J., & Mueller, C. (1986). *Handbook of organizational measurement.* Marshfield, MA: Pitman.

Thies, K., & Williams-Burgess, C. (1992). Communication as a progressive curriculum concept. *Nurse Educator, 17*(2), 39-41.

Thomas, R. (1990). From affirmative action to affirming diversity. *Harvard Business Review, 90*(2), 107-117.

Yepsen, D. (1988, October 5). Molding a candidate for the media. *The Des Moines Register,* p. 7A.

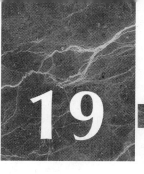

19

Motivation

Chapter Objectives

ᘒ

define and describe motivation

ᘒ

explain the need satisfaction model

ᘒ

differentiate internal and external motivation

ᘒ

explain Maslow's Hierarchy of Needs theory

ᘒ

explain Herzberg's Motivation-Hygiene theory

ᘒ

compare McClelland's three basic needs

ᘒ

differentiate Theory X from Theory Y

ᘒ

explain Hackman and Oldham's Job Characteristics theory

ᘒ

analyze motivation in organizations

ᘒ

analyze motivation in nursing

ᘒ

analyze the link between motivation and leadership and management

ᘒ

exercise critical thinking to conceptualize and analyze
possible solutions to a practical experience incident

$m$otivation is a key concept of leadership and management in nursing. The art of leading and managing groups of professionals requires creative, interesting, and continuous ways to make people feel good about what they are doing. In a service industry with professional employees, human relations variables are important for productivity, since the work is dependent on the knowledge, skill, and work effort of human beings. Motivation is important for understanding why people work, why some people are highly productive and others are not, and for comprehending complex relationships related to productivity in organizations. Organizations have a vital interest in productivity. The trend in work life is to emphasize working harder and being more effective. This requires some internal or external force to move human beings to continuous high levels of productivity. Motivation and the structures set up in organizations to motivate human beings have an effect on outcomes such as performance, turnover, and absenteeism.

DEFINITIONS

Motivation can be defined as a state of mind in which a person views any particular task or goal (see Chart 19.1). Motivation also is used as a term to describe the process of activating human behavior. The phenomenon of motivation encompasses a concern with what energizes behavior, directs or channels behavior, and maintains or sustains behavior (Steers & Porter, 1987). Thus motivation is a catalyst to move individuals toward goals. The basic unit of human behavior is an *activity*.

People vary in their ability to do an activity and in their willingness to do it. Motivation is the willingness aspect. *Motives or needs* are defined as wants, drives, or impulses within the individual. They are the drives to action and the reasons for behavior. Motives are directed toward goals and are the energizing forces that become an incentive to strive for the hoped for rewards outside the individual. The need with the greatest strength at any one time is what leads to activity (Hersey & Blanchard, 1993).

Motivation to work is defined as the degree to which members of an organization are willing to work (Price & Mueller, 1986). There are energizing forces within individuals that drive them to behave and environmental forces that trigger the drives. The idea of goal orientation means that human behavior is directed toward something. To analyze motivation from a systems orientation means to look at both forces within individuals and those in the environment that feed back to either reinforce the intensity of a drive or to discourage a course of action and redirect efforts. Thus motivation is concerned with those factors that energize, direct, and sustain human behavior (Steers & Porter, 1987). For example, motivation can appear as a result of the

CHART 19.1
～ DEFINITIONS

Motivation
a state of mind in which a person views any particular task or goal.

Activity
a basic unit of human behavior.

Motives or Needs
wants, drives, or impulses.

Motivation to work
the degree to which members of an organization are willing to work.

Data from Hersey and Blanchard (1993), Price and Mueller (1986), and from Steers and Porter (1987).

persuasive communication that occurs between leader and follower (Hersey & Duldt, 1989).

Motivation has been described as the ability to get individuals to do what you want them to do, when and how you want it done. Motivated people have a sense of forward drive as an identifying characteristic. Motivated individuals have a sense of energy, enthusiasm, and goal-directedness. The most powerful source of motivation is thought to be internal, intrinsic drives. To effectively motivate, leaders need to discover in their followers something that arouses a desire, energizes the will, and serves as a basis for action or thought (Schweiger, 1980).

BACKGROUND

Organizations that employ nurses seek to manage scarce human resources in a way that best coordinates and motivates nurses as employees. However, the best way to do this is not immediately obvious. Traditional bureaucratic organizations use close supervision and tight control of employees. Human relations or human resources models utilize limited participation or decentralization to enhance employee morale and cooperation. Because motivation is a complex yet critical element, it has been extensively investigated. There are a variety of theories of motivation. Friss (1989) categorized these as needs theory, reinforcement theory, balance theory, expectancy theory, and goal-setting theory. Lawler (1973) noted that the psychology of motivation has been approached from two different viewpoints about the nature of man: man as being driven by instinctual and unconscious drives and man as rational and behaving in ways to help achieve goals. Theories of human needs or drives are different from theories of motivation in that human needs theories specify the nature of human needs, whereas theories of motivation seek to fully explain and predict behavior.

The Need Satisfaction Model

To motivate is not an easy task. Knowledge about how individuals pursue the satisfaction of needs helps nurses understand motivation. A special process is involved with motivation. First a need is felt. For example, a felt need is something like needing to get a job or earn money. Then there is some sort of activity or behavioral response to the felt need. Then the goal either is attained or blocked. If the goal desired to reduce the feeling of need is blocked, frustration results. At this point another round of the process is initiated in an attempt to reduce the frustration. This process forms the core of the Need Satisfaction Model (Schweiger, 1980) (see Fig. 19.1). For example, a nurse assesses that a client is in pain. Comfort measures are not sufficient to alleviate

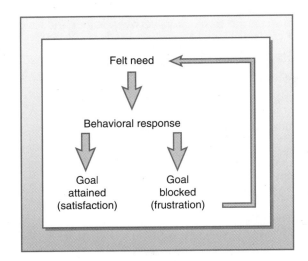

Figure 19.1
Need satisfaction model. (Data from Schweiger [1980].)

the pain or client-felt need. The nurse, in a behavioral response, contacts the physician for a pain medication order. This results in either attaining the goal if successful or in frustration if unsuccessful. If unsuccessful, new behaviors are called for as frustration has become the new felt need.

In general, motivational theories are based on the relationship of attitudes, needs, and behaviors. Motivation can be either internal or external, called intrinsic or extrinsic. *Internal* motivation is motivation that arises from within an individual and is aimed at a sense of personal accomplishment. *External* motivation is motivation that arises from outside an individual, where something or somebody becomes an incentive. External motivation is related to the application of rewards or punishments. For example, a grade given for performance on an examination is an external motivator. Weight loss, smoking cessation, and chemical dependency rehabilitation programs all deal with internal versus external motivation and the challenge of finding the right combination to overcome strong urges.

A person's attitudes and values create the internal versus external orientation. Some circumstances involve a combination of both internal and external motivators. For example, nurses may work at a rapid pace because they enjoy feeling a sense of achievement, an internal motivator, but also because they are given an external motivator in the form of a heavy assignment. Personal philosophy, values, beliefs, and assumptions are the foundations for motivation. To understand an individual's internal motivation, an understanding of his/her beliefs, values, and assumptions is needed (see Fig. 19.2).

The need satisfaction model provides insight into understanding human behavior. This model has been the basis for many theories of motivation, including Maslow's (1954) Hierarchy of Needs theory, Alderfer's (1969) ERG theory, Herzberg's (Herzberg, Mausner, & Snyderman, 1959) Motivation-Hy-

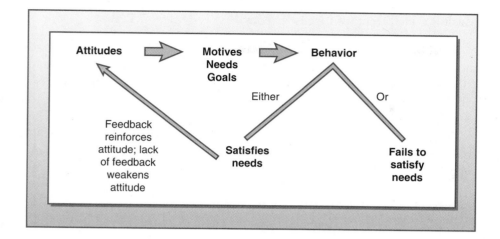

Figure 19.2
Relationship of attitudes, motives, and behavior. (Data from Schweiger [1980] and Steers & Porter [1987].)

giene theory, and McClelland's (1961; 1976) Need for Achievement theory. Some theorists have focused on specific human drives deemed to be important. Some examples are the achievement motive, the affiliation motive, the need for equity, the need for activity and exploration, the need for competence, and the self-actualization motive (Lawler, 1973).

Going beyond a description of needs is a group of motivation theories that use a cognitive premise as their base. The cognitive theories assume that individuals reason, think, and consider the consequences of their behavior. Thus the focus is on the thought and evaluative processes individuals use in participating and performing in the workplace. These theories examine the attractiveness of outcomes to individuals and are categorized as expectancy theories. Expectancy, equity, and goal-setting theories are included, although goal-setting has been viewed primarily as a technique rather than a theory. Vroom's (1964) Expectancy theory is a major example of the cognitive theories (Lawler, 1973; Steers & Porter, 1987). As applied to working in organizations, theories of motivation are discussed in connection with job satisfaction. Herzberg's theory is an example. Job satisfaction is an internal subjective state related to an affective reaction to motivated job behavior. Job satisfaction is related to organizational outcomes such as absenteeism and turnover, which are costly to organizations and influence their effectiveness (Lawler, 1973; Price & Mueller, 1981). Motivation as applied to the work environment also is the focus of Hackman and Oldham's (1979) Job Characteristics theory. Finally, McGregor's (1960) Theory X and Theory Y is discussed with motivation. Not truly a theory of human motivation, McGregor's X-Y theory is well known. It describes managerial attitudes toward employees and is more specific to assumptions about what motivates people to work. Several major motivation theories will be explained in greater detail.

Maslow's Hierarchy of Needs Theory

Maslow (1954) arrayed human needs along a hierarchy from most basic to most sophisticated. This can be thought of as stair steps or forming a pyramid (see Fig. 19.3). At the bottom or base are the most basic needs, the *physiological* drives for food, sleep, clothing, and shelter. These needs are usually associated with the survival needs for which humans seek to acquire money. The majority of an individual's activity will be at this level until the needs are fulfilled sufficiently to sustain the body. When physiological needs are fulfilled, other levels of needs emerge and dominate.

The second level is *safety and security* needs. These are needs to be free of the fear of physical harm and deprivation of basic physiological needs. Employee benefit plans are aimed at security needs. The third level is *belonging* needs that relate to needs for affiliation and love. These are social needs. In nursing, work group social support and cohesion meet some belonging needs. The next level up is *esteem and ego* needs. These are needs to achieve independence, respect, and recognition from others. Satisfaction of esteem needs results in prestige, self-confidence, power, and a feeling of usefulness. Recognition is an important motivator in nursing. The highest level of the hierarchy of needs, at the apex, is *self-actualization* needs. These relate to the need to maximize potential and achieve a sense of personal fulfillment, competence, and accomplishment. This need is individual and internal. In Maslow's theoretical framework, needs at the lower levels have to be fulfilled before those at a higher level can emerge and have energy devoted to them (Grant, 1994; Hersey & Blanchard, 1993; Maslow, 1954). Maslow's theory applies to people in general and is not specific to work or organizational behavior.

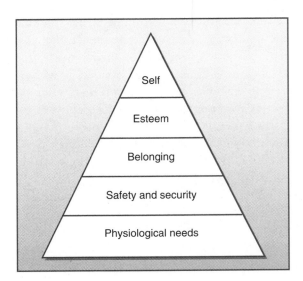

Figure 19.3
Maslow's hierarchy of human needs. (Data from Maslow [1954].)

Alderfer (1969) modified Maslow's (1954) work by collapsing the five hierarchical levels into three sets of needs: existence needs, relatedness needs, and growth needs. Existence needs would be those human needs specific to sustaining life. Maslow's physiological and safety/security needs would be included in existence needs. Relatedness needs would be needs for meaningful interpersonal relationships, similar to Maslow's belonging needs. Growth needs would be the needs for self-esteem and self-actualization, similar to Maslow's self-actualization needs. Alderfer's (1969) model has been called the ERG theory. The acronym stands for existence, relatedness, and growth needs. The ERG theory added the dimension of a frustration-regression process that occurs when higher level needs are continually frustrated. This theory also suggested that more than one need could be operating at any one time (Steers & Porter, 1987).

Herzberg's Motivation-Hygiene Theory

Herzberg (Herzberg, Mausner, & Snyderman, 1959) applied Maslow's general theory of motivation specifically to work motivation. Herzberg's Motivation-Hygiene, or Two-Factor, theory proposed that there are two different categories of needs that are independent and affect behavior in different ways: hygienes and motivators (see Fig. 19.4). The hygiene or maintenance factors are security, status, money, working conditions, interpersonal relations, supervision, and policies and administration. The hygienes are related to the environment and conditions of the job. They are not growth-producing motivators for employees, they only prevent lost productivity due to job dissatisfaction. The motivators seem to be effective in motivating toward superior performance and positively affecting job satisfaction. The motivators

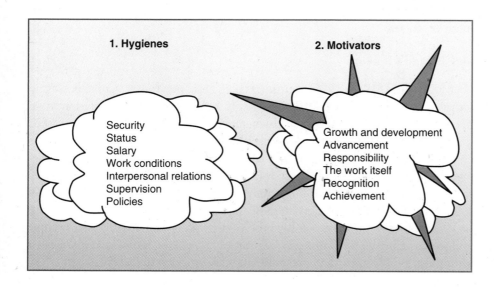

Figure 19.4
Herzberg's factors. (Data from Herzberg, Mausner, & Snyderman [1959].)

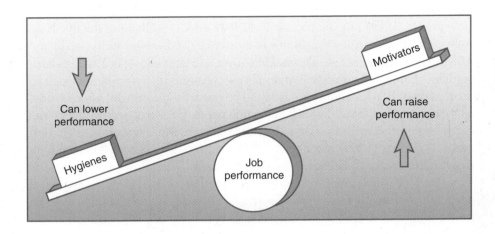

Figure 19.5
Herzberg's Two-Factor theory. (Data from Herzberg, Mausner, & Snyderman [1959].)

are related to the job itself. They are growth and development, advancement, increased responsibility for work, challenging work, recognition, and achievement (Hersey & Blanchard, 1993; Herzberg, Mausner, & Snyderman, 1959).

Work motivation was seen as composed of job satisfaction and dissatisfaction. Satisfaction is not a continuum of satisfaction on one end and dissatisfaction on the other. Rather, satisfaction and dissatisfaction were seen as two independent continuua: (1) no satisfaction to high satisfaction and (2) no dissatisfaction to high dissatisfaction. Compared to Maslow, the hygiene factors are essentially equivalent to Maslow's lower level factors, whereas the motivators are higher level factors (see Fig. 19.5). In other words, there needs to be enough of the hygienes so that the employee is not dissatisfied. Enough of the motivators need to be present to be personally rewarding. Herzberg's framework has been popular as a conceptual basis for job satisfaction studies in nursing. His theory seems to make sense as applied to the work environment of nurses.

McClelland's Theory

McClelland (1961; 1976) identified three basic needs that people possess in varying degrees (see Chart 19.2). Each person tends to have one predominant need. The needs are the need for achievement, the need for power, and the need for affiliation. The *need for achievement* means the strong desire to overcome challenges, to excel, to advance or succeed, and to grow. The need for achievement can be identified and assessed. Individuals with a high need for achievement set moderately difficult but achievable goals and like to take personal responsibility for finding solutions to problems. Included is a need for competence, or a strong desire to make a contribution or to produce some visible outcome and to do quality work. Those who exhibit high need for achievement are eager for responsibility, take calculated risks, and desire concrete feedback.

CHART 19.2
⌒ DEFINITIONS

Need for Achievement
the strong desire to overcome challenges, to excel, to advance or succeed, and to grow.

Need for Power
the need to be in control and to get others to behave contrary to what they would naturally do.

Need for Affiliation
the desire to work in a pleasant environment, and the desire for friendly, close relationships.

Data from McClelland (1961 and 1976).

The *need for power* means the need to be in control and to get others to behave contrary to what they would naturally do. Power is a drive to influence people and situations. People with a pure need for power need to control other people and the environment around them. They desire to make an impact, be influential, be in charge, and gain personal influence and prestige more than they desire productivity.

The *need for affiliation* is the desire to work in a pleasant environment, and the desire for friendly, close relationships. Affiliation is a drive to relate to people. People high on the need for affiliation seek out meaningful friendships, want to be respected and liked, avoid decisions that oppose the group, and are more interested in high morale than productivity (Hersey & Duldt, 1989; Steers & Porter, 1987; Veninga, 1982).

McClelland and Boyatzis (1982) studied individuals with long tenure in management positions and found a "leadership motive pattern" that enabled effectiveness at higher levels of an organization. The complexion of features of a leadership motive pattern are moderately high levels of the need for power and low needs for affiliation, with high levels of self-control. Absent is the need for achievement motive, which was associated with managerial success at lower management levels in non-technical areas (Henderson, 1993). Thus theories of needs motivation have been related to leadership and management by investigating which characteristics or combinations of characteristics can be used to predict job "fit" or success. Henderson (1993) found that nurse managers' and nurse executives' profiles did not fit the profile of successful managers described by McClelland and Boyatzis (1982). Specifically, about a third of respondents showed no power motive preference. There may be a variety of explanations for this, such as differences in industry versus service sector, female role socialization, the position of nurse executives in the hierarchy, individual characteristics of age or education, or the type, complexity, or culture of the setting. Measurement tools may not be precise or setting-specific enough to detect relationships. Thus theories and measures need to be evaluated as data are gathered for decision making and prediction.

McClelland's (1961; 1976) framework can be used for self-assessment and to assess and influence another person. Self-assessment is analyzing which of these types most represents an individual. Then others in the environment can be evaluated for their highest need motivation. Communication is enhanced and conflicts diminished as effective strategies are employed to meet individuals' needs. People are motivated by different needs, and understanding the basic types helps nurses to learn to work with a diversity of personalities in actual work situations. The idea is to match the individual's need structure to the assignment in the organization. To plant individuals in a place where they will grow is a key to productivity and success.

Expectancy Theories

Cognitive theories have been constructed into models about the thought processes individuals have as they engage in conscious behavior at work. Lewin (1935) described behavior as a function of characteristics in both the person and the environment. Thus motivation can be influenced by the nature of the individual and by the policies and practices of the organization. Lewin (1935) introduced the concept of valence, defined as the attractiveness of an outcome. Later theories introduced the concept of expectancy, defined as the likelihood that an action will lead to a certain outcome. The general expectancy theory framework views behavior as determined by the multiplication of valence with expectancy.

Vroom's (1964) VIE theory is the most well-known expectancy theory and is the one applied to work settings. VIE stands for valence-instrumentality-expectancy. Instrumentality is a belief about the probability that behavior will lead to other second-level outcomes. All three VIE variables are beliefs held by individuals related to what they expect will happen. Vroom (1964) postulated that behavior results from conscious choices among alternatives. The choice behaviors are related to perception and the formation of attitudes and beliefs. Humans naturally choose to maximize pleasure and minimize pain. The combinations of VIE, which Vroom represented symbolically by mathematical equations, interact to create a motivational force for action. What this means is that in the context of work, individuals will pursue the level of performance that they believe will maximize their overall best interest (Steers & Porter, 1987).

Vroom's (1964) VIE theory was refined by Porter and Lawler (1968). Porter and Lawler (1968) found that employee effort was determined jointly by two factors: the individual's assessment of the value of certain outcomes and the degree to which there is a belief that the person's effort will lead to the attainment of valued rewards. Both beliefs must be in place for further effort to be elicited. However, there is a distinction between actions and outcomes that indicates that effort may not result in job performance. Further, performance and satisfaction may or may not be related, depending upon a variety of factors (Lawler, 1973; Steers & Porter, 1987).

Nurses attempting to use VIE theory try to structure rewards on an individualized basis. However, it is difficult to assess the actual needs of employees, so their values and attitudes are assessed as a proxy. Managers work to assign personnel to jobs for which they are capable of performing. For example, nurses would operationalize this theory when delegating to unlicensed assistive personnel. Nurses' latitude of freedom may be constrained in organizations by policies and procedures, precedents, or union contracts (Steers & Porter, 1987).

Other Theories of Work Motivation

There have been a variety of ways of conceptualizing work motivation. For example, goal-setting theories like Management by Objectives (MBO), job enrichment, and organizational behavior modification theories encourage goal-setting in their implementation phases. The idea is that employee behavior is purposeful and goal directed. Conscious choice is involved in purposeful actions. Therefore, organizations need to motivate employees to direct activity toward organizational aims through voluntarily chosen purposeful actions. While needs and values are fundamental to motivation, goal setting helps to motivate employee performance since goals regulate human actions and can be influenced by managers (Steers & Porter, 1987).

Positive reinforcement and social learning theories are reinforcement-based motivational approaches. Skinner (1953) and Pavlov (1902) contributed to the understanding of conditioned and unconditioned or reflex behaviors and the stimulus-response-consequences linkage. Operant conditioning theories are less favored because the concepts of reinforcement and extinction leave out the element of conscious, rational thought (Steers & Porter, 1987). Some nurses may object to ethical issues related to the deliberate use by managers of strategies that rely on positive and negative reinforcers. However, there are circumstances in organizations where the use of behavior modification techniques provide a useful problem solving strategy for nurses managing and coordinating client care. For example, disruptive behavior in meetings, such as constantly interrupting others, may need to be handled in this manner.

In general, motivation theories have provided insight into what stimulates behavior. When applied to work behavior, the theories provide an understanding of both rewards and incentives and principles that can be applied by leaders and managers to motivate employees toward greater productivity and job satisfaction.

Job Characteristics Theory

Expanding on Herzberg's work, Hackman and Oldham's (1979) Job Characteristics theory examined more specifically the design of a job and the fit to an individual, as linked with outcomes. Five core job dimensions were identified. They are skill variety, task identity, task significance, autonomy, and feedback. Through the proper balance of the five core job dimensions, three critical psychological states occur: experiencing the meaningfulness of the work, experiencing responsibility for the outcomes of work, and knowing the actual results of work activity. These critical psychological states set up the conditions for positive personal work outcomes of high internal work motivation, high quality work performance, high satisfaction with the work, and low absenteeism and turnover. The individual's personal growth needs and the employee's satisfaction with the work context, or hygiene factors like pay and job security, moderate the core job dimensions' influence on outcomes. Guidelines for job design interventions and the development of research instruments such as the Job Diagnostic Survey are important features of this theory. Research in nursing has indicated high skill variety, task identity, and task significance, with low autonomy and feedback are features of nursing practice (Kirsch, 1988).

McGregor's Theory X and Theory Y

A manager's philosophy about people, attitudes, and assumptions play a role in his or her choice of motivational strategies. The assumptions about the nature of people that Theory X managers bring to the workplace are based on a belief that people who work for an employer are lazy. Theory X managers assume that employees dislike responsibility, prefer to be directed, resist change, and want safety. But at least employees are rational in that they can be motivated. The accompanying belief is that people are motivated by money and the threat of punishment. Thus, if the workers are lazy, management must be active. Managers need to impose structure and control and closely supervise employees, since external control is necessary to deal with unreliable, irresponsible, and immature workers. This view of human nature and motivation is called Theory X (Hersey & Blanchard, 1993; McGregor, 1960).

Challenging the conventional Theory X view of the day, McGregor (1960) proposed Theory Y (see Chart 19.3). In a democratic society, the Theory X view of human nature and the managerial practices based on it may not be correct and appropriate. Thus management approaches based on Theory X may fail to motivate individuals toward organizational goals. Theory Y assumes that people are not lazy and unreliable by nature, but rather people can be self-directed and creative if properly motivated to unleash their potential (Hersey & Blanchard, 1993).

Theory Y acknowledges that the behavior of people is complex. Under certain conditions people will accept responsibility; they are not necessarily passive; and creativity exists in all levels of the organization. Theory Y managers truly believe that motivation can be unlocked by creating and fostering an environment that is motivating. They view this as their job as a manager. They think people do like to work, can be self-directed, and will accept responsibility given an environment in which to grow, accomplish, and feel a sense of self-esteem and autonomy. McGregor's (1960) Theory X–Theory Y is not so much a motivation theory as it is a theory about managers' beliefs that then translate into the ways they choose to motivate their employees.

Motivation in Organizations

Industrial efficiency experts have been interested in determining what mix of physical conditions, work hours, and work methods are ideal to stimulate maximum productive output by workers. Unlocking the secrets of the motivation to work and the relationship between motivation and productivity has been a universal management concern.

CHART 19.3
∿ MANAGERIAL ASSUMPTIONS

Theory X
People:
- dislike work
- need control and force to make them work
- like to be directed
- lack ambition

Theory Y
People:
- like to work
- can be self-disciplined for objectives they are committed to
- will accept responsibility

Data from McGregor (1960).

In 1924, a famous experiment that came to be known as the Hawthorne studies was conducted at the Hawthorne plant of Western Electric, outside of Chicago. A team of researchers went into the plant to find out what motivated people. The purpose of the study was to test the effect of working conditions, to include lighting and pay, on productivity.

The researchers had reliable data on the production line, and they knew exactly how long it took a worker to wire a telephone. The regular production line was used as a control. For the experiments, the researchers pulled five workers off the assembly line and put them in a room, creating a mock production line so that the researchers could control and manipulate variables. The first variable was light. When more lights were added, production went up. Other variables included scheduled rest periods, company lunches, and shorter work weeks. After introduction of each variable, production went up. To test the strength of association of working conditions and productivity, all the innovations were suddenly withdrawn. Surprisingly, production went up to a new all-time high. All the researchers were able to conclude was that changes in physical working conditions alone had nothing to do with productivity. It must have been something else: specifically, productivity must be tied to the human aspects, such as the attention lavished on the workers. At this point, the research was refocused and employee interviews were conducted to explore the human relations aspects.

The Hawthorne studies resulted in a new awareness about the need to study and understand human interpersonal relationships at work. The most significant factor affecting organizational productivity was job-related interpersonal relationships, not just pay or working conditions. When informal groups identified with management and the workers felt competent, productivity increased. Further, the findings pointed to involving workers in the planning, organizing, and controlling of their own work as a way to secure workers' positive cooperation. Out of the Hawthorne studies came the phrases the "Hawthorne effect," to refer to attention paid to employees, and the "informal organization," to denote the web of interpersonal relationships beyond management control (Hersey & Blanchard, 1993). Insights gained from the Hawthorne experiments began the Human Relations era of management theory. Clearly, the behavior of people is complex. Therefore, motivation is not a simplistic matter. The motivation of human beings is not reducible to a formula as simple as "people are motivated by money." While motivating aspects can be identified and prioritized by nurses, no simple program automatically will produce motivation in nurses.

Motivation in Nursing

Motivation is a critical and recurring problem for both leadership and management. Porter O'Grady (1986, p. 39) said, "All workers expect to be rewarded consistent with their roles, responsibilities, the demands of their jobs, and their productivity... workers are looking for some evidence of fairness and appropriateness in the application of recognition of their performance." Rewards come in two basic categories: (1) *personal or professional,* such as recognition, acknowledgment, autonomy, personal esteem, and status and (2) *economic,* such as compensation via a paycheck. Employee recognition is a critical component of motivation. The research indicates that women tend to value recognition/esteem as well as pay. It is possible that men in nursing rank rewards differently than women in nursing.

Both compensation and professional recognition are rewards for service provided and are viewed as powerful motivators. Thus organizations that employ nurses can and do use both compensation and recognition as strategic methods to attract and retain nurses. Compensation clearly is an important personnel management strategy. Three levels of administrative reward strategies have been identified: (1) temporal, short-term, noncontinuing or time limited mechanisms, (2) structural features based on the recognition of professional achievements through on-going or longer term compensation, and (3) self-motivating mechanisms that more comprehensively reward the individual for meeting organizational goals. An example of a temporal reward is funding to attend a conference. An example of a structural reward is clinical ladders. An example of a self-motivating reward is profit sharing or gain sharing (Havens & Mills, 1992).

Personal and Professional Rewards

Managers need to recognize their employees' job contribution and performance. Each employee has unique skills and a unique job and some degree of initiative, creativity, enthusiasm, and skill that the leader needs to recognize in the job performance. But there also needs to be personal recognition such as recognizing the employee as a unique individual with a distinct personality. It is human nature to dislike being treated like a number or a cog on an assembly line. Recognition is a fundamental and universal need. Thus motivation goes beyond strictly the job and moves also into the relationship aspect of personal recognition from others.

It seems that there is never enough recognition. However, for recognition to be effective, it must be for an act of merit and be commensurate with the achievement. Yet even recognition for little victories can be a powerful motivation to more widespread participation in an organization, because the recognition induces further action. The leader's role is to recognize that what people need from work is to be liberated and motivated to be involved, accountable, and reaching for potential. The three steps to accomplishing this are ensure preparation, remove unnecessary and demeaning barriers, and recognize achievement (Peters, 1986).

Motivating and Mentoring

The success of the management team is achieved through experienced, creative and motivated leaders. The organizational environment must encourage participation and provide opportunities for staff to contribute their knowledge and expertise. Developing nurses for eventual positions in management begins at the staff nurse level from the moment of entry into the profession. Existing Nurse Managers must foster the management and leadership potential identified in the staff nurse and facilitate their exposure to the management process.

As a Nurse Manager with 15 years of experience in a university/teaching hospital, one of my most important roles is the development of future leaders and managers. I have been successful in this role by utilizing a process that begins at the time that I hire a nurse for a staff position on the unit. Staff nurses must possess leadership and management skills necessary to effectively manage and implement patient care. This level of skill is assessed and developed to the next level, the charge nurse role, where management and leadership duties of resource utilization, care coordination, and problem identification and resolution are tested. The nurse's ability to function in the charge nurse role is developed by a mentoring experience with the assistant nurse managers of the unit. These nurses are more experienced in the day to day operations of the area and lend their wisdom and strategies for effective problem solving. As developing charge nurses, they receive ongoing support and evaluation by the management team to enable growth in organizational and clinical skills, decision making, and interdisciplinary coordination of care. Other staff on the unit (secretary, ancillary services, and the physicians) are also excellent resources to assist the new charge nurse.

The overall culture and activity level of the unit plays a role in the transition process from novice to expert. The more challenging problems often may require senior management involvement initially to assist the charge nurse; however, this experience will greatly contribute to her or his development. Providing these opportunities for development of staff is an important part of the motivation process. Encouraging them to take the lead on special projects and committees is a method to stimulate interest and allow them to achieve the reward of a successful project. It is imperative to facilitate the scheduling of these committees or projects at convenient times for the nurses to attend and to provide replacement coverage for them on the unit.

Effective delegation and support to assistant nurse managers prepares them to assume future promotional positions in management. Providing opportunities for exposure to other departments in the organization enhances their scope of knowledge. I have found the most rewarding experiences have occurred when the assistant nurse managers provide management coverage for the unit in my scheduled absence. Debriefing with them on strategies and effectiveness of problem resolution has enabled them to gain high levels of expertise in the responsibilities of the position. Performing this role in an acting position has motivated them to continue to develop their skills.

Allowing prescheduled management times for completion of project activities also enhances the success of the projects. As the manager of the unit, I strive to maintain a culture of flexibility, maturity, and sensitivity in addition to maintaining a realistic approach to priority setting in order to foster the development of new charge nurses and assistant managers.

The following are examples of opportunities or experiences that I have provided to my staff to motivate them to contribute and participate on the management team:

• Assume responsibilities for leading and coordinating staff meetings

- Coordinate the unit's volunteer program, including orientation, hiring, scheduling, and evaluating volunteers
- Represent the unit on hospital committees and task forces
- Develop unit orientation programs for nursing staff and physicians
- Provide support for their attendance at continuing education opportunities and seminars relating to management

- Participate in the development of unit's goals and objectives, budget and capital expenditure process, and strategic initiatives

It is also important that as the manager I am viewed as approachable, caring, and supportive in my commitment to developing new leaders. There is a need to maintain a sense of humor, since the high acuity and rapid pace patient care environment is hectic and often stressful for staff. It is critical that a trusting and nurturing relationship be embraced to support and allow development, creativity, and risk taking. All these aspects encourage participation and are essential tools to maintain a motivated, creative, and experienced management team.

MARGARET SANDVIG, RN, BSN
Nurse Manager
University of Washington, Harborview
    Medical Center
Seattle, Washington

The extent to which staff feel their needs for self-esteem have been met has become important for motivation. Thus managerial displays of recognition and appreciation have a powerful motivating effect (Davidhizar, 1992). Research has shown that 92% of staff nurses ranked recognition as important to job satisfaction, yet 28% perceived that recognition was seldom or never given. The most meaningful forms of recognition are verbal feedback from the nurse manager, letter of praise, organizational award or honor, a promotion, being personally thanked during an evaluation, and a monetary bonus (Goode et al., 1993). Further analysis revealed five general types of recognition: private verbal feedback, written acknowledgment, public acknowledgment, opportunities for growth and participation, and compensation. Since recognition is important for nurse job satisfaction and retention, these types of recognition formed the basis for a management intervention protocol to provide recognition (Goode & Blegen, 1993).

The core of what motivates nurses to nurse often is the love of the work itself. This is illustrated by "Nurse . . . or Scarlet Pimpernel," one of the *AJN* reflections endpieces (Golder, 1989). The author compares herself to the literary figure the Scarlet Pimpernel (Golder, 1989, p. 154): "My cover is critical care nursing and I, too, save lives—by night, in a large metropolitan hospital." She noted that this society is impressed with entertainers, sports figures, and money handlers, whereas nurses help without acknowledgment. Clearly, the nature of the work of nursing offers a sense of competence and reward from caring for and helping others. In one survey, nurses were asked what was most important in their work as a nurse. The most important elements in order of priority were providing quality client care, caring about clients' best interests, being treated as a professional, adequate staffing, and a safe working environment (American Nurse, 1991).

Economic Rewards

The new healthcare paradigm is one of a seamless organization where the customer receives quality service from empowered employees who make decisions based on individual circumstances and desired outcomes. As hospitals move to implement self-directed teams and cross-functional workers, re-designed work, and restructured relationships, old reward structures do not fit or work as well as they did in the past. For example, compensation and pay practices, which are key to employee rewards and incentives, need to be ad-justed. Some new pay systems are base, variable, and indirect pay (see Chart 19.4). Base pay is salary for meeting non-negotiable job expectations. Variable pay includes gain sharing, bonuses, and incentive pay. Indirect pay includes benefits such as health insurance and vacation pay. Variable pay is not added to the base and thus helps control wage costs yet rewards individuals inter-mittently. Indirect pay costs can be controlled to shift resources into variable pay. Some may perceive a loss with new pay structures; others see the incen-tive of increased earning capacity with variable pay plans (del Bueno, 1993; Shuster & Zingheim, 1992). Although clearly a trend in hospitals, new pay initiatives have produced some failures when not carefully designed and im-plemented. Some label them merely a fad, while others predict they will grow in popularity and importance (Pagoaga & Williams, 1993).

Conventional wisdom in personnel management has been that wages with regular increases, benefit plans, and job security helped to motivate staff. However, employees began to view these motivators as entitlements. Follow-ing Herzberg's theory (Herzberg, Mausner, & Snyderman, 1959) nurse man-agers would need to carefully analyze compensation for its actual motivational and satisfaction effects. Pay is a hygiene, not a motivator. However, some as-pects of pay can strongly influence behavior. For example, some people count on overtime pay to supplement their income. As healthcare organizations slash overtime pay, nurses may perceive dissatisfaction. Further, demotivation may occur in team structures if an individual is highly rewarded for what the team produced. Under conditions of constrained resources, nurse managers may have little flexibility to use compensation as a strategic reward and moti-vational tool.

> **CHART 19.4**
> ∾ DEFINITIONS
>
> **Base Pay**
> salary for meeting nonnegotiable job expectations.
>
> **Variable Pay**
> includes gain sharing, bonuses, and incentive pay.
>
> **Indirect Pay**
> includes benefits such as health insurance and vacation pay.
>
> Data from del Bueno (1993) and Schuster and Zingheim (1992).

RESEARCH NOTE

Source: Goodell, T., & Coeling, H. (1994). Outcomes of nurses' job satisfaction. *Journal of Nursing Administration, 24*(11), 36-41.

Purpose

The purpose of this research was to review the research and theory base for evidence of the effects of job satisfaction on turnover, quality of care, and patient satisfaction and to report the results of a pilot study to explore these outcomes in one urban midwestern teaching hospital. Theories of motivation and job satisfaction were reviewed, including Taylor, Hawthorne experiments, Maslow, and Herzberg. Turnover literature from Lucas, McCloskey, and Tumulty were discussed. Quality of care and patient satisfaction literature were reviewed. The pilot study investigated the relationships among nurses' job satisfaction, quality of care, and patient satisfaction and identified the elements most important to nurses' job satisfaction. A stratified random sample yielded 150 usable questionnaires.

Discussion

The pilot study was unable to demonstrate any significant relationships among job satisfaction and the outcomes of quality of care and patient satisfaction. The study was limited by single institution and low-moderate response rate. There was a significant difference between high and low quality of care units on the professional status subscale of the Index of Work Satisfaction. The elements of job satisfaction were ranked in order of greatest importance by this sample of nurses as pay, professional status, autonomy, interaction, task requirements, and organizational policies.

Application to Practice

Evidence of a relationship between nurses' job satisfaction and the presumed outcome benefits from it was not demonstrated in this study. There may be many reasons for this. Perhaps there is no relationship, or the relationship may not be detectable given this design and sample. Perhaps nurses are professional enough to exclude job concerns from their delivery of care to clients. Perhaps job satisfaction in nursing is more important for outcomes not directly attributable to quality of care and client satisfaction. In order to make decisions about expensive motivation and job satisfaction programs, nurse leaders and managers need to carefully assess and consistently and individually measure variables associated with nurse satisfaction and resultant outcomes.

LEADERSHIP AND MANAGEMENT IMPLICATIONS

Just as communication is a fundamental and key aspect of leadership, so too is motivation. Leaders and managers exhibit behaviors related to motivation as a part of their role in influencing others. Leaders create a motivating climate. Managers use rewards and punishments to accomplish work through others. But what will motivate a nurse? Nurses can begin by exploring their own personal attitudes and knowledge about motivating themselves and others. For example, analyzing statements about motivation, even though they may not be the "best" descriptors, provides a basis for self-analysis and critical thinking.

To explore your personal attitudes about motivation, react to each statement in Chart 19.5 and defend your thinking. Reactions to the statements

---

CHART 19.5
∾ ATTITUDES ABOUT MOTIVATION

1. Nurses work best when money is the reward.
2. Most nurses' motivation is intrinsic or internal; therefore, the manager cannot do anything about it.
3. If nurses need feedback about how they are doing, they can ask their manager.
4. The annual performance appraisal is enough reinforcement.
5. It is uncomfortable to give praise.
6. Telling someone they are doing a good job removes their incentive to improve.

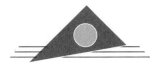

Leadership & Management Behaviors

LEADERSHIP BEHAVIORS	**MANAGEMENT BEHAVIORS**	**OVERLAP AREAS**
• enables others through high expectations	• plans motivating rewards	• motivates others
• recognizes contributions	• links rewards to performance	• provides opportunities for need satisfaction
• celebrates accomplishments	• directs others to achieve organizational goals	
• creates social support networks	• evaluates effectiveness of motivation strategies	
• fosters collaboration	• motivates subordinates	
• communicates an inspiring vision	• provides opportunities for subordinates to achieve	
• motivates followers	• provides valued rewards	
• sets an example of high motivation		
• provides opportunities for growth and development		

provide a basis for discussion and exploration of an individual's beliefs and attitudes regarding motivation.

Motivation is complex. Some people are motivated to achieve in ways that coincide with the goals of the organization, while other individuals tend to pursue their own goals. The attitudes that people hold strongly influence their behavior. Managers often feel responsible when employees appear to lack job motivation. However, a manager's job is to create an environment that fosters employee commitment to the organization's goals, not drive an individual employee with a "big stick" to motivate them. Managers may not be able to directly motivate some employees. Leaders strive for creating a climate where employees choose to perform at high levels. People tend to cooperate more when their stress level is low, when their work level is not overwhelming, when they like the individual asking for help, when they believe it is mutually beneficial, when they expect something in return, when they do not have a tightly defined job description, and when they truly believe that people are employed to serve people (Lancaster, 1985).

Motivation is related to the way individuals feel they are treated as persons. Is the manager able to convey trust? Is the manager able to convey a sense of personal recognition and job recognition? To structure an environment of achievement, the manager can take specific action to enact the following elements (Lancaster, 1985):

- explicit goals
- clear expectations
- feedback and reinforcement
- eliminate threats
- individual responsibility
- rewards
- trust

Developing techniques of motivation unlocks effectiveness. Friss (1989) suggested that leaders and managers incorporate the following principles in their motivational efforts: use rewards over punishment, use both social group processes and formal reward systems to influence behavior, tailor rewards to the individual, and give feedback frequently and consistently.

The leader and manager needs to consider all potential effects when planning a motivator. For example, some nursing organizations give a recognition reward such as a pin or button. Consider how those in a group would feel who did *not* get a pin. Then consider how those in the group would feel who *did* get a pin. Those not receiving a pin might feel disappointed or that the group's leader did not acknowledge their contribution to the group. Giving rewards creates a double-edged sword. Some employees appear embarrassed. It is possible that the reward may not meet their needs, and thus it would not be motivating. Some become hostile if they feel they deserved a reward but did not get one. Animosity may build.

Motivation and rewards are serious components of nursing. Working with nurses to help make them feel good about the work they do has a direct impact on keeping them motivated. The goal is to keep nurses in nursing and working productively over a career in the profession, despite recurrent cycles of shortage and surplus of jobs. At a personal level, each nurse needs to increase self-awareness about what is a motivator. At a group level, nurses can use research knowledge to assess and implement motivational strategies within each work group. For the profession of nursing, motivational theories combined with a knowledge of job satisfaction in nursing help leaders envision a preferred future that nurtures nurse professionals and ensures their availability to the pubic.

CURRENT ISSUES AND TRENDS

Is there some way to make nurses' work environments motivating and rewarding? Nursing's problem is to strive as a group for the motivators needed to attract and keep people interested in being a nurse. Nurses' work environments do not always nourish novices and satisfy established career people. Through research, nursing needs to identify what nurses need and then to set about deliberately structuring environments so that nurses can succeed, be satisfied, and feel that what they do is an important service to clients. One current trend is for nurses to celebrate heroine or hero stories and promote exemplars in nursing. In New York State, for example, the legislature began a program to honor "Nurses of Distinction." In 1989, eight nurses in the state of New York were identified as nursing role models and recognized as a "Nurse of Distinction" (AJN News, 1989). For each work environment, nurses should examine positive communications and the way that rewards are structured for individuals and for nursing as a profession. Having fulfilled, rewarded, and encouraged career professional nurses is a vital work environment outcome in healthcare.

Grainger (1993) offered some tips for structuring personal motivation. She suggested that personal feelings or perceptions are influenced by the way an individual might "frame" responsibilities. Thus "reframing" is under an individual's control and may be used as an internal motivator to get things accomplished. For example, examine the ever-present "to do" list. This can be restructured into three columns: the must do, the should do, and the get to do. Using "get to do" terminology may improve attitudes, perceptions, and motivation.

Motivation generates less attention in nursing during a poor economic climate or when employing institutions are laying off or downsizing RN positions. It may be that it is assumed that fear of losing a job will adequately motivate RNs during such periods. However, motivation receives greater attention during cycles of nurse shortage, when employers need to attract and retain RNs. In reality, motivation and the motivation to work should be considered important environmental and contextual variables that are consistently assessed, tracked, and evaluated. The clues provided by these data help to strengthen both leadership and management of nurses, nursing, and client care management.

SUMMARY

- Motivation is important in a service industry such as nursing.
- Motivation and human relations variables are important for productivity.
- Motivation is a state of mind in which a person views goals.
- Motivation is a process of activating human behavior.
- Motivation to work is the willingness to work.
- Motivation is a process of felt need, behavior, goal attainment/blockage, frustration, and cycle repetition.
- Motivation can be either internal or external.
- There are many theories of motivation.
- Maslow described a hierarchy of five levels of needs.
- Alderfer collapsed Maslow into three levels.

- Herzberg applied Maslow to work motivation.
- Herzberg identified hygiene and motivator factors related to satisfaction and dissatisfaction.
- McClelland identified three basic needs.
- Vroom represents the cognitive motivational theories.
- Hackman and Oldham explored the design of a job and its fit to an individual in their Job Characteristics theory.
- McGregor differentiated managers' attitudes into Theory X and Theory Y.
- The Hawthorne experiments highlighted the importance of human interaction factors in work motivation.
- Personal and economic rewards are powerful motivators in nursing.
- The core of what motivates nurses is the work itself.
- Motivation is complex.
- The manager's job is to create an environment that fosters motivated behavior.

Study Questions

1. How do you stay motivated to love nursing for the rest of your life?
2. Does loving nursing guarantee quality care?
3. What is the motivation to enter nursing as a career?
4. What is the comparison of real-world nursing practice to what motivation theories say?
5. What positive incentives are most important to nurses? To you personally?
6. What are the elements of a motivating environment?
7. Is it manipulative or Machiavellian to deliberately plan and implement rewards and incentives to get other people to perform?
8. Under cost containment pressures, what is the effect on nurses of relying on recognition as the organizational motivation strategy?

Critical Thinking Exercise

Nurse Lisa Gardner has worked at St. Anywhere's for 35 years, ever since she graduated from their former diploma program. She knows everyone and the chronological unfolding of the hospital's history. She has been the "graveyard shift" house supervisor for 25 years. Recently, a new chief nurse executive (CNE) took over with a pledge to "restructure" and "reengineer" the nursing department. The CNE has been deluged with persistent complaints that Nurse Gardner comes in late, goes home early, and has her pager turned off for long periods.

1. What is the problem?

2. Why is it a problem?

3. What should the CNE do about the problem?

4. What factors should the CNE consider before taking any action?

5. What needs motivate Nurse Gardner?

6. What needs motivate the CNE?

7. What motivational strategy(s) might be useful to the CNE? To Nurse Gardner?

REFERENCES

AJN News. (1989). New York state legislature votes for 8 "nurses of distinction" and honors them as role models. *American Journal of Nursing, 89*(10), 1362, 1384-1385.

Alderfer, C. (1969). A new theory of human needs. *Organizational Behavior and Human Performance, 4,* 142-175.

American Nurse (1991). Quality patient care tops list of what is important to nurses. *The American Nurse, 23*(8), 2.

Davidhizar, R. (1992). The path of least (staff) resistance. *American Journal of Nursing, 92*(12), 56-60.

del Bueno, D. (1993). Reflections on retention, recognition, and rewards. *Journal of Nursing Administration, 23*(10), 6-7, 41.

Friss, L. (1989). *Strategic management of nurses: A policy-oriented approach.* Owings Mills, MD: National Health Publishing.

Golder, D. (1989). Nurse . . . or Scarlet Pimpernel? *American Journal of Nursing, 89*(1), 154.

Goode, C., & Blegen, M. (1993). Development and evaluation of a research-based management intervention: A recognition protocol. *Journal of Nursing Administration, 23*(4), 61-66.

Goode, C., Ibarra, V., Blegen, M., Anderson-Bruner, J., Boshart-Yoder, T., Cram, E., Finn, L., Mills, R., & Winter, C. (1993). What kind of recognition do staff nurses want? *American Journal of Nursing, 93*(5), 64-68.

Grainger, R. (1993). Motivating ourselves. *American Journal of Nursing, 93*(5), 16.

Grant, A. (1994). *The professional nurse: Issues and actions.* Springhouse, PA: Springhouse.

Hackman, J., & Oldham, G. (1979). *Work redesign.* Reading, MA: Addison-Wesley.

Havens, D., & Mills, M. (1992). Professional recognition and compensation for staff RNs: 1990 and 1995. *Nursing Economic$, 10*(1), 15-20.

Henderson, M. (1993). Measuring managerial motivation: The power management inventory. *Journal of Nursing Measurement, 1*(1), 67-80.

Hersey, P., & Blanchard, K. (1993). *Management of organizational behavior: Utilizing human resources* (6th ed). Englewood Cliffs, NJ: Prentice-Hall.

Hersey, P., & Duldt, B. (1989). *Situational leadership in nursing.* Norwalk, CT: Appleton & Lange.

Herzberg, F., Mausner, B., & Snyderman, B. (1959). *The motivation to work.* New York: John Wiley & Sons.

Kirsch, J. (1988). *The middle manager & the nursing organization: Human resources, fiscal resources.* Norwalk, CT: Appleton & Lange.

Lancaster, J. (1985). Creating a climate for excellence. *Journal of Nursing Administration, 15*(1), 16-19.

Lawler, III, E. (1973). *Motivation in work organizations.* Monterey, CA: Brooks/Cole Publishing.

Lewin, K. (1935). *A dynamic theory of personality.* New York: McGraw-Hill.

Maslow, A. (1954). *Motivation and personality.* New York: Harper & Row.

McClelland, D. (1961). *The achieving society.* Princeton, NJ: Van Nostrand.

McClelland, D. (1976). Power is the great motivation. *Harvard Business Review, 54*(2), 100-110.

McClelland, D., & Boyatzis, R. (1982). Leadership motive patterns and long-term success in management. *Journal of Applied Psychology, 67,* 737-743.

McGregor, D. (1960). *The human side of enterprise.* New York: McGraw-Hill.

Pagoaga, J., & Williams, J. (1993). Dynamic pay initiatives. *Hospitals & Health Networks, 67*(17), 22-29.

Pavlov, I. (1902). *The work of the digestive glands* (translated by W. Thompson). London: Charles Griffin.

Peters, T. (1986, May 25). Employee recognition, no matter how slight, pays dividends. *The Cedar Rapids Gazette,* p. 3E.

Porter-O'Grady, T. (1986). *Creative nursing administration.* Rockville, MD: Aspen.

Porter, L., & Lawler, E. (1968). *Managerial attitudes and performance.* Homewood, IL: Dorsey Press.

Price, J., & Mueller, C. (1981). *Professional turnover: The case of nurses.* New York: Spectrum.

Price, J., & Mueller, C. (1986). *Handbook of organizational measurement.* Marshfield, MA: Pitman.

Schuster, J., & Zingheim, P. (1992). *The new pay.* New York: Lexington Books.

Schweiger, J. (1980). *The nurse as manager.* New York: John Wiley & Sons.

Skinner, B. (1953). *Science and human behavior.* New York: Macmillan.

Steers, R., & Porter, L. (1987). *Motivation and work behavior* (4th ed.). New York: McGraw-Hill.

Veninga, R. (1982). *The human side of health administration: A guide for hospital, nursing, and public health administrators.* Englewood Cliffs, NJ: Prentice-Hall.

Vroom, V. (1964). *Work and motivation.* New York: John Wiley & Sons.

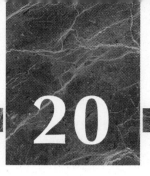

20

Power

Chapter Objectives

∾

define and describe power

∾

explain the psychological aspects of power

∾

distinguish between personal and professional power

∾

compare eight mechanisms of power expression

∾

define and discuss the five sources of power from French and Raven

∾

explain three other sources of power

∾

analyze power in organizations

∾

compare the types of power nurses have

∾

relate empowerment to organizations

∾

exercise critical thinking to conceptualize and analyze
possible solutions to a practical experience incident

*P*ower is an underlying dynamic or force in organizations, in interpersonal relations, and in all aspects of human endeavor. When viewed as a human phenomenon, power is something that happens in interpersonal moments. Power is one variable in interpersonal communication (Farley, 1987). Power can be viewed simply and directly as the ability to get others to do what we want done. Influencing others is the first step in using power. However, exerting influence over other people is really not a simple matter. In a psychological sense, power is really freedom. Power gives control over our daily lives and our personal environment. We all have power in one form or another and participate in the power around us, which takes shape in a variety of forms, such as in words and symbols.

DEFINITION

here is no total agreement about the definition of power, but generally power is the broader concept under which authority and influence are subsumed. Power connotes strength and ability. Power has different meanings: it can mean the ability to compel obedience, control, or dominate, or it can be a delegated right or privilege as occurs in the power to enact the staff nurse role. *Power* is defined as the capability of acting or producing some sort of an effect, usually associated with the ability to influence the allocation of scarce resources (Grant, 1994) (see Chart 20.1). Power also is defined as the production by some persons of intended effects on others (Price & Mueller, 1986). Other definitions identify power as the potential capacity to exert influence, characteristically backed by a means to coerce compliance.

In physics, power is defined both as the work accomplished per unit of time and as the potential for doing work. Thus power carries a connotation of being both actual and potential (Blalock, 1989). However, the use of power in nursing is as a phenomenon of interpersonal relationships. Power is a central factor in interpersonal communication. Interpersonal communication has two components: content and relationship. Power is most often found operating within the relationship component (Farley, 1987). Bennis and Nanus (1985, p. 15) called power the "basic energy to initiate and sustain action translating intention into reality." Transformative leadership would be the wise use of power. The following points clarify the definition of power (Price & Mueller, 1986):

- Basic to the definition of power is that power produces an effect or effects.
- Intended effects, either ideas or behaviors, are stressed, but actual behaviors are more typically examined.
- Force may or may not be involved.
- Face-to-face interaction may or may not be involved.
- Power is not a finite or fixed amount, indicating that for one person to gain power another does not have to give up power.

Empowerment is a corollary concept to power in groups and organizations. *Empowerment* is defined as giving individuals the authority, responsibility, and freedom to act on what they know and instilling in them belief and confidence in their own ability to achieve and succeed (Kramer & Schmalenberg, 1990) (see Chapter 4). Thus, empowerment has two meanings: the transfer of actual power and the inspiring of self-confidence. Both aspects enable others to act. Empowerment is a key leadership component.

BACKGROUND

Power is the ability to exert influence over others either by persuasion or coercion. Part of the definition of leadership is influencing other people, therefore, leadership and power are intimately intertwined. The two definitions overlap and are not mutually exclusive. Power is influence potential or the resource that enables a leader to gain both compliance and commitment from others (Hersey & Blanchard, 1993). Power also is central to concepts of autonomy and centralization. When using power, a decision is made about an approach or power strategy.

Understanding and analyzing power is a beginning strategy for knowing how to use power for positive and constructive ends. There may be a tendency to perceive power as bad or negative. However, those people who openly desire power are not necessarily power-mad or self-centered. Power is not by definition negative. Power appears to have two values attached: negative and positive. The key differentiation is that positive power exerts influence on behalf of others rather than over others (Veninga, 1982). People appear to have various orientations or attitudes toward power. The understanding and valuing of power may determine how an individual uses available power sources. Heineken and McCloskey (1985) identified six attitudes toward power (see Chart 20.2). Thus a person who believes power is good would likely use reward, expertise, and legitimate sources; the resource dependent individual would likely rely on information power; and the person who believes power is political would likely use connection sources. Skills known to facilitate power use are interpersonal skills, group communication skills, and skills in negotiation, assertiveness, and conflict resolution.

Every time power is used, people are involved in one way or another. The corollary to power is sensitivity. Being sensitive to the impact that power has on other people means there is a choice to make: if using power creates harm or hurt, we have to decide whether or not to use it (Schmidt-Posner & Schmidt, 1979).

There are some very basic human concerns involved in the interpersonal quest for power. Alone, people sometimes feel powerless. When individuals come together to pursue common goals, they begin to feel some sense of power. When aligned with others who share the same values or goals, power is attained by being a member of the group. If power is not an absolute, finite, or fixed commodity, then power can be shared, delegated, or joined together with other people's power (Schmidt-Posner & Schmidt, 1979).

CHART 20.2
✺ ATTITUDES
TOWARD POWER

Power is:
- good
- resource dependent
- an instinctive drive
- charisma
- political
- control and autonomy

Data from Heineken and McCloskey (1985).

Pleasure, love, acceptance of ideas, the respect and esteem of other people, and money all play a part in the desire for power. Psychologists view the search for power as a drive toward self-affirmation, self-assertion, and growth. Sometimes a desire for power develops as a reaction to anxiety or insecurity. Some people only can feel powerful by dominating and controlling others. Those individuals whose desire for power is based on normal drives draw from their own inner strengths. Possessing a need for achievement, they have the self-confidence to seek positions of authority. They strive to create a positive feeling about themselves so that others will join them in doing the things they want done (Schmidt-Posner & Schmidt, 1979).

The Two Forms of Power

Power takes two forms: personal power and professional power (Hamilton & Kiefer, 1986) (see Chart 20.3). McClelland (1975; 1976) viewed power as an important human need. Early work on power viewed power as the major goal of all human activity (Adler, 1930). The need for power or dominance is important for understanding organizational behavior (Steers & Porter, 1987). In managers, McClelland (1976) described two forms of power: personal power and institutionalized power. In this conceptualization, personal power-oriented individuals seek dominance for the sake of dominance and conquest. They are personal empire builders but reject loyalty to the institution. Institutionalized power-oriented individuals sacrifice their own self-interest for the good of the organization, feel a responsibility to build up the organization, and have a strong sense of fairness and justice. Employees with high needs for power tend to be superior performers, and managers with a high need for institutionalized power tend to be managing work groups that are more productive and satisfied (Steers & Porter, 1987). In nursing, these two forms of power are described as personal power and professional power.

Personal or individual power consists of the extent to which people believe that they can influence events through personal effort. This means knowing who they are, where they are going, what they want to accomplish, as well as packaging themselves as persons with power and being adaptable. There is a difference between personal power and arrogance. Arrogance is a blindness to weaknesses, a false sense of one's own power, and a belief that people will follow them no matter what. In a given situation, personal power is the ability to assess the situation in a managerial and a political sense and discern the degrees of decision freedom and the chances of being successful given any specific power strategy or leadership style. Personal power is the belief that a person can do something. Personal power also has been described as the extent to which followers respect, are committed to, and are willing to follow a leader (Hersey & Blanchard, 1993).

CHART 20.3
～ DEFINITIONS

Personal Power
the extent to which a person believes that he or she can influence events through personal effort.

Professional Power
the use of professional expertise and competence, embedded within an organization milieu, to make change or make a contribution.

Data from Hamilton and Kiefer (1986).

The other aspect is professional power. *Professional power* relates to getting the rewards from doing a job, acquiring expertise, being liked, and having charisma. It is the use of professional expertise and competence, embedded within an organizational milieu, to make change, do something good for clients, advance the profession, or make a contribution. Professional power and personal power can blend to make a package of leadership skills.

Power Mechanisms

Power is expressed through eight mechanisms (see Fig. 20.1). These mechanisms are strategies adopted to influence others to do what is desired by the power strategist. First is assertiveness. *Assertiveness* means expressing one's own position to another without inhibiting the rights of others. *Ingratiation* is trying to make the other person feel important: giving praise or sympathizing. Ingratiation is trying to make yourself look good by trying to make another person feel important. *Rationality* means using logical and rational arguments, providing pertinent information, presenting reasons, and laying an idea out in a logical, structured way. *Sanctions* are the use of threats. Positive sanctions, or rewards, are addressed within motivation mechanisms. *Exchange* means that in order to persuade, an exchange is offered, sometimes called "scratching each other's back." *Upward appeal* means appealing to a higher authority: the childhood threat of "if you don't play by my rules, I am going to go tell mom." Upward appeal simply means taking the appeal to a higher authority to arbitrate. *Blocking* means deliberately blocking others from getting their way, threatening to stop working with them, ignoring them, not being friendly, or simply attempting to make sure others cannot accomplish their aims. *Coalitions* are the result of a group of people getting together in order to speak or negotiate as one voice (Kipnis & Schmidt, 1980; Levenstein, 1982).

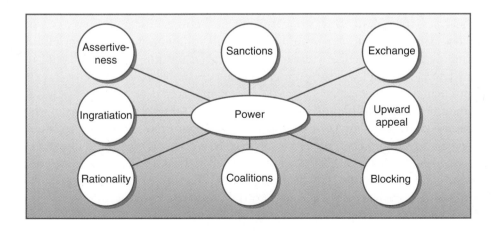

Figure 20.1
Expressive mechanisms of power. (Data from Kipnis & Schmidt [1980].)

CHART 20.4
❧ SOURCES OF
POWER

French and Raven's:
• Reward
• Coercive
• Expert
• Referent
• Legitimate

Others
• Connection
• Information
• Group decision
  making

Data from Hersey and Duldt
(1989), Liberatore et al. (1989),
French and Raven (1959), and
Raven and Kruglanski (1975).

Five Sources of Power

While at least eight mechanisms of power have been identified (see Fig. 20.1), the power base classification that is most widely accepted is French and Raven's (1959) five sources of power (see Chart 20.4). Their original conceptualization identified five power sources:

1. *Reward power* is giving something of value. For example, in nursing rewards may be a pay raise, praise, a promotion, or a day shift job. Reward power is based on the ability to deliver desired rewards.

2. *Coercive power* is force against the will. For example, in nursing coercive power can be the threat of firing, of disciplinary action, or other negative consequences. Coercive power is the power derived from an ability to threaten punishment and deliver penalties. It is a source of power used to apply pressure so that others will meet our demands.

3. *Expert power* means the use of expertise. It is knowledge, competence, communication, and personal power all combined in a reservoir of knowledge and experience. Expert power is a source of power held by those with some special knowledge, skill, or competence in a particular area. For example, the nurse with the greatest expertise in wound dressings will be sought out by other people in the work environment for this expertise. Expertise is an artful combination of skill and knowledge. It may be founded on depth of knowledge and/or psychomotor skill. In the use of knowledge and skill is power: because people need you or can benefit from your expertise, power exists. Therefore, the use of expertise can be structured to accomplish or influence movement or action toward certain goals.

4. *Referent power* is a little more difficult to understand because it is subtle. It is the use of charisma to influence others. The followers of someone with referent power respond positively to the interpersonal communication and image of the charismatic person. In organizations, this translates into an informal leadership based on liking, charisma, or personal power. Referent power comes from the affinity other people have for someone. They admire the personal qualities, style, or the dedication brought to the work. Referent power can be viewed as an inspiration power, because people's admiration for someone allows him or her to influence without having to offer rewards or threaten punishments. For example, in the political arena, occasionally there are charismatic political figures or orators. Their influence comes from their followers' liking or identification with them. An example in nursing is Florence Nightingale, who became a symbol of professional nursing. There is an emotional upsweep felt by associating with a charismatic person. Referent power is a personal liking and identification that is experienced by others. Followers attribute referent power to a leader on the basis of the leader's personal characteristics and interpersonal appeal. Physical attractiveness may contribute to referent power.

Creating Expert Power

A good manager is able to influence others, even if she or he doesn't manage personnel per se. To convince others of the need to do something, especially if that "something" is costly, inconvenient, time-consuming, or otherwise viewed negatively (or it may simply require a change from "the way we've always done it"), a manager must use persuasion skills effectively. Being viewed as an expert is critical.

Having worked in the field of hospital infection control for almost twenty years, I am frequently asked to share my knowledge with others. Approximately once a year, I present a day-long workshop on preventing and controlling infections in long-term care to nursing and administrative personnel from various long-term care settings. Many of the principles of infection control are the same in the acute and long-term care arenas, but nonetheless, I keep current with the literature in both. I teach long-term care personnel not only what is important for them to know, but also how to develop their own resources and networking opportunities.

The recent upsurge of tuberculosis in the U.S. required that health care workers become re-educated on the control measures that hospitals and other health care facilities must use to prevent transmission of tuberculosis and monitor the incidence of disease. I spend an hour and a half on these issues in the long-term care course. I discuss how old ways of thinking have changed and discover that sometimes even older, experienced nurses have a hard time understanding the reasoning behind conclusions and thought processes. But to effect change and/or influence others, one *must* understand the underlying principles and rationale of policies and practices.

This became very apparent to me approximately two weeks after I had taught the course when I received a phone call from a course participant. She had recently been assigned the role of infection control nurse in a nursing home and was telling her administrator that employees with a positive PPD skin test no longer needed to have annual chest x-rays (a practice that actually should have been discontinued years before). When her administrator asked her why, she quoted me as the expert—the teacher of the course she just took had said so. Beyond that, she couldn't explain the rationale.

She called me when it was apparent she wasn't able to change the administrator's thinking, and asked me to send her my opinion in writing. I told this nurse that her inability to influence her administrator was because she had not established any power base from which to make decisions and recommend changes. She had not yet developed her status as a credible, knowledgable, reliable, or competent expert. My opinion would likely not influence the administrator either. Why should her administrator be influenced by someone that either he knows nothing about (that is, me) or that hasn't demonstrated any expertise in the subject (that is, her)?

It was apparent that *she* needed to *be the expert*. While a nursing manager may not have any legitimate or explicit power within her workplace environment, convincing others that she can be trusted to make the appropriate decisions within her circle of expertise can create the needed expert image and thus give her inferred or presumed power. People will believe she has power and thus be much more likely to be influenced by her.

I warned her that this generally occurs with time and a thirst for knowledge that is quenched regularly. Reading relevant literature and networking with others who seem to have the power that she needs are steps to achieving the ability to use power effectively in influencing others. I suggested that she explore other ways to have her competence formally recognized by education or certification.

You need to be the expert in your facility—not some nurse from the big hospital down the street who has been around a long time—but *you.*

SANDY PIRWITZ, RN, BSN, MS, CIC
Nurse Epidemiologist and Manager of
    Infection Control
Cleveland Clinic Foundation
Cleveland, Ohio

5. *Legitimate power* means position power. It is the right to command within the organizational structure, based on the hierarchical position held. The President of the United States has power because of holding the position. Legitimate power is the most common source of power. It is what most often is called authority. Legitimate power comes from the role or position held. The authority of position gives the right to act, order, and direct others. However, leadership and influence need not be confined to those with authority. Every person possesses the ability to tap different sources of power to use in a variety of situations.

Other Sources of Power

Raven and Kruglanski (1975) and Hersey and Goldsmith (Hersey & Duldt, 1989) identified two more sources of power: connection power and information power. A third type of power has been identified (Liberatore et al., 1989): group decision making power. These three other sources of power are related to groups and organizations specifically, as opposed to French and Raven's (1959) original five sources of power that relate more to any individual.

Within organizations, the power of connections comes from networking or knowing people and from being able to go across lines laterally to gather information. For example, this occurs when a nurse knows a colleague in another hospital with whom to exchange information. For a nurse to know what effective nursing interventions are being used by other institutions helps the institution to be competitive and current. *Connection power* is one strategy to get information accurately and reliably. It also may be manifested as power based on having connections with powerful others.

Information is power. If it is given away, its power may be lost. This is especially true in situations that require negotiation. If information is used strategically, its possession can be a strong source of power. *Information power* is a source of power that can stem from any person in the organization and is based on possessing special information of value to others. Kanter's (1979) research suggested that control of resources, especially information, is a major organizational power source.

Another source of power is derived from *group decision making*. This means that there is a creative synergy and force that is created when a group comes together, makes decisions, and acts as a united front. For example, some professional groups have formed strong lobbies to influence state and national legislation. With over 2 million licensed registered nurses in the U.S., group decision making with resultant unity of action could be a powerful strategy for nurses to use to advance the group's goals.

Power and Leadership

Power and leadership are closely connected and highly intertwined concepts. This is because power is one of the vehicles by which a leader influences followers to take action. Nurses may be inclined to avoid an acknowledgement or analysis of power. However, to lead and manage, nurses need to acquire, possess, and use power.

Hersey and Blanchard (1993) described the relationships among concepts of style of leadership, readiness level of followers, and power base use. They indicated that the readiness of the followers dictates which leadership style is likely to be successful and which power base would most successfully influence followers' behavior. Combining these concepts maximizes the leader's probability of success. Thus nurses should be able to use Situational Leadership Theory (see Chapter 4) to assess and predict style choice and power source use based on the situation and readiness of followers.

Readiness is the ability and willingness of individuals or groups to take responsibility for directing their own behavior in a situation. There appears to be a direct relationship between the level of readiness in individuals and groups and the power base type that has a high probability of effectiveness for use with them (see Fig. 20.2). Readiness is a task-specific concept. At the lowest level of readiness, coercive power is most appropriate. As people move to

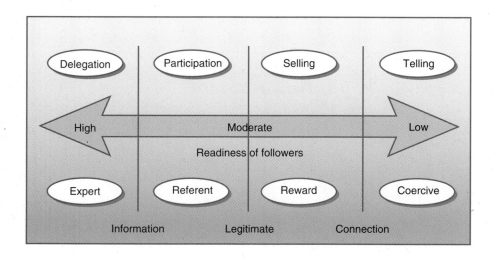

Figure 20.2
Power related to leadership. (Data from Hersey & Blanchard [1993].)

higher readiness levels, connection power, then reward, then legitimate, then referent, then information, and finally, expert power impact the behavior of people. At the highest level the followers have competence and confidence, and they are most responsive to expert power (Hersey & Blanchard, 1993).

If power is the basic energy needed to initiate and sustain action, then power is a quality without which a leader cannot lead. Power is fundamental to leadership, in that leadership may be the wise use of power. This is especially true for transformative leadership (Bennis & Nanus, 1985). Power need is highly desirable in leaders and managers. This is because power is necessary in influencing others. Assertiveness and self-confidence are associated with power and leadership. Leadership may be characterized as power in the service of others (Kouzes & Posner, 1987). For nurses, this may mean that they need to view power as an integral part of their professional roles in care management and client advocacy. Nursing leadership requires a willingness and ability to take on a power role and to expand the use of power bases.

Power in Organizations

In organizations, authority is the formal application of power; influence is the more subtle or informal aspect of power. Power, authority, and influence are intimately connected with and become the fulcrum for any change in behavior from the status quo to a new status (see Fig. 20.3). Change is difficult to bring about, especially in organizations. This is because individuals and groups resist changes that would upset their equilibrium or disadvantage them. Thus power, authority, and influence become the levers needed to energize a change and are applicable to the implementation of any organizational innovation. Change is highly threatening to human beings. Power is used to energize action despite threat and resistance (see Chapter 26).

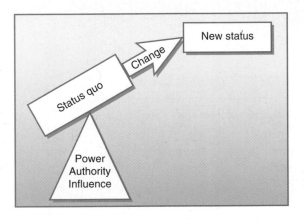

Figure 20.3
Power and change.

French and Raven (1959) identified five general sources of power for any individual. Power in organizations is slightly different because of the effect of multiple players or actors in the environment and the intersection of individual goals with organizational goals. Four different sources of power in organizations can be identified: first, *structural position,* or position power and authority; second, *personal characteristics,* or the group culture, values, and interpersonal mix; third, *expertise;* and fourth, *opportunity.*

Structural sources of power have been used to explain power in organizations. Three main structural sources of power in organizations have been identified as (Hoelzel, 1989):

- *Centrality:* being central to the major function of the organization and interconnected with its major systems
- *Control of uncertainty:* influencing organizational goal attainment by being able to cope with the organization's uncertain environment
- *Control over resources:* accessing and controlling human resources, information, and other critical organizational resources

Power factors pervade the organization and cut across all levels of the structure. Factors such as external control or regulation, individual employees' needs for power, favored fashion or trends, and organizational culture may modify the structure of an organization away from the structure that would be expected by the organization's profile of age, size, technical system, and environment (Mintzberg, 1983).

Power in organizations often is seen as the control over valuable resources. The amount of power accruing to an individual or group can be derived from two basic elements: the ability to perform important tasks or be central to solving the organization's critical problems, and the degree of discretion and visibility associated with the job, which influences the perception and reality of organizational power (Kouzes & Posner, 1987). What this means for nurses is that nurses can strengthen and empower each other by connecting to lines of information, resources, and support, working on critical organizational issues, acquiring and using discretion and autonomy, being visible, and providing recognition to nurses and nursing (Kanter, 1979; Kouzes & Posner, 1987).

Power and the effective management of organizations has been examined by two major theorists: Kanter (1977; 1979) and Kotter (1979; 1985). Kanter (1977; 1979) looked at power and opportunity as organizational structural elements affecting work effectiveness. Kotter (1985) examined power, dependence, and conflict in organizations.

Kanter's (1977; 1979) work has been called a structural theory of organizational behavior. Investigating organizational structure and its effect on employee attitudes and behaviors, she proposed that an individual's job effectiveness is influenced largely by organizational aspects of the work environment. Access to power and access to opportunity are the two structural determinants that affect work effectiveness. Those with access to power and opportunity feel empowered to contribute to the organization, participate more actively, and exhibit higher morale. Research on Kanter's theory with nurses has supported her proposed relationships (Wilson & Laschinger, 1994).

Access to power in Kanter's (1979) theory means access to support, information, resources, and the ability to mobilize these three elements from one's position in order to meet organizational goals. Access to opportunity involves providing opportunities for advancement, growth, rewards, and recognition. An individual's job effectiveness, attitudes of investment or commitment, and participation behaviors are affected by power and opportunity access. Access to power and opportunity helps employees feel empowered to contribute to the organization. Powerless jobs are often characterized by being routine, low in visibility, and removed from the core mission of the organization. Powerless employees develop behaviors that may be counterproductive to the organization (Wilson & Laschinger, 1994).

Kotter's (1979; 1985) model explored the effective management of power in organizations. A key variable is job-related dependence. Dependence refers to the degree of being influenced by others and of needing others for assistance, information, time, approval, or other resources. When two or more individuals influence and depend on each other, they are interdependent. Because leadership and management are getting work done through others, dependency increases with increasing managerial or leadership responsibility. Power is pervasive and inevitable in organizations because of its being present in all relationships and because of job dependence (Nelson, 1989).

Kotter's (1985) model explained that interdependent relationships in organizations were related to the potential for conflict. This partially is because of competition over scarce resources. Power becomes a mechanism used to resolve conflict. The effective use of power to manage conflict results in creativity, innovation, enthusiasm, and adaptiveness. The ineffective use of power to manage conflict results in power struggles, infighting, decreased efficiency, and alienated staff.

Dependence can be managed through the use of structural or position power and by developing skill in effectively engaging in "power dynamics," or the acquisition and exchange of power. Managers and leaders may want to eliminate unnecessary dependency and establish counterforce power over others. Power shifts back and forth among members of an organization and is distributed by processes of negotiation. Power in organizations can be acquired and maintained by gaining direct control over resources, controlling information, gaining access to key decision makers, cultivating favorable relationships, and controlling the impressions held by others (Nelson, 1989). Kotter's (1979; 1985) model provides insight into the interrelationships of dependence, conflict, and power in interpersonal relationships in organizations.

RESEARCH NOTE

Source: Wilson, B., & Laschinger, H. (1994). Staff nurse perception of job empowerment and organizational commitment: A test of Kanter's theory of structural power in organizations. *Journal of Nursing Administration, 24*(45), 39-47.

Purpose

The purpose of this research was to test Kanter's structural theory of organizational behavior in a nursing population. The research explored the relationship between the power and opportunity perceptions of 92 staff nurses and their commitment to the organization. Kanter's proposition that employees' perceptions of their immediate manager's power in the organization would be related to their perceptions of job empowerment also was tested. Subjects were selected randomly from six units of one large metropolitan teaching hospital and given a survey questionnaire. Data were collected on the Organizational Description Questionnaire, the Organizational Commitment Questionnaire, the Conditions for Work Effectiveness Questionnaire, and on demographics. The theoretical framework for this study was Kanter's theory, which proposed that an individual's work effectiveness is influenced largely by power and opportunity, two organizational structural determinants of the work environment.

Discussion

Of the nurses surveyed, two thirds worked in critical care areas. Nurses overall reported a belief that their environments possessed a moderate amount of empowering characteristics. Access to information was the least empowering aspect of nurses' environments. Subjects were moderately committed to the hospital organization. Nurses' overall feelings of empowerment were associated most highly with organizational commitment. Nurses' perceptions of job-related power and opportunity were significantly correlated with higher levels of perceived managerial power. Nurses' job-related empowerment scores were strongly positively correlated with the perception of empowering structural characteristics.

Application to Practice

Some nurses lack a perception of power. Kanter's theory indicated that access to power through support, information, and resources, as well as the ability to mobilize these power supplies, and access to opportunity through advancement, growth, and recognition affect the attitudes and effectiveness of employees' work behaviors. Whereas others have recommended assertiveness training to alleviate powerlessness caused by individual personal factors, Kanter argued for the impact of structural dimensions of the work environment on perceived powerlessness. Thus changing the work structures should increase job empowerment. Further, the strong relationship between empowerment and organizational commitment suggests that manipulating the work environment to increase perceived empowerment should influence nurses' commitment to the organization. It is useful to know what directions to take in developing strategies to improve nurses' work environments.

Effective Uses of Power in Nursing

Not all uses of power are successful. Many times a person comes into direct conflict with the power other people possess. These conflicts are called power moments. How a person acts when experiencing a power conflict is directly related to how they perceive the source, the nature, and the magnitude of other people's power. That perception then gives information on the strategies to use (Schmidt-Posner & Schmidt, 1979).

The various strategies adopted when a person is deliberately acting in power moments range from confrontational to cooperative. For example, *fight* is a strategy in which power is used to move against the power of another person. While it need not be physical, a fight strategy is a clear attempt to gain a power advantage. Confrontation is the hallmark of a fight strategy. *Negotiation* takes place when a mutual respect for another person's power causes the fight strategy to be abandoned and replaced with an attempt to resolve the situation. Negotiation recognizes that there may be areas where self interests converge. Therefore, each actor has some incentive to resolve the power issue. *Collaboration* takes place when an individual's power is joined with the power of others to attain common goals. Collaboration comes about because self interests converge (Schmidt-Posner & Schmidt, 1979). Thus the incentive to cooperate is the highest in a collaborative power strategy.

The effective exercise of power requires a goal or a commitment. People who capitalize on their power are typically goal driven. This means that they have a goal and the forward drive or momentum to get there. Effective power utilization requires a thorough analysis of the situation at hand and a willingness to take action, to assume power at the appropriate time. Sometimes power moments just pass by because of the fear of negative sanctions, such as losing a job. To capitalize on power bases, nurses need to see the potential of group identity and group action and to be willing to participate. Group power is diminished by an individual who feels he or she does not personally want to risk anything.

In truth, del Bueno (1987) said, nurses are never powerless. Individually, each nurse has at all times the power to reinforce image by way of dress and deportment, thus reinforcing or diminishing a positive image. For example, how do nurses introduce themselves to clients? Do they wear identification that indicates academic achievement? Nurses have power over perceptions. Burnout can be controlled to a great extent by individuals controlling their own perceptions, emotions, and reactions to events and by how they choose to handle stress.

Each nurse has the power to take a chance or a risk. Each nurse has the power to project enthusiasm, self-confidence, self-esteem, and qualities that influence others' behavior and perceptions. They have the power to conceal or reveal knowledge, feelings, opinions, and intentions. In everything done, whether it is living with another person, being part of a family, going to work every day, working in a group situation, or any of the many other activities of daily living, there is the power to obstruct or to assist, to change or not change, and to take action or remain silent. There is the power to label or praise. There is the power to withhold or confer status, give each other a positive stroke, acknowledge the good things, or simply dwell on the negative and perpetuate a negative attitude. Nurses have the power to reward or punish (del Bueno, 1987).

Perceptions and prestige are intimately related to power. For example, a perceptual image of competence enhances a power base of expertise. Part of power is having the perception of power, and part of it is the actuality of holding power. Power, lack of power, and empowerment are issues for nurses. For example, nursing has not had the esteem or prestige related to making a lot of money or being fully professional. Nurses' image is one of being concerned about service and caring. Nursing has not been identified with business prestige, yet today many nurse executives are having to fulfill the role of a business person as well as a caring professional person. Nurses need to use power sources and strategies. Concern about image may be seen as phoniness or as being deliberately structured in order to capitalize on a power base.

Nurses also derive power from the art and science of nursing practice. Power also comes from nurses being the health providers the public most respects and supports (Grayson, 1993). Benner (1984) identified six types of power exercised by nurses (see Chart 20.5). Benner's (1984) six types of nursing practice–derived power can be compared to French and Raven's (1959) five sources of power for individuals. Transformational and participative/affirmative nursing practice power types would be similar to referent power. Integrative, advocacy, healing, and problem solving types of power would be similar to expert power. French and Raven's (1959) legitimate, reward, and coercive power sources are more frequently applied to nurses as care managers than to nurses as care providers.

Individually, nurses can use power concepts to establish a power base and gain power in their work setting. For example, nurses can use information and expertise to construct powerful, persuasive arguments. Nurses can collect and analyze data that can be strategically used or controlled. Nurses can be visible and persistent in goal pursuit. Nurses can be creative and challenge the system to innovate. Nurses can use group power strategies such as networking, connecting, and collaborating to achieve professional goals.

The larger question for nursing is whether nurses will be supportive of each other as a group in nursing and capitalize on collective power in a positive, strategic, constructive way. Much depends on each individual's participation. As a group, to accumulate productive power and to capitalize on the productive power within the group, nurses need to have information, resources, and

---

CHART 20.5
⁓ POWER EXHIBITED BY NURSES IN CLIENT CARE

Transformational
the ability to assist clients to transform their self image.

Integrative
the ability to help clients return to normal lives.

Advocacy
the ability to remove obstacles.

Healing
the ability to create a healing climate and nurse-client relationship.

Participative/ Affirmative
the ability to draw strength from a caring interaction with a client.

Problem Solving
the ability through caring to be sensitive to cues and search for solutions to problems.

Data from Benner (1984).

support. Capturing information, resources, and support captures the power necessary to be highly productive (del Bueno, 1986).

RESEARCH NOTE

Source: Farley, M. (1987). Power orientations and communication style of managers and nonmanagers. *Research in Nursing & Health*, 10(3), 197-202.

Purpose

The purpose of this study was to compare orientations to power and communication styles of nurse managers to nonmanagers. The research also examined orientations to power and social style. The top nurse executive and a randomly selected staff nurse from each of 43 hospitals were surveyed for demographic data, power orientation, and social style. The Power Orientation Scale was given to assess the orientation to power on six dimensions of power as good, resource dependency, instinctive drive, political, charisma, and control and autonomy. The Social Style Profile measures social style in terms of perceived assertiveness, responsiveness, and versatility.

Discussion

Significant mean differences were found between nurse executives and staff nurses on power as good, power as political, and power as control and autonomy. Nurse executives were perceived as more assertive than staff nurses. Overall, nurse executives exhibited stronger and more positive orientations to power as good. Seeing power as good means that power is viewed as challenging and desirable. High scores for nurse executives on power as political and as control and autonomy indicate an awareness of the need to use political tactics and a valuing of power as a means of establishing control. There was a lack of difference between executive and staff nurses in their orientation to power as resource dependency.

Application to Practice

Little research has been done on the concept of power and how it is used and viewed by nurses. In this study, nurse executives held more positive orientations to power as good, political, and control and autonomy. Nurse executives were perceived to communicate more assertively than staff nurses. Power orientation and social style may influence communication behavior and the inclination to use power. Nurses need to become comfortable with power and its acquisition and use in organizations.

LEADERSHIP AND MANAGEMENT IMPLICATIONS

Leaders are power brokers on behalf of their followers (Kouzes & Posner, 1987). All people have the opportunity to exert leadership. Personal and situational sources of power vary among individuals and may be used for leader-

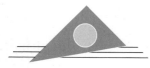 *Leadership & Management Behaviors*

LEADERSHIP BEHAVIORS	**MANAGEMENT BEHAVIORS**	**OVERLAP AREAS**
• empowers followers	• uses power to obtain resources	• uses power to achieve goals
• encourages the acquiring and use of power to accomplish group goals	• manages power and conflict moments	• uses power sources
• models the constructive use of power	• negotiates from a power base	
• mentors and supports others	• uses information strategically	
• builds connections	• gives rewards and punishments	
• enables group decision making	• exercises legitimate authority to accomplish work	
• is visible and relates to others		
• demonstrates expertise		

ship as unique situations call forth leadership behavior. Positive leadership involves empowering followers to accomplish group goals in a style that encourages them to maintain their self-esteem. Power is one of the means by which a leader influences the behavior of the followers (Hersey & Blanchard, 1993). Effective leaders and managers are aware of those factors that are relevant to their own behavior and analyze them for their impact on the use of power. Power extends into negotiation and delegation. Both negotiation and delegation are key leadership and management activities. They are tools to use in conjunction with the force of power in order to accomplish goals.

Nurses are involved in leadership and the use of power. For example, because nurses advocate for clients as a part of the staff nurse role, they have to be able to use power sources in order to influence other people to listen when changes in the client's condition occur.

A key issue in power relates to perception: power is not so much based on the reality of some absolute amount of power as it is based on the followers' perception of that power. People must perceive a leader as having power, but also as willing and able to use it. Using multiple power bases avoids the erosion of power. Leaders need to gain and exercise power. They must consciously try to build the trust and respect of coworkers. Leaders also need to develop influence with a large number of people as a way of dealing with contextual power beyond the immediate work group (Hersey & Blanchard, 1993).

In nursing, leadership is needed because of cost containment, quality concerns, and a rapidly changing turbulent environment in which new programs integrate care across healthcare settings. Decisions about what will yield high quality nursing care and be most cost effective must be addressed. If nurses allocate those decisions to physicians, hospital and health administrators, legislators who pass laws, third-party payors, or regulators such as the Joint Commission on the Accreditation of Healthcare Organizations (JCAHO), then nurses have given away a large section of the role for which they are legally and morally accountable.

How do nurses influence people? One mechanism is through power and empowerment. Another strategy is to develop and use the information power of nursing research. Without research, nurses have no data to show that they are cost effective. Healthcare payors overlook payment for the care nurses render partially because nurses have not demonstrated through research and uniform database comparisons nursing's impact on client outcomes such as cost and quality. For example, research has demonstrated that in hospital intensive care units (ICUs) there is a reduced mortality with a higher ratio of RN staff (Hartz et al., 1989). If physicians and nurses collaborate in ICUs, better client outcomes result. Nurses need to use this information in power strategies. For nursing the issue is how to influence health policy and to use power to advocate for clients.

Opportunity is an area of power in organizations that nurses have not been encouraged to analyze and develop. Opportunity includes the control of information by way of informal networking and connection power within the organization. How the stress points in organizations are handled leads nurses into real power and politics. Nursing as an occupation has relied on power that predominantly comes from the more formal sources and has not fully capitalized on other opportunities or sources. However, this may be changing as healthcare reform drives a revision of the system and as nursing matures as a profession. As organizations realize that nurses are absolutely critical to quality control and cost control because they are key people with the information that is needed for decisions, the bases and sources of power used by nurses for effectiveness may change. The following political strategies have been advocated by del Bueno (1986) for nurses to get or keep power:

- forming coalitions
- bargaining or trade-offs
- lobbying
- posturing or bluffing
- increasing visibility

Forming coalitions would develop connection power. Bargaining would involve the use of reward power. Lobbying employs a combination of information, connection, and reward sources of power. Coercive power would be involved in posturing or bluffing. Increasing visibility is a strategy to capture the effects of referent power.

CURRENT ISSUES AND TRENDS

Nurses who become expert in an area of practice may find their expertise involves them in the broader arena of healthcare issues. This may derive from the nurse's role as a client advocate and as the coordinator and manager of care. Because of their involvement in client care situations, nurses can and do become interested in larger public policy and social issues. They may seek and use power to influence professional issues, ethical issues, or national health policy.

An example of a professional power issue is whether nurses should be granted full professional autonomy. The related economic and regulatory policy issue is the right for nurse practitioners to be able to prescribe and to obtain direct third-party reimbursement. Professional autonomy implies that practitioners need to have the power to practice according to the standards of their discipline. Issues of job autonomy include whether nurses have control over working conditions. The power sought in organizations is the freedom to do the kinds of things that nurses need to do to advance the health of the public and to serve their clients. An example is nurses' work assignments. There is a controversy over whether or not nurses have the legal and the ethical responsibility to protest a work assignment considered to be inappropriate. For example, neither an obstetric nurse who is sent to work in an intensive care unit nor an intensive care nurse pulled to obstetrics is prepared for the very specialized aspects of these environments without cross-training. The cliché that "a nurse is a nurse is a nurse" has been disavowed by nurses, yet organizations shift nurses around to match the workload. This practice is exacerbated during a nursing shortage or a fiscal crisis. The concern is, to what extent do nurses have the power to determine how nursing care is practiced and delivered in organizations? At one time, the concerns about how nurses were assigned and how the skill and staff mix was structured generated a power issue about whether nurses had the right to close hospital beds. This for a time was advocated as a power strategy to encourage organizations to pay attention to the need for adequate staffing to take care of the client load. Currently, there are sporadic reports of increased unionization efforts within nursing practice in response to downsizing and staff mix issues.

Empowerment

The contemporary power issue in nursing is *empowerment,* or developing a structure and environment in which people have a strong sense of self and are motivated to excel. Empowerment combines the meanings of transferring

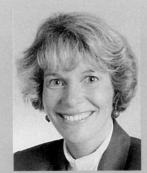

JoEllen Koerner

JoEllen Koerner Envisions Empowerment and Transformative Leadership

Executive nursing leadership involves self-expression, discovery, and reformulation of self and the world we lead. Rather than being one who objectively unravels a mystery, the caring leader sits at the loom and weaves a tapestry, while being woven into it. Through this act of mutuality we express what is within us as we reshape the world. In a reciprocal dance the world responds as we act, and both are co-created anew.

Transformative leadership emerges from an individual who is firmly planted in the rich, moist soil of strong management and leadership skills. Without it, the root system is shallow, making this leader vulnerable to being uprooted in times of turbulence. Other essential attributes needed for this leader to thrive, and not merely survive, in times of unprecedented change are the capacity to see, to hear, and to develop hardiness.

Visionary leaders see beyond themselves into a larger view of life. They stand in contact with the past and future simultaneously so the present becomes clearer and the future possible. These leaders plant seeds of possibility within the imagination of others, calling them to an enlarged version of themselves and their work. These leaders also see reality clearly without projecting their own expectations, fears, and desires onto the scene before them. Though not expecting perfection, they expect growth in self and others.

Leaders also move beyond their own small world to hear the broader needs and concerns of their constituency, nation, and universe. They hear what is in front of them—not only what is being said, but more importantly, the intent and intensity of the message. Through hearing and seeing, the leader can match unique talents and needs of the individual or group with experiences and resources that will nourish their growth and advance the work at hand.

A critical attribute of a visionary leader is the capacity of hardiness. This leader demonstrates flexibility and adaptability to survive in changing times. We must stop waiting for the world around us to be perfect in order to be happy and productive. Not what we have, but what we do with what we have determines the quality of life. Emotional maturity, essential for maintaining balance and equanimity in ambiguous times, comes when we accept the difficulty imposed upon us by others in life with patience, even temper, and persistence. Living in the moment with peaceful authenticity is the secret to a hardy and life-giving existence for self . . . and those we are privileged to serve.

JoEllen Koerner has served as Vice President of Patient Services at Sioux Valley Hospital in Sioux Falls, South Dakota, for the past 11 years. For her full biographical sketch see page 572.

power to others with a notion of enabling others to act. Transferring power to others might be accomplished by changing an organization's structure and locus of decision making. Decentralization and shared governance are examples of transferring power in organizations. Kouzes and Posner (1987) identified enabling others to act as one of the five fundamental practices of leaders who were able to accomplish extraordinary things. Exceptional leaders enable others to act because the support and assistance of others is needed to achieve success. Collaboration, team building, and empowerment are strategies to build coalitions of supporters. Empowering others makes others feel strong and capable and engenders commitment in followers. The theory is that individuals are more likely to use energy to produce exceptional results if they feel self-confident, strong, and empowered. Followers are strengthened by the leader sharing information and power and by increasing the followers' discretion and visibility (Kouzes & Posner, 1987).

There is power in the ability to problem solve and make decisions. Expert power is enhanced when nurses demonstrate the ability to better deliver care. Nurses need to help each other learn how to make decisions in a high-risk, high-stress, highly changing environment. For example, connection power can be tapped as nurses get to know their organizational leaders and serve on organizational committees. Mentoring also provides connection power and increased decision-making experiences.

Organizational power has been defined as the ability to get things done, to mobilize resources, and to meet goals. Empowerment is self-efficacy, or being free to have control over the conditions that make actions possible (Kanter, 1977). In nursing, this translates into the ability to get things done. Empowerment is a structural characteristic of the work environment. Strategies for empowerment include using analytical skills, engaging in change activities, strengthening collegiality, and extending mentorship (Gorman & Clark, 1986).

Power is enhanced in an environment that supports assertive communication, self-efficacy, and self-esteem. The willingness to take risks, a strong sense of self, the ability to make decisions, peer support, assertive communication, the vision to see problems and opportunities, and the ability to influence others all contribute to an empowering environment. This is an environment in which people feel they can do the important things for clients and for the profession of nursing rather than feeling that they are being hindered at every step. The lack of necessary support in the work environment creates an experience of powerlessness. Powerless positions demotivate workers, create powerless behaviors, increase dependence, and create frustration or panic. Self-empowerment needs to be coupled with an empowering work environment. Empowered behaviors include motivation, risk taking, achievement orientation, and high career aspiration. The concept of empowerment has been related to organizational effectiveness and group cohesiveness (Chandler, 1991).

Leadership and power are essential elements in an empowering environment. To structure an empowering environment, the power strategies employed might include:

- formation and development of alliances
- flexibility and maneuverability: not getting locked into a rigid position that obstructs the ability to adapt or change
- communication, access, and control of information
- compromise and negotiation skills
- negative timing or a withholding action, sometimes used to wait until a more opportune moment to share information
- confidence and decisiveness
- personal competence and initiative

Nursing can have a profound impact on healthcare if and only if nurses will work and speak out as a group. Power strategies can be used to promote nursing's agenda for cost-effective high-quality client care delivery.

SUMMARY

- Power is a basic element in human relations and organizational behavior.
- Power is freedom and control.
- Power is the capability to produce effects and allocate scarce resources.
- Power is the ability to exert influence over others by persuasion or coercion.
- Attitudes and values affect the use of power.
- Power is both personal and professional.
- There are eight mechanisms through which power is expressed.
- French and Raven identified five sources of power.
- Three other power sources are connection, information, and group decision making.
- Power in organizations relates to centrality, control of uncertainty, and control over resources.
- Perceptions and prestige are intertwined with power.
- Nurses derive power from nursing practice.
- Nurses can use a variety of sources of power and political strategies.
- Empowerment means developing a structure and environment where people are motivated to excel.

Study Questions

1. Pick a day in the past couple of weeks that you think of as average. Who were the people who had the most influence over you? Why were they influential?

2. Do you view power as positive or negative? Give examples.
3. Identify the kinds of power you use and the kinds of power others use on you.
4. What types of power are you most comfortable with? Which would you consider trying?
5. Think about yourself as acting with strength and power and feeling the most satisfied about it. What kinds of things would you be doing?
6. What happens in situations in which you feel powerless?
7. Does a lack of power affect the way that you feel about situations?
8. When you are trying to control a situation, what makes you feel comfortable or uncomfortable?
9. How can power principles be structured to advance nursing's professional goals?
10. What is the difference, if any, between power and manipulation?
11. How is organizational power used?

Critical Thinking Exercise

Hill 'N Dale Community Hospital has fallen on hard times. Although the surrounding community is supportive of this local hospital, the site for healthcare has shifted into the community. Multiple budget cuts have hit the hospital's departments. The nursing department first restructured and decentralized. Administrative layers were eliminated. Each nursing unit now does self-scheduling and budgeting. The hospital administration just announced that each department must cut its budget by 8%. The nurses were just told that the social work department will now provide coverage only Monday through Friday, 8 AM to 5 PM, and to turn in their pagers at other times to the central nursing office. The respiratory therapy department also announced that they will no longer do treatments. They will serve only as consultants and equipment purchasers. There is talk that housekeeping services also will be less available.

1. *What is the problem?*

2. *Why is it a problem?*

3. *Whose problem is it?*

4. *What factors do the nurses need to assess and analyze?*

5. *What should the nurses do?*

6. *What power aspects are operative in this situation?*

7. *What power strategies might be helpful to the nurses?*

REFERENCES

Adler, A. (1930). Individual psychology. Translated by S. Langer in C. Murchison (Ed.), *Psychologies of 1930* (pp. 398-399). Worchester, MA: Clark University Press.

Benner, P. (1984). *From novice to expert: Excellence and power in clinical nursing practice.* Menlo Park, CA: Addison-Wesley.

Bennis, W., & Nanus, B. (1985). *Leaders: The strategies for taking charge.* New York: Harper & Row.

Blalock, Jr., H. (1989). *Power and conflict: Toward a general theory.* Newbury Park, CA: Sage.

Chandler, G. (1991). Creating an environment to empower nurses. *Nursing Management, 22*(8), 20-23.

del Bueno, D. (1986). Power and politics in organizations. *Nursing Outlook, 34*(3), 124-128.

del Bueno, D. (1987). How well do you use power? *American Journal of Nursing, 87*(11), 1495-1498.

Farley, M. (1987). Power orientations and communication style of managers and nonmanagers. *Research in Nursing & Health, 10*(3), 197-202.

French, J., & Raven, B. (1959). The bases of social power. In D. Cartwright (Ed.), *Studies in social power* (pp. 150-167). Ann Arbor: University of Michigan, Institute for Social Research.

Gorman, S., & Clark, N. (1986). Power and effective nursing practice. *Nursing Outlook, 34*(3), 129-134.

Grant, A. (1994). *The professional nurse: Issues and actions.* Springhouse, PA: Springhouse.

Grayson, M. (1993). The power of nursing. *Hospitals, 67*(8), 10.

Hamilton, J., & Kiefer, M. (1986). *Survival skills for the new nurse.* Philadelphia: Lippincott.

Hartz, A., Krakauer, M., Kuhn, E., Young, M., Jacobsen, S., Gay, G., Muenz, L., Katzoff, M., Bailey, R., & Rimm, A. (1989). Hospital characteristics and mortality rates. *The New England Journal of Medicine, 321*(25), 1720-1725.

Heineken, J., & McCloskey, J. (1985). Teaching power concepts. *Journal of Nursing Education, 24*(1), 40-42.

Hersey, P., & Blanchard, K. (1993). *Management of organizational behavior: Utilizing human resources* (6th ed). Englewood Cliffs, NJ: Prentice-Hall.

Hersey, P., & Duldt, B. (1989). *Situational leadership in nursing.* Norwalk, CT: Appleton & Lange.

Hoelzel, C. (1989). Using structural power sources to increase influence. *Journal of Nursing Administration, 19*(11), 10-15.

Kanter, R. (1977). *Men and women of the corporation.* New York: Basic Books.

Kanter, R. (1979). Power failure in management circuits. *Harvard Business Review, 57*(4), 65-75.

Kipnis, D., & Schmidt, S. (1980). Intraorganizational influence tactics: Explorations in getting one's way. *Journal of Applied Psychology, 65*(4), 440-452.

Kotter, J. (1979). *Power in management.* New York: AMA-COM.

Kotter, J. (1985). *Power and influence.* New York: Free Press.

Kouzes, J., & Posner, B. (1987). *The leadership challenge: How to get extraordinary things done in organizations.* San Francisco: Jossey-Bass.

Kramer, M., & Schmalenberg, C. (1990). Fundamental lessons in leadership. In E. Simendinger, T. Moore, & M. Kramer (Eds.), *The successful nurse executive: A guide for every nurse manager* (pp. 5-21). Ann Arbor, MI: Health Administration Press.

Levenstein, A. (1982). Tactics of persuasion. *Nursing Management, 13*(11), 40-41.

Liberatore, P., Brown-Williams, R., Brucker, J., Dukes, N., Kimmey, L., McCarthy, K., Pierre, J., Riegler, D., & Shearer-Pedu, K. (1989). A group approach to problem-solving. *Nursing Management, 20*(9), 68-72.

McClelland, D. (1975). *Power: The inner experience.* New York: Irvington.

McClelland, D. (1976). Power is the great motivation. *Harvard Business Review, 54*(2), 100-110.

Mintzberg, H. (1983). *Structure in fives: Designing effective organizations.* Englewood Cliffs, NJ: Prentice-Hall.

Nelson, A. (1989). Analysis of power in nursing administration: Rotkovich as a case in point. In B. Henry, C. Arndt, M. Di Vincenti, & A. Marriner-Tomey (Eds.), *Dimensions of nursing administration: Theory, research, education, practice* (pp. 205-211). Boston: Blackwell.

Price, J., & Mueller, C. (1986). *Handbook of organizational measurement.* Marshfield, MA: Pitman.

Raven, B., & Kruglanski, W. (1975). Conflict and power. In P. Swingle (Ed.), *The structure of conflict* (pp. 177-219). New York: Academic Press.

Schmidt-Posner, J., & Schmidt, N. (1979). *The effective uses of power and authority.* [Film]. Del Mar, CA: CRM McGraw-Hill Films.

Steers, R., & Porter, L. (1987). *Motivation and work behavior* (4th ed.). New York: McGraw-Hill.

Veninga, R. (1982). *The human side of health administration: A guide for hospital, nursing, and public health administrators.* Englewood Cliffs, NJ: Prentice-Hall.

Wilson, B., & Laschinger, H. (1994). Staff nurse perception of job empowerment and organizational commitment: A test of Kanter's theory of structural power in organizations. *Journal of Nursing Administration, 24*(4S), 39-47.

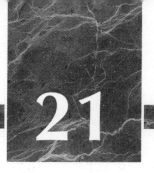

Conflict

Chapter Objectives

❧

define and discuss conflict

❧

define and discuss organizational conflict

❧

compare positive and negative aspects of conflict

❧

distinguish among three types of conflict

❧

explain the process that occurs in a conflict situation

❧

analyze sources of conflict in nursing

❧

explain methods for managing conflict

❧

analyze conflict resolution techniques

❧

analyze three conflict resolution outcomes

❧

relate collaboration to conflict

❧

relate collective bargaining to conflict in nursing

❧

exercise critical thinking to conceptualize and analyze
possible solutions to a practical experience incident

*C*onflict is always a potential part of the environment. Conflict is a part of life and arises because of the complexity of human relationships. Conflict has its origin in the fact that each person is unique and possesses a value system, philosophy, personality structure, and preferences and styles. Understanding how to maneuver around and manage conflict situations increases the ability to be more effective both in personal and professional roles.

Most people know when conflict exists because it is a part of everyday experience. The increasing complexity of healthcare institutions, specialization of roles, and the hierarchical nature of many healthcare organizations raise the potential for conflict for all healthcare providers. If the conflicts that occur within institutions are not managed appropriately, inefficiency and ineffectiveness are a result. For nurses, this is partially because in conflict situations, energy is diverted from productivity into discord. A contradiction is built into the healthcare system because, although collaboration is being promoted as a strategy, the organization of the healthcare system has not promoted true collaborative practice among healthcare professionals. In situations where the nurse's role overlaps with that of other healthcare professionals, conflicts can arise (AJN, 1987). Conflict is one factor that makes a nurse's work environment either positive or negative (Gardner, 1992).

DEFINITIONS

onflict is a natural result of self-interest behavior (Kirsch, 1988). *Conflict* is defined as a clash or struggle that occurs when a real or perceived threat or difference exists in the desires, thoughts, attitudes, feelings, or behaviors of two or more parties (Deutsch, 1973) (see Chart 21.1). Conflict exists as a tension or struggle arising from mutually exclusive or opposing actions, thoughts, opinions, or feelings. Conflict can be internal or external to an individual or group. It can be positive as well as negative. Positive effects occur when conflict results in change or growth (Henkin, Singleton, & Johnson, 1991).

Organizational conflict is defined as the struggle for scarce organizational resources (Coser, 1956; Price & Mueller, 1986). Values, goals, roles, or structural elements may be the specific locus of the struggle for scarce organizational resources. For example, two parties may be in opposition because of perceived differences in goals, a struggle over scarce resources, or interference in goal attainment. This opposition prevents cooperation (Deutsch, 1973). *Job conflict* is defined as a perceived opposition or antagonistic process at the individual-organization interface (Gardner, 1992). Conflict levels have an effect on productivity, morale, and teamwork in organizations (Gardner, 1992; Noble & Rancourt, 1991). Conflict serves to bind a group together, preserve a group by serving as a

CHART 21.1
⌒ DEFINITIONS

Conflict
a clash or struggle that occurs when a real or perceived threat or difference exists in the desires, thoughts, attitudes, feelings, or behaviors of two or more parties.

Organizational Conflict
the struggle for scarce organizational resources.

Job Conflict
a perceived opposition or antagonistic process at the individual-organization level.

Data from Coser (1956), Deutsch (1973), and Gardner (1992).

safety valve for hostility, integrate and stabilize a group, and promote growth through innovation, creativity, and change (Coser, 1956; Henkin, Singleton, & Johnson, 1991).

BACKGROUND

There are both positive and negative aspects to conflict (see Chart 21.2). The negative aspects occur when conflict is surrounded by feelings of fear, hostility, anger, threat, or lack of trust. The positive results of conflict include unification, integration, creativity, change, problem solving, and growth (Henkin, Singleton, & Johnson, 1991). Personal growth and enhanced coping ability occur because of the learning that is experienced as individuals deal with conflict. Conflict has been described as a form of socialization and necessary in forming and maintaining groups (Coser, 1956).

Conflict can be either constructive or destructive (Kramer & Schmalenberg, 1976). In constructive conflict, the issue is kept focused so direct action can be taken. For example, compromise can be an outcome of conflict. In using a compromise strategy, an effort is made to meet the needs of all parties. Open and honest communication is emphasized. Satisfaction is gained as an outcome. In destructive conflict, the issue is identified broadly and begins to escalate as reactions occur. Threats, coercion, or competition are the power strategies frequently employed. There is little attention to the responsibility to meet the needs of the other party. Misperceptions and distrust prevent honest and open communication. Frustration and dissatisfaction are the outcomes.

Some degree of conflict is inevitable in human interactions. The goal is not to drive out all conflict in the environment, but rather to manage conflict so that it is neither too low nor too high in level of intensity and so that it does not become obstructive to goal accomplishment or destructive to individuals. The constructive functions of conflict have been identified as increasing group cohesion and morale, promoting creativity, producing change and growth, improving work relations, promoting more effective problem solving, and motivating group members. The destructive functions of conflict interfere with the ideal organizational climate of stability and harmony. Thus, how conflict is viewed may influence the strategy or strategies chosen to manage it (Johnson, 1994).

Clearly, conflict is an inherent part of human growth and development. Some people say that harmony is not the absence of conflict, but rather the ability to cope with it. The more that is known about the dynamics of conflict, the better individuals will be able to handle conflicts when they occur.

Types of Conflict

There are three types of conflict: intrapersonal, interpersonal, and intergroup (see Fig. 21.1).

CHART 21.2
∽ EFFECTS OF CONFLICT

Constructive
- Defuse further conflict
- Increase effectiveness
- Increase cohesion
- Produce leaders
- Test power base

Destructive
- Decrease performance
- Fighting
- Stereotyping

Data from Kramer and Schmalenberg (1976).

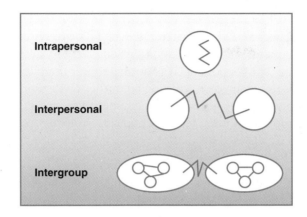

Figure 21.1
Types of conflict.

Intrapersonal means inside or internal to an individual. Intrapersonal conflict refers to the tension or stress that exists within an individual as a result of unmet needs, expectations, or goals (AJN, 1987). Intrapersonal conflict is conflict that generates from within an individual (Rahim, 1983). It often is manifested as a conflict over two competing roles. For example, a parent with a sick child who has to go to work faces a conflict: the need to take care of the sick child with the need to make a living. A nursing example occurs when the nurse determines that a client needs teaching or counseling, but the organization's assignment system is set up in a way that does not provide an adequate amount of time. When other priorities compete, then an internal or intrapersonal conflict of roles exists.

Interpersonal means conflict emerging between two or more people, such as between two nurses, a doctor and a nurse, or a nurse manager and a staff nurse. If the conflict originates between two or more individuals, it is called interpersonal (Rahim, 1983). In this case, two people have a disagreement, conflict, or clash. Either their values or styles do not match, or there is a misunderstanding or miscommunication between them. Interpersonal conflict can be viewed as happening between two individuals or among individuals within a group. To refer specifically to multiple individuals within a group, interpersonal conflict is called intragroup conflict.

Intergroup means conflict between two or more groups (Rahim, 1983). It is conflict occurring between two distinct groups of people. For example, when the American Medical Association advocated registered care technicians (RCTs) as a way to alleviate the nursing shortage of the late 1980s, the American Nurses Association disputed this as inappropriate, since nurses should determine who it is that participates in nursing practice if nurses are accountable and liable. The two groups opposed each other on the issue of an appropriate solution to the nursing shortage (AJN News, 1988; Booth, 1993). Sometimes the conflict arises between departments or units as groups. For example, hospital nurses might find themselves in conflict with central purchasing if supplies are provided that do not meet nursing's needs or are defective.

Conflict can be competitive or disruptive. *Competitive conflict* is similar to games and sports, where rules are followed and the goal is to win or best an opponent. A *disruptive conflict* is some activity designed to attack, defeat, or eliminate an opponent. It is not based in rules jointly agreed to, and its objective is not focused on winning but rather on disrupting the opponent. The feelings and actions generated by competitive conflict focus on the positive; for disruptive conflict, feelings, and actions focus on the negative (Filley, 1975).

Process of Conflict

There is a process to a conflict episode which develops over time and follows predictable stages and dynamics (Johnson, 1994; Pondy, 1967). The five stages are (Pondy, 1967):

- antecedent conditions (latent)
- perceived conflict (cognition)
- felt conflict (affect)
- manifest conflict (behavior)
- conflict aftermath (conditions)

The process begins with antecedent conditions such as unclear roles, competition for scarce resources, the quest for autonomy, or subunits with divergent goals. The process, depending on how it is handled, may be cyclical with the conflict aftermath becoming the antecedent conditions for a future conflict episode (see Fig. 21.2). The antecedent conditions form a background. This background leads to perceived conflict and then to felt conflict, which arises at an emotional level. One party senses that there is a problem and feels an emotional reaction beginning. These stages of perceived and felt conflict initiate manifest behavior. The conflict tension causes action. In this stage the individual may verbalize negativity, attack another person, or try to change the situation or the environment as a way of reducing the tension.

At the stage of manifest behavior, something happens that is visible evidence of conflict. Subsequently, either the conflict is resolved or suppressed. For example, ventilating strong emotions by verbal expression may not resolve the problem, but it calms an individual and suppresses the problem for a period of time. In the aftermath of this process, there will be new attitudes or feelings between the parties. This may be a positive feeling that coping occurred and the individual felt positive and constructive in the resolution of the conflict. However, a negative feeling may arise because of an inability to do anything to resolve the conflict or because the other person had more power. The negative feelings fester. The memory of the conflict and feelings about how it was processed linger and may provide antecedent conditions for another cycle of conflict. Thus there is an aftermath to the conflict even if it is resolved tem-

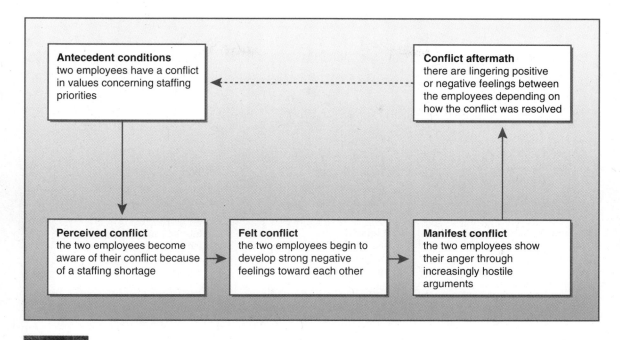

Figure 21.2
Pondy's stages of conflict. (Data from Pondy [1967].)

porarily. This is a residual effect from having had conflict or tension with which the individual invested psychological energy and emotion.

An emotional cycle of conflict was proposed as a process model of conflict by Thomas (1976) (see Fig. 21.3). He listed the five elements of the conflict process as frustration, conceptualization, behavior, interaction, and outcome. In this model, the conflict process begins as frustration, an affective-emotional trigger. Thomas' (1976) model bears a strong resemblance to Pondy's (1967) five stages. Frustration is one antecedent condition to conflict. Conceptualization is a form of cognition or perception of conflict. Frustration is an affective response, a form of felt conflict. Behavior and interaction both compare to Pondy's (1967) manifest conflict stage. Both models conclude with an outcome or aftermath conditions.

Organizational Conflict

Thomas (1976) further identified a structural model of conflict that is concerned with underlying conditions that influence the process of conflict and its resolution in organizations. This macro model, or "big picture," of conflict examines four factors that seem to influence the way conflict is handled in organizations: behavioral predispositions of individuals, social pressure in the

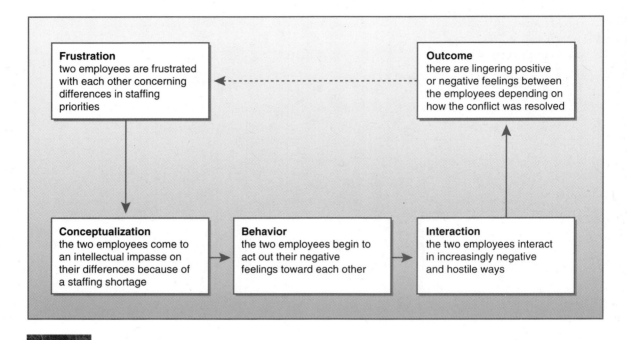

Figure 21.3
Thomas's conflict process events. (Data from Thomas [1976].)

environment, the organization's incentive structure, and rules and procedures. The different levels of power exist due to the bureaucratic hierarchy and the resultant position power.

Organizational conflict is a form of interpersonal conflict that is generated from aspects of the institution, such as the style of management, rules, procedures, and communication channels. Conflicts that arise when an individual's needs and goals cannot be met within the system are generally organizational. They also may be difficult to change (AJN, 1987). Conflict may be necessary to groups and organizations. Conflict serves to unify and bind together a group by setting boundaries and strengthening a group's identity. Conflict may help stabilize a group by serving as a test of opposing interests within the group. Conflict may help integrate a group by distributing power. Conflict may be necessary for the growth of a group and its members. Conflict serves to stimulate creativity, innovation, and change (Coser, 1956).

Organizational leadership sets a tone for conflict and conflict management (Barton, 1991). This occurs because leaders and managers model behaviors of positive or negative conflict management and choose when and how to intervene in conflict situations. Choice of intervention style and timing of conflict management are a function of the individuals' behavioral predispositions and environmental pressure coupled with the organization's reward structure and coordination and control methods.

Specifically related to organizational conflict and the focus on groups in organizations, Pondy (1967) identified three strategies to use when attempting to resolve organizational conflicts. The strategies are bargaining; using rules, procedures, and administrative control; and using a systems integrator. Bargaining might be useful when there is a conflict over scarce monetary resources. The administrative control approach might be helpful when there is a need to clarify role boundaries. The systems integrator approach might be appropriate in a matrix structure or where there is a need to coordinate personnel in vertical and horizontal structures (Booth, 1993).

There are two conflict inventories available to measure conflict. They can be used for objective measurement to determine how much conflict exists. The Rahim Organizational Conflict Inventory-I (Rahim, 1983) is designed to measure three dimensions of conflict: intrapersonal, intragroup, and intergroup. The Perceived Conflict Scale (Gardner, 1992) contains four subscales of conflict: intrapersonal, interpersonal, intergroup/other departments, and intergroup/support services. This scale is designed to measure conflict in nursing. Further, there are two conflict resolution style measures. The Rahim Organizational Conflict Inventory-II (Rahim, 1983) is designed to measure five independent dimensions of interpersonal conflict handling styles. The five measured dimensions are integrating, obliging, dominating, avoiding, and compromising. In addition, the classic Thomas-Kilmann Conflict MODE (Management of Differences Inventory) Exercise Instrument (Thomas & Kilmann, 1974) is cited as a conflict tool. However, this instrument is most properly used to diagnose styles of conflict management or resolution rather than as a conflict measuring tool.

RESEARCH NOTE

Source: Gardner, D. (1992). Conflict and retention of new graduate nurses. *Western Journal of Nursing Research, 14*(1), 76-85.

Purpose

The purpose of this research was to examine the levels and types of conflict perceived by new graduate nurses in their first year of work. The study also investigated the relationship of conflict to job satisfaction, performance, and turnover. The sample of 166 new graduate and newly employed hospital nurses from one tertiary hospital were surveyed at 6 and 12 months on the job. Demographic data, conflict, job satisfaction, commitment, turnover, and performance were measured. The Perceived Conflict Scale, McCloskey-Mueller Satisfaction Scale, and Six-Dimension Scale of Nursing Performance were the instruments administered to subjects.

Discussion

Mean conflict levels were moderate and stable overall in this sample. There were no significant differences over time. The sample proved to be highly homogeneous on demographics. Performance and turnover were not significantly related to conflict. Subjects with greater conflict had less job satisfaction at 12 months on the job. Intrapersonal conflict was the category yielding the highest mean scores and scores that increased over time.

Application to Practice

Conflict is one factor that interacts with nurses' perceptions of their work environment to create either a positive or negative impression. Conflict is pervasive in work environments. In this research, conflict had an inverse relationship to job satisfaction. Negative organizational outcomes such as performance and turnover were not directly linked with conflict but may be linked indirectly through lack of job satisfaction. Nurses need to pay attention to conflict and design administrative interventions to manage organizational conflict.

Sources of Conflict

The sources of conflict are power, communication, goals, values, resources, roles, and personalities (see Chart 21.3). Conflict arises from a variety of sources. As seen in Chapter 20, power and conflict are interrelated.

Power clashes lead to conflict. This happens if one person has more power than another. For example, in organizations there are relationships between and among individuals with unequal power.

Another source of conflict is the misunderstanding or breakdown of communication. Conflicts can be the result of clashes between deep-seated, sincere, but diametrically opposed views. Communication may be used to clarify opposing views. Since values are internalized, they are not easily changed but may be clarified by communication or become a barrier due to miscommunication. Conflict situations often arise suddenly with the awareness of conflict existing on an emotional level. Emotional intensity may be the first element communicated. The emotional reaction may include responses such as frustration or wanting to lash out with a strong verbal communication.

The roots or causes of conflict are many and varied. Other general sources of conflict are different goals, different ways to reach a goal, different values, overlapping or unclear designation of responsibility, lack of information, and personality conflicts. Some conflicts cannot be resolved (Mallory, 1981). Unresolvable conflicts will need to be carefully managed within any work group in order to balance conflict levels. For example, nurses may thrive when the conflict level is sufficient to stimulate a clash of ideas that leads to creativity and innovation or growth. However, nurses may expend energy in nonproductive activity if the conflict level is too high or becomes destructive.

CHART 21.3
∾ CONFLICT SOURCES FOR NURSES

- Power divisions
- Communication
- Personal and organizational goals and values
- Resource allocation
- Roles
- Attitudes and personalities

Conflict appears to be an inherent part of the work of nursing. Nurses are prime candidates for conflict because of the need to work collaboratively with people of varying social, ethnic, and educational backgrounds. Collaboration implies a distribution of power, yet nurses may be employed in a hierarchical system. Nurses find that working in groups creates a situation in which there are a number of different colleagues and a variety of client types and personalities with which to work. These are complex interrelationships. Added to the complexity is the fact that there are multiple providers requiring coordination and communication to manage the care for any client. For example, those involved may include physicians, nurses, nurse managers, ancillary personnel, the client, and the client's family. There is a potential for conflict to arise as a byproduct (AJN, 1987).

Within healthcare, there is interdependence among members. This situation also provides conditions ripe for conflict to arise. Multiple care providers rely on each other to carry out portions of the work. For example, physicians are dependent upon nurses in order to achieve certain client outcomes, nurses are dependent on physicians in order to achieve certain client outcomes, and both nurses and physicians are dependent on a variety of assistive or allied care workers to deliver the therapies or promote client outcomes. Nurses and physicians also have a dependence on each other's expertise. For example, nurses need the physician to write an order for pain medication if medication would be the appropriate intervention for pain. When physicians write an order for certain therapies, they rely on nurses to assess and evaluate the client, coordinate the care, get the laboratory results ordered and processed, and ensure that therapy is delivered. The complexity of the interrelationships plus the nature of interdependent work create conflict moments for nurses. This coincides with Kotter's (1979; 1985) ideas about dependency, power, and conflict in organizations. He viewed power as a mechanism to resolve conflict (see Chapter 20).

The source of a conflict can be interpersonal or organizational in nature. Further, these categories often overlap. When nurses are involved in conflict the conflict is usually one that involves nurse-nurse, nurse-doctor, nurse-assistive worker, or nurse-client and/or visitor (AJN, 1987). In some cases the conflict situation grows to involve multiple groups or pairs of groups.

Personal and organizational goals and values may clash over general policies. General policy refers to the course of action taken by an institution, department, or unit. Policies are the guidelines developed to handle specific issues. They are designed to give guidance about standardized ways to make decisions in recurring circumstances. However, professionals and care providers may approach situations with diverse viewpoints about the "best" way to handle a specific problem. Disputes between nurses, physicians, and assistive personnel arise over methods and procedures involving specific diagnostic, therapeutic, clerical, or managerial routines. Disagreements occur, for example, over paperwork, visitors' privileges, or what time is most efficient or effective to do procedures (AJN, 1987). Clashes may result at the intersection of a nurse's professional judgment as an autonomous professional with standardized policies developed by the institution and designed to produce uniform behavior.

Resource allocation is an issue associated with the definition of organizational conflict. Cost containment strategies have created conflict over scarce resources in organizations. Nurses often are placed in the center of this conflict. The scarcer the resources, the greater the potential for conflict.

Power divisions occur across both organizational and interpersonal lines to produce role conflicts. Role conflicts often manifest themselves in role overload and role ambiguity. Role overload is a common source of nursing conflict. It occurs when nurses are expected to perform the work of other employees or disciplines in addition to providing nursing care. The result of overload often is burnout. Another facet of role conflict, role ambiguity, occurs when the nurse's responsibility expands faster than is officially recognized. When roles are unclear, conflict can surface at the point where the roles intersect (AJN, 1987).

Another stress point for conflict in nursing occurs at the intersection of the individual's needs with the organization's needs and goals. Role stress and strain are a reality in the work existence of nurses. For example, other decision makers in the environment may hold one view about what the nurse's role should be, while nurses may have an entirely different view, and the two views may conflict. For example, nurses consider a part of their role to be client advocacy. When an unfavorable outcome occurs, the nurse's client advocacy role may be placed in opposition to the institution's image or legal liability needs. Further, nurses as individuals may have a need for job security, practice autonomy, or pay equity. These needs may be in conflict with the organization's needs to hold down labor costs or control the practice decisions of its largest category of workers.

Sometimes conflict stems from individuals' attitudes, personalities, and personal behavior. Personal behavior refers to style, mannerisms, or work habits. Chronic lateness is an example of a personal behavior that frequently causes conflict. Conflict comes from differences of opinions, values, and communicated understandings (AJN, 1987).

Whatever the cause, when a conflict occurs, one can expect more information to be needed to process the conflict constructively. Similar to problem solving, conflict situations need information gathering and clear problem definition. However, the conflict may be difficult to define, especially if more than one causative factor contributes to the tension. Further, the conflict may involve a covert, less obvious issue than what is presented on the surface. Conflicts often appear larger and more difficult to manage than what actually can be done about them. For example, intense or high levels of emotions are a part of conflict. Both the emotional and issues content of the conflict will need to be managed. By identifying both the areas of agreement and disagreement and then defining the extent of each party's aims, a nurse can begin the process of constructively reducing a seemingly overwhelming conflict to a manageable size (AJN, 1987).

Clearly, if not handled productively, conflicts can be a disruptive rather than a creative force. Conflict involves energy. Within an organization it usually is not effective to consistently avoid or suppress conflict because conflict can be the first process that occurs in an attempt to create changes or to innovate. If managed appropriately, conflict can motivate people to look at situations and others in new ways. It can lead to increased productivity and harmony. Modes of behavior like aggressive, hurtful competition maximize the destructive effects of conflict. Creative conflict resolution looks for ways to maximize the constructive and decrease the destructive effect of conflict (AJN, 1987). For nurses, the techniques of problem solving form a useful basis for handling conflict. However, nurses need to cultivate an understanding of conflict and an attitude of self-confidence in constructive conflict management.

LEADERSHIP AND MANAGEMENT IMPLICATIONS

Conflict Management

There are many views about conflict management. Clearly conflict is managed via the style and the strategy that is chosen by the conflict manager. There are several conflict styles and strategies, meaning that individuals have choices. The ability to select among styles and strategies if something is not working provides flexibility for the person dealing with conflict.

Managing conflict relates to whether the level is too high or too low. Assessment of levels and sources is the first step in conflict assessment. The goal of conflict management is to stimulate growth and coping behavior, but avoid reaching the point where conflict seems overwhelming. Conflict is an inherent element of change and is manifested in resistance to change. This indicates that nurses need to be alert to the predictability of resistance and conflict in any change process.

Personal styles and the interaction of styles contribute to conflict moments. The reality is that most people are more comfortable around people who are similar to them. If people are very different in terms of personality and styles, then how the styles interact contributes to conflict potential. Awareness of one's own style and the recognition of other people's styles contribute to effective management of conflict.

There are several factors to consider in conflict management (AJN, 1987). The important factors can form the basis for conflict management behaviors

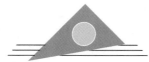

Leadership & Management Behaviors

LEADERSHIP BEHAVIORS	MANAGEMENT BEHAVIORS	OVERLAP AREAS
• enables followers to use power to manage conflicts	• plans for conflict management	• manages conflicts
• models constructive conflict resolution	• organizes the environment to decrease frustration	• resolves conflicts
• encourages growth-producing conflict	• directs subordinates in resolving conflicts	
• mentors and supports followers in conflict management	• negotiates conflict resolutions	
• builds conflict interventions	• competes and bargains for scarce resources	
• is visible in conflict situations		
• collaborates with others		

CHART 21.4
↩ CONFLICT MANAGEMENT CHECKLIST

- Identify the boundaries of the conflict, the areas of agreement and disagreement, and the extent of each person's aims.
- Understand the factors that limit the possibilities of managing the conflict constructively.
- Be aware of whether more than one issue is involved.
- Be open to the ideas, feelings, and attitudes expressed by the people involved.
- Be willing to accept outside help to mediate the conflict.

Data from AJN (1987).

needed by nurses. These behaviors have been listed in a conflict management checklist (see Chart 21.4). The checklist can be used as a review or assessment for critically analyzing conflict situations.

A companion tool is a series of systematic steps that have been recommended for nurses to use in handling conflict situations (Mallory, 1981) (see Fig. 21.4). The advantage of following a systematic approach to handling conflict is that the nurse becomes a better problem solver. This is especially important in conflict situations, which have a significant component of strong human emotions. The emotions may need to be defused before the content issues can be tackled.

CONFLICT MANAGEMENT STRATEGIES

It is important to take action as soon as a conflict surfaces so that bad feelings will not linger and grow. Conflict in groups adds the complexity of multiple parties to the conflict situation. Usually the best place for a work group to clear the air is in a group meeting. During such meetings issues can be defined and strategies worked out for managing the points of disagreement. In broad categories, the three overall frameworks or postures for conflict management are the defensive, compromise, and creative problem solving modes (AJN, 1987).

The *defensive mode* produces feelings of winning in some and loss in others. There are several conflict resolution strategies that adopt a defensive mode. Sometimes if creative problem solving and compromise fail, this may

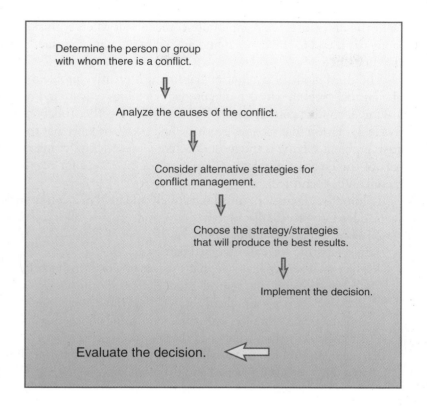

Determine the person or group
with whom there is a conflict.

⇓

Analyze the causes of the conflict.

⇓

Consider alternative strategies for
conflict management.

⇓

Choose the strategy/strategies
that will produce the best results.

⇓

Implement the decision.

Evaluate the decision. ⟸

Figure 21.4
Handling conflict situations.
(Data from Mallory [1981].)

be the only way to decrease some of the destructive effects of conflict. Or a defensive mode may be used initially to gain time to calm down or to think about how to proceed. Following are ways to defensively solve a conflict:

- Separate the contending parties. For example, people may be assigned to different shifts or teams or different days off and on.
- Suppress the conflict. For example, people may decide not to talk about their differences.
- Restrict or isolate the conflict. For example, the parties can agree to disagree about a conflict and move on to items that they do agree about.
- Smooth it over or finesse it through an organizational change. For example, sometimes it is possible to solve conflicts by restructuring around the issue.
- Avoid the conflict to diminish the destructive effects. For example, people can change the subject whenever the conflict arises or avoid the party or parties involved.

The second mode of conflict management is compromise. With a *compromise* each party wins something and loses something. In the settlement, each side gives up a part of its demands. Thus each side may "go halfway" or "split the difference." A compromise comes about when both sides want harmony or an end to the conflict and are willing to give up something to settle the difference.

The third mode of conflict management is creative problem solving. Use of a *creative problem solving* mode produces feelings of gain and no feelings of loss for all conflict participants. All parties work together collaboratively to arrive at a solution that satisfies everyone and everyone feels that they win. Creative problem solving is the most effective mode of conflict management. As part of the creative problem solving process, five steps for conflict management can be identified:

1. Initiate a discussion, timed sensitively and held in an environment conducive to private discussion.
2. Respect individual differences.
3. Be empathic with all involved parties.
4. Have an assertive dialogue that consists of separating facts from feelings, clearly defining the central issue, differentiating viewpoints, making sure that each person clearly states their intentions, framing the main issue based on common principles, and being an attentive listener consciously focused on what the other person is saying.
5. Agree on a solution that balances the power and satisfies all parties, so that a consensus is reached and everyone wins (AJN, 1987).

Conflict Resolution Techniques

Conflicts can be a source of chronic frustration, or they can lead to increased effectiveness in organizations and groups. It takes leadership and management to solve them creatively so that people exist more cooperatively with others. Leadership and management of conflict resolution has implications for work group morale and productivity. A fair proportion of a leader's or manager's time is spent on handling conflict.

Conflict management techniques stress the importance of communication, assertive dialogue, and coming from a point of empathy. Thus, when involved in conflict situations, the more that individuals look at the total situation and use positive communication techniques, the closer they will come to a path toward successful resolution. Conflict resolution techniques have been identified, described, and categorized in a variety of ways by a variety of authors. Some terms have been used interchangeably, and some terms have similar but slightly different meanings. The overall list for methods or strategies for conflict resolution (see Fig. 21.5) include (AJN, 1987; Barton, 1991; Mallory, 1981; Thomas, 1976):

Avoiding This is the strategy of avoiding conflict at all costs. Some people never acknowledge that a conflict exists. The individual's posture is, if I do

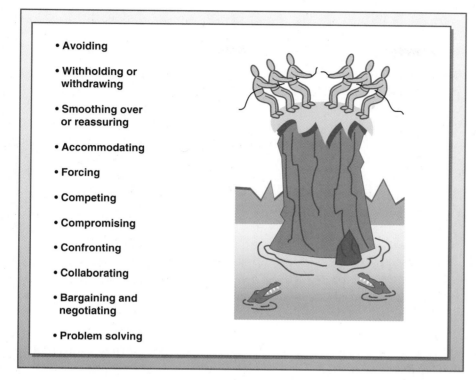

- Avoiding

- Withholding or
  withdrawing

- Smoothing over
  or reassuring

- Accommodating

- Forcing

- Competing

- Compromising

- Confronting

- Collaborating

- Bargaining and
  negotiating

- Problem solving

Figure 21.5
Strategies for conflict
resolution. (Data from AJN
[1987], Barton [1991],
Mallory [1981], and
Thomas [1976].)

not acknowledge there is a problem, then there is no problem. It is sometimes reflected in the phrase, "leave well enough alone."

Withholding or Withdrawing In this avoidance strategy, one party opts out of participation. They remove themselves from the situation. This does not resolve the conflict. However, this strategy does give individuals a chance to calm down or to avoid a confrontation.

Smoothing Over or Reassuring This is the strategy of saying that "everything will be OK." By maintaining surface harmony, parties do not withdraw but simply attempt to make everyone feel good. It is like "smoothing ruffled feathers." Smoothing over or reassuring strategies use verbal communication to defuse strong emotions.

Accommodating This strategy is used when there is a large power differential. The more powerful party is accommodated to preserve harmony or build up social credits. What this means is that the party of lesser power gives up their position in deference to the more powerful party. Accommodation may be used when one party has a vested interest that is relatively unimportant to the other party. "Kill the enemy with kindness" is the operative phrase.

Forcing This technique is a dominance move and an arbitrary way to manage conflict. An issue may be forced on the table by issuing orders or by putting it to a majority-rules vote. The hallmark phrase is, "let's vote on it." Forcing is an all-out power strategy to win while the other party loses.

Competing   This is an assertive strategy where one party's needs are satisfied at the other's expense. Competing is an all-out effort to win at any cost. It is sometimes reflected in the phrase, "might makes right." Competing strategies tend to follow rules and be similar to games and athletic contests. Applying for a job is a form of competition.

Compromising   This strategy is called "splitting the difference." It is useful when goals or values are markedly different. It is a staple of conflict management.

Confronting   This technique is called assertive problem solving that is focused on the issues. Individuals speak for themselves, but in a way that decreases defensiveness and allows another person to hear the message. It is a staple of conflict management but requires courage. "I" messages are used; "you" messages are avoided.

Collaborating   This is an assertive and cooperative strategy where the parties work together to find a mutually satisfying solution. It is invoked with the phrase: "two heads are better than one."

Bargaining and Negotiating   These strategies are attempts to divide the rewards, power, or benefits so that everyone gets something. They involve both parties in a back-and-forth effort at some level of agreement. The process may be formal or informal.

Problem Solving   This strategy's goal is to try to find an acceptable, workable solution for all parties. It is designed to generate feelings of gain by all parties. The problem solving process is employed to reach a mutually agreeable solution to the conflict.

Conflict Resolution Inventories

Of the two conflict resolution style inventories, the Rahim Organizational Conflict Inventory-II (Rahim, 1983) split styles of handling interpersonal conflict into the two dimensions of concern for self and concern for others, both in high and low degrees, to form a grid. Rahim (1983) then adapted Blake and Mouton's (1964) five types of handling interpersonal conflict (forcing, withdrawing, smoothing, compromising, and problem solving) into five styles of handling interpersonal conflict: avoiding, obliging, compromising, integrating, and dominating. The inventory measures the five identified styles.

Thomas and Kilmann (1974) also developed a style assessment and diagnosis inventory, called the Thomas-Kilmann Conflict Mode Instrument. Their grid used dimensions of assertiveness and cooperativeness on high to low degrees. Their five styles are avoiding, accommodating, compromising, competing, and collaborating. Their model blends a description of an individual's behavior on assertiveness and cooperativeness dimensions in situa-

Effective Communication

As a nurse manager I often find myself dealing with conflict between two staff members. In one situation, I had to mediate between a senior nurse and a new graduate. The senior nurse was advising the new graduate about time management skills and how to do things a bit quicker. The graduate nurse became offended by this challenge to her skills. Both nurses came to me separately for advice. I felt this problem was simply a failure to communicate and encouraged them to approach one another to try to identify the problem. When they got together, however, the situation only became worse. They would no longer speak to each other or assist each other with patient care.

I knew at that point I needed to intervene and work out the problem with them as a group. As the mediator my focus was on identifying and solving a problem, and not on finding fault with a particular person. Patience was key to overcoming any resistance to problem solving. At our meeting, each nurse explained her side of the story. I encouraged each of them to focus on the problem and not on each other. As the meeting progressed, however, it became clear that the graduate nurse was beginning to feel threatened and thinking that the other was assigning her additional duties. In fact, the senior nurse was actually trying to teach the new nurse how to delegate duties to others when the workload became overwhelming. Each one finally realized that we all needed to work together as a team and that delegation, up to a point, is sometimes necessary to help decrease the overall stress. The two nurses finally began to communicate effectively as we attacked the problem.

As the mediator of the discussion, I would restate issues brought up by each nurse to help clarify and confirm our understanding. I also explained to both of them the proper way to delegate and coordinate tasks.

In the end, the problem was resolved. Both nurses realized how important it was to communicate effectively, especially in stressful situations. They now work together as a team, and have achieved a mutual respect.

JULIE HENDERSON, RN, BSN
Nurse Manager, PICU/Pediatrics
The Cleveland Clinic Foundation
   Children's Hospital
Cleveland, Ohio

tions where the concerns of two people appear to be incompatible. The behaviors of individuals are thought to be a function of both personal predispositions and situational contingencies. Avoiding is low on both assertiveness and cooperativeness; collaborating is high on both aspects. Competing is high assertive and low cooperative; accommodating is low assertive and high cooperative. Compromising is in the middle. All modes have some use in specific situations (Barton, 1991).

Conflict Resolution Outcomes

Whatever the conflict resolution style used, the individual must be aware of the outcome that results from the strategy selected. The outcomes of con-

CHART 21.5
↪ DEFINITIONS

Win-Lose
one party exerts
dominance.

Lose-Lose
neither side wins.

Win-Win
attempt to meet the
needs of both parties
simultaneously.

Data from Filley (1975) and
Filley, House, and Kerr
(1976).

flict are what actually happen as a result of the conflict management process. There are three ways in which conflicts resolve: win-lose, lose-lose, and win-win (Filley, House, & Kerr, 1976) (see Chart 21.5).

A *win-lose* situation is one in which one party's views, ideas, or opinions predominate and the other side's are ignored. Putting something to a majority vote creates a win-lose situation where the majority wins, the minority loses. A *lose-lose* situation is one in which the conflict deteriorates to the point where both parties end up losing. Strategies of averaging, using bribes, using a third-party to arbitrate, or trading may result in a lose-lose outcome. The *win-win* outcome is an attempt to make sure that each party gains something and that there is a solution acceptable to all parties. Problem solving, consensus building, and integrative decision making are techniques that are aimed toward a win-win outcome.

Managing clients or other nursing personnel places the nurse in many conflict resolution situations. The leader's role is to use positive communication techniques and alternatives to come to a resolution of conflicts. Many institutions have no officially sanctioned way to handle hostility among their members. A participative leadership style contains a means for dealing with some conflict sources (Glennon, 1985). Effective conflict management techniques establish a common etiquette to lessen conflict tension, increase mutual respect, engender confidence, and increase power through willing collaboration in the endeavors of the organization.

The need for nurses to have professional autonomy in order to practice as professionals can become a source of conflict. The employee status of most nurses enhances what Kramer (1974) called the professional/bureaucratic role conflict. Nurses are educated and socialized into accepting professional values. To be autonomous, nurses need to have the amount of authority that goes along with the responsibility and accountability that is being delegated. The reality of the work setting is that there are many constraints: policies and procedures and a lack of resources are in conflict with the concept of professional autonomy. Bureaucratic goals may conflict with a nurse's professional sense of what is appropriate care. This may be manifested as a conflict between humanistic service values and business values of cost reduction. Thus values and role beliefs may conflict and create tension that challenges the leader and manager to resolve in a win-win manner (Storlie, 1982).

CURRENT ISSUES AND TRENDS

It is important to understand conflict and its management in healthcare. Conflict forms a framework for understanding current issues and trends. Healthcare reform has meant a major shift in thinking about, organizing, structuring, and financing healthcare. Conflict is inevitable in any change.

Healthcare reform has resulted in a variety of different organizational structures being developed. When structures change, roles change. Nursing's role is not as clear cut as it used to be, and this can cause stress and frustration. There are time demands on nurses, requiring that they figure out new ways to improve productivity while decreasing costs. One method is to use assistive personnel in their work. Layoffs and the downsizing of nursing positions create stress because nurses feel they already lack time to do the work in a way that they feel is most appropriate for their clients and because it directly attacks their sense of job security. These job stresses further contribute to organizational conflict.

Two current trends are receiving increased attention in nursing: the conflict resolution technique of collaborating and the re-emergence of collective bargaining issues as an outgrowth of labor-management conflict. Both issues arise at the intersection of power and conflict in nursing practice within organizations.

Collaboration has been called the most effective strategy for managing conflict to achieve long-range benefits. However, a wide differential in power, as traditionally has existed between nurses and physicians, diminishes the probability that collaboration will occur. Rather, with wide differences in power where one group predominates, compromise and accommodation tend to be the most frequently used strategies. Thus power disparity has been an impediment to nurse-physician collaboration (Johnson, 1994). There are indications that this will change with reform-driven healthcare system changes. As nursing assumes a greater role under healthcare reform, the power disparity may diminish, and nurse-physician collaboration may become more common.

Collaboration is the basis for team building in healthcare. Work redesign, restructuring, and reengineering depend on collaboration, cooperation, and group accomplishment. Proactive conflict resolution in work groups is the essence of building successful teams. Successful teams work cooperatively rather than competitively, are flexible and adaptable, and have a high degree of trust and communication. A team is characterized by (Neubauer, 1993):

- a common goal
- interdependence
- cooperation
- coordination of activities
- task specialization
- division of effort
- mutual respect

Team building is defined as a deliberate process of creating and unifying a group into an effective and efficiently functioning work unit in order to accomplish specified goals (Farley & Stoner, 1989). Diplomacy, negotiation, and the use of power-based strategies or alliances are the skills needed for team building. Facilitation skills allow for sharing knowledge and maintaining positive communication among peers, both necessary for team leadership and reduction of high levels of conflict. Group process provides a framework for understanding team development and, by extension, team collaboration (Farley & Stoner, 1989). Interdisciplinary collaborative practice groups are projected to be a prime strategy in healthcare to meet future needs (Velianoff, Neely, & Hall, 1993).

Collective bargaining issues have re-emerged in nursing. They are a manifestation of nurses' conflicts with employing organizations over economic and nursing welfare issues. In the decade of the 1970s, collective bargaining was a prominent issue in nursing. The debate focused on collective bargaining versus collective action. Collective bargaining was associated with unionization and labor-management negotiations. However, since the air traffic controllers' (PATCO) strike and resultant union breakup in the early 1980s, labor union influence in the United States has been diminishing. A resurgence in interest in collective bargaining within nursing has been triggered by the externally driven redesign of the work of nursing prevalent in the mid-1990s. Connected to work redesign are the dual issues of a dramatic alteration in staff mix to drastically reduce the number of RNs and a corollary rise in the use of non-nurse assistive personnel. Nurses argue that such externally-induced rapid changes compromise client safety. Administrators and consultants argue that nurses are merely job-threatened and are looking only to preserve their employment, not assist the fiscal needs of the organization. The conflict level has escalated around these workplace issues.

The National Labor Relations Act (NLRA) (The Wagner Act) was passed in 1935. Not-for-profit hospitals were excluded from all provisions of this act and the 1947 Taft-Hartley amendments. In 1974, however, further amendments to the Taft-Hartley act removed the exemption on not-for-profit hospitals. Thus, hospital employees, including nurses, could engage in federally protected labor union activity. This allows nurses to collectively bargain over wages, benefits, working conditions, and professional/client care concerns (Grant, 1994). During the 1970s and 1980s a number of state legislatures also adopted laws extending collective bargaining rights to nurses at publicly owned hospitals.

The 1990s are a time of considerable change in the healthcare delivery system. While organizations are realizing that they are in partnership with their workers in delivering healthcare, work redesign, downsizing, closures, reengineering, altering staff mix, and take-overs have threatened nurses' long-term job security and benefits (Porter-O'Grady, 1992). Untenable working conditions have contributed to a flurry of organizing activities. Staff cuts have sparked unionizing drives (AJN Headlines, 1993). Collective bargaining exists to limit employers' ability to take unilateral action (Cohen, 1989). Triggered by job and security threats, a growing number of hospital, nursing home, and rehabilitation workers are joining labor unions in search of job security and a voice in healthcare reform (Tomsho, 1994). Further, there are indications that reengineering that results in layoffs and downsizing does cut expenses in the short term but may be unsuccessful in achieving hoped-for productivity results and may actually be a waste of time and energy. The destructive effects range from anger and fear in demoralized workers to job burnout. Thus currently popular efforts at reengineering have become a fad adopted in many places without a full consideration of the consequences (Associated Press, 1994).

In a recent labor relations development, the United States Supreme Court ruled that nurses who oversee lower level personnel are supervisors and, therefore, not protected by federal laws on collective bargaining under the NLRA. This is a reversal of the traditional holding of nurses under the NLRA. The decision narrows the definition of who can participate in an RN collective bargaining unit. Eligibility will be decided locally. The American Nurses' Association's argument that there is a distinction between an RN's direction of other employees in the exercise of professional judgment in the care of clients and the exercise of supervisory authority in the interest of the employer was not upheld. The question becomes, when does a professional become a supervisor (Ketter, 1994)? While the answer may lie with the Wagner Act (NLRA), the interpretation and reinterpretation of the NLRA through subsequent rulings has a local and national impact on nurses and nursing. This conflict has challenged nurses as a collective body.

Both movements, toward collaborative interdisciplinary teams and toward collective bargaining in nursing, are conflict issues for nursing. Nurses are challenged to strike a balance among competing needs and values in order to create and maintain a positive work climate and quality client outcomes.

SUMMARY

- Conflict is a part of life and everyday experience.
- Conflict is a clash when threat or difference exists among people.
- Organizational conflict is a struggle for scarce resources.
- There are both positive and negative aspects to conflict.
- The goal is to learn how to manage and adapt to conflict.
- The three types of conflict are intrapersonal, interpersonal, and intergroup.
- Conflict can be competitive or disruptive.
- There are five stages to the conflict process.
- There are many sources of conflict, but power clashes are at the root of conflict.
- Conflict is an occupational hazard for nurses.
- There is power in managing conflict.

* Nurses can follow a series of steps in handling conflict situations.
* There are three general strategies for conflict management.
* There are ten different conflict resolution techniques.
* Conflict outcomes are win-lose, lose-lose, or win-win.
* Collaboration/team building and collective bargaining are current conflict issues.

Study Questions

1. What was the most recent conflict you experienced?
2. What types of conflict are common in nursing students?
3. What sources of conflict are most common in nursing practice?
4. What is your usual way of handling conflict?
5. What is the usual way nurses handle conflict?
6. Does the way your immediate superior handles conflict help or hinder you?
7. Is there one best way to handle the conflicts most common to nursing practice?
8. Do advanced practice nurses experience different conflicts? If so, what are they?
9. What organizational factors are related to unionization activity?

Critical Thinking Exercise

Nurses Brandon Nau and Sally Smith work for a large community health-care agency. The agency has been inundated with new clients, and several new programs are badly needed in the community. All of the nurses are faced with increasing workloads, and tensions are rising as they are stressed to meet demands. Today, Nurse Nau asked to call a staff meeting to discuss a proposal. He wants to purchase and introduce portable computerized laptops and communication devices for the nurses to carry and use on home visits and at distance sites. Upon hearing this, Nurse Smith verbally exploded, accusing Nurse Nau of trying to make the nurses' jobs "impossible."

1. What is the problem?

2. Why is it a problem?

3. What antecedent conditions may have contributed to the problem?

4. What should nurse Nau do? What should Nurse Smith do?

5. What conflict resolution strategy(s) might be helpful in this situation?

6. What power aspects need to be considered?

7. What conflict handling style might each nurse consider using?

REFERENCES

AJN. (1987). *Conflict management.* [Video-tape]. New York: American Journal of Nursing Company.

AJN Headlines. (1993). Staff cuts are sparking unionization drives. *American Journal of Nursing, 93*(9), 9.

AJN News. (1988). AMA meets growing opposition to the "RCT". *American Journal of Nursing, 88*(9), 1265,1286,1288.

Associated Press. (1994, July 7). Does downsizing really work? *The Des Moines Register,* pp. 7S-8S.

Barton, A. (1991). Conflict resolution by nurse managers. *Nursing Management, 22*(5), 83-86.

Blake, R., & Mouton, J. (1964). *The managerial grid.* Houston, TX: Gulf Publishing.

Booth, R. (1993). Dynamics of conflict and conflict management. In D. Mason, S. Talbott, & J. Leavitt (Eds.), *Policy and politics for nurses: Action and change in the workplace, government, organizations, and community* (2nd ed.) (pp. 149-165). Philadelphia: Saunders.

Cohen, A. (1989). The management rights clause in collective bargaining. *Nursing Management, 20*(11), 24-34.

Coser, L. (1956). *The functions of social conflict.* New York: The Free Press.

Deutsch, M. (1973). *The resolution of conflict: Constructive and destructive processes.* New Haven: Yale University Press.

Farley, M., & Stoner, M. (1989). The nurse executive and interdisciplinary team building. *Nursing Administration Quarterly, 13*(2), 24-30.

Filley, A. (1975). *Interpersonal conflict resolution.* New York: The Free Press.

Filley, A., House, R., & Kerr, S. (1976). *Managerial process and organizational behavior.* Glenview, IL: Scott Foresman.

Gardner, D. (1992). Conflict and retention of new graduate nurses. *Western Journal of Nursing Research, 14*(1), 76-85.

Glennon, T. (1985). Practitioner vs. bureaucrat: Professions in conflict. *Nursing Management, 16*(3), 60-65.

Grant, A. (1994). *The professional nurse: Issues and actions.* Springhouse, PA: Springhouse.

Henkin, A., Singleton, C., & Johnson, M. (1991). Functions of conflict: Perceived utility in the emergent professions. *Journal of Research in Education, 1*(1), 35-43.

Johnson, M. (1994). Conflict and nursing professionalization. In J. McCloskey and H. Grace (Eds.), *Current issues in nursing* (4th ed.) (pp. 643-649). St. Louis: Mosby.

Ketter, J. (1994). Ruling questions NLRA protection for nurses. *The American Nurse, 26*(6), 10,13.

Kirsch, J. (1988). *The middle manager & the nursing organization: Human resources, fiscal resources.* Norwalk, CT: Appleton & Lange.

Kotter, J. (1979). *Power in management.* New York: AMA-COM.

Kotter, J. (1985). *Power and influence.* New York: Free Press.

Kramer, M. (1974). *Reality shock: Why nurses leave nursing.* St. Louis: Mosby.

Kramer, M., & Schmalenberg, C. (1976). Conflict: The cutting edge of growth. *Journal of Nursing Administration, 6*(10), 19-25.

Mallory, G. (1981). Believe it or not conflict can be healthy once you understand it and learn to manage it. *Nursing 81, 11*(6), 97-101.

Neubauer, J. (1993). Redesign: Managing role changes and building new teams. *Seminars for Nurse Managers, 1*(1), 26-32.

Noble, K., & Rancourt, R. (1991). Administration and intradisciplinary conflict within nursing. *Nursing Administration Quarterly, 15*(4), 36-42.

Pondy, L. (1967). Organizational conflict: Concepts and models. *Administrative Science Quarterly, 12,* 296-320.

Porter-O'Grady, T. (1992). Of rabbits and turtles: A time of change for unions. *Nursing Economic$, 10*(3), 177-182.

Price, J., & Mueller, C. (1986). *Handbook of organizational measurement.* Marshfield, MA: Pitman.

Rahim, M. (1983). *Rahim organizational conflict inventories: Experimental edition: Professional Manual.* Palo Alto, CA: Consulting Psychologists Press.

Storlie, F. (1982). Surviving on-the-job conflict. *RN, 45*(10), 51-53, 96.

Thomas, K. (1976). Conflict and conflict management. In M. Dunnette (Ed.), *The handbook of industrial and organizational psychology* (pp. 889-935). Chicago: Rand McNally.

Thomas, K., & Kilmann, R. (1974). *Thomas-Kilmann conflict mode instrument.* Tuxedo, NY: Xicom.

Tomsho, R. (1994, June 9). Mounting sense of job malaise prompts more health-care workers to join unions. *The Wall Street Journal*, pp. B1, B6.

Velianoff, G., Neely, C., & Hall, S. (1993). Developmental levels of interdisciplinary collaborative practice committees. *Journal of Nursing Administration, 23*(7/8), 26-29.

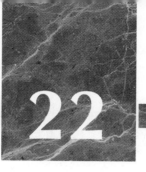

Persuasion and Negotiation

Chapter Objectives

❧

define and discuss persuasion

❧

distinguish among five reasons to exert influence at work

❧

analyze persuasion techniques

❧

analyze persuasion in leadership and management

❧

define and discuss negotiation

❧

compare three criteria for true negotiation

❧

explain four elements of negotiation

❧

describe ten steps of a negotiation process

❧

compare terms related to negotiation

❧

analyze negotiation strategies

❧

analyze collective bargaining and negotiation issues

❧

exercise critical thinking to conceptualize and analyze
possible solutions to a practical experience incident

onflicts are pervasive in groups and organizations. Both persuasion and negotiation are power and conflict interventions. Fundamentally, there are two ways individuals can get what they want: coercion or persuasion. If the person lacks the power to coerce or is unwilling to exercise coercion because of ethical concerns or practical concerns about its effects, then persuasion is used as an influence strategy. Bargaining and negotiation are twin influence techniques employed to persuade others to resolve conflicts or share resources. These concepts are common in everyday experiences of satisfying needs and wants; they also are an inherent part of human interactions at work. Thus nurses will find that persuasion and negotiation penetrate into work situations and become useful techniques for implementing decisions and gaining resources for quality client care and care management.

PERSUASION

DEFINITION

ersuasion is defined as a human communication activity designed to influence another to modify attitudes or alter behaviors by using argument, reasoning, or entreaty (see Chart 22.1). Persuasion emphasizes skill, knowledge, creativity, values, and unity (Hersey & Duldt, 1989). Unless a change is accomplished by using a purely directive strategy, nurses will use persuasion as a major technique for accomplishing goals. Persuasion is a basic, dynamic process of politics. It is the art of getting people to share a similar perception of the truth so they can work together (Curtin, 1991). It is founded on human psychology and the strengths and limitations of communication and personal status at any given point in time (Baker, 1986).

A prime objective of persuasion is generally action or activity. The persuader seeks to control others' perceptions of reality through the use of language to convince others that one option is more desirable than another (Hersey & Duldt, 1989). People respond negatively to the concept of persuasion because it sounds manipulative and, therefore, negative. Persuasion is neither bad nor good. It can be neutral or used for positive or negative purposes. Ideally, it leaves the receiver with some perception of choice (Rappsilber, 1982).

BACKGROUND

Persuasion, rather than force, is the appropriate action to use when the course of events need to be controlled for any length of time. Persuasion is indicated in at least two circumstances. First, whenever those involved have equivalent or complementary resources in terms of knowledge, skill, or authority. In other words, persuasion may need to be used when dealing with a peer. Second, whenever those involved in the interaction have common or even conflicting interests in the outcome of an activity, persuasion is used (Baker, 1986). As nurses work in collaborative, interdisciplinary teams, persuasion becomes an important skill for gaining objectives.

Persuaders assess the various motives of their targeted audiences. The most common appeals are for self-preservation, money, romance, and recognition (Baker, 1986). While advertising and marketing are the best examples of common persuasive appeals, nurses can apply persuasive appeals to their work environment. For example, nurses use persuasion in economic and general welfare issues or when proposing new programs.

Persuaders engage the attention of the audience and maneuver to speak to issues, needs, and values. Persuaders arouse feelings as a way of overcoming resistance and inertia. Persuaders challenge the audience to motivating actions (Hersey & Duldt, 1989). Effective persuaders include every listener by voice modulation, eye contact, gestures, and movements. They try to identify themselves with their audience, and they compliment and enlist their audience's attention (Baker, 1986). First a persuader has to penetrate the listener's defenses. This is done by identifying with the listener and trying to get the listener to identify with the persuader. This identification process creates feelings of trust and openness to listening to the persuader's message. Then the persuader will clarify the issue at hand as concretely as possible, because only then can the persuader maneuver into a position to negotiate an understanding of values. Technique and timing are vital, and credibility is essential. Persuaders will time their technique so as to lower the listener's defenses, compliment and enlist the listener's intelligence, clarify the issue at hand, and deliver a message (Baker, 1986).

Three aspects are crucial to the success of a persuasive communication: commitment, imagination, and trust (see Fig. 22.1). Commitment sparks arousal of feelings in the audience. Imagination paints a desired picture of reality. Trust is the key factor in eliciting followership (Hersey & Duldt, 1989). For example, a nurse who plans and develops a proposal to implement a new program to provide better access to healthcare for clients generally will need to obtain funding approval. Either a grant proposal document or an oral presentation may be used for persuasive communication. Commitment, imagination, and trust are essential aspects of success in persuasive communications. Similarly, persuasive communications are needed in the process of applying for a job.

A number of social science disciplines have been interested in aspects of persuasion. Speech communication views persuasion as rhetorical skills that process messages. Psychology's interest in persuasion is for its relationship to motivation. Sociology examines persuasion and the social/cultural environ-

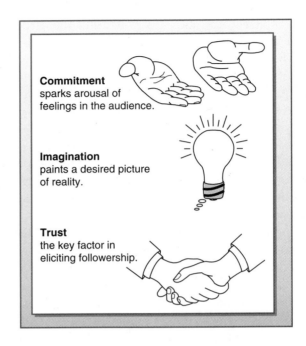

Commitment
sparks arousal of
feelings in the audience.

Imagination
paints a desired picture
of reality.

Trust
the key factor in
eliciting followership.

Figure 22.1
Elements of persuasive communication. (Data
from Hersey and Duldt [1989].)

ment. Public relations and politics emphasize creating favorable public images. Marketers apply methods to arouse or trigger buying/consumption.
Healthcare applies persuasion to client care and health services (Rappsilber,
1982). For example, nurses try to persuade clients to adopt wellness behaviors.
Nurse managers try to persuade nurses to work collaboratively with each other
and with other care providers.

Research about the ways people at work influence their colleagues has indicated five basic categories of reasons to exert influence (Kipnis & Schmidt,
1980):

- to obtain assistance with one's own job
- to get others to do their job
- to obtain personal benefits
- to initiate a change in work
- to improve the individual's job performance.

Eight categories of influence tactics have been identified: assertiveness, ingratiation, rationality, sanctions, exchange, upward appeal, blocking, and coalitions. The status of the person the persuader is trying to influence tends to be
the most decisive factor determining which tactic is chosen (Levenstein,
1982) (see Chapter 20).

Techniques of persuasion can be thought to be aimed at changing existing
attitudes and behaviors. In some persuasion techniques, the persuader seeks to
increase identification with himself or herself and reduce interpersonal dis-

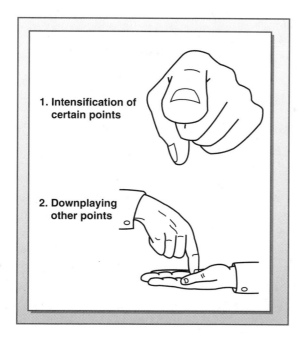

1. **Intensification of certain points**

2. **Downplaying other points**

Figure 22.2
Two major persuasion tactics. (Data from Rappsilber [1982].)

tance. Threats and fear are avoided; rational explanations are used to help change attitudes into actions. The two major persuasion tactics often employed are intensification of certain points and the downplaying of other points (see Fig. 22.2). Intensification uses repetition to imprint a way of responding on the receiver's mind, association or linking of one idea with something held in esteem, and contrasting of one idea to a less desirable one. Downplaying uses tactics of omission, diversion, and confusion. Key information can be withheld or concealed. Jargon and technical language can be used to create miscommunication and can be overwhelming in a way that makes people reluctant to ask questions. Effective change strategies and practical persuasive success are linked to choice of technique, audience attributes, effort, ethics, and evaluation (Rappsilber, 1982).

There has been some interest in how effective persuaders are so effective. The question arises as to why some individuals can seem to be able to sell anything, yet others are unable to be successful at sales. For example, neurolinguistic programming is a communication model dealing with ways to establish rapport. It is based on the study of effective communicators. Effective communicators establish intense rapport. Rapport is facilitated through structuring breathing patterns, body position, and language to mirror those of the other person. Individuals have different ways of patterning their thought processes and their concepts of the world. Part of understanding persons targeted for persuasion is to understand their patterning. A basic rule of persuasion is that speaking to another person in his or her language will increase the comfort and trust he or she feels, so the persuader is more likely to be successful (Knowles, 1983).

LEADERSHIP AND MANAGEMENT IMPLICATIONS

Persuasion is one technique for obtaining personal benefit, persuading others to cooperate, or satisfying organizational goals (Levenstein, 1982). Persuasion enters into interactions with roommates, spouses, or parents, and in most situations where there is a need that has to be fulfilled through other people. For example, in job interviews, the applicants are trying to persuade an organization to hire them. Applicants will talk positively about themselves. It takes an estimated four seconds to form an opinion about a person during the first meeting. That is, the average human being forms a lasting impression about another in four seconds. Therefore, the content of what the applicant has to say is likely to be less persuasive than more impressionistic aspects like body language, dress, and the image presented.

Strategies of persuasion are one of the tools available for nurses to use to accomplish client care goals. Part of the ability to be effective is having an expanded repertoire of strategies and tactics as alternative solutions when problems arise. Theories and techniques of persuasion can be applied to problems of client education, adherence to medical regimens, and functioning of health services (Rappsilber, 1982).

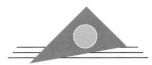 *Leadership & Management Behaviors*

LEADERSHIP BEHAVIORS	MANAGEMENT BEHAVIORS	OVERLAP AREAS
• persuades followers to accomplish goals	• persuades subordinates to accomplish organizational goals	• persuades others
• models collaborative behavior	• uses reasons to persuade employees to reach organizational goals	• negotiates with others
• communicates a vision persuasively	• bargains for scarce resources	
• convinces followers to work together	• exchanges ideas and plans	
• invites agreement and commitment	• negotiates agreements and contracts	
• negotiates common understandings		
• exchanges ideas		

One technique used for interpersonal effectiveness in groups, collaborative teams, and interdisciplinary work situations is persuasion. The tactics of persuasion are useful if the leadership situation is such that an authoritarian leadership style is not appropriate, but rather the situation is one where the nurse has to convince colleagues to work together.

Hersey and Duldt (1989) noted that communication is the core of leadership. If leadership is defined as a process of influencing, then the process of influencing is achieved through the type of communication called persuasion.

Harvey (1990) suggested that skillful, positive questioning can persuade people to accept change. People are more willing to commit themselves when they see personal benefits. Positive questioning capitalizes on this to establish hopeful, affirmative attitudes. In other words, problems can be approached from either a negative or a positive attitude. This is analogous to the classic question of whether a glass is half full or half empty. Inviting agreement, commitment, and realization of benefits facilitates necessary changes. Leadership and management styles vary. However, setting a positive and cooperative tone within a work group is each member's responsibility. Nurses frequently may find themselves in situations in which they need to persuade others to cooperate. Influencing others will take strategies of persuasion and negotiation.

NEGOTIATION

DEFINITION

Negotiation is defined as a process of give-and-take exchange among persons aimed at resolving problems or conflicts in a way that is acceptable to all parties (see Chart 22.2). *Bargaining,* a closely related term, is the exchanging of favors or trading activity. Negotiation uses a communication process and attempts to settle a problem or a conflict or gain more resources. Both bargaining and negotiating are strategies to divide up the areas of contention so that each party gains something. To reach a level of agreement, a back-and-forth process occurs in which the parties have sequential rounds of offering their position on terms and conditions for settlement. This process is called negotiation.

Negotiation has been described as getting what you want. It is a life process (Laser, 1981). Every desire and need is a potential occasion for negotiation. Exchanging ideas with the intention of changing relationships and conferring for agreement are negotiations. Negotiation focuses on gaining favor with parties from whom we want something (Cohen, 1980). Negotiation is the process that occurs when individuals engage in resolution to reach an agreement with stated conditions and expectations (Booth, 1993). Negotiation is used when both parties have strong feelings or conflicting views, and when there is a need for agreement, resolution, or compromise.

CHART 22.2
◠ DEFINITIONS

Negotiation
a process of give-and-take exchange among persons aimed at resolving problems or conflicts in a way that is acceptable to all parties.

Bargaining
the exchange of favors or trading activity.

Negotiation can be applied specifically to labor-management disputes and unionization. Nurses may work in settings in which the RNs and/or ancillary workers are unionized. In unionized settings, the term negotiation takes on a specific collective bargaining connotation. *Collective bargaining* is a prescribed realm of negotiation in which there are specific laws and rules that govern the negotiating activity. Negotiation becomes more narrowly defined as a process in which the terms and conditions of work are resolved between the employer and the organized representatives of the employees. Collective bargaining exists to limit employers' ability to take unilateral action (Cohen, 1989) (see Chapter 21).

BACKGROUND

Negotiation is a tool, strategy, or a technique useful to avoid head-on competition or a win-lose conflict outcome. Negotiation employs communication, interpersonal skills, persuasion, the ability to articulate a point of view, and the acknowledgement of the other person's position. Learning to negotiate is a way to acknowledge each party's needs and to reach a win-win conflict solution.

To contrast the strategies of influence, there is a difference between win-win and win-lose conflict outcomes. Negotiation for conflict resolution can be one of two basic types: competitive (only one party wins) or cooperative (all parties win). The objective in both cases is to achieve agreement (Smeltzer, 1991). Competitive negotiation brings about a win-lose or lose-lose result and is more associated with persuasion and compromise. However, negotiation as a strategy is more closely associated with cooperative negotiation. Cooperative negotiation is a strategy of pursuing common goals, acknowledging the other party's needs and goals, and incorporating them in resolutions. Satisfaction is the medium of exchange during a negotiation. Win-lose means solely attaining one party's goals, without regard to the other parties or their needs. In a problem solving modality, participants negotiate to equalize power, whereas in a win-lose modality one side emphasizes its own power and independence by trying to force its position on somebody else. The win-lose strategy incorporates an all-or-nothing posture. Negotiation uses trust as opposed to exploitation of the other party. Thus successful negotiation provides satisfaction to both parties (Laser, 1981).

Successful negotiation involves identifying the needs of the other party. Identifying the other party's needs puts an adversary in a better position to exchange and negotiate by acknowledging that other party's need and incorporating it into a solution. Recognizing personal ambitions and interests and then establishing a constructive dialogue about how to satisfy those needs is a beginning to negotiation. This requires a basic understanding of human interaction and reaction and the possible strategies for negotiation.

The Process of Negotiation

Nurses will find situations arising in which negotiation takes place. For example, nurses negotiate with physicians about client care management needs. Nurses negotiate with each other for distribution of the workload or administration of the work group. Sometimes nurses negotiate over vacation time off or coverage of the unit. Negotiations follow a process. First, three criteria need to be met for true negotiation to occur (Nierenberg, 1973; Smeltzer, 1991): the issue must be negotiable, the negotiators must be interested in both giving and taking, and the parties must trust each other and the negotiating process. Thus nurses can evaluate each negotiation circumstance for the presence of these three criteria. Any negotiation has four elements (Laser, 1981):

1. *Goals* that are both conflicting and nonconflicting
2. *Values* that vary as to urgency and priority as information is exchanged
3. *Mutual victory* when both sides realize satisfaction and feel something has been won
4. *Incomplete information* since parties never reveal all information and thereby shift the negotiating power

The negotiation process occurs as a back-and-forth dance that is triggered by one party attempting to alter the current relationship with another party. Despite the issues, it is desirable to maintain the relationship, hence negotiation. However, the climate surrounding a negotiating incident may vary from the parties being defensive to the parties being supportive. In a defensive milieu, there are feelings of superiority and strategies of controlling. In a supportive environment, feelings are focused on the problem issue and strategies are sincere and problem-focused. Poor listening, inaccurate communication, strong reactions to stress, or failure to disclose information or feelings may contribute to a defensive environment (Nierenberg, 1973; Smeltzer, 1991).

The process of negotiation may proceed through a series of steps. The ten steps to most negotiation processes are (Smeltzer, 1991):

1. Preparing for negotiation
2. Communicating a general overview of what is to be accomplished
3. Reviewing why negotiation is required
4. Redefining the issue or issues
5. Selecting when issues will be addressed
6. Encouraging discussion throughout the process
7. Addressing the fall-back or compromise position for both parties on each issue
8. Agreeing in principle during the settlement stage
9. Recapping and summarizing the agreement
10. Monitoring compliance with the agreement after settlement

Nurses should expect negotiations to follow steps similar to the ones presented here. However, the more formal the negotiation process, the more closely the steps will be used in a systematic manner. Nurses preparing to initiate a negotiation will find a review of these steps helpful.

Formal negotiations also use a specific language. A review of terms will clarify the meaning of the language of negotiation. Some terms used in the process of negotiation are (Laser,1981):

- issues: the things to be negotiated or resolved.
- deadlock or stalemate: what occurs when no agreement can be reached by the parties.
- impasse: what occurs when an issue cannot be resolved to the parties' mutual satisfaction. Impasse occurs first, then deadlock.
- concession: what is given to provide satisfaction to the other party in order to advance toward a settlement.
- power: the ability to influence the other party's behavior.

There are numerous strategies available for use by nurses in the process of negotiation. The most effective use of a technique occurs when it is deliberately planned or consciously used. Laser (1981) identified four significant strategies for negotiation (see Chart 22.3). Awareness of strategies enhances a nurse's ability to choose alternative approaches and enhance effectiveness.

If the end result is obtaining what you want, then successful negotiation will incorporate the following points (Kippenbrock, 1992; Kirk, 1986):

- Open the parameters to negotiate as a way of controlling the framing of the issues and areas.

CHART 22.3 ∾ LASER'S FOUR NEGOTIATING STRATEGIES

The Flinch
to flinch is to draw back or wince at the initial proposition or opening position of the other party. This uncovers whatever doubt or uncertainty exists in the other party and opens a negotiation dialogue potential.

The Deadline
deadlines produce results and are advisable for every negotiation. However, negotiate the deadline.

The Nibble
a nibble is a small something extra that is sought and obtained after a settlement is apparently reached. The nibble relies on the impatience to conclude a negotiation and the ease of obtaining small decisions after a large decision has been made.

The Concession
concessions that are valuable to the other party but are of little or no value to you are possible in almost every negotiation. They should be identified and used strategically. Make sure the other party understands that this is a concession. Avoid making the first major concession. Keep track of concessions exchanged.

Data from Laser (1981).

- Prepare thoroughly and completely.
- Dress carefully and be aware of body language and nonverbal aspects.
- Use talking and listening skills for good communication.
- Maintain a positive tone.
- Take calculated risks.
- Work toward a solution that everyone can support.

The strategies of negotiation that are chosen in any situation may depend on whether the climate for negotiation is supportive or defensive. Defensive environments can lead to negotiation mistakes such as poor listening and mismanagement of issues. Progress should be monitored throughout the negotiation to avoid communication blocks and to overcome deadlocks. Needs, power, and timing are the essential components of negotiating (Smeltzer, 1991). Information becomes a critical resource in any negotiation process. Information about a party's needs and awareness can be a strategic power resource and becomes an input to decision making. Both verbal and nonverbal cues are important in negotiating. Information may be altered, filtered, given selectively, or withheld as an advantage-gaining power strategy (Cohen, 1980; Smeltzer, 1991).

Experts also suggest that any negotiator always maintain room to maneuver. It is essential that opening positions contain enough latitude so that both parties can win, yet concessions not drop below minimum requirements (Laser, 1981). Nurses may need to be encouraged to build an experiential base in negotiation. Confidence and skill are built through practice in negotiation in low risk areas. It is important to remember the influence of information power in negotiation. Foolishly assuming that all the facts are known overlooks the secret agenda, or unspoken and purposely concealed position, that is presumed to exist in a negotiation. Loss to the negotiating party may occur. Thus nurses may need to build careful assessment and healthy skepticism into negotiations.

LEADERSHIP AND MANAGEMENT IMPLICATIONS

The work of successful nurses and managers depends upon the ability to negotiate. Nurses need to be able to articulate needs, positions, and justification for resources. The different techniques of conflict resolution and influencing in nursing include bargaining and negotiation as one method of gaining power and persuading others to grant autonomy by using individual and collective action. The use of collective action at both the work group and the larger profession levels can make a difference in terms of autonomy in professional practice, job satisfaction, and a general positive feeling about the profession of nursing (see Leadership and Management table, p. 436).

Human interaction issues are the general arena in which leaders and managers spend most of their time. Power and conflict become important focal points of human interactions in organizations that may need management or resolution through persuasion or negotiations. Both conflict resolution and negotiation techniques can and should be used to manage change. As nurses are confronted with the impact of mergers, downsizing, restructuring and reengineering, and alterations in skill mix, negotiation skills are needed. Negotiation techniques can help improve relationships and can aid managers to function in their designated roles. Negotiation is useful to educate clients and other professionals about nurses' roles and contributions, to get a fairer exchange in decision making autonomy, to interact with vendors, to deal with client complaints, to interact with integrated health systems and group healthcare purchasers, to deal with unionized employees, to respond to the media, and to negotiate with medical staff and managed care groups to consolidate contracts (Sherer, 1994).

CURRENT ISSUES AND TRENDS

Negotiation skills are being used by nurses in debates on national healthcare policy, uncompensated care issues, and standards of care development. Negotiation skills also are used in legal actions and malpractice suits, as well as with collective bargaining negotiations (Sherer, 1994).

The year 1992 marked the end of a period of significant wage gains for nurses. It appeared to mark yet another swing in nursing's chronic shortage-surplus cycles. First, pay gains slowed to about half their pace of the previous two years. Then a new wave of structural changes in hospitals occurred via alterations in staff mix, not filling some vacancies, phasing out RN positions, and downsizing to reduce costs. This activity echoes a cycle begun 15 years ago: shortage in the late 1970s boosting salaries, then downsizing triggered by Diagnosis-related Groups (DRGs) and the implementation of prospective reimbursement for healthcare financing in the mid-1980s (Brider, 1993).

Tension and resistance have been mounting between healthcare unions and employers who respond to cost containment with staff reductions. As noted in Chapter 21, the 1990s are a time of change and restructuring in healthcare. Since 1992, nurses have experienced threats to their long-term job security and benefits. Layoffs and reductions in hours are becoming more common; incentives are being slashed; and a growing trend is to cease across-the-board pay raises and substitute one-time or "merit" raises. Strike tactics, the labor union's major power strategy to persuade management to negotiate with workers, have lost some effectiveness as employers were willing to do without workers. However, in 1992, data showed that those nurses who were organized maintained a competitive edge in pay and benefits over those who were not unionized (Brider, 1993).

Exemplar 22.1

Renegotiating Advanced Practice Roles

Our five-level, Benner-based, nursing clinical ladder at the University of Virginia Medical Center recognizes advanced practice at the fourth and fifth tiers. The role elements of advanced practice are recognized as follows: clinical practice, education, research, consultation, and management. Initially, at the implementation of the clinical ladder, the clinician 4 role was primarily that of direct patient care. At the clinician 4 level, registered nurses were providing staffing coverage 75% of their scheduled hours. The focus of the remaining 25% of their time was to be negotiated with the unit manager.

Our Surgical Service Center encompasses the surgical intensive care unit—two acute surgical units serving general surgery, trauma, transplant, urology, and surgical subspecialty patients—and a Wound Care Center serving burn and plastic surgery patients. There are four unit-based clinician 4s currently in the service center. Recent changes in our organizational structure, service center development, and the healthcare environment at large have led us to look closely at advanced practice roles.

The outcomes we plan to achieve through the renegotiation of these roles are:

- improved patient outcomes via care coordination, early planning, multidisciplinary communication, and education
- improved patient satisfaction
- reduction in length of stay
- reduction in cost per case

To accomplish these outcomes, we had to prepare to exclude the clinician 4s from daily staffing. Each would shift his or her focus to a discrete patient population within our service line. Advanced clinicians are ideal persons to effect these outcomes in our setting: they have the expert knowledge of the clinical needs of these patients as well as an awareness of the complex system issues that influence the patients' experience and overall outcome.

All of the advanced clinicians had reservations about this shift in approach to their role. Their concerns varied from fear of losing their highly valued clinical skills of direct care delivery to issues of role identity and acceptance on the part of the other staff. They agreed they saw benefit in this approach but were concerned about the personal impact it would have on them. This was clearly a situation in which persuasion and negotiation were indicated.

We began with discussions about the benefits and goals of this patient-centered approach. We also discussed the ever changing, competitive healthcare environment and the need to drive down our costs of caring for these complex surgical patients. By increasing the level of their understanding of the situation we faced, the group was persuaded to move the discussion forward to developing and negotiating the actual responsibilities of the role. Negotiations occurred between the advanced clinicians and manager and among the individual clinicians. The patient groups were identified as trauma, transplant, general surgery, and plastic surgery. These would be the first patient groups the clinician 4s would focus on. It was up to them to negotiate for which group of patients they would align themselves. They managed this process very effectively. This required open-mindedness and willingness to compromise, as it was not possible for all clinicians to have the patient population of their choice.

Next we negotiated how much if any of their time would be spend in direct patient care. We agreed that they would support patient care on an as needed basis but that they would not be scheduled for any routine patient care time at the outset. Because this required the addition of full-time employees to our units, much time and attention was needed for the organization and implementation of these new roles. A third negotiable point was which projects, from previously negotiated roles, could remain a part of new responsibilities. For example, one member of the group had been the principal investigator on a clinical research project. We would clearly want to continue to support this research with the time necessary to see it through to its completion.

The final step of our negotiations was to decide on outcome measures and the way in which we would evaluate the implementation and success of this role change. Measures of success would include patient satisfaction, staff satisfaction with the role, length of stay, and cost per case. We are presently at the point of implementation.

DONNA W. MARKEY, RN, MSN
Patient Care Service Manager
Transplant and Surgical Subspecialties
University of Virginia Health
 Sciences Center
Charlottesville, Virginia

Tensions in healthcare downsizing have sparked a resurgence of interest in collective bargaining negotiations and labor union activity in nursing. Staff cuts have sparked unionizing drives in Florida and a fight to set staffing ratios and bar unlicensed workers from performing procedures requiring nursing skills by the California Nurses Association (AJN Headlines, 1993; Brider, 1993). Job cuts continued to be reported as hospitals merged, and nurses began speaking out against inadequate staffing (AJNNewsline, 1994a; 1994b).

Since the Taft-Hartley amendments of 1974 opened federally protected labor union activity to nurses, two Supreme Court decisions have had a profound effect on nurses' collective bargaining. A 1991 Supreme Court decision upheld specialized all-RN bargaining units by recognizing small, homogeneous units of employees such as nurses and physicians. The issue had been vigorously opposed by the American Hospital Association, who feared unionization (AJN News, 1991).

A major Supreme Court ruling occurred in 1994. The Court held that nurses who supervise lesser-skilled personnel should be considered supervisors and, therefore, are not protected by the National Labor Relations Act (NLRA) that allows non-supervisory workers to organize and bargain (see Chapter 21). Such "supervisory" nurses' rights to join organized activity about client care concerns and employment issues under NLRA are jeopardized. The decision was triggered by a case involving LPNs who were fired from a nursing home for complaining about working conditions. The LPNs were deemed supervisors because they assigned and monitored aides' work. Although professionals are expressly covered by NLRA, and every professional's work involves some degree of directing the work of others, the long-standing definition of a supervisor as one who hires, fires, disciplines, assigns and rewards other employees was not applied to nurses. The distinction between employees who have the control that places them in management and those who perform highly skilled work with incidental supervisory activity was not upheld by the majority decision (AJNNewsline, 1994c).

With healthcare being a service industry that comprises a large segment of the U.S. economy, labor-management conflicts spark negotiating activity. As nurses feel job security threats and stress due to workload, negotiations take on a greater importance and become more common.

RESEARCH NOTE

Source: Buerhaus, P., (1992). Nursing, competition, and quality. *Nursing Economic$*, *10*(1), 21-29.

Purpose

Negotiation and persuasion are nursing strategies useful in competitive situations. The purpose of this article is to analyze changing economic incentives under market-driven competition that create challenges and opportunities as compared to regulatory control of healthcare services. Regulation failed to control costs and ensure quality of care. Economic competition is projected to develop more fully in healthcare in the 1990s. Economic competition implies strong incentives to minimize production costs in order to be competitive in pricing products and services. Capital and labor costs need to be minimized while quality is maintained or improved. Consumers have choices, and providers conduct market research to assess consumer preferences. Nurses will face intensifying pressures for low-cost, high-quality care.

Discussion

Challenges and opportunities for nursing include pressures to reduce costs, pressures to change regulations governing nursing practice, opportunities to increase nursing's value by quality of care, pressures to integrate nursing's quality management with the larger organization, and opportunities to understand what purchasers want from nursing. Persuasion can be used to enhance the strength of nursing's reputation. Outcomes data can be used in resource-related negotiations. Nurses need to be aware of tensions surrounding spending resources to improve satisfaction at the expense of spending them to improve quality.

Application to Practice

The healthcare future is likely to include elements of greater competition. The challenge to nurses is to seek resolution of cost and quality concerns. Persuasion can be used in conjunction with traditional marketing efforts. Negotiation is a tool for bargaining within a competitive environment and for negotiating contracts for services. Nurses need to be prepared to meet the challenges and opportunities afforded by economic competition. Rewards will come to those who offer a quality product, take risks, and innovate.

SUMMARY

- Persuasion and negotiation are influence techniques.
- Persuasion is human communication designed to influence another to modify attitudes or alter behaviors by using argument, reasoning, or entreaty.
- Persuasion is used to generate action or activity.
- Persuasion is used to control the course of events.

- Persuaders use appeals and engage their audience's emotions.
- Successful persuasive communication uses commitment, imagination, and trust.
- There are five categories of reasons to exert influence.
- There are eight types of influence tactics.
- Intensification and downplaying are two common persuasion tactics.
- Persuasion is used both for obtaining personal benefit and to satisfy organizational goals.
- Communication is the core of leadership; influencing is achieved through persuasion.
- Negotiation is a give-and-take exchange to resolve conflicts.
- Negotiation often is applied to collective bargaining.
- Negotiation is used to avoid a win-lose outcome.
- Three criteria set the framework for true negotiation.
- There are four elements to the negotiation process.
- There are ten steps to the negotiation process.
- Four negotiating strategies are the flinch, the deadline, the nibble, and the concession.
- The work of a manager depends on the ability to negotiate.
- Negotiation is used to manage change and in labor union activities.

Study Questions

1. What persuades nurses to become a nurse?
2. What feelings are associated with an interview for a nursing position?
3. What was the last issue you negotiated?
4. What behaviors contribute to cooperative and productive negotiation?
5. What words or actions indicate competitive negotiation?
6. What approaches or strategies of negotiation are most effective for nursing?
7. What factors are facilitators or barriers to collaboration among professionals?
8. Does collective bargaining increase professionalism in nursing?
9. What organizational factors are associated with unionization?
10. Is positional power eroding in nursing? With what forms of negotiation can nurses replace positional power?

Critical Thinking Exercise

The Friendly Visitor Home Health Agency wants to negotiate a contract for services with a regional Health Maintenance Organization (HMO). The HMO decides to contract with providers based on some mix of cost and quality parameters. The Friendly Visitor nursing director does not know exactly what tips the decision. The staff at Friendly Visitor have begun the planning for a contract proposal. They have their costs projected on a spreadsheet.

1. Is there a problem?

2. What is the problem?

3. Why might Friendly Visitor have a problem(s)?

4. What should the Friendly Visitor staff do next?

5. What information will be important for persuasion?

6. What information will be important for negotiation?

7. What strategies might the Friendly Visitor staff adopt?

REFERENCES

AJN Headlines. (1993). Staff cuts are sparking unionizing drives. *American Journal of Nursing, 93*(9), 9.

AJN News. (1991). Unanimous Supreme Court vote for all-RN units ignites a major campaign to organize nurses. *American Journal of Nursing, 91*(6), 95, 103-104.

AJNNewsline. (1994a). Huge job cuts loom in Massachusetts as HMOs take over. *American Journal of Nursing, 94*(7), 69, 74-75.

AJNNewsline. (1994b). Fired for speaking up, an RN wins Supreme Court's support for a trial. *American Journal of Nursing, 94*(7), 69-70.

AJNNewsline. (1994c). Striking at bargaining rights, Court says RNs are supervisors. *American Journal of Nursing, 94*(7), 67, 70-71.

Baker, D. (1986). Persuasion: The power is in the art. *Nursing Management, 17*(11), 59.

Booth, R. (1993). Dynamics of conflict and conflict management. In D. Mason, S. Talbott, & J. Leavitt (Eds.), *Policy and politics for nurses: Action and change in the workplace, government, organizations, and community* (2nd ed.) (pp. 149-165). Philadelphia: Saunders.

Brider, P. (1993). Where did the jobs go? *American Journal of Nursing, 93*(4), 31-40.

Cohen, H. (1980). *You can negotiate anything.* Secaucus, NJ: L. Stuart.

Cohen, A. (1989). The management rights clause in collective bargaining. *Nursing Management, 20*(11), 24-34.

Curtin, L. (1991). Leaders: The organization's pacemakers. *Nursing Management, 22*(3), 6-8.

Harvey, K. (1990). The power of positive questioning. *Nursing Management, 21*(5), 94-96.

Hersey, P., & Duldt, B. (1989). *Situational leadership in nursing.* Norwalk, CT: Appleton & Lange.

Kippenbrock, T. (1992). Power at meetings: Strategies to move people. *Nursing Economic$, 10*(4), 282-286.

Kipnis, D., & Schmidt, S. (1980). Intraorganizational influence tactics: Explorations in getting one's way. *Journal of Applied Psychology, 65*(4), 440-452.

Kirk, R. (1986). Negotiations: Getting what you want. *Journal of Nursing Administration, 16*(12). 6-9.

Knowles, R. (1983). Building rapport through neuro-linguistic programming. *American Journal of Nursing, 83*(7), 1010-1014.

Laser, R. (1981). I win-you win negotiating. *Journal of Nursing Administration, 11*(11/12). 24-29.

Levenstein, A. (1982). Tactics of persuasion. *Nursing Management, 13*(11), 40-41.

Nierenberg, G. (1973). *Fundamentals of negotiating.* New York: Hawthorne.

Rappsilber, C. (1982). Persuasion as a mechanism for change. In J. Lancaster and W. Lancaster (Eds.), *The nurse as a change agent: Concepts for advanced nursing practice* (pp. 132-145). St. Louis: Mosby.

Sherer, J. (1994). Resolving conflict {the right way}. *Hospitals & Health Networks, 68*(8), 52-55.

Smeltzer, C. (1991). The art of negotiation: An everyday experience. *Journal of Nursing Administration, 21*(7/8), 26-30.

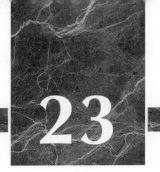

Staffing and Scheduling

Chapter Objectives

❧

define and describe staffing

❧

define and describe scheduling and staff mix

❧

define nursing resources, nursing workload, acuity and intensity

❧

compare four essential elements of a staffing program

❧

explain suggested steps for developing staffing patterns

❧

analyze workload measurement and patient classification systems

❧

define and discuss differentiated practice

❧

analyze staffing issues and economic pressures

❧

analyze the use of nurse extenders

❧

exercise critical thinking to conceptualize and analyze
possible solutions to a practical experience incident

*n*ursing is one of the occupations that comprise the healthcare delivery system. Nursing care delivery is a service industry whose product is client care and client outcomes. A service industry relies on service providers. For nursing, this means registered nurses and the assistive personnel who work with nurses. Whether in hospitals, community nursing organizations, long-term care, or other settings, the delivery of nursing services to clients is founded on having the right skill mix of providers in the right numbers at the right place and properly prepared to render care. Regulatory agencies like the Joint Commission on Accreditation of Healthcare Organizations (JCAHO) identify a standard that calls for a sufficient number of qualified registered nurses to be on duty at all times to give clients nursing care that requires the specialized skill and judgment of an RN (Cleland, 1990). Registered nurses can be considered a scarce human resource critical to the provision of healthcare because the availability of RN services to clients may be limited by financial reimbursement issues. Further, healthcare facilities limit the number of RN positions and overtime work when they tightly control labor budgets. Thus nurses are a human resource that may be sparsely deployed.

DEFINITIONS

Staffing is defined as human resources planning to fill positions in an organization with qualified personnel (see Chart 23.1). Short-term plans involve filling existing positions. Long-term plans are concerned with determining the gap between the present and a desired future human resources status (Jernigan, 1988). Staffing is the process of creating a plan to determine how many and what types of personnel will be needed for a given unit for each shift (Barnum & Mallard, 1989). The determination should be made based on production requirements: client needs, program goals, and/or set standards.

Scheduling is defined as the ongoing implementation of the staffing pattern by assigning individual personnel to work specific hours and days and in a specific unit or area (Barnum & Mallard, 1989). Scheduling generally means the actual preparing of work hour assignments according to the staffing plan and mix. Staff mix is defined as the skill level of individuals delivering the required care (Kirby & Wiczai, 1985).

The term nursing resources refers to the number and types of employees designated to provide nursing services to clients (Brett & Tonges, 1990). There are many ways to distribute resources within any organization. Nursing workload is defined as the nursing care needs of clients. It refers to the nursing resources required for individuals or groups of clients. Nursing workload is a measurement of the nursing work activities and the dependence of the clients on nursing care. Nursing workload in a hospital is a function of two variables: the number of patient days and the hours of nursing care required per patient day (Kirby & Wiczai, 1985). Workload is the use of time, and time is the basis of nursing workload measurement.

Acuity is defined as the severity of illness or client condition. Acuity can translate into volume (census, visits, or encounters) or severity or intensity.

CHART 23.1
∽ DEFINITIONS

Staffing
human resources planning to fill positions in an organization with qualified personnel.

Scheduling
the ongoing implementation of the staffing pattern by assigning individual personnel to work specific hours and days in a specific unit or area.

Data from Barnum and Mallard (1989).

CHART 23.2
↩ FOUR MAJOR
DIMENSIONS OF
NURSING INTENSITY

- Severity of illness (the medical condition and how ill the person is in relationship to abnormality and instability of physiological parameters)
- Client dependency (need for assistance with activities of daily living)
- Complexity of nursing care
- Time (the hours of direct and indirect care received by a client)

Data from Prescott (1991).

Nursing intensity is defined as both the amount of care and the complexity of care needed by patients in hospitals. Prescott (1991) identified four major dimensions to nursing intensity (see Chart 23.2). The four components of severity of illness, client dependency on nursing, complexity, and time are related to each other and have been combined into a 10 item nursing intensity scale, called the Patient Intensity for Nursing Index (PINI) (Soekin & Prescott, 1991). Intensity is usually a composite measure of the amount of work or time involved with a level of complexity of the care required (Detwiler & Clark, 1995).

A *nurse extender* is defined as an individual who assists in the care of clients and enables the nurse to provide a larger volume of services (Gardner, 1991). Nurse extenders include both licensed and unlicensed assistive personnel (UAPs). Both nursing assistants and technicians fall in the UAP category (Barter, McLaughlin, & Thomas, 1994).

BACKGROUND

Staffing and scheduling are two aspects of human resources management and the allocation of scarce and expensive personnel resources. To increase the chance of successful and appropriate allocation of resources, the administrative function of planning is involved in staffing and scheduling. The planning may be simple or complex. It may be as simple as deciding what is wanted and then as complex as determining what must be done to obtain it. In some cases sophisticated analytical and informatics tools may be employed to derive a model of what is needed. Staffing and scheduling have obvious budgeting and costing implications. This linkage of an expensive labor supply to the fluctuations in client care needs and revenue income absorbs considerable managerial time and effort in nursing. The effort is especially intense under conditions of tight budgets and cost containment pressures.

Staffing Decisions

Considerable preliminary work precedes staffing and scheduling decisions. Following are the four elements essential to a staffing program are (Ramey, 1973):
1. A statement of philosophy for the unit, department, and institution that defines values and beliefs
2. Objectives general for the department and specific for each unit
3. Job descriptions for each type and level of personnel
4. A determination of the frequency with which nursing care is to be provided and who will provide it

It is thought that the quality of a staffing program is related to the philosophy and objectives. Staffing by patient census in a hospital usually ignores nursing's philosophy, objectives, and job descriptions in predicting staffing. This in turn complicates efforts to evaluate or measure progress toward objectives and standards (Arndt & Huckabay, 1980).

Staffing decisions usually are based on some measure of volume and/or time. Staffing may be the result of methods of time sampling, work sampling, continuous sampling of time or work, or self-report. The measurement of the staff's workload in many instances is not done through an ongoing compilation of what actually occurs. Rather, a workload measure is devised as a proxy. For example, the mean direct care time can be determined for an "average client." Averages, or means, are sensitive to outliers. This means that unusually high or low numbers throw the mean value off from the typical case. Thus changes in average direct care times or shifts within severity of illness categories may have a substantial impact on staffing. Averages do not allow individualization to a client's care experience and subsequent linkage to outcomes at the level of an individual client. Staffing decisions are setting-specific, based on some combination of minimum external standards; outcomes for clients, staff, and the organization; risk factors; and organizational revenue.

An intense focus on measuring and quantifying the time spent in nursing activities, usually by means of time-and-motion studies, makes nurses uncomfortable. This is because of the similarity to models of industrial efficiency. Discomfort is further generated when nursing's psychosocial work aspects and valuing time being with and interacting with clients and families are not taken into account. It is difficult to justify the reduction of professional nursing care to repetitive tasks and procedures.

Nurse staffing in some settings may be based on standardized volume measures (see Table 23.1). For example, a home health agency may set a minimum

---

Table 23.1

Standardized Volume Measures

VOLUME MEASURE	SETTING
Number of visits	Home health agency
Core staff	Emergency department
Patient days or occupied beds	Inpatient hospital unit
Client encounters	Ambulatory care clinic
Covered lives	Capitated reimbursement system in a health maintenance organization (HMO)
Births	Labor and delivery
Operations	Operating room surgical services
Exercise sessions	Wellness program

Some data from Kirk (1988).

of five visits per day as the norm for staffing. In a small community hospital's labor and delivery unit, the staffing pattern may be two RNs as a standard. These and other forms of staffing ratios based on volume measures such as patient census or client encounters ignore important factors related to planning nurse staffing. Other factors include amount of travel or downtime, type of equipment available to facilitate the staff's work, ease of communication, the physical design of a unit, proximity to related resources, the availability of specialists, and individual client complexity. Clearly, knowledge of the nursing time needed to care for different types of clients is valuable in determining staffing (Arndt & Huckabay, 1980). However, simplistic workload measures and many patient classification systems do not yield the type of data needed to make the leap between workload data and staffing plans. The numbers may be calculated, but they are not helpful to nurses for comfortable and perceived workable staffing decisions. The lack of an easy fit between workload data and staffing plans creates a level of stress and tension in the work of nursing.

Staffing Methods

Nursing provides a service. The common denominator for identifying and measuring activities for quality and quantity is the unit of service. The unit of service is a volume measure. The unit of service may be patient days, treatments, visits, encounters, births, operations, exercise sessions, or client contact. Time is measured in "hour per . . . ," for example, hours per patient day (HPPD). Averages or standards may be derived and entered into staffing planning and calculations (Kirk, 1988). Activities related to client care are evaluated in relation to the consumption of staff labor per hour. For example, inpatient nursing units have calculated the HPPD as a productivity measure. If a generic productivity equation divides work inputs by work outputs, then the nursing application of this productivity standard divides nursing hours required by the unit of service (such as patient days) to result in HPPD (Soule & Dobson, 1992). Calculating the HPPD is an example of a direct method of patient classification related staffing (DeGroot, 1994). Using HPPD alone as a productivity system assumes a direct relationship between HPPD and salary expense per patient day (SEPPD), a measure of cost. Research indicates that HPPD alone is insufficient for either accurate staffing projections or for monitoring and controlling labor budgets (DeGroot, 1994; Soule & Dobson, 1992).

Although there are various calculations and ways to determine nurse staffing, no completely satisfactory method has been identified. Kirby and Wiczai (1985) noted that the credibility of nursing leadership and management may be tested, since staff nurses question the appropriateness and fairness of the distribution of resources, and hospital administration questions nursing's ability to manage costs.

Two general methods of nurse staffing are the traditional fixed staffing and controlled variable staffing (see Chart 23.3). With fixed staffing, staffing is built around a fixed projected maximum workload requirement, and the plan is based on maximum workload conditions. With variable staffing, units are staffed below maximum workload conditions and staff then supplemented as needed. Supplementation may be done by creating a "float pool" or by using supplemental staffing agencies. This is a system of flexible resource management (Bennett, 1981). Fixed staffing based on historical census trend data and projections results in predictable staffing and scheduling that is handy for budgeting. However, real world occurrences of workload fluctuations, both high and low, result in overtime, short staffing, or periods of idleness, all with budget and satisfaction implications. Kirk (1988) listed a semiflexible system as a third type of nurse staffing system. In this system, about 10% to 15% of staff are fixed, while the rest are flexible and the volume is adjusted to match the need.

If variable staffing is to be used, then a system is needed that accurately measures workload. In an accurate system, effective staffing would result from matching resources to the workload. The system needs to be responsive to fluctuations in workload, simple to use, and credible with both nurses and administration (Kirby & Wiczai, 1985).

Steps in Developing a Staffing Pattern

Since the majority of nurses have been working in acute care inpatient hospital settings, staffing patterns have been more elaborate for hospital nursing staffing. Ramey (1973) suggested eleven steps for developing hospital staffing patterns:

1. Select criteria to classify clients into severity of illness categories. Survey the unit at intervals to establish percentages.
2. Record all direct and indirect activities, the number of times performed, and the total time needed for performance for a specified period.
3. Collect data on a representative number of clients to determine valid averages by classification.
4. Collect data in several ways.
5. Average the number of minutes required to accomplish each nursing activity to equal an average performance time.
6. Determine the average performance time for new functions to be instituted.
7. Note the skill level of personnel required to perform each nursing activity per severity of illness category.
8. Calculate the average amount of nursing time required by each client in each severity of illness category by the percentage of time devoted to them by both professional and nonprofessional nursing personnel by shift.

9. Obtain the projected patient days on the unit for the year.
10. Calculate the total number of nursing hours needed annually for the unit. Compute the hours worked in a year by professional and non-professional staff, discounting time off.
11. From the average amount of nursing time required and the total number of nursing hours needed annually, derive the number of persons required on each shift. An additional calculation is needed to determine the number of personnel needed to cover inservicing, unit administration, orientation, and research or professional development activities.

LEADERSHIP AND MANAGEMENT IMPLICATIONS

Workload Measurement and Patient Classification Systems

Patient classification means grouping patients or clients according to a standard assessment of their nursing care requirements over a specified period of time (Reitz, 1985). Patient classifications systems provide a quantified measure of the nursing time and effort required to care for clients (Giovannetti, 1979). Nurse managers seek ways to quantify nursing resource requirements. Three ways to accomplish this quantification are by time-and-motion techniques, work sampling techniques, and acuity estimation or patient classification systems.

Time-and-motion studies are aimed at developing time standards for specific nursing activities. In time-and-motion studies, nurses are observed to determine actual activities performed and the amount of time devoted to each task. Average or mean times are derived per task and a uniform standard time per task is established. Many patient classification systems use this informa-

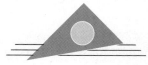 *Leadership & Management Behaviors*

LEADERSHIP BEHAVIORS	MANAGEMENT BEHAVIORS	OVERLAP AREAS
• integrates philosophy, values, and beliefs in staffing plan	• develops a staffing plan	• plans staffing
• enables followers to self-schedule	• makes out a schedule	• communicates about staffing and scheduling
• communicates the need for the staff mix	• allocates labor resources	
• collaborates with others in staffing and scheduling	• determines job descriptions	
• encourages discussion of workload issues	• matches client needs to available staff	
	• negotiates staff coverage	
	• evaluates workload data	
	• communicates the staffing method	

tion in deriving standard times for the average client. Although the practice of nursing is central to a healthcare organization's products, no generally accepted standards of nursing time exist (Mowry & Korpman, 1986).

Work sampling is used to sample work activities by observation at regular intervals over random times. Activities are classified by types, and probability and statistics are used on the work activities observations to generalize to all nursing care. The information needed to classify activities, however, may not be clear or distinct. The concepts of time-and-motion and work sampling became the foundation for systems of patient classification based on nursing time requirements and labor costs. The various patient classification systems have been used to project staffing and scheduling (Mowry & Korpman, 1986).

Patient classification systems are developed to group or categorize clients according to some assessment of their nursing care requirements over a specified time period. There are a variety of patient classification systems that vary in terms of their degree of specificity and comprehensiveness of scope. Patient classification systems have been designed to tackle the management problems of the proportion of RNs to unlicensed assistive personnel, the proper use of nursing resources under cost containment, and realizing improvements in the delivery of care (Mowry & Korpman, 1986). Research in nursing has indicated that medical care-based systems such as Diagnosis-related Groups (DRGs) do not reflect nursing care intensity and, therefore, like standard hours of care based on census, do not become useful to categorize clients according to nursing care requirements. The medical care-based systems are not workable to bridge the gap between client categorization and nursing resource consumption prediction. Current efforts focus on categorizing clients according to their anticipated and actual requirements for nursing care.

There are three broad types of patient classification systems (Mowry & Korpman, 1986; Reitz, 1985) (see Chart 23.4):

CHART 23.4 ❧ TYPES OF PATIENT CLASSIFICATION SYSTEMS

Prototype
Prototype is based on average care times for groups of clients defined by broad categories and typical characteristics.

Factor
Critical indicators are used to describe individual elements of direct care requirements. Adjustments are made for indirect care. Each indicator is rated, relatively valued or weighted, and the combination of these ratings determines the score and category.

Computerized Real-Time Factor
Actual times of all direct and indirect nursing care activities are recorded. These time computations and acuity ratings are automatically calculated and updated in real time.

Data from Mowry and Korpman (1986) and Reitz (1985).

1. *Prototype systems* are based on average care times for groups of clients defined by broad categories and typical characteristics. Categories are hierarchical for amount of care required. Clients are classified by being compared to the described prototype. Prototypes are often called subjective systems whose reliability is questioned.

2. *Factor systems* use critical indicators to describe individual elements of direct care requirements. For example, time-and-motion studies may be conducted to derive those elements of the job that are critical to work accomplishment. Adjustments are added for indirect care. The indicators are each rated, relatively valued or weighted, and combined to determine a score and category. Factor systems are heavily based on tasks and specific activities. Their ability to capture the nursing process is questioned.

3. *Computerized real-time factor systems* record the actual times of all direct and indirect nursing care activities. Time computations and acuity ratings are automatically calculated and updated in real time. If all activities are documented, the computer captures actual activity performed for the client, rapidly and automatically calculates data, and determines acuity and staffing while avoiding subjectivity and information delay.

Overall, patient classification systems attempt to identify acuity that can approximate workload and become the basis for staffing and budgeting. The systems have been criticized for reliability, validity, and comparability across settings. Some are not practical; some do not lend themselves to evaluation. The need for nation-wide standardized definitions and classifications for standardized input data has been suggested to avoid "managing without facts." Some believe that resources are allocated to nursing based on hospital revenues and financial issues rather than being based on acuity systems. Thus acuity systems may be of use to nurses but ignored by organizational financial administration (McManus & Pearson, 1993). Since nurses devote considerable time and energy into developing and maintaining patient classification systems, it is important to analyze whether the time is well spent. Are valid and reliable data generated that are useful to nurses and nursing? Should the effort be abandoned because political decisions allocate resources, not data-based decisions? Nurses need to assess and analyze their work settings to determine the best way to manage acuity and workload.

RESEARCH NOTE

Source: Schade, J., & Austin, J., (1992). Quantifying ambulatory care activities by time and complexity. *Nursing Economic$*, *10*(3), 183-192.

Purpose

Ambulatory care settings have experienced an explosion of increased volume and acuity. A valid and reliable patient classification system is needed to better match nursing resources with client care needs. The purpose of this article is to describe the development of an instrument to measure ambulatory care clients' nursing care requirements and to quantify care in time and complexity dimensions. The instrument developed in this study was the Ambulatory Care Patient Classification Tool (ACPCT). The tool was developed and tested by four ambulatory care nurses using 30 pediatric clinics. Both time and complexity weights were established for each patient care activity by means of a series of Delphi surveys of ambulatory care staff.

Discussion

The instrument was tested in this study on 444 patients in 32 ambulatory care pediatric clinics. Total mean scores for time and complexity were determined for each patient, then aggregated. The total hours of care from the classification tool were compared to actual nursing time worked, and a variance index was computed. Based on the results, the ACPCT instrument adequately described and measured the time and complexity variables of tasks related to ambulatory care nursing.

Application to Practice

The ACPCT was a useful tool to measure nursing care time and complexity needs in ambulatory settings. This measure of intensity, with refinement, could form the basis for staffing and costing decisions. Efforts to increase the precision of the match of nursing resources to patient needs will help to provide an environment in which nurses deliver cost-effective, high quality client care.

Differentiated Nursing Practice

Differentiated Nursing Practice is a term used to refer to the sorting of the roles, functions, and work of registered nurses according to some identified criteria, usually education, experience, and competence—or some combination. Differentiated nursing practice is associated with many other terms such as entry into practice, new roles, restructuring, delegation, staff mix, case management, care delivery models, assistive personnel/nurse extenders, redesign, and all-RN staffing. Differentiated practice has been described as a philosophical construct addressing the multiple levels of educational preparation for, and the resulting multilevel conceptual framework of, nursing as a practice (Primm, 1990).

Differentiated practice came into use three decades ago as a way to use associate (technical) and BSN degree graduates in nursing service. The basic premise for differentiated nursing practice revolves around the idea that the hospital environment can be restructured in such a way as to increase RN productivity and satisfaction without jeopardizing client care. Roles and functions of nursing personnel should be based on education, experience, and competence, and nurses should be compensated accordingly (NCNIP, 1989).

There are several rationales given in the literature for implementing and utilizing differentiated nursing practice. These rationales can be divided into two basic arguments:

1. *Organizational benefits:* Focusing on decreasing costs and increasing efficiency, the organizational benefits argument describes better utilization of nursing resources and restructuring for efficiency.

2. *Professional benefits:* Focusing on professional satisfaction and role clarification, the professional benefits argument says that there needs to be an intensified focus on deciding what nursing is and what it is not. To support the transfer of non-nursing responsibilities and eliminate the substitution of RNs *for* other healthcare workers and *by* other healthcare workers, the professional benefits arguments suggest that nurses must accelerate the development of assistive roles and split RN roles into two levels of managing routine care progression and handling complex interactions or changes. What this argument means is that if nursing is a profession, then the profession of nursing is the proper body to establish the control of practice by identifying the roles and functions of nurses.

Nursing is described by its roles, functions, and work. The practice of nursing can be envisioned as ranging along a continuum (see Fig. 23.1). The "difference" in differentiation is the role the nurse assumes. Four tiers for differentiation for practice can be identified:

1. General healthcare aide
2. Nurse professional: handles developing patterns
3. Nurse professional: handles complex changes
4. Nurse professional: conducts research and develops knowledge base

Provision of care, communication, and management of care are the three domains of the role of the nurse (Primm, 1987; 1990). The nurse's two-fold role was identified as caregiver and integrator (McClure, 1991). Caregiver functions are dependency, comfort, education, therapeutics, and monitoring. The monitoring function of the caregiver role links to the integrator role. The integrator role is a complementary function developed so that the work output of differentiated professionals can be put together to create a product such as client outcomes through a process of linking, synthesizing, and integration.

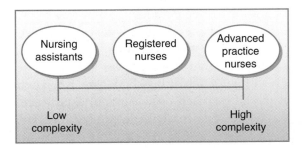

Figure 23.1
The nursing continuum of practice.

Integration falls to the one position in the structure that has the knowledge to perform as an integrator. In healthcare, this is nursing's traditional function.

While nurses can identify their roles and functions and ways that criteria of education, competence, and experience can be used to differentiate nursing practice roles, the implementation of differentiated nursing practice has been controversial. Nursing contains a group of care providers diverse in educational background (diploma, ADN, BSN) and in level of licensure (LPN, RN). There are philosophical differences that prevent consensus within nursing, as well as issues of licensing and credentialing, supply and demand, economics, and management/deployment. Further, tensions exist between what nurses may decide about nursing and what employers will do to structure employment positions. These controversies continue to swirl and affect issues related to staffing and scheduling.

The nurse leader and manager will find staffing and scheduling to be a critical, core function. The decisions have broad impact. Staffing and scheduling are a fine balance of competing interests and needs. There are predetermined standards, budget constraints, personal preferences, legal aspects, and individuals to please. Tenure versus equity may need to be balanced. For example, nurses may need to confront individual and collective philosophies about whether experience and time in a job are the decision factors in staffing and scheduling or whether experience and tenure are weighted with or replaced by a balance of needs of both newer and longer employed unit members. Shared governance may include self-staffing as an aspect of autonomy. Legal changes such as the Family Leave Bill may create challenges to ongoing staffing and scheduling at the specific unit level.

CURRENT ISSUES AND TRENDS

Management of human resources is one of the most important components of a healthcare service. Personnel costs have been the single largest healthcare expense item, estimated at 60% to 80% of a hospital or healthcare organization's operating budget. In a typical hospital, about half of the personnel have been employed in nursing service. Thus 20% to 40% of a hospital's operating budget traditionally has not been subjected to cost analysis and cost identification, nor have revenues been recouped by nursing services. Labor expenses are a logical target for cost containment, and nursing service became the visible and obvious area to cut in poor economic times (Mowry & Korpman, 1986).

Two cycles of economic pressures have occurred recently: the mid-1980s with the implementation of DRGs and prospective reimbursement, and the mid-1990s with healthcare reform and restructuring. The immediate responses were to slash budgets and lay off nursing personnel. Many nursing positions became in effect part-time jobs as forced time off occurred. Staff mix rapidly changed. As acuity rose and lengths of stay were reduced in hospitals, the RN role also changed. Workload measurement standards and acuity systems came under review. The roles and functions of advanced practice nurses were reviewed and revised (Mowry & Korpman, 1986).

Several general issues were triggered. Layoffs and downsizing created short-term economic gains for employers, but these actions caused threats to job security and resultant low morale. They established a difficult climate for recruitment and retention when the inevitable nursing shortage cycled around again. A predisposition to unionization was sparked by employers' actions. Nursing's roles, functions, and skill mixes were affected in ways that appeared to follow fads instead of research knowledge. Thus over time, nursing practice appears to be driven more by employer-determined job descriptions and positions than by nursing-determined parameters of practice. It is not clear what the effective and efficient mix of RNs and unlicensed assistive personnel is or should be. Thus the role of the nurse is unclear. Staffing and scheduling become more complicated without clear standards and guidelines. If the number of RNs in the skill mix drops too low, a backlash of concern over client safety can be expected. This may eventually result in an equilibrium that balances the needs of all parties.

Use of Nurse Extenders

The restructuring or redesign of nursing care often is triggered by the rapidly accelerating pressures to reduce healthcare costs (Bostrom & Zimmerman, 1993). One aspect of the economics-driven focus on restructuring nursing care delivery has been an experimentation with changed configurations of staff mix and the roles and functions of each category of worker in nursing (Gardner, 1991). The use of nurse extenders is a system reconfiguration that impacts on many related areas of nursing practice (see Fig. 23.2). Nurse extenders may be licensed or unlicensed assistants to nurses who enable nurses to handle a larger volume of client services.

The redesign of nursing care delivery ("new models" of care delivery) usually includes the introduction of some type of nurse extender and the alteration of the skill mix to include unlicensed personnel who are added to the registered nurse staff with a subsequent increase in the RN to client ratio. The Tri-Council for Nursing's Statement on Assistive Personnel to the Registered Nurse (1990) affirmed that unlicensed personnel historically have assisted RNs to deliver client care and continue to do so today. Ehrat (1990) noted that healthcare organizations historically have used substitute labor to meet client care needs because of nurses' failure to define or capitalize on their special contribution to client outcomes.

A classic study of nurse staffing and scheduling was done by Aydelotte and Tener (1960). Since then, studies have looked at the value and cost of staffing

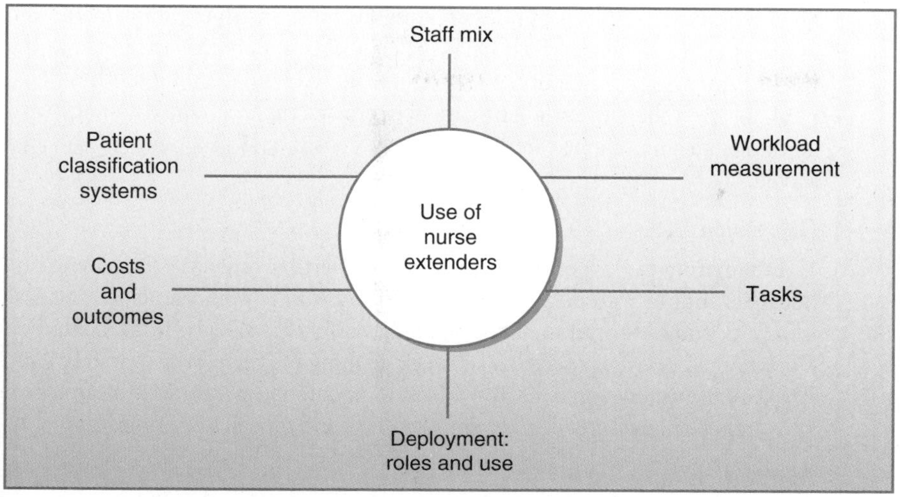

Figure 23.2
Impact of nurse extender use.

with an all RN staff, evaluating and testing primary nursing, and identifying core nursing tasks and the associated costs of various skill mix ratios. Evaluative efforts have been sparse and not of sufficient rigor to document that the use of nurse extenders is justified on cost, satisfaction, and quality bases (McCloskey et al., 1994). Thus nurses have not validated that quality will not suffer with the implementation of nurse extenders.

In any setting, staffing a nursing service is difficult. Cycles of nursing shortage-surplus create labor force instability. Rising acuity levels in hospitals, varying census, and varying admissions make predictions hazardous. A lack of good information and the diversity of educational preparation in nursing contribute to a high level of frustration in attempting to staff and schedule nurses to match the workload (Mowry & Korpman, 1986). Shifting the setting of care delivery away from hospitals and into the community will highlight the same staffing issues but with a new twist: much of the literature derived from a hospital setting-specific focus may not apply to alternative settings and, therefore, not be as useful as those developed to apply directly to an alternative setting. Staffing and scheduling remain challenges for nurses as they manage and deliver care to clients.

RESEARCH NOTE

Source: Fritz, D., & Cheeseman, S. (1994). Blueprint for integrating nurse extenders in critical care. *Nursing Economic$*, *12*(6), 327-331, 326.

Purpose

Hospitals are using techniques of work restructuring to change skill mix in order to control costs. The purpose of this article was to describe the analysis process and the outcomes of roles and responsibilities with the implementation of Patient Care Specialty Technicians (PCST), a form of nurse extender, in the ICU setting. A cross-functional team from the ICU units of one southern hospital analyzed the current client care delivery system and related systems variables of staff mix, client care hours, acuity, census, and geography of the area served.

Discussion

Eliminating the use of agency nurses and overtime and adjusting client care hours per shift by introducing a new healthcare worker would generate cost savings. The 100% RN staffing ratio was reduced to 75% RNs by introducing PCSTs who had been exposed to a six week training program. Both physician and RN "buy in" were secured. Early evaluation of outcome measures indicated positive trends on pressure ulcer, client teaching, and satisfaction indicators.

Application to Practice

Communication, teamwork, education, and a comprehensive plan for change encouraged successful integration of nurse extenders in the ICU units. Thus ICU units were able to effectively and economically alter the nursing skill mix. Essential staff and physician input was obtained prior to the change. Implementing the PCSTs served to control costs, maintain quality of care, and preserve client satisfaction. The change depended on planning, commitment and patience.

SUMMARY

* Delivery of nursing services is founded on staffing, scheduling, and skill mix determinations.
* Staffing is a process of planning to fill positions with qualified personnel and allocate scarce resources.
* Scheduling is implementing the staffing plan by preparing work hours.
* Nursing workload is the time determination of the nursing care needs of clients.
* Acuity and intensity measure the volume of care and the complexity of care needed.
* Staffing decisions are complex and based on volume and/or time.
* Methods of time sampling, work sampling, continuous sampling, or self-report are used to decide on staffing.
* Standardized volume measures may be used for staffing.
* Staffing systems may be fixed, controlled variable, or semiflexible.
* Patient classification systems group clients according to nursing care requirements of time and effort.
* The three types of patient classification systems are prototype, factor, and real-time factor.

- Differentiated nursing practice is the sorting of nursing work into roles based on criteria.
- Differentiated nursing practice may have organizational and professional benefits.
- Human resource management is influenced by economic pressures.
- The use of nurse extenders is a current issue in nurse staffing and scheduling.

Study Questions

1. Should nursing services be staffed to the minimum, maximum, or mean? Why?
2. What is the influence of the budget on staffing and scheduling?
3. To what extent should staff preferences determine staffing and scheduling?
4. What is the role of the patient classification system for staffing and scheduling? Does this vary by setting of care?
5. Should a manager do the schedule or should staff schedule themselves?
6. What is the "right" mix of RNs and assistive personnel?

Critical Thinking Exercise

Nurse Sean Danielson was just promoted to a case manager position in an integrated healthcare network of hospitals, long-term care facilities, and home health agencies. At first his caseload seemed reasonable. He worked hard to coordinate care needs and maintain a high level of communication. Now he feels the strain of putting in more and more time. His clients are dispersed over a wide geographic area and across multiple facilities. Client severity of illness and dependency needs are increasing. Today, Nurse Danielson sat down in his office to draw up a plan to avoid submerging in the workload.

1. What is the problem?

2. Why is it a problem?

3. What should Nurse Danielson do first?

4. What information does Nurse Danielson need? What variables should be measured?

5. What staffing issues are involved?

6. What scheduling issues are involved?

7. What further actions should Nurse Danielson plan for?

REFERENCES

Arndt, C., & Huckabay, L. (1980). *Nursing administration: Theory for practice with a systems approach* (2nd ed.). St. Louis: Mosby.

Aydelotte, M., & Tener, M. (1960). *An investigation of the relation between nursing activity and patient welfare*. Iowa City, IA: University of Iowa.

Barnum, B., & Mallard, C. (1989). *Essentials of nursing management: Concepts and context of practice*. Rockville, MD: Aspen.

Barter, M., McLaughlin, F., & Thomas, S. (1994). Use of unlicensed assistive personnel by hospitals. *Nursing Economic$, 12*(2), 82-87.

Bennett, T. (1981). Operations research and nurse staffing. *International Journal of Biomedical Computing, 12*, 433-438.

Bostrom, J., & Zimmerman, J. (1993). Restructuring nursing for a competitive health care environment. *Nursing Economic$, 11*(1), 35-41, 54.

Brett, J., & Tonges, M. (1990). *Resource allocation in managing the nursing shortage* (Monograph 3) (pub #154182). Chicago: American Hospital Association.

Cleland, V. (1990). *The economics of nursing*. Norwalk, CT: Appleton & Lange.

DeGroot, H. (1994). Patient classification systems and staffing: Part 1, problems and promise. *Journal of Nursing Administration, 24*(9), 43-51.

Detwiler, C., & Clark, M. (1995). Acuity classification in the urgent care setting. *Journal of Nursing Administration, 25*(2), 53-61.

Ehrat, K. (1990). *Administrative issues and approaches* (Monograph 2) (pub #154182). Chicago: American Hospital Association.

Gardner, D. (1991). Issues related to the use of nurse extenders. *Journal of Nursing Administration, 21*(10), 40-45.

Giovannetti, P. (1979). Understanding patient classification systems. *Journal of Nursing Administration, 9*(2), 4-9.

Jernigan, D. (1988). *Human resource management in nursing*. Norwalk, CT: Appleton & Lange.

Kirby, K., & Wiczai, L. (1985). Budgeting for variable staffing. *Nursing Economic$, 3*(3), 160-166.

Kirk, R. (1988). *Healthcare staffing & budgeting: Practical management tools*. Rockville, MD: Aspen.

McCloskey, J., Maas, M., Huber, D., Kasparek, A., Specht, J., Ramler, C., Watson, C., Blegen, M., Delaney, C., Ellerbe, S., Etscheidt, C., Gongaware, C., Johnson, M., Kelly, K., Mehmert, P., & Clougherty, J. (1994). Nursing management innovations: A need for systematic evaluation. *Nursing Economic$, 12*(1), 35-44.

McClure, M. (1991). Introduction. In I. Goertzen (Ed.), *Differentiating nursing practice: Into the twenty-first century* (pp. 1-11). Kansas City, MO: American Academy of Nursing.

McManus, S., & Pearson, J. (1993). Nursing at a crossroads: Managing without facts. *Health Care Management Review, 18*(1), 79-90.

Mowry, M., & Korpman, R. (1986). *Managing health care costs, quality, and technology: Product line strategies for nursing*. Rockville, MD: Aspen.

NCNIP. National Commission on Nursing Implementation Project. (1989). *Nursing practice patterns (differentiated practice)*. Milwaukee, WI: National Commission on Nursing Implementation Project.

Prescott, P. (1991). Nursing intensity: Needed today for more than staffing. *Nursing Economic$, 9*(6), 409-414.

Primm, P. (1987). Differentiated practice for ADN- and BSN- prepared nurses. *Journal of Professional Nursing, 3*(4), 218-225.

Primm, P. (1990). Approaches and strategies. In American Organization of Nurse Executives (Ed.), *Current issues and perspectives on differentiated practice* (pp. 17-34). Chicago: American Hospital Association.

Ramey, I. (1973). Eleven steps to proper staffing. *Hospitals, 47*(6), 98-104.

Reitz, J. (1985). Toward a comprehensive nursing intensity index: Part 1, development. *Nursing Management, 16*(8), 21-30.

Soeken, K., & Prescott, P. (1991). Patient intensity for nursing index: The measurement model. *Research in Nursing & Health, 14*(4), 297-304.

Soule, T., & Dobson, J. (1992). SEPPD and HPPD: More effective control of nursing care costs. *Nursing Economic$, 10*(3), 205-209.

Tri-Council for Nursing. (1990). *Statement on assistive personnel to the registered nurse*. Washington, DC: American Association of Colleges of Nursing.

PART VI

Evaluation and Control in Nursing Administration

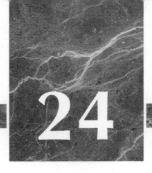

Computer Applications in Nursing Administration

Chapter Objectives

∾

define and describe computer applications in nursing administration

∾

define and describe nursing informatics

∾

define and describe management information systems

∾

analyze information needs in healthcare

∾

explain computer software application categories
that support nursing administration

∾

analyze nursing's data needs

∾

distinguish between two aspects of nursing informatics

∾

explain effectiveness research and nursing informatics

∾

compare the relationship of costs to data needs

∾

analyze the need for a standardized and retrievable management data set

∾

exercise critical thinking to conceptualize and analyze
possible solutions to a practical experience incident

*C*ritical data and information to support nursing decision making is essential in order to address issues of quality, effectiveness, and client outcomes. Nursing administration is concerned with leadership and management elements, derived from the setting in which nursing care is delivered to clients, that have an intervening effect on client outcomes. Nursing's data are important to client outcome determinations. The wave of the future is to computerize data so that analysis is possible and swift. Therefore, data will be available to manage better and to improve quality. As payors of healthcare costs require financial and evaluative data, it is rapidly becoming unfeasible to continue to hand tabulate data and manually keep track of records. Both are extremely slow and inefficient ways of handling data. Further, the Joint Commission on the Accreditation of Healthcare Organizations (JCAHO) has encouraged hospitals to have a computerized data retrieval system and has included standards about information management.

The automation of all aspects of information flow seems a virtual certainty in the healthcare delivery system. Nurses are central and key to the processing of healthcare data (Mowry & Korpman, 1986). Nurses have served as documenters and data collectors as reflected in complaints about the volume of paperwork. Nurses may need to do more data analysis functions in the future.

DEFINITIONS

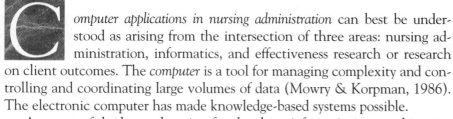

*C*omputer applications in nursing administration can best be understood as arising from the intersection of three areas: nursing administration, informatics, and effectiveness research or research on client outcomes. The *computer* is a tool for managing complexity and controlling and coordinating large volumes of data (Mowry & Korpman, 1986). The electronic computer has made knowledge-based systems possible.

As a part of the larger domain of technology, *informatics* is a combination of computer science with information science. *Nursing informatics* is defined as the management and processing of nursing data, information, and knowledge to support the practice of nursing and the delivery of nursing care (Graves & Corcoran, 1989) (see Chart 24.1). Nursing informatics involves the use of information management technologies to facilitate nursing practice, education, administration, and research (Schwirian, 1986). *Effectiveness research* is defined as the study of relationships among healthcare problems, interventions, outcomes, and costs, generally by analyzing large data bases or using epidemiologic methods.

A *management information system* (MIS) is defined as an integrated system for collecting, storing, retrieving, and processing a collective set of data. The data are

---

CHART 24.1
∾ DEFINITIONS

Nursing Informatics
the management and processing of nursing data, information, and knowledge to support the practice of nursing and the delivery of nursing care.

Management Information System
an integrated system for collecting, storing, retrieving, and processing a collective set of data. The data are transformed from storage into knowledge that is directly useful and applicable in the process of directing and controlling resources and their application to the achievement of specific management objectives.

Data from Ein-Dor and Segev (1978), Graves and Corcoran (1989), and Hanson (1982).

transformed from storage into knowledge that is directly useful and applicable in the process of directing and controlling resources and their application to the achievement of specific management objectives (Ein-Dor & Segev, 1978; Hanson, 1982). A management information system essentially is a system that provides information that managers use in decision making processes. Applications may process, store, and retrieve information, may estimate the outcomes of alternative decisions, or may assist in communicating decisions (Peterson & Hannah, 1988). The ten criteria, or desirable characteristics, for a good MIS are informative, relevant, sensitive, unbiased, comprehensive, timely, action-oriented, uniform, performance-targeted, and cost effective (Austin, 1979).

BACKGROUND

Curtin and Zurlage (1991) noted that every sector of healthcare is scrambling for state-of-the-art information. Healthcare reform, medical effectiveness, and outcome-oriented quality are current topics. Curtin and Zurlage (1991) described this practically: healthcare professionals want to know what works, what will/will not be reimbursed, and what this means for the running of their organizations and the actual delivery of healthcare services.

The information collected in healthcare generally is used to establish reimbursement, determine access to healthcare, define services, monitor the quality of care, direct healthcare policy, and affect the standard of care delivered (Lang & Marek, 1992). Nurses devote nursing time to documentation. Yet nurses have not systematically explored the rationale for each part of this activity: What are the essential data elements *for nursing?* Who should do the work of *organizational* documentation? Who uses the data, and how? Who benefits? This indicates that nurses may function as data gatherers but may not collect and use nursing data for nursing care management needs.

The initial motivation for the development and implementation of computerized hospital information systems was financial and administrative (Hannah & Shamian, 1992). More recently there have been strides in medical data collection and analysis, but nursing lags behind medicine in developing data support mechanisms due to a lack of agreement about how nursing knowledge should be represented and how nurses make decisions (Moritz, 1990; Ozbolt, 1987). Hannah and Shamian (1992) noted that it is impossible to overemphasize the need for a common nursing language so that nursing data can be stored, retrieved, and electronically compared.

Nursing has entered an era in which the use of data and information is critical and urgent. Nurses contribute much, and they have an obligation to capture and measure that contribution. For nursing this has meant pressure being brought to bear on nurses to identify and standardize nursing's data for information systems (Grobe, 1992).

Nursing has about a 20 year history of computer usage that demonstrates that information technology can be helpful. The major advantage is the ability to process more data at a greater speed. Unfortunately, the programs vary widely in ease of use, functionality, and adaptability to local needs (Grobe, 1992). The challenge is to process data in a useful and relevant form.

Information systems that support nursing administrative practice and provide essential decision support also are being developed and utilized. As computer software applications in nursing advance, nursing management applications have come to support decision making and strategic planning (Peterson & Hannah, 1988). For example, Cleland, Forsey, and DeGroot (1993) described a test of a differentiated pay structure model that used computer simulations to analyze data from two hospitals. Staffing and scheduling systems, patient acuity systems, quality monitoring results, precise cost information, fiscal resource management, workload measurement, personnel management, and utilization reports are examples of data and systems that support administrative decision making (Fralic, 1992).

Nursing's Data Needs

Nursing's data needs fall into four domains. Nurses need data about client care, provider staffing, administration of care and the organization, and knowledge-based research. The first three are distinct areas, whereas research interacts with all of the other three. The four areas and the source for the data are:
1. *Client:* Client care/clinical care and its evaluation, clinical data, and client outcomes. *Source:* The client record
2. *Provider:* Professional data, caregiver outcomes, and decision maker variables. *Source:* Personnel records, national data banks, and links to client records
3. *Administrative:* Management and resource oversight, administrative data, system outcomes, and contextual variables. *Source:* Executive/managerial data and fiscal and regulatory data
4. *Research:* Knowledge base development. *Source:* Existing and newly gathered data and relational databases

Table 24.1 displays examples of outcomes and variables to be measured in relation to the three distinct domains of nursing's data needs. For example, in the client domain, cost of care to the client is an important outcome for which data are needed to manage care. Intensity of nursing care is one variable that may be measured to monitor and control costs.

The collection and analysis of data is a critical thrust of current health services research. Data analysis is aimed at cost, quality, and effectiveness outcomes. McCormick (1988) acknowledged the significant contribution computer technology can make to the documentation of nursing practice.

Table 24.1

Outcomes and Variables in Three Domains of Nursing Data Needs

	DOMAINS		
	CLIENT	**PROVIDER**	**ADMINISTRATIVE**
OUTCOMES	Client satisfaction	Job enrichment	Costs
	Achieved care outcomes	Job/work satisfaction	Productivity
	Costs	Physician satisfaction	Turnover
	Access to care	Job stress	Income
		Intent to leave	
VARIABLES	Attitudes/beliefs	Attitudes, beliefs	Agency philosophy
	Diagnosis, gender, age	Education	Priorities
	Marital status	Years of experience	Organizational structure
	Support system	Age	Fiscal data
	Satisfaction	Work excitement	Climate
	Level of dependency		Policies and procedures
	Severity of illness		Conflict
	Intensity of nursing care		

However, this contribution rests on structuring the input logically, providing adequate processing and memory, and assuring valid and reliable output. Clear definition, valid linkage between data sets, and clear coding of input are essential in securing meaningful output that has utility. The aggregation of information over time and how this aggregation affects the quality of information is especially important to uniform data sets. Similarly, the reliable and valid aggregation of nursing management information is important for policy and resource allocation strategies in nursing administration.

RESEARCH NOTE

Source: Flarey, D. (1993). Quality improvement through data analysis: Concepts and applications. *Journal of Nursing Administration, 23*(12), 21-30.

Purpose

Flarey quotes Deming as saying, "In God we trust. All others must use data." The purpose of this article was to review and explain commonly used data analysis tools with a focus on applications such as quality improvement in nursing practice. After performance and outcomes are measured, data analysis begins. Reliable data used to drive process improvements produce the most long-lasting results. Quality improvement comes from measuring process elements that lead to outcomes and then using the data to better manage client care processes. Statistical methods are used to hone in on variations and process dysfunctions.

Discussion

Commonly used quality improvement tools are flow charts, histograms, Pareto charts, cause-and-effect or fishbone diagrams, scatter diagrams, trend charts, control charts, run charts, force field analysis, selection grids, and affinity diagrams. Many of the tools are relatively simple. They identify common causes of variation. Data analysis and display tools organize data and visually display collected data in a logical fashion.

Application to Practice

Many data analysis and display tools are applicable to nursing practice because nurses need to collect, analyze and communicate to others about care management. Quality improvement is one outcome of the manipulation of nursing data. Inefficiencies, redundancies, and misunderstandings can be identified and targeted for improvement through process or system redesign. A visual display will highlight problems and areas for further study. Deming emphasized the necessity of collecting, measuring, and analyzing data to improve work processes.

Nursing Informatics

Two primary aspects of informatics in nursing were identified by Grobe (1992):

1. *Engineering aspect:* the application of technology to performing a function; using computers for very specific functional purposes.
2. *Scientific inquiry:* the determination of what data and information are needed and how this information should be captured, represented, processed, and stored so that it provides:
   a. A realistic reflection of practice
   b. Adequate support of decision making
   c. Effective management of resources and knowledge
   d. Sound hypothesis testing

Some general principles for informatics in nursing administration can be identified and used by nurses as they come to a consensus about what variables are important to measure. First, nursing needs accurate, reliable, real-time, discipline-specific data that are gathered, stored, retrievable, and analyzed into useful information. Second, nursing's data will become visible when nurses agree on uniform, standardized data elements and collect these across settings and sites. And third, data need to be collected in each of the four domains—client, provider, administrative, and research—in order to round out nursing's data availability.

Effectiveness Research

Effectiveness research is a growing area of inquiry due to the considerable variation in clinical decision making and in healthcare delivery, resulting in variation in clinical outcomes. The lack of consistency found within therapeutic decisions, intervention strategies, and resulting outcomes has led to a national effort to evaluate clinical care.

Effectiveness research uses large databases and epidemiologic methods to examine the relationships among problems, interventions, outcomes, and costs. For nursing this means the relationships among nursing diagnoses, interventions, outcomes, and contextual variables in the environment of client care (Ozbolt, 1992).

Success in improving outcomes can only come from blending nursing information back into integrated databases that support care delivery and shared responsibilities (Stevic, 1992). This may take the form of a longitudinal client record connecting information stored in departmental systems (nursing, pharmacy, lab, radiology, billing) with data held in management information systems (Hospitals, 1993). Some feel that the next wave of evaluative data will need to provide predictive information (Stevic, 1992). In order for progress to occur, nurse administrators might take the perspective that information technology is an asset, not an overhead expense.

The need for large data sets and evaluative information abound in healthcare. Two recent examples are:

1. The Institute of Medicine's initiative on a *Computer-based Patient Record (CPR)*, which is designed to:
   a. Provide a longitudinal account of care, since more and more care is being given outside of the hospital
   b. Meet the need for an information system that allows tracking of care to nursing home, retirement home, or client's private residence
   c. Move away from an emphasis on episodes of care and move to measurement of care across settings and across time (JONA, 1993)
2. *Nursing Information System (NIS)*: the American Nurses Association and the National Council of State Boards of Nursing (NCSBN) with a Robert Wood Johnson Foundation grant are developing an NIS, an unduplicated count of RN and LPN licensees plus characteristics such as employment status, educational preparation, and clinical specialty. The NIS effort is targeted at nursing's need to picture the nation's nursing supply more accurately, as a resource for researchers and planning groups, and an efficient mechanism to check credentials (AJN News, 1993).

There are some restraining forces that may slow the growth of large data sets. McClure (1991) identified two problems associated with the collection, analysis, and dissemination of large data sets:

1. Instances in which data are gathered concerning the performance of institutions and agencies, for example, the annual release of corporate mortality reports by the Health Care Financing Agency (HCFA). There may be flaws in the methodology and in the interpretation of the

data as quality indicators. However, flawed or not, institutions do not want a hint of tarnish to their image or reputation. Therefore, these data are very sensitive.

2. The collection of data related to the practices of particular individuals. For example, the National Practitioner Data Bank (NPDB) was created to collect and release information related to the professional competence of certain healthcare practitioners. McClure (1991) believed that there is a potential for a big-brother-is-watching-you environment that could become corrosive and punitive over time. In all aspects of automated healthcare information, the issues of privacy and confidentiality of records remain serious concerns (Milholland, 1994).

LEADERSHIP AND MANAGEMENT IMPLICATIONS

How do we keep score? With the costs of healthcare escalating to a crisis proportion, how do nurses and nurse managers manage the cost aspects of nursing care delivery, given a political environment of cost shifting and resource constriction? The answer lies in computerized nursing management information, standardized language, and the development of and access to uniform nursing management data sets that would enhance the collection, retrieval, analysis, and comparison of nursing's "invisible" data. Nurses at all levels need to collect data and analyze it to demonstrate that nursing outcomes are cost-effective. The first step is to understand the need for data. Nurses need to ensure that the organizations they work for provide nurses with

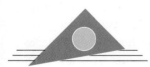 *Leadership & Management Behaviors*

LEADERSHIP BEHAVIORS

- envisions a structure to capture data needs
- projects data needs
- enables followers to use data and information
- models knowledge-based practice
- uses electronic data management resources
- uses data and information for power and political advantage

MANAGEMENT BEHAVIORS

- identifies needed data
- plans for the collection of data
- organizes data collection
- uses electronic resources
- analyzes data
- uses information strategically

OVERLAP AREAS

- identifies data and information needs
- uses electronic resources
- uses information

the tools for data management and analysis. Strategic planning and leadership vision are needed. Nurses can then continually improve their knowledge base about how to analyze and report data in a persuasive presentation. This requires that nurses approach data management from the perspective of its use as a nursing tool as opposed to only assuming the function of documenting and data entry to satisfy organizational maintenance.

Many factors influence the effectiveness of clinical interventions, including the client, the clinician/provider, the organization, and other contextual factors. Contextual and organizational factors influence nursing practice. The impact of nursing practice may be more evident in some settings than in others, e.g., nursing homes, home care agencies, and nurse-managed clinics where nursing personnel are the predominant formal caregivers. It is important that the client record reflect all providers who are giving care so that their independent and collective clinical influences can be considered. Management practices and organizational designs (the internal contextual covariates or factors) impact on nurses, the delivery of nursing care to clients, and client outcomes.

At the systems level, outcome measurement may include variables such as length of stay, cost, client satisfaction, complications, variance analysis, intensity, quality, access, and satisfaction. Both the cost of care and the quality of care are measurable and can be compared. Therefore, there will be continuing emphasis on the development of huge national databases for the purposes of integrating collected information from a variety of sources related to utilization and outcomes of healthcare (Curtin & Zurlage, 1991).

If nursing's data are not included in these large data sets, the impact of nursing care will remain largely unmeasured and invisible (Mallison, 1990). Therefore, nurses have to start identifying and collecting their data for inclusion and analysis. Nurses no longer have the luxury of maintaining a local, provincial perspective about nursing. Cost pressures and healthcare changes have forced a national perspective about healthcare. Nursing needs to be at the political table, armed with data. Ozbolt (1992) noted that nursing data have been excluded from large databases such as the Uniform Hospital Discharge Data Set, not because of any discrimination against nursing but rather because of nursing's failure to agree upon and offer a set of clearly defined, valid, reliable, and standardized data elements for inclusion. Thus nurses must focus their energies on nursing data and their use for nursing. This means defining, validating, standardizing, measuring, and analyzing nursing's data.

Mattera (1992) has asked how care can be planned or reimbursed when there are no sets of uniform national codes to plug into computers to capture and analyze nursing's data. Nurses will not be able to play a significant role as first-line healthcare providers if the computers do not have a data set for the payment of nurses for the work they do. Perhaps other providers are being credited and reimbursed for work nurses perform.

Nursing's data have been described as being "invisible." This makes nursing care all but invisible and undervalued within the healthcare delivery system. A search of all the federal databases revealed that none contained nursing information, leading nurse leaders to describe nursing care, in the context of healthcare generally, as a huge black box. Resources such as money, nursing care delivery time, and nursing skills and interventions go in, and a client exits with a physician's bill and a hospital/healthcare organization's bill.

Yet nurses know that something happens in the process. Nurses and nursing personnel constitute the largest number of healthcare providers, and the nursing budget is the largest labor budgetary item in most healthcare organizations. Despite the fact that nurses have been documenting for a very long time, only two charges visibly result, identifying and rewarding physicians and hospitals for healthcare services. Further, others capture reimbursement for the work nurses do. Ott, Griffith, and Towers (1989) found that nurses perform many of the services for which physicians have been reimbursed. An examination of the Current Procedural Terminology (CPT) codes revealed that nurses perform many of the services listed, yet the CPT coding system acknowledged only physicians as providers of all the coded services. Nurses were encouraged to identify explicitly the value of the nursing component involved in each physician service.

Nurses and nurse managers both will need solid basic computer skills and the ability to work with computer programmers. The most important skill is to know what data are essential and what analyses need to be done. Inservices can be set up for skills acquisition, and consultants can be used for advice about data management.

CURRENT ISSUES AND TRENDS

Nursing Management Minimum Data Set (NMMDS)

As nurses have been participating in the automation of healthcare data and the integration of nursing data within information systems, a realization of the need for agreed-on definitions of the appropriate elements describing clients and their care came to light (Grier, 1984; Moritz, 1990). Werley and Lang (1988) have identified and described the need for a standardized data set in nursing, the Nursing Minimum Data Set (NMDS). Adoption of the NMDS would allow for on-going collection of data that can be compared across settings and client populations for clinical and administrative decision making. According to the Study Group on Nursing Information Systems (1983), computerizing the data facilitates the management and use of the information by standardization, organization, and automation to produce timely and comprehensive information. The NMDS provides the structure for electronic storage of nursing data, and the unified nursing language provides the substantive data definitions to be stored in that structure (Hannah & Shamian, 1992).

Nurses have not yet agreed upon those factors that comprise the basic, core data elements needed by nurse administrators to manage nursing services. The NMDS has been proposed as the standardized data set for the collection of comparable nursing data. However, the NMDS omits some essential service-related variables. DeGroot, Forsey, and Cleland (1992) found that the NMDS does not contain nursing practice and personnel data about individual nurses, thus restricting the ability to answer crucial cost and quality questions faced by nurse administrators. Further problems related to inaccessible or unavailable data elements were uncovered in their research, including lack of uniform collection practices within and across hospitals.

Awareness of the need for standardized, uniformly collected, retrievable, and comparable service-related management data elements, combined with the awareness of their unavailability in practice, was the impetus for the research to develop and test a Nursing Management Minimum Data Set (NMMDS) (Huber et al., 1992) (see Table 24.2). The NMMDS identified elements potentially critical to evaluating the impact of nursing interventions on client outcomes. Further, the NMMDS work has the potential of facilitating the linking and augmenting of the other minimum health data sets by providing information uniquely important to nursing administrative decisions and thus to the evaluation of nursing services for cost and quality outcomes of care delivery. Mattera

Table 24.2

The 18 Proposed NMMDS Elements

FOR EACH NURSING UNIT	FOR THE INSTITUTION
Type of nursing unit	Medicare case mix
Method of care delivery	Occupancy (total admissions, ambulatory activity, observations/holds)
Nurse manager characteristics	Staff mix
Unit of service or workload unit	Budget
Size of nursing unit (licensed, operational, and occupied beds)	Revenues (gross and net)
Cost (direct and indirect)	Satisfaction (patient, nursing staff, and physician)
Nursing resources (productive and non-productive full time equivalents, and productive employees)	Achievement of accrediting body standards (number met, number of recommendations, and subject of focused review)
Nursing unit budget (budget, direct, indirect, nonlabor, and revenue)	Nursing administration complexity
Average intensity of nursing care	Nursing demographic elements across the institution (turnover, vacancy rate, education, tenure, experience, and certification of staff)

(1992) noted that the very reason clients go to hospitals is because they need the services nurses provide. Yet none of the uniform data sets now available captures what nurses do for clients. Clearly, when nurses identify and standardize their unique critical variables, these variables can be included in the data bases already set up to collect healthcare information. Then the data will be available for analysis and use.

Building on the NMDS, the NMMDS specifically identified variables essential to nurse managers for decision making about nursing care effectiveness. For example, the NMMDS can be linked to the nursing care elements of intensity/staff mix to provide an enhanced assessment of the consumption of healthcare resources to produce specific client care outcomes for a specific age cohort, racial/ethnic group, or geographic region. Linkage to the NMDS service elements, specifically the expected payor of the bill, would assist in isolating budgetary elements.

Nursing needs a standardized data set that will facilitate decision making and policy development in such areas as job satisfaction, turnover, costs of nursing services, allocation of nursing personnel, and comparison of nursing care delivery models. Such a data set would foster data collection, retrieval, analysis, and comparison of nursing management outcomes across settings, populations, time intervals, and geographic regions. Using a core of variables captured by computerized information systems, data essential to nursing care delivery management can be analyzed and used to meet nursing's goals and objectives. Management information systems join large data base development efforts and other information software applications to enhance nursing leadership and management. The future points to further developments and refinements to augment the practice of nursing. The future will hold more computer power, portable computers and handheld terminals, voice input, videodisk technology, expert systems, artificial intelligence, and more advanced decision support and modeling systems. There will be greater connectedness and outreach linkages. Computing is the medium of communication in the future; information is the message that needs to be delivered (Ball & Douglas, 1988).

SUMMARY

- Critical data and information to support nursing decision making are essential.
- The wave of the future is to computerize data so that analysis is possible and swift.
- Computer applications in nursing administration can best be understood as arising from nursing administration, informatics, and effectiveness research.

- Nursing informatics is the management and processing of nursing data, information, and knowledge to support the practice of nursing and the delivery of nursing care.
- A management information system (MIS) is an integrated system for collecting, storing, retrieving, and processing a collective set of data from storage into knowledge.
- The information collected in healthcare is used to establish reimbursement, determine access to healthcare, define services, monitor the quality of care, direct healthcare policy, and affect the standard of care delivered.
- Information systems that support nursing administrative practice and provide essential decision support are being developed and utilized.
- Nursing's data needs lie in the areas of the client, the provider, administrative, and research.
- Nursing informatics has an engineering aspect and a scientific inquiry aspect.
- Effectiveness research uses large databases and epidemiologic methods to examine the relationships among nursing diagnoses, interventions, outcomes, and contextual variables in the environment of patient care.
- Nursing's data have been described as being "invisible."
- Computerized nursing management information, standardized language, and the development of and access to uniform nursing management data sets would enhance the collection, retrieval, analysis, and comparison of nursing's "invisible" data.

Study Questions

1. What role do computers play in nursing care?
2. Who uses nursing's data?
3. What are the data used for?
4. What difference do nurses who manage health care services make and under what circumstances?
5. What are the cost, quality, and satisfaction outcomes that nurses are mainly responsible for?
6. Which data need to be client specific, nurse specific, or organization specific?

Critical Thinking Exercise

Nurse Aminta Gonzalez works in a community health clinic in the inner city of a large urban area. The clinic serves mostly indigent or homeless clients. The clinic building is old and needs renovation. Clinic attendance has been rising and clients have long waits for service. Staffing was increased recently to meet the demand. However, clients now endure long wait times for intake and exit processing. Nurse Gonzalez has drawn up a plan for computer equipment purchase. Now Nurse Gonzalez needs to identify software, relational databases, and staff inservicing needs.

1. *What problems does Nurse Gonzalez face?*

2. *Why are they problems?*

3. *What should Nurse Gonzalez do first?*

4. *What factors does Nurse Gonzalez need to assess and analyze?*

5. *What data needs might Nurse Gonzalez anticipate?*

6. *What can Nurse Gonzalez do to form a persuasive data management plan?*

REFERENCES

AJN News. (1993). ANA, NCSBN move to mend data gaps. *American Journal of Nursing, 93*(3), 97.

Austin, C. (1979). *Information systems for hospital administration.* Ann Arbor, MI: Health Administration Press.

Ball, M., & Douglas, J. (1988). Integrating nursing and informatics. In M. Ball, K. Hannah, U. Jelger, & H. Peterson (Eds.), *Nursing informatics: Where caring and technology meet* (pp. 11-17). New York: Springer-Verlag.

Cleland, V., Forsey, L., & DeGroot, H. (1993). Computer simulations of the differentiated pay structure model. *Journal of Nursing Administration, 23*(3), 53-59.

Curtin, L., & Zurlage, C. (1991). Cornerstones of healthcare in the nineties: Forging a framework of excellence—A report on a landmark conference. *Nursing Management, 22*(4), 32-43.

DeGroot, H., Forsey, L., & Cleland, V. (1992). The nursing practice personnel data set: Implications for professional practice systems. *Journal of Nursing Administration, 22*(3), 23-28.

Ein-Dor, P., & Segev, E. (1978). *Managing management information systems.* Toronto: Lexington Books.

Fralic, M. (1992). Into the future: Nurse executives and the world information technology. *Journal of Nursing Administration, 22*(4), 11-12.

Graves, J., & Corcoran, S. (1989). The study of nursing informatics. *Image, 21*(4), 227-231.

Grier, M. (1984). Information processing in nursing practice. In H.H. Werley & J.J. Fitzpatrick (Eds.), *Annual Review of Nursing Research, 2,* 265-287.

Grobe, S. (1992). Nursing service administration and the future: View from a nursing informatics perspective. In B. Henry (Ed.), *Practice and inquiry for nursing administration: Intradisciplinary and interdisciplinary perspectives* (pp. 48-51). Washington, DC: American Academy of Nursing.

Hannah, K., & Shamian, J. (1992). Integrating a nursing professional practice model and nursing informatics in a collective bargaining environment. *Nursing Clinics of North America, 27*(1), 31-45.

Hanson, R. (1982). Applying management information to staffing. *Journal of Nursing Administration, 12*(10), 5-9.

Hospitals. (1993). All connected: Infrastructure is path to IS growth. *Hospitals, 67*(4), 31.

Huber, D.G., Delaney, C., Crossley, J., Mehmert, M., & Ellerbe, S. (1992). A nursing management minimum data set: Significance and development. *Journal of Nursing Administration, 22*(7/8), 35-40.

JONA. (1993). Panel urges nurses to take active role in information systems decisions. *Journal of Nursing Administration, 23*(2), 7-8.

Lang, N., & Marek, K. (1992). Outcomes that reflect clinical practice. In NCNR (Ed.), *Pa-*

tient outcomes research: *Examining the effectiveness of nursing practice: Proceedings of the state of the science conference* (pp. 27-33). Washington, DC: DHHS/NIH/NCNR #93-3411.

Mallison, M. (1990). Access to invisible expressways. *American Journal of Nursing, 90*(9), 7.

Mattera, M. (1992). Learn a new language. *RN, 55*(8), 1.

McClure, M. (1991). The uses and abuses of large data sets. *Journal of Professional Nursing, 7*(2), 72.

McCormick, K. (1988). Conceptual considerations, decision criteria, and guidelines for the nursing minimum data set from a research perspective. In H. Werley & N. Lang (Eds.), *Identification of the nursing minimum data set* (pp. 34-47). New York: Springer.

Milholland, D. (1994). Privacy and confidentiality of patient information: Challenges for nursing. *Journal of Nursing Administration, 24*(2), 19-24.

Moritz, P. (1990). Information technology: A priority for nursing research. *Computers in Nursing, 8*(3), 111-115.

Mowry, M., & Korpman, R. (1986). *Managing health care costs, quality, and technology: Product line strategies for nursing.* Rockville, MD: Aspen.

Ott, B., Griffith, H., & Towers, J. (1989). Who gets the money? *American Journal of Nursing, 89*(2), 186, 188.

Ozbolt, J. (1987). Developing decision support systems for nursing. *Computers in Nursing, 5*(3), 105-111.

Ozbolt, J. (1992). Strategies for building nursing data bases for effectiveness research. In NCNR (Ed.), *Patient outcomes research: Examining the effectiveness of nursing practice: Proceedings of the state of the science conference* (pp. 210-218). Washington, DC: DHHS/NIH/NCNR #93-3411.

Peterson, M., & Hannah, K. (1988). Nursing management information systems. In M. Ball, K. Hannah, U. Jelger, & H. Peterson (Eds.), *Nursing informatics: Where caring and technology meet* (pp. 190-205). New York: Springer-Verlag.

Schwirian, P. (1986). The NI pyramid—A model for research in nursing informatics. *Computers in Nursing, 4*, 134-136.

Stevic, M. (1992). Patient-linked data bases: Implications for a nursing outcomes research agenda. In NCNR (Ed.), *Patient outcomes research: Examining the effectiveness of nursing practice: Proceedings of the state of the science conference* (pp. 198-202). Washington, DC: DHHS/NIH/NCNR #93-3411.

Study Group on Nursing Information Systems. (1983). Computerized nursing information systems: An urgent need. *Research in Nursing & Health, 6*, 101-105.

Werley, H., & Lang, N. (Eds.) (1988). *Identification of the nursing minimum data set.* New York: Springer.

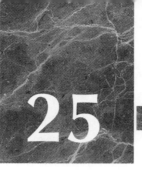

Quality Improvement and Risk Management

Chapter Objectives

ᐧᐧ

define and describe quality

ᐧᐧ

define and describe quality assurance and improvement

ᐧᐧ

define TQM and CQI

ᐧᐧ

analyze the development of quality assurance programs

ᐧᐧ

analyze the development of TQM and CQI

ᐧᐧ

explain key principles of CQI

ᐧᐧ

explain the process of quality monitoring

ᐧᐧ

analyze regulatory agency impacts

ᐧᐧ

review ANA standards

ᐧᐧ

explain quality measurement

ᐧᐧ

define structure, process, and outcome standards

ᐧᐧ

compare methods of quality assessment

ᐧᐧ

differentiate between research and quality methods

∾

analyze trends in quality improvement

∾

define and explain risk management

∾

exercise critical thinking to conceptualize and analyze
possible solutions to a practical experience incident

*t*rading off between cost and quality is one of the dilemmas facing the
healthcare system in this country. Nurses, as providers, become embroiled
in the controversies that relate to quality and how to define, measure, and improve it. Quality improvement is linked to evaluation and accountability to
society. However, quality improvement is complex and time-consuming. It involves data gathering, statistics, and analysis.

People evaluate all the time. This is a process that comes naturally to human beings. For example, evaluation cards at restaurants or hotels or patient
satisfaction questionnaires from a hospital are ways of evaluating or getting
feedback. Evaluation surveys are done to elicit the perceptions of customers
and to determine how satisfied they are with the service. The evaluation of
quality may appear simple. However, as internal and external pressures to deliver high quality care at a lowered cost impinge on the healthcare delivery
system, major quality transformations will be required to compete successfully.
The industrial model of quality through inspection is being replaced with the
prevention approach of improving systems on the front end by designing quality into the service (Marszalek-Gaucher, 1992).

CHART 25.1
∾ DEFINITIONS

Quality
refers to characteristics
of and the pursuit of
excellence.

Quality of Care
the degree to which
health services for in-
dividuals and popula-
tions increase the like-
lihood of desired
health outcomes and
are consistent with
current professional
knowledge.

Some data from Institute of
Medicine (1990).

DEFINITIONS

 uality refers to characteristics of and the pursuit of excellence. Excellence may be established by determining whether or not the
outcomes compare favorably to the standards that were set (see
Chart 25.1). *Quality of care* was defined as the degree to which
health services for individuals and populations increase the likelihood of desired health outcomes and are consistent with current professional knowledge
(Institute of Medicine, 1990).

Quality has been defined in many ways. There is no single definition of
quality (Donabedian, 1980; Gardner, 1992). The core of a definition of quality is the balance of health benefits and harms to a client (Donabedian, 1980).
Quality can be described in terms of effectiveness and efficiency, benefits and
harm, or appropriateness of care. In a service setting, quality is concerned with

effectiveness, efficiency, and appropriateness. Thus quality exists to the degree that service is efficient, well executed, effective, and appropriate (Stetler, 1992). Quality has been described as consisting of two interdependent parts: quality in fact and quality in perception. Quality in fact is conforming to standards and meeting one's own expectations. Quality in perception is meeting the customer's expectations (Omachonu, 1990). Within the framework of continuous quality improvement, quality is defined as meeting or exceeding customer requirements (Marszalek-Gaucher & Coffey, 1990).

Assurance means achieving a state of accomplishment and implies a guarantee of excellence. *Quality assurance* generally refers to an organization's effort or ability to provide services according to accepted professional standards and in a manner acceptable to the client (see Chart 25.2). Quality assurance has been defined as a process of evaluation that is applied to the healthcare system and the provision of healthcare services by RNs (Stetler, 1992). Quality assurance builds on quality assessment, the measurement of quality, by taking evaluative action to ensure a designated level of quality (Lang & Clinton, 1984).

A *quality improvement program* in an organization is an umbrella program that extends into many areas for the purpose of accountability to the consumer and payor. The program is a continuous, ongoing measurement and evaluation process that includes structure, process, and outcomes. The quality improvement process uses pre-established criteria and standards, and then follows with an appropriate change for the purpose of improvement.

Total quality management (TQM), sometimes called the *total quality process*, is a way to ensure customer satisfaction by involving all employees in the improvement of the quality of every product or service (see Chart 25.3). All systems and processes are evaluated and improved. TQM aims to reduce the waste and cost of poor quality (Marszalek-Gaucher, 1992). TQM has been defined as a structured system for involving an entire organization in a continuous quality improvement process targeted to meet and exceed customer expectations (Triolo, 1994).

Continuous quality improvement (CQI) is a process of continuously improving a system by gathering data on performance and using multidisciplinary teams to analyze the system, collect measurements, and propose changes. The four main principles are a customer focus, the identification of key processes to improve quality, the use of quality tools and statistics, and the involvement of all people and departments in problem solving (Bohnet et al., 1993; Miller & Flanagan, 1993).

BACKGROUND

Four driving forces that underlie healthcare system policies and decisions are cost, equity, access, and quality. Thus quality is one factor that is impor-

CHART 25.2
∾ DEFINITIONS

Quality Assurance
generally refers to an organization's effort to provide services according to accepted professional standards and in a manner acceptable to the client.

Quality Improvement Program
an umbrella program that extends into many areas for the purpose of accountability to the consumer and payor. It is a continuous, ongoing measurement and evaluation process that includes structure, process, and outcomes.

CHART 25.3
∾ DEFINITIONS

Total Quality Management
a way to ensure customer satisfaction by involving all employees in the improvement of the quality of every product or service. All systems and processes are evaluated and improved.

Continuous Quality Improvement
continuous improvement of a system by gathering data on performance and using multidisciplinary teams to analyze the system, collect measurements, and propose changes.

tant in public policy regarding healthcare delivery (Hodges, Icenhour, & Tate, 1994). Some trace quality assessment and quality assurance in nursing to 1855 and Florence Nightingale's efforts during the Crimean war. She gathered data and developed standards for noise, food, cleanliness, and bed position. The "modern era" of quality assurance began between 1952-1966, when the American Nurses Association (ANA) established committees and divisions to develop standards of nursing care. The standards were to be used for developing quality assurance programs (Dean-Baar, 1994; Reiley, 1992; Smeltzer, 1988).

Quality assurance became a familiar term in nursing. However, problems arose with the definition and measurement of quality, research knowledge dissemination, controversies over standards, the impact of cost containment, prospective payment, TQM/CQI innovations, regulatory agencies, and the shift from process to outcome measurement.

Regulatory and licensing agencies mandated quality and accepted quality assurance programs that contained relatively arbitrary thresholds that defined minimum expectations and identified problems. Lacking was a mechanism for finding causes or areas for improvement. Thus quality was maintained, but systems were not improved. Quality assurance was based on a collection of information about incidents or errors; the systems affecting errors and the processes for improvement were not identified (Cohen & Cesta, 1993). Over time the term quality assurance was replaced with quality assessment, quality management, TQM, CQI, and outcomes measurement.

Clearly, the approach to healthcare quality improvement is undergoing rapid change. Since the late 1980s, it has evolved from a problem-focused approach to one that emphasizes ongoing monitoring and improvement. Regulatory agency criteria require a facility to be able to demonstrate that an ongoing, systematic monitoring and controlling process is in place for both the quality of the care and the appropriateness of the care. Further, there must be documentation to reflect these efforts.

In the recent past, the measurement of quality has been focused on process. The process argument suggests that if nurses do things right, there is quality care as a result. However, regardless of whether the right process is followed, the client's outcomes may not be positive. Nursing is beginning to draw out care linkages to look more closely at what happens in terms of nursing care and how it affects client outcomes.

In the past few years, the emphasis has shifted from the assurance of quality to quality assessment (its measurement) and continuous quality improvement (its management). However, the fundamental focus for quality still remains the pursuit of excellence (Stetler, 1992).

The evolution of quality assurance programs has included a number of changes. Some important changes include programs to develop unit-based quality assurance, quality circles or quality councils, concurrent monitoring, interdisciplinary quality assurance, client satisfaction, automation of data sources, performance/competence, TQM, and CQI (Bohnet et al., 1993; Marszalek-Gaucher, 1992; Reiley, 1992). Not all programs are implemented in all healthcare institutions.

A resurgence of interest in quality has been traced to a National Broadcasting Corporation (NBC) documentary in June of 1980, where W. Edwards Deming compared Japanese and U.S. productivity. His message was that quality commitment and listening to customers had contributed to Japanese marketplace predominance (Marszalek-Gaucher, 1992). Nursing efforts at that time were focused on quality assurance. Unit-based quality assurance was the focus. Unit-based quality assurance was described as decentralized quality assurance and as a method of accountability in nursing practice (Schroeder, Marbusch, Anderson, & Formella, 1982). Quality circles or quality councils were groups of employees focused on a quality-related project. This idea crept into nursing practice after being borrowed from business and industry but soon died down. As the financial crisis in healthcare grew, a number of changes were triggered. Deming's ideas began to disseminate. The customer-centered approach of TQM and CQI began to invade healthcare settings.

TQM is more closely associated with Deming's philosophy (Aguayo, 1990; Flarey, 1993; Marszalek-Gaucher, 1992). Deming changed the prevailing approach to quality from activities of inspection to activities that build quality into the process used to produce the product or service. Deming was a statistician who applied statistical thinking, inference, and prediction to science and technology. He placed a strong emphasis on the collection, measurement, and analysis of data in order to use data to improve processes (see Chapter 24). Deming's perspective saw profit as generated by loyal customers. Continually improving quality improves productivity and produces loyal customers. Therefore, increasing the quality of a service leads to higher productivity and profitability. Further, increasing quality was seen as decreasing costs. Knowledge of variation and the use of statistical process control are powerful methods of quality process improvement (Aguayo, 1990; Flarey, 1993).

CQI is a more general term used to refer to all variations of a customer-centered approach and total organizational commitment to quality. TQM/CQI are seen as a strategic priority and the way to survive in a competitive economic environment (Bohnet et al., 1993). The key principles that form the core of CQI are (Mitchell, 1994):

- commitment of the organization as a whole to quality
- commitment to understanding the customer's individual needs and expectations
- a continuous effort to improve the process
- empowering employees to improve the process through granting authority, training, and resources
- organizational commitment to providing high-quality services and products

- integral use of information and data collection
- commitment to quality by the organization's top management
- commitment by the organization to learning from the best practices, called "benchmarking"
- forming long-term relationships with a few suppliers who can deliver a quality product

CQI has been called a paradigm shift from a focus on providers' values to a focus on customers' values. This means a pervasive shift in the prevailing model used as a framework for organizing healthcare to meet customers' needs over providers' needs. CQI attempts to transform a traditional bureaucracy into a system that uses a multidisciplinary framework driven by managerial leadership to focus on quality as accountability for both process and outcomes (Mitchell, 1994).

The Process of Quality Monitoring

Quality monitoring follows an identifiable process (see Fig. 25.1). The first step in the quality improvement process is to establish the standard by which to evaluate. This is called standards setting. Then the methods to be used to meet the standards are identified. With this information a tool is developed to measure the existing practice. Subsequently, the practice that occurred is compared to the standard using the measurement tool. The data produced by these previous steps must then be analyzed and interpreted, and any deficiencies that have been identified are corrected by intervention actions (Sliefert, 1990).

A quality improvement program should pervade the entire organization, throughout multiple levels. At the level of an individual nurse and client, the

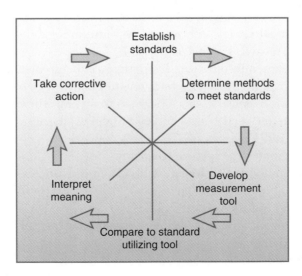

Figure 25.1
The quality monitoring cycle. (Data from Sliefert [1990].)

quality improvement process is an appraisal of how the nurse is performing in taking care of clients. At the individual level, a performance appraisal controls and monitors quality. At the unit level, the nursing unit or program audit, whether concurrent or retrospective, may be used to examine the process and outcomes of care. At the nursing department level, a quality improvement program is established for the nursing department as the quality mechanism. Each unit's or program's data are compiled and compared. Quality improvement projects for the department of nursing may be conducted across units via multidisciplinary teams. At the organizational level, the accrediting body's standards drive the quality improvement mechanism or process. Looking at the whole organization, there is a circular process of standards, appraisal against standards, and goal setting for improvement.

Regulatory Agency Impacts

There are three ways standards setting occurs outside of the professional arena: the federal government via Medicare/Medicaid reimbursement regulations, state licensure, and private accreditation. All are concerned with quality, usually at minimum standards (Mitchell, 1994). The Joint Commission on Accreditation of Healthcare Organizations (JCAHO), the accrediting body for hospitals and healthcare organizations, is a private, not-for-profit organization. Since its founding in 1951, JCAHO has become the principal standards setter for healthcare facilities. It accredits in the following areas: ambulatory, long-term care, psychiatric, home care, and hospitals. JCAHO accreditation is technically voluntary (AONE, 1992). JCAHO requires quality improvement and, therefore, any organization accredited by the JCAHO must have a quality improvement program. Medicare or Medicaid reimbursement will not be paid to healthcare organizations that are not accredited. Although JCAHO accreditation technically is voluntary, capturing payment makes it in effect mandatory. There are hospitals in which Medicare/Medicaid payments are between 40% and 60% of the entire organization's budget, and accreditation is important to them.

The JCAHO has outlined a ten-step process of quality assurance for institutions. There must be (JCAHO, 1990):
1. Clear assignment of responsibility
2. A delineation of the scope of care for each practitioner
3. An identification of the important aspects of care
4. Specific indicators of care
5. Establishment of thresholds for evaluation
6. Collected and organized data to monitor important aspects of care
7. Evaluation of care
8. Actions taken to solve problems and improve care
9. Assessment of those actions and documented improvement

10. Communication of relevant information to the organization-wide quality assurance program

The JCAHO is a powerful private accrediting agency. At least since the 1970s, they have required quality assurance planning. Currently, the whole area of quality management, quality assurance, and quality improvement has been changing. There has been greater pressure on assuring quality as a way of controlling and monitoring the way that professionals deliver care.

In community health nursing there are three voluntary accrediting agencies: the JCAHO, the National HomeCaring Council, and the Community Health Accreditation Program (CHAP) of the National League for Nursing. The National HomeCaring Council has established standards and addressed quality in paraprofessional services since 1962. The National League for Nursing established standards and accreditation for community health nursing programs in 1961, which became the full independent subsidiary CHAP in 1987 (Rooney, 1992).

In long-term care, JCAHO accreditation is voluntary. The standards are modeled on hospital standards and not weighted toward resident outcomes. Nursing homes are required to meet state and federal licensing standards. The regulatory process was deemed inadequate to protect residents. Therefore, federal Medicare/Medicaid certification procedures were reformed by legislation (OBRA) in 1987. Federal and state surveys and regulatory activities have increased (Harrington, 1992).

RESEARCH NOTE

Source: Sherman, J., & Malkmus, M. (1994). Integrating quality assurance and total quality management/quality improvement. *Journal of Nursing Administration*, 24(3), 37-41.

Purpose

Hospitals need to demonstrate quality improvement. The challenge is to integrate JCAHO standards into hospital quality assurance (QA) processes. The purpose of this study is to describe a pilot program to combine total quality management/quality improvement (TQM/QI) with QA in a cost-effective and efficient blend. Quality assurance and TQM/QI were identified as a duplication of parallel but separate processes due to their different origins and separate structures and processes. TQM/QI was implemented independent of the already existing QA in one hospital. A pilot program was initiated in the postanesthesia care unit (PACU) of this hospital to integrate the two programs at the nursing unit level.

Discussion

The PACU's QA and TQM/QI teams were combined to integrate responsibility for quality improvement activities. The team combined the preexisting

JCAHO 10-step process for QA with the multidisciplinary team effort of FOCUS-PDCA (find, organize, clarify, understand, select, plan, do, check, act) cycle. Thus an established data collection methodology was combined with a continuous, integrated approach. PDCA corresponded to steps 7 to 10 of the JCAHO 10-step process. The team involved other departments, outlined customer requirements, created a flow chart, used problem-solving methods, and determined the data needed to identify and evaluate process improvements.

Application to Practice

TQM/QI and more traditional QA can be integrated to avoid duplication and focus all efforts in a more efficient manner into one goal of quality of care. Improved cooperation and communication can result. This creates a better use of resources and less confusion about responsibility for quality activities. A high level of commitment contributed to integration of functions in the PACU.

ANA Standards of Nursing Practice

Standards of quality are critically important and are the first step of a quality improvement program. The people who decide the standards are the people who have the most power over the system of quality improvement. If nurses accept the obligation and responsibility to set nursing standards, even though it takes work, thought, time, and effort, then nurses are controlling the practice of nursing.

Standards are authoritative statements. They describe a common level of care or performance by which the quality of practice can be determined. Standards define professional practice. Standards reflect the profession's values. Standards of care describe an acceptable level of client care. Standards of professional performance describe an acceptable level of professional nurse role behavior (Dean-Baar, 1994). This means, for example, that standards of care address the nursing process and the care management process used by the nurse in providing and managing care. Standards of professional performance speak to professional nurse role aspects such as nurse education, ethics, collegiality, research, and resource utilization.

Patterson (1988) defined quality as a numerical ratio of the degree of adherence between the nursing standard of care and observed client outcomes. Quality is thus founded on generally recognized standards compliance and outcomes as measured against criteria derived from standards. She noted that a *standard of care* focuses on the client, is outcome oriented, and relates to what the client can expect. A *standard of practice* focuses on the nurse as provider, is process oriented, and relates to what is expected of the provider to achieve the standard of care.

The American Nurses Association (1991) has formulated general standards and guidelines for nursing practice (see Fig. 25.2). The original document was

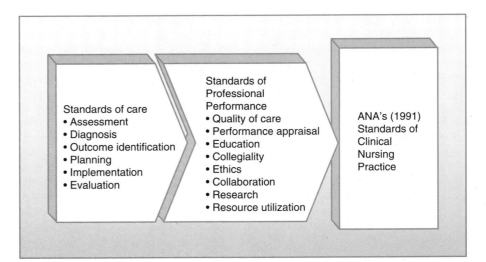

Figure 25.2
Nursing standards. (Data
from American Nurses
Association [1991].)

published in 1973 (ANA, 1973) and set the foundation for professional nursing practice. The standards were based on the nursing process and were general to any setting or specialty. The nursing standards of practice evolved as they were used to derive criteria against which care was measured for quality assurance purposes. Reevaluation of the nature and purpose of standards of nursing practice led to the ANA's (1991) Standards of Clinical Nursing Practice, which contained two parts: standards of care and standards of professional performance. The 1991 document was substantially different from previous standards due to the development of a combined framework for standards of nursing practice and nursing practice guidelines. The framework can provide direction for nursing practice, a means to evaluate practice, and a way for nursing to be accountable to the public (Dean-Baar, 1994; Gardner, 1992).

The ANA also publishes standards for many specialty areas. For example, there are standards of community health nursing practice, hospice nursing practice, college health nursing practice, home health nursing practice, nursing practice in correctional facilities, school nursing, gerontological nursing, maternal/child nursing, perinatal nursing, medical/surgical nursing, oncology nursing, rehabilitation nursing, and perioperative nursing. The standards of practice can be used as the basis on which a nursing program or unit develops standards of nursing care. Standards of care are pervasive and fundamental to and should be the basis for job descriptions and the standards of nurses' practice. They should relate intimately to the client acuity and assignment system and they should give guidance to orientation and inservice. Evaluation is based on initial standards and goal setting. If evaluation is to be continuous and ongoing, then documentation should form the basis of the continuous and ongoing monitoring.

Measurement of Quality: Structure, Process, and Outcomes

The measurement of quality is founded on several principles (Hodges, Icenhour, & Tate, 1994):
- Quality can be measured.
- Quality measures a standard or some degree of excellence.
- Excellence is determined either by validating standards of care or by measuring professional actions in caring for clients.

Standards essentially define quality, against which outcomes and performance are measured. Therefore, standards setting is absolutely critical. Standards are arbitrary, since there is no absolute answer to the question, what is quality? In actuality, standards establish the baseline against which an evaluation is conducted.

How is quality measured? Are the measures that determine if the standards are met reliable and valid? The methods used to measure quality against the standards can be described in three basic approaches: structure, process and outcome. Donabedian (1980) developed the initial theoretical framework that quality can be measured by structure, process, and outcome.

Structure Standards Structure standards, or structural measures, focus on the internal characteristics of the organization and its personnel (see Chart 25.4). They answer the questions, is the structure in place that will allow quality to exist, and is the structure of the organization set up to allow quality of care? For example, a structural standard for a long-term care facility might be having enough nurses on site to ensure that quality of care is delivered. For specialized areas, are there enough specialists to ensure quality care? The presence of certain committees, policy statements, rules and regulations, or manuals, forms or contracts may be needed. Structure standards regulate the environment to ensure quality. Human resources, organizational resources, physical resources, standards of practice, and environmental characteristics are addressed in structure standards.

CHART 25.4 ∾ DEFINITION

Structure Standards
focus on the internal characteristics of the organization and its personnel. They regulate the environment to ensure quality. They answer the question, is the structure in place that will allow quality to exist?
Examples:
- Nursing department provides inservice and opportunities for staff development.
- There is a computerized system for recording accurate and objective observations of clients in the clinical record.
- Agency will staff at least one RN for every five client visits.

CHART 25.5 ～ DEFINITION

Process Standards
focus on whether the activities within an organization are being appropriately conducted. They focus on behavior, activities, interventions, and the sequence of caregiving events.
Examples:
• A nursing assessment will be done for each client within 24 hours of initial client contact.
• Music therapy and other nursing measures are used as possible alternatives for medications.
• Vital signs will be taken q. 1 h.

CHART 25.6
～ DEFINITION

Outcome Standards
refer to whether the services provided make any difference. They address physical health status, mental health status, social and physical function, health attitudes/knowledge/behavior, utilization of services, and the client's perception of quality care.
Examples:
• Breath sounds are clear (free of rales and rhonchi).
• Client will stop smoking within six months.
• Resident will assist in feeding activity.
• Ambulates without assistance.
• Mother will breastfeed baby.

Process Standards   Process measures focus on whether the activities within an organization are being appropriately conducted (see Chart 25.5). Process measures focus on the behaviors of the nurse. The ANA standards have been process standards. They relate to what the nurse will be doing, and the process the nurse should follow in order to assure quality of care. Process standards look at activities, interventions, and the sequence of caregiving events. Process standards typically are assessed by an audit.

Outcome Standards   Outcome measures refer to whether the services provided by the organization make any difference (see Chart 25.6). They answer the question, is it accurate to say that the services nurses provide make a difference to the clients or to the health status of the population? Outcome standards address physical health status, mental health status, social and physical function, health attitudes/knowledge/behavior, utilization of services, and the client's perception of quality care. Outcome refers to a change in the current or future health status attributed to antecedent healthcare and client attributes of healthcare. Outcome standards present the possibility of measuring the effectiveness, quality, and time allocated for care. In addition, measurement of nursing care outcomes as related to cost would assist in establishing the value of nursing care (Hodges, Icenhour, & Tate, 1994).

•   •   •

Donabedian's (1980) framework of structure, process, and outcomes quality domains is the most well known and used in research. However, as an integrative approach an alternative model that incorporates the cost of nursing care into evaluation has been proposed. In this integrative approach, the inputs are services rendered. For example, an input might be an hour of nursing care. Inputs lead to intermediate outputs or products such as tests and procedures. In nursing, an example would be Foley catheter care or instruction on foot care for diabetics. These lead to final outputs, called the episode of care. An example in nursing is completion of a teaching program. Efficiency is measured between inputs and intermediate outputs. Effectiveness is measured between the intermediate outputs and the final outputs. This model moves beyond measurement to focus on the efficiency and effectiveness comparisons of productivity (Fetter & Frieman, 1986).

In measuring quality, both structure and process parameters are important, but not sufficient. Did the care make a difference? For example, did the client learn, recover, or get healthier? Some say neither structure nor process matter as long as the client improves. What is important is that the care makes a difference and that it is not above a certain cost.

To summarize, structure standards describe the structure needed to reach the outcome, and they focus on the environment. Process standards describe the process needed to reach the outcome, and they focus on the nurse as a provider. The outcome standards describe the outcome desired, and they focus on the client and specific client behaviors.

Methods of Quality Assessment

A variety of approaches to the assessment and measurement of quality are available. Some components embedded in the total organizational umbrella quality improvement program include accreditation audits, practice documentation, utilization review, client care studies, performance appraisals, client satisfaction surveys, length of stay studies, cost analyses, and epidemiological studies. Examples of some methods that are used to obtain quality improvement data include observation, checklists, rating scales, time-and-motion studies, questionnaires, peer review, and chart audits (see Chart 25.7).

The audit is probably the most common technique of quality improvement assessment. Nursing audits can be prospective, retrospective, or concurrent. With a prospective audit, there is a determination before care occurs. For example, for gerontological clients the risk for altered levels of awareness or falls can be anticipated; therefore, a program can be set up so that each client is assessed against a checklist. Concurrent means ongoing at the time of the client encounter. Thus the quality audit would be conducted in "real time" while the client is in the care process. This may be accomplished, as an example, when a computerized program detects variances from a critical path and alerts the caregivers. Retrospective means an audit of the chart is done after discharge to determine if the documentation indicated a record of quality care. The retrospective audit typically uses a random sample of charts of clients previously served. One method of peer evaluation uses a random sample review of the charts of the clients the nurse has cared for to form one element of a performance appraisal.

A retrospective audit may form the core of quality management efforts. For example, if outcomes are looked at as the criteria, and the nurse simply charts

CHART 25.7
∿ SELECTED
EXAMPLES OF
METHODS USED TO
OBTAIN DATA

- Peer review
- Chart audit: prospective, concurrent, and retrospective
- Observation
- Checklists
- Rating scales
- Time-and-motion studies
- Questionnaires

that the client reported pain and a pain medication was given with no documentation of the client's response to the medication, then there is no evidence of what happened and no ability to assess that a difference was made. Completeness and accuracy in documentation are critical. Nurses need to document what was done, assure that the care was rendered in a timely and a comprehensive manner, and demonstrate evidence of complete discharge of duties. If it is not documented, it is not considered to be done. This is a legal standard of accountability.

Other methods of quality assessment include the data analysis tools advocated by Deming for quality improvement. Reliable data are needed for process improvements to have the most long-lasting effects (Flarey, 1993). Computerized systems can be used for data collection, storage, retrieval, and analysis (see Chapter 24). However, nurses need to know how to analyze critical variables.

Using statistical methods, Deming advocated the identification of critical variables and the analysis of variations. Commonly used quality improvement techniques from Deming include control charts, flow charts, and fishbone or cause-and-effect diagrams. Other tools for quality improvement are histograms, Pareto charts, scatter diagrams, trend charts, run charts, force field analysis, selection grids, and affinity diagrams. These tools may be relatively simple and useful for identifying the causes of variations. Visual displays help to organize and present data in a logical fashion (Aguayo, 1990; Flarey, 1993).

Three commonly used tools are flow or control charts, fishbone diagrams, and Pareto charts. A flow or control chart visually outlines and displays the steps involved in any process. Thus they clearly present the flow of an activity. A control chart contains three lines: average, upper control limit, and lower control limit, each derived from data. For example, client wait time in a clinic could be mapped for flow on a flow chart and aggregate data on wait times displayed on a control chart. Flow charts can be constructed to show the ideal or the real occurrence of work (Aguayo, 1990; Flarey, 1993).

Fishbone diagrams look like charts used to diagram sentences. All processes feeding into the outcome are placed on diagonals and flow from left to right. The problem or outcome is at the far right end of a horizontal line placed in the middle of the diagram. All major categories of causes, such as people, materials, methods, and equipment, are listed on the diagonals along with relevant feeder processes to each major cause. The result is a clear and explicit display of causes and effects that can be used to brainstorm improvements (Aguayo, 1990; Flarey, 1993).

A Pareto chart is a graphic tool that was made famous by a nineteenth century economist who showed that 80% of the wealth was held by 20% of the people. This "80-20" rule was found to have wide applicability. For example, 80% of all problems or errors result from 20% of all causes or individuals. Thus improvement needs to be targeted at the problematic 20%. A Pareto chart is a modified form of a histogram or graph that plots two significant variables contributing to a problem. In a Pareto chart, causes are graphed as a percentage of the total and displayed in descending order from left to right on the graph. A quality improvement team can construct and use flow charts, control charts, fishbone diagrams, and Pareto charts for analysis and investigation of data for quality improvement.

Quality Improvement and Research Studies

Research and quality assessment and management both rely on evaluation and are applications of the problem solving process. However, the conduct of research and the conduct of quality management and improvement are distinct and different processes. Highly controlled experimental research is on one end of a continuum of rigor; day-to-day quality assessment evaluation is on the other (Stetler, 1992).

Research studies manipulate variables, may introduce new nursing procedures, and may not have an immediate application to practice. In quality improvement studies, however, an intervention is not withheld to see if it made a difference. In a quality improvement study an intervention that is not commonly accepted would not be introduced. What exists is measured. Quality improvement studies are necessary for the institution's client care management. They are not designed to manipulate variables, withhold interventions, or introduce new techniques. That is the area of research. Quality improvement is designed for measuring what exists with the idea of determining how it measures against standards, so that client care can be managed and improved. The purpose of nursing research is generalizable knowledge; the purpose of quality assurance is determining effectiveness, efficiency, and appropriateness of care (Stetler, 1992).

Research utilization and other research activities can contribute to quality improvement. This occurs through the generation of knowledge, methods, and instruments and through increasing the analytical skills of nurses. The contribution of quality assessment to the research process is through problem identification. A key challenge is to integrate research, clinical practice, and evaluation methods. Incorporating components of the research process into the quality improvement program strengthens the measurement and evaluation of care delivery. The research process may provide alternatives to an audit for data collection in quality assessment. Data collection instruments and principles of data analysis and interpretation can strengthen quality methods (Driever, 1992; Stetler, 1992).

Research utilization can contribute to the evaluation of the effectiveness of nursing care interventions. One quality assurance model using research

(QAMUR) was described as containing two tracks: research utilization and research conduction as problem solution paths. The QAMUR model promoted increased rigor in quality assessment studies (Watson, Bulechek, & McCloskey, 1987).

LEADERSHIP AND MANAGEMENT IMPLICATIONS

Staff nurses are intimately involved in quality improvement. Staff nurses often are considered the prime quality monitor because of their presence with the client and their consistent monitoring function. Nurses control many implementation decisions. For example, the choices about the supplies that are used, the choices about how to facilitate client care, the information flow, and the coordination of care are decisions made by nurses.

The management process involves planning, organizing, directing, and controlling. The controlling phase is similar to the evaluation phase of the nursing process. The controlling functions of the management process complement the planning functions. A manager develops plans and establishes goals and objectives during the planning phase. In the control phase, the manager assesses the progress toward goal achievement. The idea is to control the process through evaluation so as to be able to assure quality. This is similar to the nursing process in that the manager is looking for deficiencies or omissions in the planning and

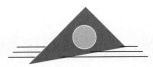 *Leadership & Management Behaviors*

LEADERSHIP BEHAVIORS

- builds a culture of quality
- models quality care management
- encourages electronic systems for quality management
- envisions high quality care
- collaborates across disciplines to enhance quality
- is visible in quality management activities
- enables interdisciplinary quality improvement
- evaluates quality of care

MANAGEMENT BEHAVIORS

- plans for quality in care delivery
- organizes a quality-driven service
- directs others to achieve quality
- monitors quality of care
- evaluates quality of care
- participates in ongoing quality management

OVERLAP AREAS

- evaluates quality of care
- injects quality into care delivery and management of care

delivery of care, and takes action to rectify any deficiencies that occur. Professionals and managers of client care have a legal and ethical obligation to rectify deficiencies and obtain continued improvement in practice.

There is a shift in terms of quality improvement from an emphasis on process to an emphasis on outcomes. Researchers are trying to determine what the important client outcomes are and who affects those outcomes. Nursing has been slower than medicine to develop its database and thereby have the ability to demonstrate a unique effect on client care. Nurses need to be able to demonstrate a causal link between nursing actions taken to identify a problem, indicate a plan, and choose an intervention based on research that has a high probability of solving the problem or remediating the situation and a subsequent change in the client's health status. Outcomes of interest are client satisfaction, the quality of the care delivery, functional status improvement, quality of life improvement, costs, and morbidity/mortality improvement. Nursing needs to show a demonstrable link between what nurses do and what happens to the client and to show to which elements of client outcomes nurses contribute significantly. Outcomes assessment, measurement, and evaluation are a current major thrust of health services research.

CURRENT ISSUES AND TRENDS

A key feature of a profession is that it monitors its own practice. The argument for a profession like nursing is that only another like professional has the expertise to truly evaluate nursing performance and determine the quality of care from the providers' perspective. Therefore, nurses have an obligation to monitor the quality of nursing practice.

The public is concerned about quality. Consumers and payors seek assurances that nurses are monitoring and evaluating the quality of nursing practice. One measure of how well the professions regulate themselves is the number of disciplinary proceedings processed by a state board of nursing in a year. In nursing the misuse of chemical substances is a major category of disciplinary action and subsequent loss of licensure. Consumers also raise concerns over reports that non-profit hospitals are making large amounts of profit. Quality concerns arise over the cost of transplants or other expensive leading-edge therapies as well as who has control and access to them. The ANA's (1980) Social Policy Statement noted that there are two routes to regulation: either the group monitors itself, or society, through laws such as licensure through state boards of nursing, imposes restrictions. The National Council of State Boards of Nursing also functions to protect consumers. An issue for nurses is how to monitor and control within the profession, so that there are mechanisms to ensure to consumers that practicing nurses are functioning, prepared, and competent.

Development and Implementation of a Pain Management Protocol

An oncologist and a surgeon voiced their very different perspectives about optimal pain management during a quality of care meeting in the spring of 1992. This discussion inspired appointment of a task force charged with developing a monitor for successful pain management that could be used throughout our academic medical center.

I was asked to organize the task force and to recruit adequate representation from other disciplines and departments. At the first meeting, all concurred that no tool could be useful unless the outcomes it measured were agreed upon as valid. Moreover, we identified the need for a consistent definition of both pain and effective pain management. The task force acknowledged that any prescription for medical practice would be rejected and that no single protocol for pain management could be developed that would be applicable to all clinical and social situations. We came to understand that successful completion of our charge could change the culture at our institution by making excellent pain management an overriding principle for all medical and nursing care providers.

The task force adopted the International Association for Study of Pain definition of pain as an unpleasant sensory and emotional experience associated with actual or potential tissue damage or related to such damage. We accepted the Agency for Health Care Policy and Research's (AHCPR) Guidelines that had been published in February, 1992, as a framework to develop a "philosophy" or "Approach to Pain Management" and "Standards for Pain Management." These were widely disseminated.

Next we developed tools to measure current performance with a goal of establishing a baseline, identifying weak areas, and making changes in practice that would improve pain management for our patients. Consistent with the definition of pain that we had accepted, our tools for measuring effective pain management were based on patient perceptions, using physiologic indicators for preverbal, nonverbal, and comatose patients.

We constructed a broad outcome monitor: "How satisfied were you with the way your pain was managed during your last hospitalization (or clinic visit)" for inclusion in the Patient Satisfaction Telephone Survey conducted by our Patient Relations Department. Over a one year period, scores on this retrospective survey improved from 74% to 80% of patients surveyed being "very satisfied" with pain management. Moreover, dissatisfaction with pain management decreased from 6% to 5% over the same period. A more sensitive concurrent outcome monitor was developed and is given to representative samples of patients on each nursing unit near the time of discharge. This tool measures consistency of the patient's experience with the standards for pain management we set for ourselves.

We have identified that doctors and nurses don't often tell patients that their experience of pain is important to us and that we want to know when pain is present. We often fail to listen to patients' ideas about management of their pain. We don't often enough explain why we address pain in the ways we do and not in some other way the patient may feel would be better. Simply conducting these monitors has changed the way nurses administer and document the effectiveness of ordered pain medication and has improved collaboration among nurses, physicians, and pharmacists when a patient's pain is not being effectively relieved.

The third level of monitoring was developed as a practice monitor. Use of this monitor is triggered when patient satisfaction monitoring indicates a problem, when patients complain about pain management to the Patient Assistance representative, or when pain control has been particularly difficult to achieve. The Interdisciplinary Practice Monitor is a tool for chart review to determine whether our pain management standards were followed in assessing, prescribing, dosing, and teaching relative to pain.

During the period of this project, intermittent prn dosing has decreased. Around the clock dosing, use of continuous IV drips, patient-controlled analgesia pumps, epidural analgesia, and nonpharmacologic interventions (including counseling and pastoral care) have all dramatically increased. These changes correspond to measured improvement in patient satisfaction with pain management.

The charge of the task force has been completed. A new interdisciplinary Pain Policy and Education Committee has been created that examines institutional barriers to excellent pain management and makes recommendations for changes in the medical school curriculum and in hospital policy relative to pain management. A modest project developed to "assure quality" has changed both culture and practice in our academic medical center.

SHARON E. MELBERG, RN, MPA
Assistant Director, Hospital and Clinics
University of California Davis Medical
 Center
Sacramento, California

One related aspect of quality improvement is the professional issue of mandatory continuing education. Continuing education is related to quality by its effect on improving competence. Mandatory continuing education means that by law nurses must continue their education. This is not in force in every state in the union. Therefore, nurses need to know the law in the state in which they practice. The state's Nurse Practice Act identifies whether that state requires mandatory continuing education for relicensure. There are rules and regulations that vary by state to govern mandatory continuing education. Continuing education affects nursing license endorsement. Continuing education is considered a major vehicle for professional development and is also considered important for quality because refreshing practice by acquiring more knowledge places a professional in a position to better assure quality.

Continuing education is used to address the competency issue: how do nurses stay competent? Is a nursing license for life, and nurses never need to demonstrate ongoing learning? Practice is changing so rapidly that obviously that is not viable. Employees are morally, and in some states legally, responsible for practicing to current standards and for their own personal and professional development. On the other hand, the employing organization is legally responsible for orientation and inservice. Continuing education is considered to be beyond routine inservicing: it is one component of career development and professional improvement.

A second related aspect of quality improvement is the development and use of critical paths and variance analysis (see Chapters 16 and 17). Generally developed as a component of managed care or case management programs, critical paths map out the expected care pattern and outcomes for a client encounter or episode of care. Variance from the map triggers a review and analysis. Alterations in the plan of care may result. These activities generally occur concurrent to care delivery and trigger immediate quality management.

Risk Management

Risk management is an extension of quality improvement in a service profession like nursing. An employing organization is concerned about the kinds of risks that reasonably might be foreseen and, therefore, are preventable. Risk management is embedded within the managerial process of control. The idea is to prevent undesirable events from happening and minimize the impact of unpreventable risks.

Some interventions, such as assessing the situation and alerting appropriate authorities, need to occur when there is a specific policy, procedure, rule, or regulation that has been or is likely to be violated. When there is danger to clients or staff, when a subordinate is not able to carry out his or her delegated duties, or when there is a threat to the property of the institution, then intervention ought to occur. Monitoring, surveillance, and assessment are possible intervention strategies for protecting staff and client safety. Corrective actions include disciplinary action, which is an attempt to point out behavioral deficiencies and prevent the recurrence, and counteractive measures that are taken to remediate the immediate situation. For example, if an employee is rude or abusive to a client, a counteractive action tries to remediate the current situation. A disciplinary action tries to prevent recurrence. Thus the employee may be instructed to apologize for rudeness (counteractive) and may receive a verbal warning (disciplinary).

A *risk management program* is defined as an organization-wide program to identify risks, control occurrences, prevent damage, and control legal liability (see Chart 25.8). The term has arisen since the 1970s, triggered by the quality assurance movement and malpractice claims. Risk management is a process whereby risks to the institution are evaluated and controlled in order to reduce or prevent future loss. The main purpose is the controlling of financial loss due to malpractice claims (Culp, Goemaere, & Miller, 1985). The JCAHO has required a risk management program for the entire organization as a part of quality assurance efforts. A risk management program is structured to identify, analyze, and evaluate risks, accompanied by a plan for reducing the frequency and severity.

There are certain known risk-prone areas in healthcare. For example, the risks and liability associated with needle stick injuries has changed dramatically with the onslaught of AIDS and awareness about blood borne pathogens. Needle sticks are a known risk and an occupational hazard in healthcare. Hospitals put systems into place to prevent occurrences. Assessment of the risk focuses on the cause of the problem. Actions are initiated to try to reduce occurrences to an irreducible minimum. Another example is the risk for falls in

CHART 25.8
～ DEFINITION

Risk Management
an organization-wide program to identify risks, control occurrences, prevent damage, and control legal liability. It is a process whereby risks to the institution are evaluated and controlled.

elderly or disoriented clients. Hospital risk management programs focus on finding a method of identifying who is at risk for falls, so as to create a planned surveillance program to try to prevent occurrences.

Risk management programs are one part of quality improvement because of the prevention of known risk factor activities. New areas of focus relate to employee wellness and prevention of injury due to back strain, repetitive stress injuries or carpal tunnel syndrome, and poor health practices that put the employer at risk for paying the healthcare costs of ill or injured employees.

The monitoring system may include incident reports, audits, review of committee minutes, a process for monitoring client and visitor complaints, and client satisfaction questionnaires. Actions include analyzing risk categories, reviewing and appraising the safety elements, monitoring the laws and the regulations to be in compliance with legal parameters and legal mandates, trying to eliminate and reduce risks, identifying the educational needs of the staff, and evaluating the risk management program itself so as to create ongoing, continuous monitoring.

The purpose of an incident report is to provide a permanent record of an incident to assist in refreshing the participant's memory in case he or she is called on to recount the incident sometime later. The incident report also alerts the person who is designated to be in charge of the risk management program that there may be a possible malpractice or lawsuit claim. Incident reports usually are kept by the central administration in a locked file. The incident reporting system allows for timely investigation by giving the administration an opportunity to investigate immediately any serious situation. Incident reports are compiled, reviewed, and used for statistical analysis. A statistical profile of the kind of incidents that are occurring is prepared and used for consideration in the organization's risk prevention program.

For nurses, a key element in leadership and management is what decisions and actions to take when there is a sudden realization that something has gone wrong. Since the goal is to protect the safety of the client, reporting and remediation must occur as quickly as possible. The reporting mechanisms set up in the system need to be followed. An incident report needs to be filled out to document appropriately and show evidence of discharge of duty in a timely and thorough manner, and with concern for the client. The combination of detailed risk management programs with ongoing continuous quality improvement efforts can combine to create a level of quality of care that creates a positive service to clients, enhances the organization's esteem, and minimizes legal liability.

SUMMARY

* Quality is one key dimension of healthcare.
* Nurses are key players in ensuring quality healthcare.

- Quality refers to characteristics of and the pursuit of excellence.
- Quality assurance is an organization's effort to provide services according to accepted professional standards and in a manner acceptable to the client.
- TQM is a way to ensure customer satisfaction by involving all employees in quality improvement.
- CQI is a process of continuously improving a system.
- The approach to healthcare quality improvement is undergoing rapid change.
- The emphasis has shifted from the assurance of quality to quality assessment (its measurement) and continuous quality improvement (its management).
- Quality monitoring follows an identifiable process.
- A quality improvement program should pervade the entire organization.
- Three ways standards setting occurs outside of the professional arena: the federal government via Medicare/Medicaid reimbursement regulations, state licensure, and private accreditation.
- The JCAHO has outlined a ten-step process of quality assurance for institutions.
- Standards of quality are critically important and are the first step of a quality improvement program.
- The American Nurses Association has formulated general standards and guidelines for nursing practice.
- Evaluation is based on initial standards and goal setting.
- Standards essentially define quality, against which outcomes and performance are measured.
- Structure, process, and outcome are the methods used to measure quality against standards.
- A variety of approaches to the assessment and measurement of quality are available.
- The audit is probably the most common technique of quality improvement assessment.
- Nursing audits can be prospective, retrospective, or concurrent.
- Research studies manipulate variables.
- Quality improvement studies are necessary for the institution's client care management.
- There is a shift in terms of quality improvement from an emphasis on process to an emphasis on outcomes.
- A key feature of a profession is that it monitors its own practice.
- The public is concerned about quality.
- Risk management is an extension of quality improvement.
- A risk management program is an organization-wide program to identify risks, control occurrences, prevent damage, and control legal liability.

* There are certain known risk-prone areas in healthcare.
* The purpose of an incident report is to provide a permanent record of an incident to assist in refreshing the participant's memory and for reporting data to insurance carriers.

Study Questions

1. Whose responsibility is quality management?
2. What are the differences between institutional and professional responsibilities for quality? Why does this occur?
3. How is quality defined? How is it measured?
4. How is the implementation of TQM/CQI affected by healthcare reform?
5. What components of CQI are easiest/hardest to implement? Why?
6. How are research and quality management related? Can they be combined in one program?
7. What is the relationship of payment to level of quality?

Critical Thinking Exercise

The nurses from 5 North have gathered with other nurses from the hospital for the monthly department-wide nursing staff meeting. The Director of the department of nursing leads the meeting. At agenda item 3 the Director of the Dietary Department rises to speak to the group. The Dietary Director tells the nurses that JCAHO has mandated that nutrition screening be provided as a program. All patients will need to be screened for nutrition deficits. Consequently, Dietary has developed a nutrition screening form that will need to be filled out for each patient. The outcome should be improved quality in the care of clients. However, someone needs to fill out the screening form, notify Dietary of high risk patients, and ensure that alteration in nutrition is documented on the nursing care plan. Under questioning by the nurses, the Dietary Director admits she came to nursing first, before assessing duplicate sources of patient information, computerized relational databases, or interdisciplinary care plans.

1. *What is the problem?*

2. *Whose problem is it?*

3. *Why is it a problem?*

4. *What should the 5 North nurses do?*

5. *What elements of quality and cost should be investigated?*

6. *What data and methods of analysis might be useful?*

7. *How can the new standard be incorporated into TQM or CQI?*

REFERENCES

Aguayo, R. (1990). *Dr. Deming: The American who taught the Japanese about quality.* New York: Lyle Stuart/Carol Publishing.

ANA (The American Nurses' Association). (1973). *Standards of nursing practice.* Kansas City, MO: American Nurses' Association.

ANA (The American Nurses' Association). (1980). *Nursing: A social policy statement.* Kansas City, MO: American Nurses' Association.

ANA (The American Nurses Association). (1991). *Standards of clinical nursing practice.* Kansas City, MO: American Nurses Association.

AONE (The American Organization of Nurse Executives). (1993). Nursing management and JCAHO. *Nursing Management, 23*(5), 26-32.

Bohnet, N., Ilcyn, J., Milanovich, P., Ream, M., & Wright, K. (1993). Continuous quality improvement: Improving quality in your home care organization. *Journal of Nursing Administration, 23*(2), 42-48.

Cohen, E., & Cesta, T. (1993). *Nursing case management: From concept to evaluation.* St. Louis: Mosby.

Culp, B., Goemaere, N., & Miller, M. (1985). Risk management: An integral part of quality assurance. In C. Meisenheimer (Ed.), *Quality assurance: A complete guide to effective management* (pp. 169-192). Rockville, MD: Aspen.

Dean-Baar, S. (1994). Standards and guidelines: How do they assure quality? In J. McCloskey & H. Grace (Eds.), *Current issues in nursing* (4th ed.) (pp. 316-320). St. Louis: Mosby.

Donabedian, A. (1980). *Explorations in quality assessment and monitoring: The definition of quality and approaches to its assessment* (Vol. 1). Ann Arbor, MI: Health Administration Press.

Driever, M. (1992). Quality assessment from a research perspective. *Western Journal of Nursing Research, 14*(1), 106-108.

Fetter, R., & Frieman, J. (1986). Product line management in hospitals. *Academy of Management Review, 11*(12), 41-54.

Flarey, D. (1993). Quality improvement through data analysis: Concepts and applications. *Journal of Nursing Administration, 23*(12), 21-30.

Gardner, D. (1992). Measures of quality. *Series on Nursing Administration, 3*, 42-58.

Harrington, C. (1992). Quality in nursing home care. *Series on Nursing Administration, 3*, 132-149.

Hodges, L., Icenhour, M., & Tate, S. (1994). Measuring quality: A systematic integrative approach. In J. McCloskey & H. Grace (Eds.), *Current issues in nursing* (4th ed.) (pp. 295-302). St. Louis: Mosby.

Institute of Medicine. (1990). *Medicare: A strategy for quality assurance* (Vol. 1). Washington, DC: National Academy Press.

JCAHO (The Joint Commission on Accreditation of Healthcare Organizations). (1990). *Quality assessment and improvement: Proposed revised standards.* Chicago: Joint Commission on Accreditation of Healthcare Organizations.

Lang, N., & Clinton, J. (1984). Quality assurance: The idea and its development in the United States. *Recent Advances in Nursing, 10*, 69-88.

Marszalek-Gaucher, E. (1992). Total quality management in health care. *Series on Nursing Administration, 3*, 105-118.

Marszalek-Gaucher, E., & Coffey, R. (1990). *Transforming healthcare organizations.* San Francisco: Jossey-Bass.

Miller, S., & Flanagan, E. (1993). The transition from quality assurance to continuous quality improvement in ambulatory care. *Quality Review Bulletin, 19*(2), 62-65.

Mitchell, M. (1994). How can we assure health care quality? In J. McCloskey & H. Grace (Eds.), *Current issues in nursing* (4th ed.) (pp. 287-294). St. Louis: Mosby.

Omachonu, V. (1990). Quality of care and the patient: New criteria for evaluation. *Health Care Management Review, 15*(4), 43-50.

Patterson, C. (1988). Standards for patient care: The Joint Commission focus on nursing quality assurance. *Nursing Clinics of North America, 23*, 625-638.

Reiley, P. (1992). Quality assurance programs. *Series on Nursing Administration, 3*, 71-85.

Rooney, A. (1992). Community nursing care and quality. *Series on Nursing Administration, 3*, 119-131.

Schroeder, P., Maibusch, R., Anderson, C., & Formella, N. (1982). A unit-based approach to nursing quality assurance. *Quality Review Bulletin, 8*, 10-12.

Sliefert, M. (1990). Quality control: Professional or institutional responsibility? In J.

McCloskey & H. Grace (Eds.), *Current issues in nursing* (3rd ed.) (pp. 234-241). St. Louis: Mosby.

Smeltzer, C. (1988). Evaluating a successful quality assurance program: The process. *Journal of Nursing Quality Assurance, 2*(4), 1-10.

Stetler, C. (1992). Nursing research and quality care. *Series on Nursing Administration, 3*, 191-207.

Triolo, P. (1994). TQM/CQI: What is it? Does it work? In J. McCloskey & H. Grace (Eds.), *Current issues in nursing* (4th ed.) (pp. 321-326). St. Louis: Mosby.

Watson, C., Bulechek, G., & McCloskey, J. (1987). QAMUR: A quality assurance model using research. *Journal of Nursing Quality Assurance, 2*(1), 21-27.

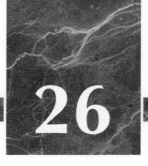

Management of Change

Chapter Objectives

❧

define and describe change

❧

define planned change and a change agent

❧

analyze four major areas of rapid change in healthcare and nursing

❧

explain the process of planned change

❧

distinguish between Lewin's steps in the process of planned change

❧

explain a force field analysis

❧

compare Roger's five phases to the adoption of change

❧

compare Lippitt's and Havelock's elements of the process of change

❧

analyze emotional responses to change

❧

define and discuss resistance to change

❧

analyze effective change

❧

synthesize the concepts of change and innovation

❧

exercise critical thinking to conceptualize and analyze
possible solutions to a practical experience incident

Change has been described as inevitable, constant, universal, and powerful (Workman & Kenney, 1988). Some common sayings reflect the pervasiveness of change: "nothing is sure but death and taxes," "the more things change, the more they stay the same," and "let's go back to the good old days." Change is a pervasive element of society, of today's healthcare environment, and of life. Upon reflection, growth and development is a process of change: life is a sequential pattern of inevitable change. Professional growth and development also are highlighted by periods of growth and change. Change is an inevitable part of nursing and, if planned, can be used as a leadership and management strategy.

DEFINITIONS

hange is defined as an alteration to make something different. Change has been categorized as haphazard or planned (Duncan, 1978) and as developmental, spontaneous, or planned (Lancaster, 1982; Sampson, 1971) (see Chart 26.1). *Planned change* is defined as a process of intentional intervention. In general, it is a process by which an invention of new ideas is created and developed, diffused through communication, and results in consequences of adoption or rejection (Lancaster, 1982). Planned change involves careful thought and action, problem solving, decision making, and interpersonal competence (Welch, 1979).

From an organizational perspective, planned change is a decision to make a deliberate effort to improve the system. Lippitt, Watson, and Westley (1958) added to the definition of change the obtaining of the help of an outside agent in making a deliberate effort to improve the system. A *change agent* is the outside helper used to plan and implement the change process. The term has come to mean a person who functions as a change facilitator.

BACKGROUND

Change occurs on a continuum from haphazard drift to structured planned change. Change can occur by drift as things and people unilaterally change in an uncontrolled fashion. At the other end of the continuum, change can be deliberate and planned, such as occurs when an organization identifies a plan to adopt and implement total quality management. This is a conscious decision that is implemented through a planned change process. In the middle are ad hoc or active approaches to change based on strategies of education, emotional arousal, or coercion. These three strategies of organizational change are called rational-empirical, normative-reeducative, and power-coercive respectively (Bennis et al., 1976). Change in an organization may require generat-

> **CHART 26.1**
> ✍ DEFINITIONS
>
> **Change**
> an alteration, haphazard or planned, to make something different.
>
> **Change agent**
> the outside helper used to plan and implement the change process.
>
> Some data from Duncan (1978).

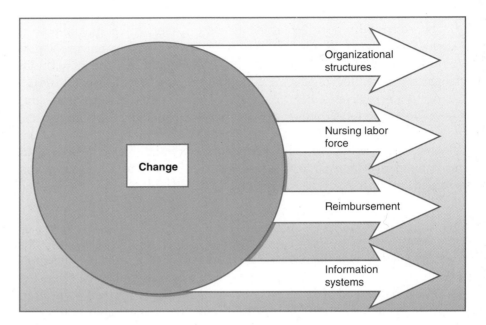

Figure 26.1
Areas of major change in
healthcare and nursing.

ing a push for change from the bottom of the organization and then persuasion of the key leaders at the top of the organization of the need for change.

What is changing in healthcare and nursing? To give a perspective about
the scope of change surrounding nursing, four areas of major change can be
identified. They are organizational structures, the nursing labor force, reimbursement, and information systems (see Fig. 26.1). First of all, organizational
structures are changing and reconfiguring in response to the environment and
financial pressures. For example, case management, shared governance, decentralization, and total quality management (TQM) or continuous quality
improvement (CQI) are elements reflecting change in regard to client care
systems redesign. Bureaucratic systems endured for a long time, but were not
well suited to the work of professionals. The empowerment of staff to result in
the outcome of quality is what the new quality imperatives are designed for.
Clearly, national healthcare reform is an issue creating uncertainty and
change throughout the healthcare delivery system and its organizations.
Changes also are occurring in healthcare generally as integrated networks
form and care increasingly is moved to community settings.

Second, the labor force issues related to a nursing shortage seem to be in
flux. For example, since the 1940s there have been cycles of shortage and surplus in the United States. The future projected demand for nurses is tied to an
increase in chronic illnesses and an increasingly geriatric population. Salaries
in nursing have been increasing, although compensation is sensitive to eco-

Jim O'Malley Envisions Change . . . More Change . . . and Change Again!

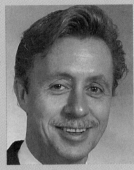

Jim O'Malley

Experience with change has shown that it can ruthlessly destroy those who refuse to adapt. Change does not have a conscience. It doesn't single out people or organizations. Strange as it may seem, change is rapidly becoming the only stabilizing factor in our environment. The massive transformation that is systematically reordering all we thought we knew demands new approaches and new rules for success. It is becoming clear that what we know about change and the ways we created and managed change in our recent past may well be detrimental as we look to the future.

It is an illusion to think that dimensions of change can be isolated. Implementing a vision usually involves the management of change along multiple dimensions simultaneously. Once we have reframed our thinking and broadened our options, it becomes easier to answer the primary question: Can our culture change so that we can survive in a world of competition and rapid change . . . and more importantly will we give our bureaucratic structures and traditional cultures permission to change?

Initiation of change is not without risk, and there are no right answers or easy solutions. People follow leaders who undertake meaningful changes connected to a strategy and who recognize that the ability to change depends largely on effective followership. Change is always a journey and often leaders must drive for action while tolerating inaction. Implementing change involves retaining accountability which creates ownership and responsibility but surrenders control. We will have to constantly challenge the present in order to create the future. We must change our assumptions, invert problems, and invent solutions in order to survive in today's turbulent environment.

Jim O'Malley, MSN, RN, NP, CNS, is Senior Vice President of Nursing Services at Allegheny General Hospital, Pittsburgh, Pennsylvania. See page 15 for the complete biographical note.

nomic and political forces, and salary compression occurs over a work career. The demographics of the workforce are changing. There are new configurations of nurse extenders, ancillary workers, and unlicensed assistive personnel, reflecting a struggle with what is the proper balance of staff mix. It is felt that an all-RN staff is too costly, but beyond that the "ideal" mix is unknown. Job security has lessened as fiscal constraints tighten. There has been some discussion about whether staff nurses could be empowered to make all the management decisions if true decentralization were implemented, and then the role of the nurse manager could be eliminated. Certainly leadership at the unit level is crucial. However, staff mix determination and the role of the nurse are undergoing further experimentation and change.

Another area of important change in healthcare is reimbursement. For example, reimbursement (the payment) for physicians has been changing, driven by the federal government's relative value units determinations. Reimbursement for nurse practitioners now is allowed under Medicare/Medicaid. Payment reforms are likely to continue and to change. The cost areas are physician payment, already being ratcheted down, pharmaceutical costs, and equipment/technology costs. The government will continue to review and explore the amount of dollars spent and the way those dollars are spent in an effort to reduce a huge national budget deficit fueled in part by healthcare costs. An increase in governmental intervention and regulatory control can be predicted in healthcare.

Future changes will bring an increasing use of information systems. Computerization is the wave of the present and the future. For example, there is a national practitioner's data bank which was created from quality concerns. Any physician or nurse who has been party to a lawsuit must have that information reported to the national practitioner's data bank. Large national databases of all licensed nurses also are being compiled. Powerful computers and sophisticated software programs go through updates and generational changes within a few years or less (see Chapter 24).

The amount of change and the rapidity of the pace of change disrupt and disorganize human beings. The perception by some people is that history is what occurred two years ago, and ancient history refers to five years ago. Obsolescence occurs before people have had a chance to adapt to the last round of changes. Stress is an inevitable result. These dynamics affect nurses in their roles as care providers and care managers.

Planned Change

The use of planned change is a nursing management intervention strategy. The nurse uses diagnosis and intervention in clinical practice: the nurse assesses, diagnoses, develops a plan for the client's care needs, and selects an intervention that is matched to that assessment and diagnosis. Managers also as-

Creation of a Dedicated AIDS Unit

Our medical center began seeing patients with acquired immune deficiency syndrome (AIDS) in 1982. The epidemic was in its infancy, as was our understanding of how best to deal with the progression of symptoms, protect healthcare workers from infection, and connect the patient to what little community support existed. Care for patients admitted with what was then variously called HTLV-III, or GRID, or gay men's disease, was haphazard and carried out in an atmosphere of fear, judgment, and isolation.

As we learned more about the disease's transmission factors, clinical manifestations, treatment, and progression, it became evident from care conferences, staff meetings, and patient interviews that we needed a space where specialized doctors and nurses, armed with the knowledge they needed to overcome fear, could provide total care for patients so they could learn to live with a debilitating disease, to fight for as long as they chose, and to die in a place of comfort and support where people knew their names and their stories. Concerns for establishing an appropriate market niche, obtaining adequate reimbursement, and supporting school of medicine research, education, and clinical programs all had to be addressed.

Planning for an AIDS unit took nearly three years and was carried out by an informal team of physicians and nurses who occupied positions of influence within the medical center. Initially we tried to identify everyone who would be impacted positively or negatively by the creation of an AIDS unit and determine his or her role in the decision. We assessed attitudes and knowledge about AIDS and homosexuality among our staff. We arranged AIDS education for the nursing and medical staff and began work that eventually led to universal precautions, HIV testing and provision of AZT for employees with needlesticks, and a needleless IV system for protection of healthcare workers. We searched the literature, visited the AIDS unit at San Francisco General Hospital, and established connections to outside agencies that were beginning to provide AIDS-related services. We publicized these activities within the hospital to stimulate interest and uncover objections.

We prepared a formal proposal to the Hospital Director that included a request to take two inpatient beds out of service to create a day room for the AIDS unit. This room would provide a tangible focus for community attention as well as the private space needed for pa-

tient and family conferences. We prepared a cost-revenue analysis that recognized the low percentage of cost reimbursement anticipated from public payors but highlighted the importance of having the only AIDS unit in our city, linking it to our ability to attract privately funded patients. We projected the cost savings of a case management approach that kept patients out of the hospital longer and reduced readmissions by providing practical education for the patient and significant others and maximizing referrals and placement options.

We hired an AIDS clinical resource nurse to plan care and guide development of nursing expertise on the AIDS unit. Nurses with a specific interest in working with AIDS were hired for the unit, and other nurses from the internal medicine unit or elsewhere in the hospital were floated in as census and acuity required. Some employees expressed concern about exposing their children to HIV. Pregnant nurses were particularly worried about blood and body fluid exposures, and some employees had to deal with the anger and fear of their sexual partners. Use of gloves for handling all blood and body fluids, masks, and goggles to prevent splashing, and counseling from Employee Health Services were provided. Concerns were voiced that an AIDS unit would stigmatize patients housed there and that any patient admitted to the internal medicine unit would be thought to have AIDS. Some believed they would be judged homosexual by working on an AIDS unit. Each concern was addressed individually and in group discussions. Some employees chose to leave the internal medicine unit; some others requested transfer to work there.

Members of the "Fairy Godfathers" and "Hand-to-Hand" volunteers were solicited to provide emotional support and friendship. Their presence and open attitude helped to desensitize some staff to issues of homosexuality and to dispel fear. Pastoral care and social services were arranged. The day room was furnished and decorated using funds contributed by the gay community. Plaques of appreciation and recognition were awarded and hung in the day room. Fundraisers provided money for activities and diversional materials and advertised the unit to the community. A media event and open house announced the official opening of the AIDS unit. Influential members of the gay community, legislators, and community physicians working with AIDS were well represented. These activities instilled pride among the nursing staff and helped assure the long-term success of the AIDS unit.

Successful implementation of the AIDS unit has provided an avenue for bedside nurses to develop teaching and public speaking skills that have taken them into the community as experts. Changes in healthcare reimbursement, especially capitation, have made Medicare/MediCal coverage a more desirable funding source in 1995 than it was in 1989 when the AIDS unit officially opened. Case management of AIDS patients has decreased healthcare costs while maintaining quality. This organizational change has been positive for our patients, our professional nursing practice, our hospital, and our community.

SHARON E. MELBERG, RN, MPA
Assistant Director, Hospital and Clinics
University of California Davis Medical
  Center
Sacramento, California

sess, diagnose, and plan interventions to meet organizational needs and goals. They look at resource allocation and the deployment of people in using planned change as a management intervention. Planning and managing the change process may focus on any or all of the following situational elements: the organizational structure, people, or resources.

Lippitt, Watson, and Westley (1958) identified four types of systems that become the focus for change: individuals, face-to-face groups, organizations, and communities. Change can be thought of as change in an individual or change in a group. Hersey and Blanchard (1993) viewed change from four levels: knowledge, attitudes, individual behavior, and group or organizational behavior or performance (see Fig. 26.2). These levels of change can be graphed from high to low according to the difficulty and the time involved in making a change. The lowest difficulty and shortest time to make a change occurs with knowledge changes. Attitudes are more difficult to change because of being emotionally charged. Individual behavior is the next most difficult and time-intensive change. Group behavior and performance changes are the most difficult and take the longest time.

For nurses with clients and nurses managing other people, the intervention to change someone's knowledge is to teach them. Changing individual behaviors takes more time and is more difficult. For example, in working with

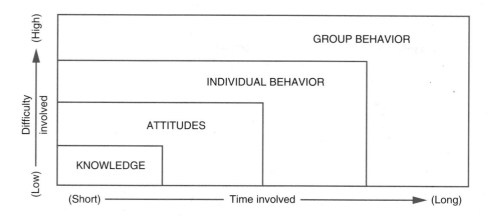

Figure 26.2

Implementing change: time and difficulty. (From Hersey, P., and Blanchard, K. [1993]. MANAGE-MENT OF ORGANIZATIONAL BEHAVIOR: Utilizing Human Resources, 6/E. Englewood Cliffs, N.J.: Prentice Hall, p. 4, and from 4/E. Reprinted with permission from the Center for Leadership Studies.)

clients with diabetes, understanding health principles is easier and takes less time than does demonstrating a change in their behaviors such as selecting foods based on size, quantity, and balance of nutrients. It is even more difficult to change group behaviors among staff. This may be partially a function of dealing with two entities simultaneously, because the group does not change unless individuals first change. For example, if a group is having communication difficulties and conflict is occurring, a change in knowledge can be attempted by an explanation of the destructive behavior. Sensitivity training could be used to change attitudes. The group may understand perfectly, but getting them to change their behavior takes more time and is more difficult. Changing individual and group behavior is not impossible, but it involves time and a large investment of effort.

The Planned Change Process

LEWIN'S FORCE FIELD ANALYSIS

The basic concepts of the change process were outlined by Lewin (1947; 1951). A successful change involves three elements: unfreezing, moving, and refreezing (see Fig. 26.3).

Lewin's (1947; 1951) theory of change uses ideas of equilibrium within systems. Unfreezing is the first stage of change and can be characterized as a process of thawing out the system and creating the motivation or readiness for change. An awareness of the need for change occurs. This first stage is cognitive exposure to the change idea, diagnosis of the problem, and work to generate alternative solutions. A change agent needs trust, respect, and rapport to

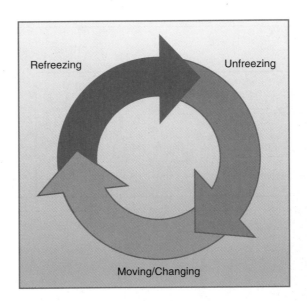

Figure 26.3
Elements of a successful change. (Data from
Lewin [1947] and Lewin [1951].)

effectively unfreeze individuals and groups. Awareness of the need for change
is generated from:
- unmet expectations (lack of confirmation)
- discomfort about action/inaction (guilt/anxiety)
- removal of an obstacle to change (psychological safety).

The unfreezing stage is complete when those involved understand and accept
the necessity of change (Lancaster, 1982; Welch, 1979).

The second change stage is moving. It means moving to a new level of behavior, implying that the actual change occurs in this stage. When the individuals involved collect enough information to clarify and identify the problem, then the change itself can be planned out and initiated. Lewin (1951)
felt that a process of "cognitive redefinition," or looking at the problem from
a new perspective, occurs. In the moving stage, the change can be pretested
and a transition period launched (Lancaster, 1982; Welch, 1979).

The final change stage is refreezing. In this stage, new changes are integrated and stabilized. Reinforcement of behavior is crucial as individuals integrate the change into their own value systems. Techniques of positive feedback, encouragement, and constructive criticism reinforce new behavior
(Olson, 1979).

Lewin's (1947; 1951) planned change process bears similarity to the nursing process and the problem solving process (see Table 26.1). Unfreezing is
like assessing in the nursing process and problem identification and definition
in the problem solving process. Moving is like planning and implementing in
the nursing process and problem analysis and seeking alternative solutions in

Table 26.1

Similarities of Change, Nursing Process, and Problem Solving

CHANGE	NURSING PROCESS	PROBLEM SOLVING
Unfreezing	Assessing	Problem identification
Moving	Planning and implementing	Problem analysis and seeking alternatives
Refreezing	Evaluation	Implementation and evaluation

Data from Workman and Kenney (1988).

the problem solving process. Refreezing is like evaluation in the nursing process and implementation and evaluation in the problem solving process (Workman & Kenney, 1988).

Individuals naturally strive for equilibrium. Lewin (1951) saw this as a balance between driving forces that promote change and restraining forces that inhibit change. Both driving and restraining forces impinge on any situation. The relative strengths of these forces can be analyzed. To create change, the equilibrium is broken by altering the relative strengths of driving and restraining forces. A force field analysis facilitates the identification and analysis of driving and restraining forces in any situation. Unfreezing occurs when disequilibrium is introduced into the system to disrupt the status quo. Moving is the change to a new status quo. Refreezing occurs when the change becomes the new status quo, and new behaviors are frozen.

The process of change may flow back and forth among stages. It is not a simple linear process where one step follows the preceding step. The process may move rapidly, or it may get stuck in any one phase. The goal of planned change is to plan, control, and evaluate the change.

Lewin's (1947; 1951) work forms the classic foundation for change theory. Other change theorists have elaborated further understandings and applications of change theory. Rogers (1962) identified that the background of the individuals involved in a change plus the environment of the change are antecedents to change. He identified five phases to the adoption of change: awareness, interest, evaluation, trial, and adoption. Individuals need to be interested in the innovation and be committed to making change occur. The outcomes of change are two:

1. The change is accepted or adopted.
2. The change is rejected.

If the change is accepted, it can either be continued or eventually dropped. If the change is rejected, it can remain rejected or be adopted later in some other form. Rogers' (1962) theory described change as more complex than Lewin's (1947; 1951) three stages (Lancaster, 1982; Welch, 1979). Further work led to the identification of five factors that determine successful planned change (Rogers & Shoemaker, 1971; Welch, 1979):

1. Relative advantage: the change is thought to be better than the status quo.
2. Compatibility: the change is compatible with existing values of the individuals or group.
3. Complexity: simple techniques are more readily adopted.
4. Divisibility: changes tried out on a small scale (trial) have a greater chance of succeeding.
5. Communicability: the easier the change is to describe, the more likely it will spread.

Lippitt (1973) expanded Lewin's (1947; 1941) work to identify seven phases of the change process:

1. Diagnosis of the problem
2. Assessment of motivation and capacity to change
3. Assessment of the change agent's motivation and resources
4. Selecting progressive change objectives
5. Choosing an appropriate role for the change agent
6. Maintaining the change once it is started
7. Termination of the helping relationship with the change agent

The first three steps compare to Lewin's (1947; 1951) unfreezing. Steps 4 and 5 match to moving, and steps 6 and 7 compare to refreezing. Similar to Lippitt (1973), Havelock (1973) listed six elements to the process of planned change:

1. Building a relationship
2. Diagnosing the problem
3. Acquiring relevant resources
4. Choosing the solution
5. Gaining acceptance
6. Stabilization and self-renewal

The first three correspond to the unfreezing stage of change, the fourth and fifth correspond to the moving stage, and the last relates to refreezing. The various conceptualizations of the stages of the process of change bear similarity to one another but vary in emphasis (see Table 26.2).

Change agents can follow a number of steps in the process of change. The steps include:

- articulating a clear need for the change
- getting the group participating by leaving details to those people who have to implement the change
- getting reliable information and the details to those who are to implement the change
- motivating through rewards and benefits to help the change along
- not promising anything that cannot be delivered

Table 26.2

Comparison of the Process of Change Theories

Lewin:	Unfreezing	Moving	Refreezing
Rogers:	Awareness, interest, evaluation	Trial	Adoption
Lippitt:	Steps 1, 2, 3	Steps 4, 5	Steps 6, 7
Havelock:	Steps 1, 2, 3	Steps 4, 5	Step 6

For example, when implementing a planned change to shared governance, the change agent would need to be clear about the need for and benefits of the change. This might include greater autonomy for nurses. The details of implementation should be left to the group, but only after reliable and detailed information is communicated to them. Rewards and benefits, not threats to performance appraisal, should be the basis of the motivation to change. Participation itself may be motivating. Promised benefits from the change should be limited to what the change agent can deliver.

RESEARCH NOTE

Source: Finkler, S., Kovner, C., Knickman, J., & Hendrickson, G. (1994). Innovation in nursing: a benefit/cost analysis. *Nursing Economic$*, *12*(1), 18-27.

Purpose

In the 1980s a nursing shortage triggered the implementation of a variety of innovative projects aimed at restructuring the work environment of nurses and attempting to better use nursing resources. However, hospitals did not know the true costs of the implementation of these innovations. The purpose of this study was to analyze the cost-benefit ratio of nurse recruitment and retention projects at 37 hospitals that participated in New Jersey's Nursing Incentives Reimbursement Awards Program (NIRA). The innovations were broadly grouped into categories of case management, reorganization of nursing activities, computer projects, shared governance, and education.

Discussion

Data were collected on costs for both computer-based and non-computer-based projects. The average project costs ranged from $1,029 per bed for shared governance to $8,399 per bed for computer projects. An average of 1,800 hours of personnel time were devoted to implementation activities on a typical 30 bed unit for a non-computer project. Overall, implementation of an innovation cost more than was expected. A cost/benefit analysis demonstrated that potential savings due to decreased length of stay were about $3,015 for each $1,000 of investment in one-time implementation costs spent per bed.

> *Application to Practice*
>
> This study provided information about how much implementation of various innovations cost hospitals. Clearly, project costs varied widely based on the type of project. Costs may be one-time or incremental. A major element of the cost of implementing an innovative project is the cost of personnel time. Hours are spent on planning and training. Managerial decisions were aided by cost/benefit analysis ratios concerning the value of the investment, the adequacy of the benefit, and the level of cost.

Emotional Responses to Change

Within nursing, Perlman and Takacs (1990) focused on how individuals cope with change and work through the changes that affect them. Although individuals must devote personal resources and energy to accomplish change, organizations tend to overlook the human emotions associated with an organizational change. Using the death and dying literature as a foundation, Perlman and Takacs (1990) described ten stages to the emotional voyage of the process of change:

1. Equilibrium: there is a sense of balance and inner peace before change occurs.
2. Denial: energy is drained by denial of the reality of a change.
3. Anger: energy is used to ward off the change.
4. Bargaining: energy is used in an attempt to eliminate the change.
5. Chaos: energy is diffused, with a loss of identity and direction.
6. Depression: no energy is left to produce results.
7. Resignation: energy is expended to passively accept change.
8. Openness: renewed energy is available.
9. Readiness: there is willingness to use energy to explore new events.
10. Reemergence: energy is rechanneled, producing empowerment.

Individuals proceed through the emotional stages at various rates. Somewhere between stage 7, resignation, and stage 8, openness, the individual begins to heal and cope with the change. Any organizational change process involves continual letting go of the status quo and emotional grief reactions. Change is more successful as the intellectual and emotional issues involved in the change phases are recognized and dealt with.

Resistance

Resistance to change also is to be expected as integral to the whole process of change. Resistance occurs because people are afraid of being disorganized or of having their routines interrupted. Some may have a vested interest in the status quo. Change may diminish the status of some people, or their web of interpersonal relationships may be disrupted.

Almost all changes encounter some resistance. Resistance seems to arise from fear. For example, some individuals fear expenditure of the energy

Exemplar 26.2

Motivating and Promoting Staff to Take Ownership of the New CDU

The clinical decision unit (CDU) is a 24-hour observation unit that is an extension of the emergency department (ED), where patients are further treated, diagnosed, and stabilized and a disposition is made for either discharge to home or admission to the main hospital.

The CDU is a 20-bed unit, ideally staffed by experienced ED RNs, patient care technicians, and respiratory therapists. The ED physicians follow the patients' care and are responsible for both admission and discharge orders.

Opening a new unit usually creates normal stress with all patient care delivery systems; however, what we needed to keep in mind was that we were introducing a new unit concept with new practice standards for all ED staff. The main focus of the ED is constant turnover of patients, while the CDU focuses on further diagnosis and treatment with a length of stay greater than four, but less than 24, hours. This concept is totally new in the practice of ED medicine. The hardest task was to make the staff believe that this was not a regular nursing floor but truly an extension of the ED.

The staff did not know or understand what the needs of the patients would be in the CDU. The concerns voiced were that these patients are not always as acute as an ED patient, so what will we do for them in an 8 to 12 hour shift? An ED nurse's focus is treating and releasing patients. The CDU is extended treatment, with longer lengths of stay. Ideally, every manager wants an effective and knowledgeable staff. The CDU was not a desired career choice for all of our core staff, but by counterbalancing the desire to remain an ED nurse and managing the unit in an innovative and shared governance style, the staff have taken ownership of the unit.

First, we established committees that not only would help the unit become operational but also would allow staff members the opportunity to choose a committee that would be of interest to them. The four committees selected were the documentation committee, policy and procedures committee, quality assurance and quality indicators committee, and communications committee.

It was a requirement that each staff member sign up for one committee. To our surprise, the staff did more than the expected and became members of multiple committees. The staff realized that we supported them by allowing them to design the committees to meet their needs according to their schedules and then offered them office time during their schedules.

Working on the committees made the staff realize that their input was valued by management and that their suggestions were implemented for the good of the unit. As the committees' ideas developed and took shape, we could see the positive attitudes from the staff and the fact that they were becoming proud of the unit.

Scheduling and education committees were added at the staff's recommendation. The education committee is simple and self-motivated. A three-ring notebook possessing medical articles is available to the staff at all times for reading. Staff members are encouraged to add any articles that will enhance their nursing practice. One of the committee members will be conducting an inservice on electrocardiograms for contact hours, which will be presented to the entire department.

There were negative attitudes toward the original ED scheduling committee and a general restructuring was indicated. One of the staff nurses volunteered to be the representative for the CDU. Her responsibilities include not only core staff scheduling but also scheduling PRN staff members, overtime posting, and accountability for schedule changes. In addition, she has collected data for statistics (i.e., how many weekends were worked and the variance between 8-hour and 12-hour shifts).

By empowering this nurse, the opportunity for self-governance was identified for the entire unit. The staff realizes that the needs of the unit must come first, and they consistently make the necessary ad-

justments to the schedule when peers request time off from the unit.

In the short period of time that the unit has been open, we can see the camaraderie and the ownership that the staff have for the unit. They make recommendations, offer constructive comments, and identify avenues for improvement. Because of their belief in the unit and their quest for quality patient care, managers applaud their diligent and pro-

fessional approach to nursing care and look forward to what we, as a unit, can accomplish in the future.

ANDREA WASDOVICH, RN, BSN, BA
Nurse Manager, Clinical Decision Unit
Emergency Department
Cleveland Clinic Foundation
Cleveland, Ohio

ELIZABETH KEMPE, RN, BSN, CEN
Assistant Nurse Manager, Clinical Decision
Unit
Cleveland Foundation
Cleveland, Ohio

needed to cope with change. Some fear a loss of status, power, control, money, or their job. Resistance generally occurs for two reasons: because of the nature of the change and because of misconceptions and inaccurate information about what the change might mean. Not all resistance is bad. It may be a warning to the change agent to reevaluate the change, clarify the purpose, or increase communication. The change agent needs to anticipate resistance, determine why it is occurring, and decipher what the person who is resisting is trying to protect (Lancaster, 1982).

Asprec (1975) identified four ways in which resistance to change may be manifested (see Fig. 26.4):

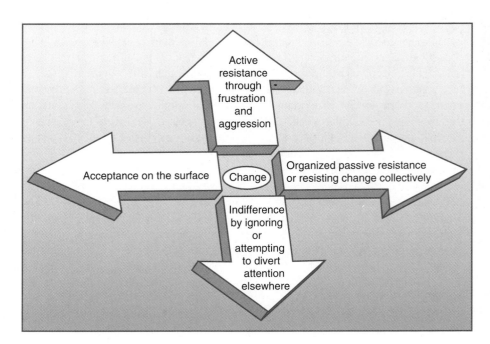

Figure 26.4
Four manifestations of resistance to change. (Data from Asprec [1975].)

1. Active resistance through frustration and aggression
2. Organized passive resistance or resisting change collectively
3. Indifference by ignoring or attempting to divert attention elsewhere
4. Acceptance on the surface or by not openly opposing a change

When initiating a planned change, it is advisable to test the waters to see if individuals or groups are mobilizing organized resistance. There can be a variety of ways in which the resistance surfaces. For example, attendance may drop at meetings. Individuals may withhold information. Individuals or groups may attempt to block the change by refusal to participate or by trying to stop implementation activities. Assessing the quality and the character of resistance will help in making decisions about how to proceed through the process of planned change by identifying interventions and strategies to use.

LEADERSHIP AND MANAGEMENT IMPLICATIONS

Change is implied in the definition of leadership. If leadership is defined as influencing others, then the activity of influencing is directed toward some change. The ability to envision and communicate a changed future is part of the definition of leadership. Leadership has been described as an essential intervention for change (Salmon, 1994). Hersey and Blanchard (1993) noted that change is an inevitable fact of life, but leaders and managers can cope by developing strategies to plan, direct, and control change. The elements of effectiveness that are needed are good diagnostic skills, adapting the leadership style to the situation, and changing some or all of the situational variables.

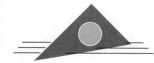 *Leadership & Management Behaviors*

LEADERSHIP BEHAVIORS

- envisions a changed future
- enables change to progress constructively
- models healthy adaptation to change
- influences followers to change and innovate
- communicates the need for change
- plans changes
- evaluates the impact of change and innovation

MANAGEMENT BEHAVIORS

- plans changes
- organizes the group and the environment to implement change
- directs planned change
- adapts to change
- influences subordinates to change
- evaluates planned changes
- communicates the need for planned change

OVERLAP AREAS

- plans changes
- influences others to change
- evaluates changes
- communicates the need for change

It is possible for leaders and managers to plan and implement large scale organizational change without the use of outside consultants. Change can be designed from the inside with (Cauthorne-Lindstrom & Tracy, 1992):

- a clear vision of what the change is to look like
- an organizational culture of trust
- the presence of a champion(s)
- intense involvement of the people who must carry out the change

Both leaders and managers can be effective in implementing organizational change. Anyone in the organization can be the focal point for making appropriate and effective change, but the employees at the bottom of the organization may need to enlist the cooperation of the administrative hierarchy.

Effective Change

Ineffective responses to change do not allow the change process to move along. They include being defensive, giving advice, and premature persuasion. The way to deal with emotionality is to allow people to express themselves while avoiding action based on the emotionality. Trying to immediately persuade people cuts off their ability to vent emotions. Without venting, they may not be able to work through the stages. Censuring, controlling, or punishing probably drives resistance underground. The more that a planned change is driven by authoritarian actions, the more that the seeds of future discontent are sown. The most effective managers possess self-confidence, knowledge of the change process, and the interpersonal skill to help participants to accept, allow, and see the process of change as natural.

Change cycles can be either participative or directive. In a participative change, new knowledge is made available to participants to trigger change. Personal power is used to trigger knowledge, attitude, individual behavior, and group behavior change. Directive change occurs when a change is imposed by some external force. Position power is used to trigger group behavior, individual behavior, attitudes, and knowledge change (Hersey & Blanchard, 1993) (see Chapter 20).

The probability of effectiveness of the change process can be increased through several techniques:

- Explain the rationale for a change so that individuals cognitively understand it.
- Allow emotions to be worked out.
- Give participants a lot of information.
- Help individuals to cope with change.

Actions to be avoided when implementing a change within an organization are to:

- simply announce a change without bothering to lay a foundation.
- ignore or offend powerful people in the organization.
- violate the authority and communication lines in the existing organization.
- rely only on formal authority in implementing a change.
- overestimate your formal authority.
- make a poor decision about what change is needed and do not be open to people critiquing the decision.
- communicate ineffectively.
- put people on the defensive.
- underestimate the perceived magnitude of the change.
- do not deal with the people's fears about insecurity or change of status.

Concerns, insecurities, and resistance are predictable as a part of change. Effectiveness and success are increased as these reactions are anticipated and strategies to cope are developed.

How is change effective? A positive and constructive group process needs to be established: interpersonal relationships are very important. Given the number of changes going on in the environment, empowerment involves using change successfully. Successful change empowers participants. Nurses are empowered when change increases their responsibility, authority, and accountability, and gives them the mechanisms to make decisions to be able to affect client care. Nurses must not only change but must lead the changes as well (Curtin, 1989).

CURRENT ISSUES AND TRENDS

As identified in the background section, there are many changes occurring in healthcare. The healthcare environment has been described as turbulent because of the rapid rate of change and the perceived constancy of change. However, change can be growth-producing, renewing, and invigorating for individuals and organizations. This occurs as individuals and organizations enlist creativity to derive an innovation that improves the environment or client care delivery.

An *innovation* is defined as something new: the introduction of a new process or new way of doing something. Drucker (1985, p. 23) defined innovation from an economic perspective as a change in the yield of resources or as "changing the value and satisfaction obtained from resources by the consumer." According to Drucker (1985) change provides the opportunity for new and different things and processes. A purposeful and organized search for change is the basis for systematic innovation. A careful analysis of the opportunities for change is the best hope for successful economic or social innovation. This occurs because successful innovations exploit change. Thus, Drucker (1992) came to describe innovation as the systematic use of opportunity from changes in the economy, technology, and in demographics. He noted that the challenge today is to make institutions capable of innovation. This can be approached from the viewpoint of innovation as systematic and hard work having little to do with genius and inspiration. Innovation, Drucker (1992, p. 340) noted, depends on "organized abandonment." This is a process of eliminating the obsolete and the no longer productive efforts of the past. Clearly, there needs to be a willingness to view change as an opportunity.

Drucker (1985; 1992) identified seven sources for innovation opportunities: the unexpected, incongruity, process needs, changes in industry or market structure, demographics, new knowledge, and changes in perceptions or moods. He likened the seven sources to windows on a building. In an information-based organization where innovation needs to be systematized, the leader or manager will find four skills important: get outside the organization for facts and perspective, take responsibility for one's own information needs, focus for effectiveness, and build learning into the system.

Change and innovation are companion terms. In nursing, theories of planned change and nursing research utilization are used for conceptualization and research on innovations. In one analysis of the nursing literature, Lewin's (1947; 1951) change theory and Rogers' (1983) diffusion theory were the most frequently cited theories (Tiffany, Cheatham, Doornbos, Loudermelt, & Momadi, 1994). However, popular change theories may be incomplete or inadequate to meet the needs of nurse change agents in practice. This is because popular theories overlook social systems problems or focus on analyzing and watching change rather than being theories of change planning (Tiffany et al., 1994).

Innovation has been differentiated from change. Change is a disruption; innovation is the use of change to provide some new product or service (Romano, 1990). Innovation also has been viewed as the use of a new idea to solve a problem (Kanter, 1983). Organizational innovation is a change from previous practices or the first appearance of a change in an institution (Hess, 1994). The idea of an organizational innovation can be extended to include the imitation or replication of an original innovation if it is perceived as new when adopted (Evan & Black, 1967).

The diffusion of innovations is a term derived from Rogers' (1983) work that is used to discuss the adoption of a new idea or process. Innovations create consequences. To move a new idea to the level of dissemination and adoption requires information, enthusiasm, and authority (Romano, 1990). Innovations diffuse through separate stages in an organization: identification of a performance gap, idea forming or initiating, solution development, implementation, and diffusion (Rogers, 1983). Four elements to consider in an innovation diffusion are the innovation itself, communication channels, time, and the members of the social system (Romano, 1990).

Individuals will react to any change. An individual may adopt one of several roles: innovators, early adopters, early majority, late majority, laggards, or rejectors (Rogers, 1983; 1992). In nursing, Bushy and Kamphuis (1993) used this adoption of innovations model to anticipate negative responses to the introduction of a change in a healthcare institution. A similarity to change reaction styles can be found in problem solving styles as viewed by the Kirton Adaption-Innovation Theory (Kirton, 1989). Innovators use a problem solving style that seeks solutions to problems in original, creative, and innovative ways (see Chapter 6).

Hess (1994) analyzed shared governance and found it to be a further innovation in governance in specific hospitals. McCloskey et al. (1994) analyzed organizational and management changes in nursing. They (McCloskey et al., 1994, p. 36) defined management innovations as "new strategies, structures, or processes for the organization, delivery, and financing of quality care." They identified five categories of nursing managerial innovations: the introduction of new technology, personnel development, changes in the organization of work, changes in rewards/incentives, and implementation of quality improvement mechanisms. In times of constant change and with pressures for cost containment and quality enhancement, nurses need to be able to evaluate innovations for effectiveness and efficiency. No systematic evaluation method currently exists. Therefore, innovations lack the systematic analysis element advocated by Drucker (1985; 1992) and may be adopted primarily following managerial fashion trends.

While healthcare continues to be enmeshed within a changing environment, nurses can learn to cope with change. Beyond coping, nurses can creatively capture change opportunities to improve client care management and service delivery. The result is greater effectiveness and staff and client satisfaction.

SUMMARY

* Change is a pervasive element of society, of today's healthcare environment, and of life.
* Change is defined as an alteration to make something different.
* Planned change is defined as a process of intentional intervention.
* A change agent is the outside helper used to plan and implement the change process.
* Change occurs on a continuum from haphazard drift to structured planned change.
* The amount of change and the rapidity of the pace of change disrupt and disorganize human beings.

- The use of planned change is a nursing management intervention strategy.
- Four systems become the focus for change: individuals, face-to-face groups, organizations, and communities.
- Lewin's theory of change uses ideas of equilibrium within systems.
- A successful change involves Lewin's three elements: unfreezing, moving, and refreezing.
- Unfreezing is the first stage of change and can be characterized as a process of thawing out the system.
- The second change stage is moving to a new level of behavior.
- The final change stage is refreezing new changes so that they are integrated and stabilized.
- Both driving and restraining forces impinge on any situation.
- To create change, the equilibrium is broken by altering the relative strengths of driving and restraining forces.
- Rogers identified five phases to the adoption of change and five factors that determine successful planned change.
- Lippitt identified seven phases of the change process.
- Havelock listed six elements to the process of planned change.
- Perlman and Takacs describe ten stages to the emotional voyage of the process of change.
- Almost all changes encounter some resistance.
- Resistance comes from two general sources: nature of the change and misconceptions and inaccurate information.
- The ability to envision and communicate a changed future is part of the definition of leadership.
- Ineffective responses to change do not allow the change process to move along.
- Change cycles can be either participative or directive.

Study Questions

1. How do individuals in organizations get the information resources that they need in order to effect change?
2. How can informal leaders be used for successful change?
3. What changes need to take place in nursing? Why?
4. How does resistance manifest itself?
5. How can nurses' perceptions be changed to result in empowerment? Why is this important?
6. How should nursing education change? Why?
7. Do we have too much change? What can be done about this?

Critical Thinking Exercise

University Hospital has been feeling the pressure of reimbursement changes to capitation, the effects of being a teaching hospital, and the integration of competitive networks in the area. To improve quality and contain costs, the nursing department has decided to implement case management as a care delivery model. This decision was made after the Chief Nursing Executive had attended a conference and found out that many other hospitals were implementing case management. After the change was announced, a number of staff nurses began to grumble. They did not see how such a change would improve care or how it would work. "Real" nursing care would suffer. Upon hearing about these complaints, the Chief Nurse Executive first tried to persuade the nurses to cooperate, then she called in the most vocal dissenters to tell them why the change was needed and to advise them to be supportive.

1. *Is there a problem?*

2. *What is the problem?*

3. *Whose problem is it?*

4. *What should the nurses do?*

5. *What should the Chief Nurse Executive do?*

6. *What change theory might be useful?*

7. *How might planned change help implement this innovation?*

8. *What emotional responses to change might be anticipated?*

REFERENCES

Asprec, E. (1975). The process of change. *Supervisor Nurse, 6*, 15-24.

Bennis, W., Benne, K., Chin, R., & Corey, K. (1976). *The planning of change.* New York: Holt, Rinehart & Winston.

Bushy, A., & Kamphuis, J. (1993). Response to innovation: Behavioral patterns. *Nursing Management, 24*(3), 62-64.

Cauthorne-Lindstrom, C., & Tracy, T. (1992). Organizational change from the "mom and pop" perspective. *Journal of Nursing Administration, 22*(7/8), 61-64.

Curtin, L. (1989). The sweet smell of success is changing. *Nursing Management, 20*(11), 7-8.

Drucker, P. (1985). *Innovation and entrepreneurship: Practice and principles.* New York: Harper & Row.

Drucker, P. (1992). *Managing for the future: The 1990s and beyond.* New York: Truman Talley Books/Plume.

Duncan, W. (1978). *Essentials of management* (2nd ed.). Hinsdale, IL: Dryden Press.

Evan, W., & Black, G. (1967). Innovation in business organizations: Some factors associated with success or failure of staff proposals. *Journal of Business, 40*, 519-530.

Havelock, R. (1973). *The change agent's guide to innovation in education.* Englewood Cliffs, NJ: Educational Technology Publications.

Hersey, P., & Blanchard, K. (1993). *Management of organizational behavior: Utilizing human resources* (6th ed). Englewood Cliffs, NJ: Prentice-Hall.

Hess, Jr., R. (1994). Shared governance: Innovation or imitation? *Nursing Economic$, 12*(1), 28-34.

Kanter, R. (1983). *The change masters: Innovation for productivity in the American corporation.* New York: Simon & Schuster.

Kirton, M. (1989). *Adaptors and innovators: Styles of creativity and problem solving.* London: Routledge.

Lancaster, J. (1982). Change theory: An essential aspect of nursing practice. In J. Lancaster & W. Lancaster (Eds.), *The nurse as a change agent: Concepts for advanced nursing practice* (pp. 5-23). St. Louis: Mosby.

Lippitt, G. (1973). *Visualizing change: Model building and the change process.* La Jolla, CA: University Associates.

Lippitt, R., Watson, J., & Westley, B. (1958). *The dynamics of planned change: A comparative study of principles and techniques.* New York: Harcourt, Brace & World.

Lewin, K. (1947). Frontiers in group dynamics: Concept, method, and reality in social science; social equilibria and social change. *Human Relations, 1*(1), 5-41.

Lewin, K. (1951). *Field theory in social science: Selected theoretical papers.* New York: Harper & Row.

McCloskey, J., Maas, M., Huber, D., Kasparek, A., Specht, J., Ramler, C., Watson, C., Blegen, M., Delaney, C., Ellerbe, S., Etscheidt, C., Gongaware, C., Johnson, M., Kelly, K., Mehmert, P., & Clougherty, J. (1994). Nursing management innovations: A need for systematic evaluation. *Nursing Economic$, 12*(1), 35-44.

Olson, E. (1979). Strategies and techniques for the nurse change agent. *Nursing Clinics of North America, 14*(2), 323-336.

Perlman, D., & Takacs, G. (1990). The 10 stages of change. *Nursing Management, 21*(4), 33-38.

Rogers, E. (1962). *Diffusion of innovations.* New York: Free Press.

Rogers, E. (1983). *Diffusion of innovations* (3rd ed.). New York: Free Press.

Rogers, E. (1992). *Social change in rural societies.* Englewood Cliffs, NJ: Prentice-Hall.

Rogers, E., & Shoemaker, F. (1971). *Communication of innovations: A cross cultural approach.* New York: Free Press.

Romano, C. (1990). Diffusion of technology innovation. *Advances in Nursing Science, 13*(2), 11-21.

Salmon, M. (1994). Leadership for change in public and community health nursing. In J. McCloskey, & H. Grace (Eds.), *Current issues in nursing* (4th ed.) (pp. 232-240). St Louis: Mosby.

Sampson, E. (1971). *Social psychology and contemporary society.* New York: John Wiley & Sons.

Tiffany, C., Cheatham, A., Doornbos, D., Loudermelt, L., & Momadi, G. (1994). Planned change theory: Survey of nursing periodical literature. *Nursing Management, 25*(7), 54-59.

Welch, L. (1979). Planned change in nursing: The theory. *Nursing Clinics of North America, 14*(2), 307-321.

Workman, R., & Kenney, M. (1988). The change experience. In S. Pinkerton & P. Schroeder (Eds.), *Commitment to excellence: Developing a professional nursing staff* (pp. 17-25). Rockville, MD: Aspen.

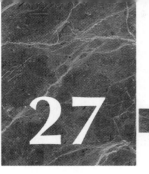

Performance Appraisal

Chapter Objectives

❧

define and describe performance appraisal

❧

define peer review

❧

explain the role of values in evaluation

❧

distinguish among the purposes of performance appraisal

❧

analyze the performance appraisal process

❧

explain performance measurement tools

❧

define and differentiate common evaluator errors

❧

analyze effective performance appraisal

❧

relate leadership and management to performance appraisal

❧

analyze current trends

❧

exercise critical thinking to conceptualize and analyze
possible solutions to a practical experience incident

*P*erformance appraisal is an activity that individuals do informally all the time. For example, restaurants and hotels solicit client feedback. For employees in an organization, part of a manager's job is to formally appraise the performance of employees. The process of managerial control includes doing evaluations. They are done for multiple purposes. The reason for the management step of evaluating and controlling is to measure the quality and effectiveness of nursing activities. Conventional performance appraisal systems are designed to measure nursing performance and motivate personnel toward greater achievement (Albrecht, 1972).

Further, managers need to determine the competency of staff personnel. It is not sufficient to assume that because nurses are licensed they are competent. Assessing the competency of staff is done to demonstrate that staff are competent practitioners as one element of quality care. Certainly to payors and consumers the quality of care providers is an issue. Regulatory agencies are beginning to require proof of competency assessment. They look for evidence of staff inservice and the range of nursing skills attained.

DEFINITION

P erformance appraisal and evaluation in nursing are concerned with measuring the efficiency, determining the competency, and measuring the effectiveness of the nursing process and activities used by the individual nurse in the care of clients. *Performance appraisal* means evaluating the work of others. Albrecht (1972) defined *conventional performance appraisal* as a systematic, standardized evaluation of an employee by the supervisor, aimed at judging the perceived value of the employee's work contribution, quality of work, and potential for advancement (see Chart 27.1). The employee's work is measured against standards, and in that sense it is very much like the quality assessment process. Standards, whether explicit or not, are applied to what ought to be or to what is superior, excellent, average, or unacceptable performance. *Peer review* is defined as the examination and evaluation of practice by a nurse's associates (Christensen, 1990).

BACKGROUND

Performance is determined by two elements: ability and motivation. Ability is made up of a collection of physical and mental capacities that enable a person to exhibit a skill or set of skills. Thus ability is an innate capacity that is molded by experience and training. Motivation is a willingness to work and a desire to achieve. Motivation influences the vigor and diligence with which an individual applies his or her capability to a task (Nauright, 1987). Mager and Pipe (1970) outlined ability and motivation as two paths to take to analyze performance and performance problems. Ability deficits are remediated through careful assignments and training. Lack of motivation can be identified in four situations when:

* it is punishing to perform as desired (e.g., volunteering for extra work with no extra compensation)

CHART 27.1
∿ DEFINITIONS

Conventional Performance Appraisal
a systematic, standardized evaluation of an employee by the supervisor, aimed at judging the value of the employee's work contribution, quality of work, and potential for advancement.

Peer review
the examination and evaluation of practice by an employee's associates.

Data from Albrecht (1972) and Christensen (1990).

- nonperformance is rewarded (e.g., someone who is chronically late to work)
- it makes no difference whether or not there is performance (e.g., no feedback)
- there are obstacles to performance (e.g., lack of supplies or time)

Motivation problems can be remediated by changing the conditions or consequences causing nonperformance (see Chapter 19 for further discussion of motivation).

The most direct goal of any performance appraisal system is the improvement of performance. Nauright (1987) identified four integral components of a comprehensive performance appraisal system (see Chart 27.2). Some examples of the tools and methods used in performance appraisal are job descriptions, personnel selection, staff development, and the reward system.

The basic assumption of performance appraisal systems is that being told about positive qualities and any shortcomings lets the employee know "where they stand." Knowing their status will stimulate improvement in performance (Albrecht, 1972). Performance feedback has been rated by employees as the strongest nonfinancial reward that produces motivation, satisfaction, and remediation (Graham & Unruh, 1990; Haas, 1992).

Values and Evaluation

Evaluation by definition is subjective. The word value is a segment of the term evaluation. The evaluator's perception and interpretation of events drives the evaluation. There really is no such thing as performance in a vacuum. Therefore, no performance appraisal system is absolutely objective. The key to being effective is figuring out the evaluator's expectations and value system and realizing the natural element of subjectivity inherent in performance appraisal. Individuals may be able to narrow the discrepancy between the evaluator's perception and their own perception of what performance occurred. For example, much of nurses' performance occurs within the client-nurse interaction, when the nurse may be alone with the client. Thus a nurse's best work may occur in isolation and may not be visible to an evaluator who is not present at the time. What is visible is the documentation, and performance may be judged on such a byproduct of work. Further, supervisors and peers may personally observe only a select sample of a nurse's work, not the totality of it. Thus performance may be judged on a sample of work output.

The evaluator has a set of values, beliefs, and biases and an experiential base that filters what is evaluated as performance. Therefore, since image, appearance, and attitude make an impression, they also make a difference. Fair or not, that is human nature and reality. Deportment, dress, grooming, and attitude are nonverbal communication modes that make an impression and a difference in how others make a judgment (see Chapter 18). This occurs not

CHART 27.2
∽ COMPONENTS OF COMPREHENSIVE APPRAISAL SYSTEM

- Determine the ability required (job description).
- Match abilities of the employee to job requirements (personnel selection).
- Improve employees' abilities (staff development).
- Enhance employees' motivation (staff development and the reward system).

Data from Nauright (1987).

only with clients but also in the way an individual is perceived by peers, superiors, and other people who will be evaluating performance. Although it may be preferable to have an objective performance appraisal tool and process, the reality of human nature is that performance appraisal is more complex and interpersonal than that and much more tied to perceptions, biases, values, attitudes, and appearance.

If the point of performance appraisal is to improve performance, then the evaluator can make a positive difference by making a point of evaluating behavior as opposed to concentrating on personal characteristics. Evaluating behavior gives a basis for focused improvement. Individuals can change what they do and how they behave. Thus in the work environment the choices made can make a difference in terms of both performance and performance appraisal.

A key concept to remember is that clients, peers, and superiors always are evaluating a nurse's performance. Whether done well or poorly, and regardless of the process used, evaluation is constantly occurring. The performance appraisal information will vary as to whether or not it is written, given as feedback, and communicated in a constructive way. Individuals who do not anticipate this dynamic may be surprised about organizational evaluations and rewards.

Performance Appraisal Purposes

In healthcare, performance appraisal generally is done as a part of overall quality assessment and to promote the best possible client care. Performance appraisal also is done to maintain, improve, and motivate employee behaviors. In a service industry, quality and efficiency are a reflection of the performance of personnel. As employee performance improves, productivity is expected to increase (Bushardt & Fowler, 1988). As noted in Chapter 25, Deming's ideas and total quality management or continuous quality improvement (TQM/CQI) are being instituted to improve the quality of systems. At the level of the individual nurse and client interaction, performance appraisal is the mechanism used to assess and improve quality of care. Thus it is done for both quality and motivation purposes. At the level of teamwork, performance appraisal is focused on the outcomes obtained, including efficiency, effectiveness, efficacy, and performance (see Chapter 28).

In nursing, performance appraisal may be conducted through three mechanisms (see Fig. 27.1): personal, peer, or managerial evaluation. Administrative or managerial performance appraisal is done to ensure organizational success, improve performance, and let employees know how well they are performing (Veninga, 1982). Two purposes of managerial performance appraisal are evaluative and judgmental or developmental. An evaluation approach puts the

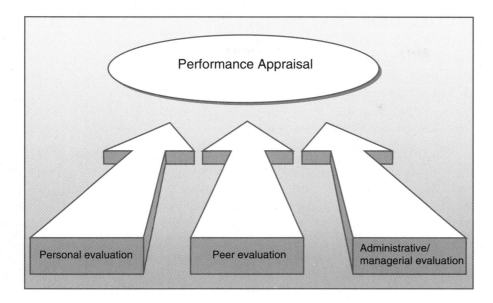

Figure 27.1
Mechanisms for performance appraisal in nursing.

manager in a judgmental role. The evaluation aspect results in data for making administrative decisions about the perceived value of an employee to the organization. A reward approach requires that the manager make a judgment about the person's performance and determine a raise or other rewards. For example, in facilities where across-the-board increases in salary are given, the reward approach would be used for promotions or other awards. The focus of the *evaluative or judgmental* purpose is past performance, with the objective of improving performance by linking it to rewards (Nauright, 1987).

The *developmental* purpose puts the manager in the role of counselor. Related activities include counseling about areas for improvement, the resources available for improvement, and the intermediate goals to accomplish improvement. The focus of the developmental purpose is on the individual's potential for performance. Improvement of performance is attempted through self-learning and growth stimulated by feedback and leading to knowledge and skill development (Nauright, 1987).

Two judgment standards exist. First is an *absolute standard* that is internal to the manager. The absolute standard means that the evaluative standard is the manager's own biases and opinions about what ought to be. For example, consider ways of grading college courses. If the scale is 71 to 80 = C; 81 to 90 = B; 91 to 100 = A, then an internal standard is being used that is arbitrarily decided by the instructor. This internal standard is the instructor's decision that 71 to 80 acquired points equals C level accomplishment. Second is a *comparative standard*. A comparative standard is used to evaluate an individual in relative standing compared to other people. For example, in a course where students' scores are arrayed from high to low and then grades are assigned based on rank compared to the other people in the class, a comparative standard is being used because individuals are compared to other people in the same group. With an absolute standard, it is possible for all students to get an A. This would not likely occur using a comparative standard.

The Process of Performance Appraisal

The process of performance appraisal includes assessing needs and setting goals, establishing the objectives and the time frame, assessing the progress and evaluating the performance, and then starting over again (see Fig. 27.2). At the start of a new job, an employee is assessed as to knowledge and skills. In the orientation program, progress will be assessed and tracked and then evaluated periodically throughout employment.

The performance appraisal process is both informal and formal. The informal process includes day-by-day supervision or coaching to moderate, modulate, or refine small parts of performance. Coaching is an approach to developing people in an organization that is described as falling somewhere between preceptoring and mentoring (Haas, 1992). The term coach invokes a sports metaphor. Every team relies on a coach to help the athlete(s) reach full potential. Coaching as a management tool is ongoing, face-to-face collaboration and influencing to improve skills and performance. The formal performance appraisal should include written documentation and a formal performance appraisal interview with follow-up.

The employee's work is measured against some standard for the purposes of determining the level of quality of job performance. The guides to evaluation criteria include governmental standards, such as Medicare/Medicaid regulations, professional standards published by the American Nurses Association, nursing care audits, opinion polls, client feedback in various forms, and departmentally-developed standards. Ideally, a performance appraisal measures

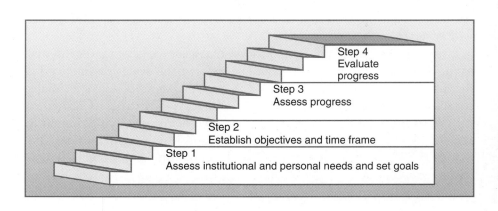

Figure 27.2
Four steps of a performance appraisal.

performance and motivates the person. However, performance appraisal is not the only or major source of motivation for most nurses (see Chapter 19). Measuring performance is not at all easy, and motivating someone else is an art. To combine those things in a performance appraisal that may have negative connotations is a challenging endeavor.

In nursing, standards may be developed around areas of performance. For example, to capture components of professional nursing practice for the purpose of staff nurse evaluation and performance appraisal, one performance appraisal tool was constructed around the following five areas of nursing practice:

1. Nursing process
2. Collaborative practice
3. Leadership
4. Management
5. Professional development and continuing education

In this example, standardized objectives established consistent criteria for evaluation (Behrend et al., 1986).

Both the job description and the performance evaluation tool, if they are well-constructed, should reveal what is considered most important by nursing management. For example, an organization that says its philosophy, purpose, and goals are teaching, research, and service should have job descriptions and performance appraisal tools that address teaching, research, and service. Both documents need to be clear and distributed to employees.

Performance appraisal can have positive outcomes. It can be an opportunity to set goals. Performance appraisals can and should:

- improve performance
- improve communication
- reinforce positive behavior
- be one method employed to communicate about and ultimately to correct negative or less than optimal behaviors
- provide a basis for rewards, which also is a basis for motivation
- provide a basis for termination if necessary
- identify learning needs and develop personnel

Within the performance appraisal process, constructive problem solving focuses on the positive aspects first by describing the positive things that have occurred over the course of the evaluation period in order to lay a groundwork. Positive elements can be found in almost everybody's behavior and performance. The individual should be encouraged to continue positive behaviors. Then the areas of deficiency or problems that need be to worked on can be reviewed and discussed. Be specific. Focus on the actual behaviors that need to change and identify a behavior-oriented outcome target. Ideally there is a process in which both strengths and weaknesses are identified, and then there is a plan identified for augmenting or developing the person in his or her areas of less strength. Setting targeted outcome goals and timeframes improves performance by directing energy toward desired results.

Ten useful research-based principles for performance appraisal are (Sashkin, 1982):

1. Managers need to be rewarded for developing subordinates.
2. Managers need skill and training in using appraisal tools effectively.
3. Job descriptions need to be tied to the appraisal mechanism.
4. Employees who are involved in the appraisal process consistently perform better and are more satisfied.
5. Mutually agreed upon performance goal setting increases worker performance.
6. A problem solving focus to appraisal counteracts defense-avoidance behaviors.
7. Separating a counseling or developmental appraisal from an administrative appraisal allows more discussion and problem solving.
8. Paperwork and administrative support to carry out the performance appraisal process need to be matched to organizational goals.
9. The appraisal process must match the specific expectations of the job.
10. The performance appraisal system needs to generate useful and accessible information for administrative decisions.

Performance Measurement Tools

Performance is measured from collected data. There are various methods and tools used (Veninga, 1982). *Anecdotal notes and critical incident descriptions* are written records of observation about behaviors and attitudes (see Chart 27.3). For example, when an incident arises where something untoward occurs, notes are written by the individual personally, to textually describe what happened. Included are facts about who was there, what time it occurred, what happened, and what the individual did and said. Managers use anecdotal notes as a way of compiling a record, since their memory is not perfect. A running log may be established. At the end of an evaluation period, the log provides a platform for discussion about performance and specific instances. Anecdotal notes are one tool for systematic performance appraisal.

Other tools for performance appraisal include *open-ended essays*. They are descriptions of the perception of performance written by an evaluator in an essay form. At the opposite end of structured formats for evaluation, structured *checklists* also are used for performance appraisal. They are lists of desired characteristics or behaviors. The evaluator checks off if behaviors are present or absent. For example, a psychomotor skills evaluation lists psychomotor skills and asks if the individual has done them, with a yes or no response. Check-

CHART 27.3
∾ DEFINITIONS

Anecdotal Notes
written records of observation of behaviors and attitudes.

Open-ended Essays
descriptions of the perception of performance written by an evaluator in essay form.

Checklists
lists of desired characteristics or behaviors.

Rating Scale
Likert-type scale within a range of numbers such as 1 to 5 for assessing characteristics such as quality of work and initiative.

Behaviorally Anchored Rating Scales
scales that focus on behaviors to increase objectivity of the appraisal.

Data from Veninga (1982).

lists do not address how well the individual is able to use the skills, rather they merely determine the level of basic skill attainment.

A *rating scale* may be used to locate behavior on a Likert-type scale within a range of numbers, such as one to five. For example, a nurse might be asked to evaluate a peer or subordinate on a scale of 1 to 5 on characteristics of quality of work, initiative, dependability, cooperation, appearance, concern for others, and emotional stability. These items are global and related more to personality and appearance than to specific individual performance behaviors. Rating scales are used as a way to assess performance, but a question arises as to whether the ratings can be defended. The evaluator may be challenged on, for example, the difference between a 3.5 and a 4. Rating scales are faster for the evaluator to fill out than are essays.

Finally, there are *behaviorally anchored rating scales*. These scales attempt to move toward performance appraisal objectivity by focusing on documentation of behaviors (Bushardt & Fowler, 1988). One well-known behaviorally anchored scale that also is used as a research instrument asks about specific nurse behaviors. It is the Schwirian Six-Dimension Scale of Nursing Performance (Schwirian, 1978).

Clearly, there is a range of performance appraisal tools from anecdotal notes, to rating scales, to research-based instruments. The level of structure and the sophistication of these performance appraisal tools vary widely, as does how specifically performance is determined and measured.

Many performance appraisal tools categorize performance into levels. The number of levels varies. Seven levels have been identified as (Nauright, 1987):

1. Completely unacceptable
2. Marginally unacceptable
3. Marginally acceptable
4. Adequate
5. Good
6. Very good
7. Exceptionally good

For behavioral descriptions of nursing performance, a range of categories includes (Bushardt & Fowler, 1988):

1. Unacceptable
2. Poor
3. Average
4. Good
5. Excellent

There are various ways to collect evaluative data. First, sample behavior needs to be collected over time, remembering that direct observation is probably the best data source. There are ranges of and different ways of doing di-

Staff Evaluations

For a nurse manager, annual staff evaluations are a natural part of the job. Nurse managers, however, cannot always identify the positive and negative attributes of all members of the staff. I found this out in my first year as a nurse manager, when I had to write the annual evaluations for the entire staff.

The difficulty I encountered was in being able to describe the individual's performance throughout the year. I kept a log in which every two to three weeks I would write down my observations of staff members' performance. I would also note any comments from families and feedback from peers. Nurses, however, can sometimes be overly critical of their coworkers. Whenever something went wrong, as when a nurse did not follow a doctor's order, someone would make sure I was the first to know. If something positive happened, as when a nurse acted as a patient advocate or handled a difficult situation, I was usually the last to be informed. Thus, when it came time to write the evaluation, I had the data to write constructive criticism but was unable to include positive feedback or cite that special incident with a patient or family. Pointing out where a nurse excels is necessary so that the positive feedback can promote a healthy and hopeful work environment.

The following year I tried a different approach, peer evaluation, which I found to be more reliable. I gave each staff member two blank evaluations with a peer's name on each, so that each nurse wound up evaluating two other nurses. Each nurse also received a blank evaluation form for self-evaluation. Guidelines for evaluation were provided and posted in the unit. Performance ratings were exceeds expectations, achieves expectations, or needs improvement. Staff members were instructed to cite examples of their peer's performance to support one of the three ratings. Matching up those being evaluated with those doing the evaluation required much planning on my part to avoid the bias that might arise from two nurses who were close friends.

As the staff turned in the evaluations I reviewed the self-evaluation along with the two peer evaluations. I also continued to maintain my own log of observations and incidents. I used these to write my final evaluation for each staff member for the annual performance appraisal. Confidentiality was essential for the peer evaluations and self-evaluations, so that the feedback could be as honest and constructive as possible.

In the administration of the annual evaluations the staff would ask me what others thought of their performance. This would give me the opportunity to relay the positive qualities that their peers identified, which really helped to create a better team by clarifying everyone's expectations. Peer evaluations also helped identify suggestions for improvement and strategies for achieving it—such as a seminar on how to deal with difficult people.

The self-evaluations and peer evaluations often had similar comments. For example, one nurse had difficulty communicating with physicians. Both the nurse herself and her peers identified this problem, and her peers suggested how she might improve this skill. Together the nurse and I set goals for the upcoming year and focused on her communication skills. Throughout the year the rest of the staff and I worked with this nurse and noticed a marked improvement.

Peer and self-evaluations seem to have been successful in our unit by giving the staff a change to think about the quality of performance and to critique their peers on a professional level.

JULIE HENDERSON, RN, BSN
Nurse Manager, PICU/Pediatrics
The Cleveland Clinic Foundation
    Children's Hospital
Cleveland, Ohio

rect observation. For example, using powers of observation to scan the environment and see behaviors is a way to gather data. Reviewing charting is direct observation of documentation and a way of observing one piece of total performance. Talking to others who also observe behavior is another way to gather data. Although the element of bias due to perception is a consideration, this can be balanced by using multiple data sources for input and analysis and to create a more balanced picture.

Common Evaluator Errors

Performance appraisal is an interpersonal process. All evaluation contains an element of subjectivity. Further, individuals are prone to certain common errors in perception. Nauright (1987) identified a number of evaluator rating errors (see Chart 27.4). The first rating error is the *halo effect*. The halo effect is a tendency for the rater to assume that if the person does well in several known areas, he or she will do well in all areas. Just because someone can make a bed quickly and with perfect corners does not necessarily mean that he or she is proficient in another area, such as in dealing with psychosocial aspects. Sometimes a rater is not able to sample all ranges of behavior. Therefore, if the person is very good in certain areas, it is assumed that he or she must be good in all areas, and this becomes the input data used to appraise performance.

Another error is the *recency effect*. This means that the rater only recalls or uses recent data. For example, if in a performance appraisal the only point of evaluation is the most recent negative incident, then the evaluator is focusing only on the most recent behavior and not on the range of behavior over time. This creates an unbalanced perspective of the person. It generally benefits poorer performers, who can alter behavior toward the positive for a short time prior to known evaluation. Anecdotal notes are a useful tool to offset the recency effect.

Problem distortion means that one negative event is remembered more than multiple positive ones. That one negative event could have occurred 20 years ago, and yet it keeps showing up on a performance evaluation. The evaluator cannot get past that incident. The possibility of growth and change are overlooked by the evaluator.

The *sunflower effect* means that a rater rates everybody high because they belong to a "great team." This is wonderful for the person being rated, because everyone likes to have a high rating. However, it does nothing in terms of developing the individual. The evaluator decides that everybody here is perfect: there are no problems because this is the best team. Employees are not helped to see areas in which they could grow or develop. Some evaluators do not want to face the fact that they should tell someone to improve. However, employees are denied the opportunity for individual achievement to be recognized and thereby acquire a form of motivation and satisfaction.

CHART 27.4
〰 EVALUATOR
RATING ERRORS

Halo Effect
the rater assumes that if the person does well in several known areas, he or she will do well in all areas.

Recency Effect
the rater only recalls or uses recent data.

Problem Distortion
the rater remembers or uses one negative event more than multiple positive ones.

Sunflower Effect
rater scores everyone high because they are a great team.

Central Tendency Effect
the rater marks everyone average.

Rater Temperament Effect
different raters tend to score more strictly or leniently.

Guessing Errors
rater is apathetic or overloaded and does not really collect the necessary evaluative data.

Data from Nauright (1987).

The *central tendency effect* is one in which the evaluator marks everybody average, especially if the evaluator is unsure of the actual performance. This is the opposite of individually looking at each employee and knowing what his or her performance really is. It is the path of least resistance to list employees as average because the evaluator really does not know very much about them or has not taken the time to fully assess strengths and weaknesses.

The *rater temperament effect* occurs when different raters rate strictly or leniently. People vary in terms of the strictness with which they appraise performance. Thus an individual's performance appraisal may vary for the same performance depending on the rater. In research methodology, interrater reliability is computed to assess a similar type of bias.

Guessing errors occur with apathetic or overloaded evaluators who do not really collect the necessary evaluative data. They simply guess at the performance. Guessing leaves open a wide path for error. The halo effect incorporates an element of guessing error.

The chief concern with all forms of evaluator errors is how to establish equity and fairness. The biases of evaluators are a practical reality. Performance appraisal, although it is subjective, ought to be done with equity and fairness, and with encouragement for people to grow and develop. Therefore, performance appraisal activities need to be as comprehensive, equitable, and accurate as possible.

Effective Performance Appraisal

To be effective, a performance appraisal system needs to provide objective assessment of the knowledge, skills, and abilities of employees and also must enhance staff development (Albrecht, 1972). Developing skill in assessment and interview techniques is a key to effective performance appraisal. Asking questions can elicit important evaluative data. Using a coaching process means studying present behavior and developing planned, purposeful change strategies or intermediate multiple small steps to bring performance closer to what is desired. A process of the employer and employee establishing mutual goals contributes to improved performance.

From the employee's perspective, documentation is a strategy to use in performance appraisal. This is one portion of a process of personal or self-evaluation. One technique is to accumulate one's own documentation, particularly the positive events over the course of an evaluative period. Knowing that an annual performance appraisal occurs, the employee can submit a profile or portfolio ahead of the scheduled formal performance appraisal. For example, a self-analysis should be done to review prior accomplishments and to set personal goals. This can then be presented along with documentation of accomplishments. Submitting positive documentation may structure a more positive

appraisal experience. From the evaluator's perspective, he or she can anticipate areas of potential disagreement or those that may create an emotional response. Equity, fairness, and trust are built by encouraging two-way communication, choosing the time carefully, and using a private setting so that the
person feels that confidentiality is protected. A comfortable setting aids in establishing rapport. The evaluator should decrease or avoid interruptions. A
problem solving climate facilitates a positive experience. Setting mutual goals
provides a structure so that each party is clear about expectations. At the end
of the performance appraisal process the evaluator needs to ask the person
about his or her perceptions of what occurred to try to elicit feedback.

In some institutions, peer evaluation is a part of the performance appraisal
process. For example, peer evaluation may be mandated as a part of a clinical
ladder program. A specified number of peers, perhaps two or three, review
charts and other compiled portfolio materials to appraise an employee's performance. As a part of a unit's appraisal system a nurse will hold roles of both
evaluator and evaluatee in the course of an appraisal cycle. However, like personal or self-evaluation, peer evaluation provides another important perspective to the evaluation of performance to add to the mandated administrative
or supervisor review of performance.

LEADERSHIP AND MANAGEMENT IMPLICATIONS

In nursing, performance appraisal occurs in different ways. One example
would be a code blue review. This occurs after a cardiopulmonary resuscitation (CPR) event, when there is an evaluation or post-hoc review of how
well the code was run. The performance of the nurses, physicians, communications system, respiratory therapists, electrocardiogram technicians, and
anyone else involved is reviewed and critiqued, and areas for improvement
are identified.

Managers universally complain about performance appraisal, usually because of the uncomfortable interpersonal relationship aspects (Albrecht,
1972). It takes appropriate interpersonal skills and practice to present constructive criticism in a way that encourages the person to grow. Employees
may have had experiences with less-than-positive performance appraisals, becoming conditioned to fear and hate them. They bring those feelings into the
next performance appraisal. Behaviors like bargaining, crying, anger, or a personal attack may occur. The way the individual was parented conditions feelings and reactions. Focusing on the positive benefits of performance appraisal,
especially improved performance and communication, helps a manager to develop a more positive attitude toward this task. Subordinates also should be
given the opportunity to appraise managers' performance (McGee, 1992).
This is the idea of reverse performance appraisals, which can be built into the

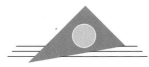

Leadership & Management Behaviors

LEADERSHIP BEHAVIORS	MANAGEMENT BEHAVIORS	OVERLAP AREAS
• enables high level performance	• evaluates performance	• evaluates performance
• inspires high performance in individuals	• conducts performance appraisals	• takes corrective actions
• models desirable performance characteristics	• coaches subordinates	
• evaluates performance	• analyzes performance problems	
• counsels followers with performance problems	• corrects performance problems	
• motivates followers to improve knowledge and skills	• disciplines employees	
	• validates clinical competence	

overall performance appraisal and quality improvement system. However, trust and anonymity need to be guarded and preserved.

CURRENT ISSUES AND TRENDS

In the first nursing job, the nurse may not have a performance appraisal for the first year. This is a shock to many people who are used to constant feedback in their educational experiences. Then suddenly it may be a long time before an evaluator appraises performance and they receive feedback to reassure them about progress.

Nurses may face uncomfortable issues in clinical practice that require action based on informal performance appraisal. For example, if nurses are in the unfortunate situation in which they observe inferior care or an unsafe action by another nurse, they automatically become involved in the process of performance appraisal. First of all, the judgment is made that the behavior was unsafe, then the nurse has to make a decision about what to do about it. Ethical implications are involved in difficult decisions.

The most fruitful evaluation process for any individual might be a personal review of progress and performance. In the process of doing a personal evaluation, an individual spends time figuring out how he or she is doing and in what areas improvement is needed. In some places peer evaluation is institutionalized in clinical ladders. Their promotion tracks include mandatory evaluation of a nurse's performance by her or his peers. Peer review through auditing can become the foundation of constructive communication among staff and promotes professionalism and autonomy (Christensen, 1990). However, administrative or managerial evaluation is part of the manager's job.

Concern about a nurse's level of competence has gained renewed interest as accountability for the delivery of safe and effective care emerges from healthcare delivery system pressures. Professional competence is defined as the degree to which a nurse uses the knowledge, skills, abilities, and judgment associated with nursing to perform effectively in the nurse-client interaction. The methods used in nursing to assess the degree of clinical competence have been performance testing and objective testing. Performance testing uses checklists and skill inventories, peer evaluation, and audits. Objective testing includes licensure and certification exams. With the current litigation and regulatory environment, clinical competence evaluation will remain an important issue (Yocom, 1994). In some places, job descriptions have become broader in scope. Performance appraisal in such circumstances is more difficult and time-consuming. The focus may need to shift to the evaluation of outcomes as the standards used to evaluate performance.

With the advent of TQM and CQI programs, the use of multidisciplinary teams has been expanded. If quality problems are seen as system problems to be tackled by all in the system, then an interesting wrinkle to individual performance appraisal occurs. Perhaps individual performance appraisal should be abolished. To create integrated teams, the team needs to be evaluated as a team on its performance. Evaluating individual contributions becomes nearly impossible and counterproductive. However, many systems and regulatory agencies are driven by the individual performance appraisal as a quality measure. This tension is likely to be an ongoing issue.

RESEARCH NOTE

Source: Fitzpatrick, M. (1994). Performance improvement through quality improvement teamwork. *Journal of Nursing Administration, 24*(12), 20-27.

Purpose

Improving Organizational Performance is the title of the chapter of the 1994 Joint Commission on the Accreditation of Healthcare Organizations (JCAHO) standards that focuses on quality. The 1994 standards include nine dimensions of organizational performance. The purpose of this article was to discuss a framework for documentation and communication of a team's performance that used JCAHO terminology. One organization developed a framework for process design; performance measurement, assessment, and improvement; and the maintenance of stability that applied JCAHO terminology in a meaningful way to nursing planning activities. A multidisciplinary team was used as a collaborative strategy for process improvement.

Discussion

Performance measurement is the first step in a systematic approach to performance improvement. Problematic processes were described as they exist. They became opportunities for improvement. The second step is performance assessment, undertaken to determine where performance should be. A comparison was made to standards and customer satisfaction. A quality improvement team then began to work on quality improvement. Flow charts and fishbone diagrams were used for analysis. Plans for performance improvement were developed around the identified improvement goal. Data gathering, education and awareness, and systems improvement were used as implementation strategies. A team report form was designed to reflect the stages of process/performance improvement described by JCAHO. The team report form communicates the group's work.

Application to Practice

The performance measurement, assessment, improvement, and maintenance model presented in this article was described as useful, adaptable, and applicable to healthcare organizations. Its close adherence to JCAHO accreditation standards makes it attractive to nurses. This article highlights the integration of JCAHO standards with quality assurance (QA), quality improvement (QI), TQM, or CQI and the use of multidisciplinary teams. Rather than focusing on an individual's performance, this article highlights team performance and teamwork to improve organizational performance. A useful report form was displayed and described.

SUMMARY

* Conventional performance appraisal systems are designed to measure performance and motivate personnel.
* Peer review is an examination and evaluation of practice by a nurse's associates.
* Performance is determined by two elements: ability and motivation.
* The most direct goal of any performance appraisal system is the improvement of performance.
* Evaluation by definition is subjective.
* In healthcare, performance appraisal is done as a part of overall quality assessment.
* Performance appraisal may be conducted through personal, peer, or administrative/managerial evaluation.
* The process of performance appraisal includes assessing the needs and setting goals, establishing the objective and the time frame, assessing the progress and evaluating the performance, and then starting over again.

- The performance appraisal process is both informal and formal.
- Performance appraisal can have positive outcomes.
- Performance is measured from collected data. There are various methods and tools used.
- There are a variety of ways to collect evaluative data.
- There are a number of evaluator rating errors.
- To be effective, a performance appraisal system needs to provide objective assessment of the knowledge, skills, and abilities of employees and also must enhance staff development.
- Clinical competence evaluation will remain an ongoing issue.

Study Questions

1. What experiences have you had in the past with performance appraisals? Have those experiences been positive or negative? Why?
2. Why does the handling of the performance appraisal process leave an aftermath of feelings?
3. Think about those times when you were evaluated in a positive and constructive manner. Why was that a good experience?
4. How do you feel when you are expected to evaluate others? Why?
5. How are performance appraisal and quality improvement related?
6. How should pay, promotions, and other rewards be tied to performance and its evaluation?
7. How do you evaluate the performance of a team?

Critical Thinking Exercise

Nurse Lindsey Benavides is a staff nurse in an ambulatory primary care clinic. The clinic is a clinical teaching site for the local nursing education program. Faculty come with a group of students for hands-on experiences. The students are paired with the staff nurses to learn client care. Nurse Benavides has a problem. The nursing student assigned to her today has a strong and overpowering body odor. The student appears neat and clean except for a wrinkled uniform, although the student acts tired and sluggish. Nurse Benavides is having difficulty handling the odor in close quarters and fears the effect on the clients. The faculty instructor isn't immediately available.

1. What is the problem?

2. Why is it a problem?

3. *Whose problem is it?*

4. *What should Nurse Benavides do?*

5. *What aspects of performance appraisal apply?*

6. *Should this incident affect the student's educational evaluation/grade?*

7. *How should the problem be handled with the student?*

REFERENCES

Albrecht, S. (1972). Reappraisal of conventional performance appraisal. *Journal of Nursing Administration, 2*(2), 29-35.

Behrend, B., Finch, D., Emerick, C., & Scoble, K. (1986). Articulating professional nursing practice behaviors. *Journal of Nursing Administration, 16*(2), 20-25.

Bushardt, S., & Fowler, A. (1988). Performance evaluation alternatives. *Journal of Nursing Administration, 18*(10), 40-44.

Christensen, M. (1990). Peer auditing. *Nursing Management, 21*(1), 50-52.

Graham, G., & Unruh, J. (1990). The motivational impact of nonfinancial employee appreciation practices on medical technologists. *Health Care Supervisor, 8*(3), 9-17.

Haas, S. (1992). Coaching: Developing key players. *Journal of Nursing Administration, 22*(6), 54-58.

Mager, R., & Pipe, P. (1970). *Analyzing performance problems.* Belmont, CA: Pitman Learning.

McGee, K. (1992). Making performance appraisals a positive experience. *Nursing Management, 23*(8), 36-37.

Nauright, L. (1987). Toward a comprehensive personnel system: Performance appraisal-Part IV. *Nursing Management, 18*(8), 67-77.

Sashkin, M. (1982). Appraising appraisal: Ten lessons from research for practice. *Journal of Nursing Administration, 12*(1), 21.

Schwirian, P. (1978). Evaluating the performance of nurses: A multidimensional approach. *Nursing Research, 27*(6), 347-351.

Veninga, R. (1982). *The human side of health administration: A guide for hospital, nursing, and public health administrators.* Englewood Cliffs, NJ: Prentice-Hall.

Yocom, C. (1994). Validating clinical competence: Old and new approaches. In J. McCloskey & H. Grace (Eds.), *Current issues in nursing* (4th ed.) (pp. 336-341). St. Louis: Mosby.

28

Productivity and Costing Out Nursing

Chapter Objectives

ॐ

define and describe productivity

ॐ

define effectiveness

ॐ

define efficiency

ॐ

define costing out nursing services

ॐ

analyze nursing productivity

ॐ

distinguish among four areas for productivity increases

ॐ

explain productivity measures

ॐ

discuss costing out nursing services models

ॐ

analyze leadership and management and current issues
in productivity and costing

ॐ

exercise critical thinking to conceptualize and analyze
possible solutions to a practical experience incident

*r*aising the productivity of service industry professionals has been called
the single greatest challenge facing managers (Drucker, 1991). Competition in the healthcare delivery system is derived from changes in financial re-

imbursement and healthcare reform initiatives, including related elements of managed care and capitated payment.

Historically, healthcare providers have provided the client care which they determined to be necessary and were then paid either directly by the client or more often by a third party payor, most likely an insurance company. The insurance company looked at the likelihood of expenditures for those covered clients they represented and charged a premium estimated to sufficiently provide the insurer with the funds to pay the healthcare providers for their efforts, plus a profit. The payments to the providers were based on a dollar amount determined appropriate for a procedure performed or for hospitalization felt necessary for the diagnosis category to which the client was assigned.

Capitated payment refers to the per person rather than per procedure or per diagnostic grouping payment by managed care organizations to providers who provide a package of services to an enrollee at a fixed rate for a contract period (Grimaldi, 1995). Under such arrangements the provider may become the insurer as well as the healthcare provider, since the arrangement calls for the provider to estimate the amount of care that will be necessary and to develop a charge based on that estimate. Competition forces an evaluation of costs and prices. Facilities able to increase productivity levels will be able to deliver a larger volume of care for the same amount of resources, thus making them competitive on price and better able to capture market share. As constraints on resources increase, productivity becomes more important (Ward, 1988).

Nurses are the critical input in producing nursing care (Cleland, 1990). Since nursing costs account for a substantial portion of total inpatient labor expenses in hospitals, improvement in nursing staff productivity is a natural area for cost savings. A short term measure would be to precisely adjust staffing to workload. Longer range strategies focus on the cost effectiveness of the staff mix and the nursing care modality used to deliver care. This is because labor efficiency is directly related to the cost of the service. As a part of productivity examination, the job tasks and the use of time by each skill level of personnel are carefully examined for potential productivity improvements through reengineering (Mowry & Korpman, 1986). In nursing, the direct applications relate to staffing, scheduling, and budgeting.

DEFINITIONS

or service workers such as nurses, quality and quantity together constitute performance (Drucker, 1991). *Productivity* is defined in the management literature as the ratio of output to input in an organization (see Chart 28.1). This is described as the amount of output derived from a unit or quantity of resource (Ward, 1988) and the relationship between inputs and outputs within a system (Jordan, 1994). Productivity is a variable index that is relative to increases or decreases in the inputs as related to the

---

CHART 28.1
⌇ DEFINITIONS

Productivity
the ratio of output to input in an organization.

Effectiveness
the accomplishment of quality outcomes.

Efficiency
the accomplishment of objectives with the lowest expenditure of resources.

Costing Out Nursing Services
a method of determining the specific costs of the nursing services provided to clients.

Data from Barnum and Mallard (1989), Eckhart (1993), McCloskey (1989), Price and Mueller (1986), and Ward (1988).

outputs. The way to increase productivity is to either decrease inputs or increase outputs. For example, in nursing this would mean decreasing nursing hours per patient day or increasing patient days per nursing hour. *Output* means the goods and services produced. Output is some measure of the product. *Input* means the resources used to produce the outputs. In nursing inputs are resources such as personnel hours, supplies, or equipment. The more output produced for a given input, the greater the productivity. The less input needed to produce a given level of output, the greater the productivity. The mathematical formula for productivity is $P = I/O$ (Barnum & Mallard, 1989; Mayberry, 1991).

Effectiveness is defined in the business literature as success or the financial viability of an organization (Price & Mueller, 1986). In nursing, the definition of effectiveness primarily relates to quality outcomes being achieved (Barnum & Mallard, 1989). Effectiveness is concerned with doing the right things (Drucker, 1973). Effectiveness has been described as the degree to which the care is provided in the correct manner to achieve the desired client outcome (JCAHO, 1993b). *Efficiency* is defined as the accomplishment of objectives with the lowest expenditure of resources. It may be translated into how fast or cheaply a product is produced (Barnum & Mallard, 1989). Efficiency is a minimum condition for survival and is concerned with doing things right (Drucker, 1973). Efficiency has been described as the relationship of outcomes of care to resources used to deliver care (JCAHO, 1993b). *Efficacy* has been described as the degree to which client care can be shown to accomplish desired outcomes (JCAHO, 1993b). Thus, effectiveness focuses on quality, efficiency focuses on cost, and efficacy focuses on meeting outcome goals.

Productivity and the concept of working harder may become confused. Personnel can work hard yet not be very productive. Clerical work under a manual system as compared to an automated system is one example. Currently the term "working smarter" is equated with productivity. This means improving the way jobs are structured: streamlining, reducing redundancy, and using technology to support human effort (Ward, 1988).

Costing out nursing services is defined as the determination of the costs of the services provided by nurses. It is performed as a method of determining the specific costs of the nursing services provided to clients (Eckhart, 1993; McCloskey, 1989). Costing out nursing services is done to monitor finances in nursing and identify the outcomes of nursing care relative to its cost. The client could then be billed for nursing care according to the services required and received (see Chapter 9).

BACKGROUND

Productivity is an important healthcare issue. Barnum and Mallard (1989) noted that when resources are in scarce supply it becomes more urgent to get the most out of every available resource. In nursing, productivity can be thought of as the input of nursing care hours and the output of nursing care services. This would be only one simple productivity index, because other inputs, or costs, such as supplies and overhead, are not included. However, in this index of productivity an increase in productivity could be captured if the same nursing care services were provided by fewer nursing hours (increase the nurse to client ratio) or if the same nursing care hours delivered more nursing care services (get more done per hour or see more clients per hour) (Barnum & Mallard, 1989).

Healthcare organizations feel the need to improve internal efficiency and cut costs. Nursing productivity is being scrutinized and analyzed. Inputs in healthcare are tangible human resources, capital equipment, supplies, and facilities. The outputs, however, are intangible client outcomes. The outputs are more difficult to quantify than the inputs. The proxy measures that have been used to measure outputs include morbidity and mortality rates, medical diagnoses or diagnosis-related groups (DRGs), surgical outcomes, return for services rates, case mix measures, nosocomial infection rates, volume of services, and patient days or length of stay. Nursing has struggled to quantify its outputs. Acuity, or patient classification, is the proxy most commonly used to measure nursing care. One nursing output proxy measure is the required hours for nursing care activities, which can be converted to a monetary value based on average nursing salaries. Defining productivity in monetary terms has been advocated for analyzing performance elements of staff mix and efficiency of care delivery systems (Jordan, 1994).

There are at least four areas where employee productivity might be increased (Sibson, 1976):

- substitution of equipment for human effort
- improved methods of work
- removal of unproductive practices
- improved management of human resources

Efforts under total quality management or continuous quality improvement (TQM/CQI) and restructuring or reengineering nursing care delivery are targeted at these four productivity improvement areas. For example, computers can substitute for some human work effort. Critical paths may be used to improve methods of work. Bringing x-ray examinations to the hospitalized client removes unproductive transporting practices. Altering staff mix is designed to improve the management of human resources.

Productivity Measures

The recommended measure of productivity is cost per unit of output, calculated as the cost incurred divided by the unit of output (Price & Mueller,

1986), although there are various ways to calculate productivity (see Chart 28.2). Inputs and outputs are measured in dollars and work hours. For nursing, translating outputs and inputs into quantifiable monetary terms has been difficult because acuity measures are not standardized, indirect and direct nursing care costs are defined differently, and various formulas for calculating nursing costs are used (Jordan, 1994).

The oldest nursing productivity index is the measure called nursing hours per patient day (HPPD). The input is the nursing hours worked. The number of hospitalized patient days is the output. Unfortunately, this index was imprecise, because of the wide variation in client acuity and intensity that made the measure "patient days" not equivalent. A variety of data sources and productivity indices can be used. For example, staffing, calculated as the total number of work hours of a given staff for a given time period, can be compared to client volume or census. This is the ratio of staff to census, or patient days. If the staff hours are held constant while the volume or number of clients increases, the productivity ratio is better (Barnum & Mallard, 1989).

In nursing, productivity has been tightly linked with staffing numbers through measurement of workload. This translates into a linkage of productivity to task completion, thus reducing nursing to a task-driven process. Outcomes are ignored when nursing productivity is equated with functional performance. Task-based work is associated with manual skill work, not knowledge-based work. To be efficient and effective, knowledge-based workers need to be able to use knowledge and skill to make decisions and act on their own initiative within their area of expertise. This is how quality is maintained by the knowledge-based worker (Manthey, 1991). Standards of care, time and motion studies, and client care requirements form the basis of tools used to collect nursing workload data. No one tool adequately measures the work of nursing. Therefore, matching the number of staff to the clients' needs is difficult. In one Veterans Administration hospital, the percent of productivity was calculated by dividing the staff required from the acuity tool by the staff on duty ([required ÷ on duty] × 100). The resulting percent of productivity was then accumulated and graphed. The graphing process identified trends and maldistribution phenomena. The data can then be analyzed more effectively (Cromwell, 1993).

Productivity measures need to be evaluated critically and with caution. Price and Mueller (1986) advocated using cost per unit of output as the preferred measure because other measures may not take into account all costs related to producing the output. Not including all costs skews the data about total productivity and clouds the inferences or conclusions about costs derived from analysis. For example, labor productivity indices such as HPPD ignore the costs of supplies, overhead, and unit administration. Thus the cost contributions of all employees are not included, as only direct care providers are analyzed (Price & Mueller, 1986).

CHART 28.2
〜 METHODS FOR CALCULATING PRODUCTIVITY

Productivity (P) = Cost per unit of output

$$P = \frac{\text{Input}}{\text{Output}}$$

$$P = \frac{\text{Cost}}{\text{Unit of output}}$$

$$P = \frac{\$}{\text{Work hours}}$$

$$P = \frac{\text{Nursing hours worked}}{\text{Number of hospital patient days}}$$

$$P = \frac{\text{Number of nursing staff}}{\text{Census or patient days}}$$

CHART 28.3
∾ FINANCIAL
MODELS FOR
PRODUCTIVITY

**Cost-Effectiveness
Model**
compares the costs of
two or more methods
to achieve desired
outcomes.

Cost-Benefit Model
compares different
programs whose
objectives also differ.

**Required for Either
Model**
• careful collection
  and statistical analy-
  sis of data used to
  measure productivity.
• standardized
  measures and
  comparisons.

Data from Barnum and Mal-
lard (1989).

Financial models for productivity include the cost-effectiveness model and the cost-benefit model (Barnum & Mallard, 1989) (see Chart 28.3). The cost-effectiveness model is a goal-driven model of productivity. The cost-effectiveness model compares the costs of two or more different methods or means to achieve desired goals or outcomes. For example, a nurse might be considering ways to achieve the goal of a promotion. Returning for more education and conducting a unit-based project are two alternative methods that may be considered to achieve the goal. Criteria such as time investment and costs are weighed in the decision process. As opposed to the goal-driven comparison of alternative methods, the cost-benefit model is a resource-driven model. The cost-benefit model compares different programs or projects whose objectives also differ. Thus different programs are compared for their different input costs and their different outcome benefits. For example, a program to provide food to the homeless might be compared to a medical services program for the homeless. A careful collection and statistical analysis of data are used to measure productivity. However, such analyses need to be based on standardized measures and comparisons. A clear identification of what is being measured and whether or not the measure is a proxy will aid in efforts to monitor productivity and use the results to improve practice.

The cost of the staff mix used in providing care is the basis of the computation of the cost of nursing care. Without standardized measures, comparisons become meaningless (see Chapter 24). For example, differences in case mix, staff mix, setting, and amount and type of support services may invalidate cross-setting or site comparisons. Further, in measuring client outcomes, numerous categories of caregivers are involved, as well as the client and their family. It is difficult to sort out the various contributions to outcomes (Cleland, 1990).

Productivity measurement is complex for three reasons (Edwardson, 1989): measuring nursing care outcomes is difficult and controversial, the relationships among care processes and nursing outcomes are not well understood, and the most efficient combination of resources for performing care processes is not known. Work on outcomes measurement is progressing. It is thought that outcomes measurement will provide a useful adjunct to the purely financial measures of healthcare productivity.

Nurses need to control costs and justify program or departmental budgets. To do this, productivity is defined in monetary terms. Then staff mix is analyzed, and care delivery systems are explored and critiqued for contributions to efficiency. Jordan (1994) used Omachonu's (1988) model for nursing productivity that compared nursing costs to the portion of DRG reimbursement attributable to nursing care. This amount was estimated by dividing total nursing costs by total hospital costs. Total nursing costs equal direct nursing costs plus indirect nursing costs. Direct nursing costs were the labor costs of RNs, LPNs, and NAs providing direct nursing care. Indirect nursing costs were labor costs for secretarial, supervisory, and administrative activities. Both direct and indirect nursing costs are inputs; the portion of DRG reimbursement attributable to nursing care is the output. Nursing productivity was calculated as total DRG reimbursement for a specific DRG, times total inpatient hospital nursing costs divided by total inpatient hospital costs, all divided by the sum of direct nursing costs for a specific DRG plus indirect nursing costs for a specific DRG.

The productivity calculations were done for comparison purposes. However, comparisons across hospitals are difficult due to variability across facilities. Comparisons of nursing productivity can be used within a facility or unit and to track a unit or DRG over time. Nursing productivity is impacted by variables beyond nurses' control, such as by overhead costs, physician practice patterns, and the efficiency and productivity of other departments (Jordan, 1994).

RESEARCH NOTE

Source: Jordan, S. (1994). Nursing productivity in rural hospitals. *Nursing Management, 25*(3), 58-62.

Purpose

Costs are more problematic for small rural hospitals because they often do not have access to the economies of scale available to larger facilities. The purpose of this study was to compare nursing productivity in two rural hospitals and to discuss extraneous factors that have an effect on nursing productivity. Data were collected from two small rural hospitals in Ohio on patients with DRGs 89, 96, 127, and 140: pneumonia, bronchitis, heart failure, and angina. Omachonu's productivity model was used for examining productivity variables. Variables measured were total nurse hours per day (NHPD), length of stay (LOS), direct nursing costs, and indirect nursing costs.

Discussion

Productivity was defined as the ratio of DRG reimbursement attributable to nursing care (estimated by dividing total nursing costs by total hospital costs) to the sum of direct nursing costs plus indirect nursing costs per DRG. After data collection and productivity calculation, the results showed that productivity was higher in Hospital B. For DRG 127, productivity was significantly higher in Hospital B. Nursing productivity for individual patients varied widely across DRGs and within DRGs. This method of productivity calculation was useful to compare different units within a hospital or for tracking over time and monitoring costs.

Application to Practice

Although nursing needs to be productive while accomplishing optimal outcomes, nursing productivity is complex to calculate. Nursing productivity does not stand alone: overhead costs, physician practice patterns, workload distribution, and the efficiency of other departments directly impact on nursing productivity but are not under nursing's control. Staffing patterns, scheduling practices, staff mix, skill mix, and educational levels influence the efficiency and effectiveness of nursing care delivery. Further work needs to be done on accurate productivity formulas.

Costing Out Nursing Services

Productivity can be approached from the perspective of effectiveness or efficiency. The effectiveness perspective emphasizes the measurement of outcomes and the assessment and improvement of quality (see Chapter 25). However, the focus for productivity more often is efficiency. This perspective uses financial analyses and management and emphasizes costs. Nursing has been unable to adequately address costs and efficiency insofar as data on the actual costs of nursing services were unavailable to nurses. Nurses have become interested in costing out nursing services for the purposes of productivity analysis (see Chapter 9).

Ideas about costing out nursing services arose in the mid-1980s, coinciding with the implementation of DRGs. The importance of determining costs is compelling. The purposes of costing out nursing services are to facilitate health policy and for reimbursement decisions. Costing out nursing services provides data for productivity comparisons. Acuity, or patient classification, is the most frequently used tool for collecting nursing's cost data. A variety of acuity tools are used. The definitions of direct and indirect costs vary among reported studies. The calculations of nursing time per intensity level often are not reported in the literature (McCloskey, Gardner, & Johnson, 1987).

Two models for costing out nursing services have been identified (McCloskey, 1989). The first model reflects the general trend of the literature: the amount of nursing time per intensity level as related to a specific DRG is multiplied by the nurse's average hourly salary-benefits and added to an indirect cost amount to determine the total nursing cost per DRG. Since the first model has some limitations and lacks an ability to define what nursing activities are provided for the cost, it only yields nursing cost per DRG or intensity level. A second model was developed to yield nursing cost per nursing intervention or nursing diagnosis. In the second model, medical diagnosis and nursing diagnosis both initiate nursing interventions. To measure the costs of nursing interventions, direct costs (nursing time multiplied by average salary, plus equipment) and indirect costs are added to derive total nursing costs (see Chapter 9 for further detail).

LEADERSHIP AND MANAGEMENT IMPLICATIONS

Careful scrutiny of productivity has become equated with survival in healthcare organizations. Management techniques emphasize control of expenses such as hours, costs, overtime, and other resources. However, organiza-

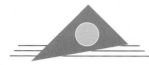 *Leadership & Management Behaviors*

LEADERSHIP BEHAVIORS	MANAGEMENT BEHAVIORS	OVERLAP AREAS
• plans strategy for productive use of resources	• plans resource allocation to improve productivity	• plans for productivity
• envisions a productive group output	• organizes the environment to enhance productivity	• influences others toward productivity
• enables followers to be productive	• calculates costs and productivity indices	
• influences followers to increase productivity	• monitors cost factors	
• enables release of followers' potential	• controls resource expenditure	
• creates a productive environment	• communicates the need for productivity	
• communicates values that enhance productivity	• evaluates productivity patterns	
	• influences subordinates to be productive	
	• justifies departmental budget	

tional leadership may be the key to productivity by focusing on the release of employee potential. One key aspect is enabling employees to work together effectively and focus on the accomplishment of mutually derived organizational goals (McNeese-Smith, 1992).

The nurse leader and manager will be directly involved in the aspects of nursing work that are projected to most directly affect labor productivity: motivation, work methods, and control through work measurement and scheduling. However, as the nurse is challenged to measure and manage productivity, it is difficult to identify a useful and meaningful definition of output. The result is that proxy measures are used that may not deliver an acceptable level of precision (Edwardson, 1989).

Nursing managerial and clinical decision making both include a concern about the impact of nursing practice on costs to clients (Gardner, 1992). Nursing's efforts to cost out nursing services and obtain third party reimbursement places nursing in an arena of money, power, and influence control. Knowledge of the issues is important. Characteristics of assertiveness, determination, and political savvy will be needed by nurse leaders and managers (McCloskey, 1989). Nursing's financial future is based on nurse leaders' abilities to firmly control and clearly determine nursing's costs (Eckhart, 1993) (see Chapters 9 and 24).

Because productivity has taken on an association with perceived survival in healthcare, both leadership and management can be tapped for productivity improvement. Management takes the perspective of control of costs, hours, or supplies. Leadership takes the perspective of releasing the potential in followers to be more productive. The leadership perspective seeks to enhance productivity by enabling and enlisting the involvement of followers in the processes and outcomes of effective and productive client care. Whereas management efforts may be concentrated on cost containment, leadership efforts are concentrated on enabling followers to work together efficiently and effectively in order to accomplish goals with the least wasted effort (McNeese-Smith, 1992). Leadership is important for productivity. Productivity is important in nursing because of its relationship to employee job satisfaction and organizational commitment (McNeese-Smith, 1992).

CURRENT ISSUES AND TRENDS

Productivity and performance are judged in part by the value of a service to clients. The value of a service to the users is equal to the quality of the service divided by the cost of the service. Good value becomes desired quality at a reasonable cost (JCAHO, 1993a) (see Chart 28.4). Nurses may fear that increased productivity automatically means decreased quality (Edwardson, 1989).

Nurses are feeling an urgent need to demonstrate nursing's contribution to health and medical care, so that nursing's value is more visible to clients and payors. As managed care and care management become a greater force in healthcare delivery, nurses are challenged to demonstrate their cost and quality outcomes with data. As managed care providers seek to contract with agencies to provide primary healthcare, nurses are asked to produce evidence and to negotiate contracts from a cost basis. Many nurses are baffled about how to do this.

With the current prominence of advanced practice nurses, specifically nurse practitioners, in the healthcare reform debate, costing out nursing services is seen as one element promoting efforts to secure third party reimbursement by nurses. Although capitated reimbursement is being considered to be the reimbursement wave of the future, third party reimbursed fee-for-service is still available to certain healthcare professionals. For those providers able to capture fee-for-service, personal income under a fee-for-service plan is much higher than it is for salaried employees.

Currently, physicians are paid for many services that nurses routinely provide (Griffith & Robinson, 1993; Ott, Griffith, & Towers, 1989). Careful examination and analysis of nursing's costs may raise fears in those who currently hold power in the healthcare delivery system. Some fear that nursing's independence and reimbursement will diminish their power and income. Some fear raised healthcare costs, triggered by nurses' demands for salary increases as the cost-effectiveness and subsidization of others becomes known. However, there are reasons why nursing's efforts to cost out nursing services might benefit clients and should be pursued (McCloskey, 1989).

CHART 28.4
∾ CONSUMER
VALUE DECISIONS

$$\text{Value} = \frac{\text{Quality}}{\text{Cost}}$$

Data from JCAHO (1993a).

SUMMARY

* Raising the productivity of knowledge and service workers has been called the single greatest challenge facing managers.
* Labor effectiveness is directly related to the cost of nursing services.
* Productivity is defined as the ratio of output to input in an organization.
* Effectiveness is defined as achieving quality outcomes.
* Efficiency is defined as the accomplishment of objectives with the lowest expenditure of resources.
* Costing out nursing services is defined as a method of determining the specific costs of the nursing services provided to clients.
* Nursing productivity is being scrutinized and analyzed.
* There are at least four areas where employee productivity might be increased.
* The recommended measure of productivity is cost per unit of output.
* The oldest nursing productivity index is the measure called nursing hours per patient day.
* Productivity measurement is complex.
* Two models for costing out nursing services have been identified.
* As managed care and care management become a greater force in healthcare delivery, nurses are challenged to demonstrate their cost and quality outcomes with data.

Study Questions

1. Why would quality of care suffer when nursing care hours are reduced?
2. Do more experienced nurses work more productively? Why or why not?
3. Why should nurses worry about productivity?
4. What issues in productivity are most urgent? Why?
5. How do nurses determine if their care is effective and efficient?
6. Why should nurses cost out their services?
7. How can nurses control healthcare costs? Nursing costs?
8. What is the ideal ratio of nurses to clients?

Critical Thinking Exercise

Nurse Lydia Trader has been Nursing Director of an ambulatory clinic for the past six months. The hospital with which the clinic is affiliated recently has been experiencing some downsizing and reengineering of its nursing department. Fortunately for Nurse Trader and her staff, clinic visits have been increasing and are projected to continue to increase. However, Nurse Trader has returned from an administrative meeting in which the healthcare organization's fiscal crisis was explained along with the message that financial reversions will have to come from each area's budget, including the profitable ambulatory clinic. Nurse Trader has a problem. She has been using an all-RN staff. Reversions will likely need to come from her department's labor budget. Nurse Trader sits down to calculate productivity and costs in order to develop a budget plan and justification to meet the required reversions.

1. What is the problem?

2. Why is it a problem?

3. What should Nurse Trader do first?

4. What data does she need? Why?

5. What calculations should she make?

6. Should Nurse Trader argue effectiveness or efficiency?

7. What model might assist Nurse Trader in her deliberations?

REFERENCES

Barnum, B., & Mallard, C. (1989). *Essentials of nursing management: Concepts and context of practice*. Rockville, MD: Aspen.

Cleland, V. (1990). *The economics of nursing*. Norwalk, CT: Appleton & Lange.

Cromwell, T. (1993). Productivity presented graphically. *Nursing Management, 24*(4), 73-78.

Drucker, P. (1973). *Management: Tasks, responsibilities, practices*. New York: Harper & Row.

Drucker, P. (1991). The new productivity challenge. *Harvard Business Review, 69*(6), 69-79.

Edwardson, S. (1989). Productivity measurement. In B. Henry, C. Arndt, M. Di Vincenti, & A. Marriner-Tomey (Eds.), *Dimensions of nursing administration: Theory, research, education, practice* (pp. 371-385). Boston: Blackwell.

Eckhart, J. (1993). Costing out nursing services: Examining the research. *Nursing Economic$, 11*(2), 91-98.

Gardner, D. (1992). The CNS as a cost manager. *Clinical Nurse Specialist, 6*(2), 112-116.

Griffith, H., & Robinson, K. (1993). Current procedural terminology (CPT) coded services provided by nurse specialists. *Image, 25*(3), 178-186.

Grimaldi, P. (1995). Capitation savvy a must. *Nursing Management, 26*(2), 33-34.

JCAHO (The Joint Commission on the Accreditation of Healthcare Organizations). (1993a). Defining performance of organizations. *Journal on Quality Improvement, 19*(7), 215-221.

JCAHO (The Joint Commission on the Accreditation of Healthcare Organizations). (1993b). *1994 accreditation manual for hospitals*. Oakbrook Terrace, IL: JCAHO.

Jordan, S. (1994). Nursing productivity in rural hospitals. *Nursing Management, 25*(3), 58-62.

Manthey, M. (1991). Staffing and productivity. *Nursing Management, 22*(12), 20-21.

Mayberry, A. (1991). Productivity and cost-effectiveness measures: Factors in decision making. *Nursing Administration Quarterly, 15*(4), 29-35.

McCloskey, J. (1989). Implications of costing out nursing services for reimbursement. *Nursing Management, 20*(1), 44-49.

McCloskey, J., Gardner, D., & Johnson, M. (1987). Costing out nursing services: An annotated bibliography. *Nursing Economic$*, 5(5), 245-253.

McNeese-Smith, D. (1992). The impact of leadership upon productivity. *Nursing Economic$*, 10(6), 393-396.

Mowry, M., & Korpman, R. (1986). *Managing health care costs, quality, and technology: Product line strategies for nursing*. Rockville, MD: Aspen.

Omachonu, V. (1988). *A methodology for assessing hospital nursing unit productivity using DRG measures as output*. Unpublished Doctoral Dissertation, Polytechnic University (University Microfilms International Dissertation Information Service No. 8805231).

Ott, B., Griffith, H., & Towers, J. (1989). Who gets the money? *American Journal of Nursing, 89(2)*, 186-188.

Price, J., & Mueller, C. (1986). *Handbook of organizational measurement*. Marshfield, MA: Pitman.

Sibson, R. (1976). *Increasing employee productivity*. New York: American Management Association.

Ward, Jr., W. (1988). *An introduction to health care financial management*. Owings Mills, MD: National Health Publishing.

29

Managing a Stressful Environment

Chapter Objectives

∽

define and describe stress in nursing

∽

define and describe occupational or job stress

∽

define and describe burnout

∽

explain a general model of stress

∽

distinguish between stress mediators

∽

analyze sources of stress in nursing

∽

analyze coping and adaptation in nursing

∽

relate stress to leadership and management

∽

exercise critical thinking to conceptualize and analyze
possible solutions to a practical experience incident

*n*urses are healers. Nurses focus on activities related to caring in the diagnosis and treatment of human responses to health and illness phenomena. However, inherent in this caring occupation are numerous sources of built-in stress that become occupational hazards for nurses. For example, dealing with human illness and suffering, life and death situations, clients who are demanding or in pain, making critical judgments about interventions and treatments, and balancing work and family commitments become forces that realistically generate stress in nurses (Aurelio, 1993). Further, the organizations that employ nurses may become stressful environments within which to practice nursing. For example, organizational cultures may devalue nurses, policies and deployment practices may prevent nurses from using knowledge and skills, and job and professional autonomy may be restricted (Aurelio, 1993).

Under conditions of restructuring and reengineering, layoffs and downsizing, nurses feel job threatened and concerned about personal security of employment. Further, perceived short staffing and increasing workloads raise concerns about client safety and the nurse's ability to cope and deliver adequate service to clients. Like the concept of conflict (see Chapter 21), stress needs to be neither too high nor too low. Thus moderate levels should be the target. At levels that are too low, nurses may become apathetic or nonproductive. At too high a level, energy is absorbed in trying to deal with stress and is, therefore, diverted from productivity. Performance drops as stress reaches high levels. Clearly, both nurses and their employers have a stake in managing stress and stressful environments.

DEFINITIONS

Stress is one concept that links and examines the effects of behavior on health (Fagin, 1987). *Stress* is defined as "a physical, mental, psychological, or spiritual response to a stressor" (Narasi, 1994, p. 73) (see Chart 29.1). A *stressor* is defined as an experience in a person-environment relationship that is evaluated by a person as taxing or exceeding resources and threatening the sense of well-being (Dietz, 1991; Lazarus & Folkman, 1984).

Selye's (1965) General Stress theory forms the theoretical background for understanding stress. According to Selye (1965; 1976), stress is a nonspecific state that is composed of a variety of induced changes in the human biological system. Thus stress is a syndrome with a characteristic set of symptoms. Stress also is described as a personal response and phenomenon that occurs inside a body as a reaction to the stimulus of a stressor. The body's emotional and physical response is a result of a "fight-or-flight" syndrome (Woodhouse, 1993).

The concept of stress has been applied from Selye's (1965; 1976) biophysiology framework to psychosocial states in individuals. For example, stress has been viewed as something that occurs when individuals interact with their environment such that they are presented with a demand, constraint, or opportunity for behavior (McGrath, 1976).

CHART 29.1
⌘ DEFINITIONS

Stress
physical, mental, psychological, or spiritual responses to any stressor.

Stressor
an experience in a person-environment relationship that is evaluated by a person as taxing or exceeding resources and threatening the sense of well-being.

Occupational or Job Stress
a tension arising in a person related to the demands of the role or job.

Burnout
responses to chronic emotional stress that have three components: (1) emotional and/or physical exhaustion, (2) lowered job productivity, and (3) overdepersonalization.

Data from Dietz (1991), Grant (1993), Hinshaw and Atwood (1983), Lazarus and Folkman (1984), Narasi (1994), and Perlman and Hartman (1982).

Within nursing, research has been focused increasingly on the variable of stress. A variety of conceptual frameworks has been used to study stress, stressors, reactions to stress, and ultimate outcomes for clients (Lowery, 1987). Stress has been seen as a stimulus, a response, or a transaction (Lyon & Werner, 1987).

Occupational or job stress is defined as a tension arising in a person related to the demands of the role or job (Grant, 1993; Hinshaw & Atwood, 1983). Job stress, or "disquieting influences," can accumulate into levels that are too high and reach burnout (Hinshaw & Atwood, 1983). *Burnout* is defined as "a response to chronic emotional stress with three components: (1) emotional and/or physical exhaustion, (2) lowered job productivity, and (3) overdepersonalization" (Perlman & Hartman, 1982). Burnout in nursing is described as being the terminal phase of the individual's failure to resolve work stress or the accumulated inability to cope with day-to-day job stresses (Smythe, 1984). Levels of job stress that are too low or too high decrease individual productivity (Benson & Allen, 1980; Cleland, 1965; Hinshaw & Atwood, 1983).

RESEARCH NOTE

Source: Blegen, M. (1993). Nurses' job satisfaction: A meta-analysis of related variables. *Nursing Research, 42*(1), 36-41.

Purpose

Turnover is an ongoing nursing professional concern. The purpose of this research was to describe the strength of the relationships between nurses' job satisfaction and frequently associated variables. The purpose also was to determine the factors most important to job satisfaction, using meta-analysis to describe the strength and consistency of relationships. From 250 studies, 48 articles met inclusion criteria. Sample sizes of studies ranged from 30 to 1597. The meta-analysis total sample size was 15,048, with 79% of the nurses employed in hospitals.

Discussion

Of the 13 variables often linked with nurses' job satisfaction and identified in this study, four were personal attributes of age, education, years of experience, and locus of control. The other nine were organizational variables of stress, commitment, supervisor communication, autonomy, recognition, routinization, peer communication, fairness, and professionalism. The two variables with the strongest relationship to job satisfaction were stress and commitment. Satisfaction was measured by 21 different instruments across the studies, possibly contributing to the variation among studies.

Application to Practice

Meta-analysis is a useful technique to quantitatively summarize a large body of literature because the analysis is performed on pooled results. The results indicated that nurses' job satisfaction is most strongly related to stress (higher satisfaction with lower stress) and commitment (higher satisfaction with higher commitment). Human service workers such as nurses are susceptible to job stress and burnout. Stress appears to have a strong association with job satisfaction and ultimately turnover. Moderating job stress is clearly an important intervention strategy useful in nurses' work environments.

BACKGROUND

From the work of Selye (1965; 1976), stress is known to have biophysiological effects on humans. However, stress is most often applied in nursing practice to a discussion of the psychosocial state of persons as they interact with their environment. Demands, constraints, and opportunities occur (McGrath, 1976).

One general model of stress portrays stress along a continuum from potential stressor to consequences or outcomes (Elliott & Eisdorfer, 1982). At one end is a potential stressor such as a demanding client. Then come mediators such as social support, coping behaviors, or defense mechanisms; the individual's psychological reactions such as emotional states of anxiety or fear; biological reactions such as an increase in catecholamines. Finally, there are consequences or outcomes such as physical illness, burnout, or coping. In this model, stress is pictured as a dynamic process across a continuum and the result of an interaction between an individual and the environment (Lowery, 1987) (see Fig. 29.1).

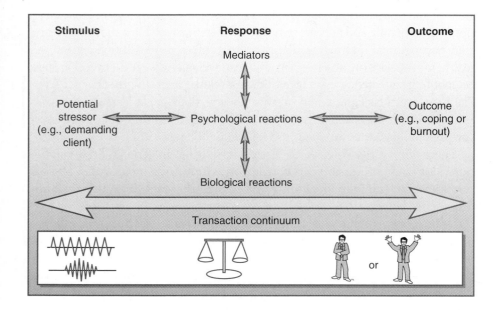

Figure 29.1
General model of stress. (Data from Elliott & Eisdorfer [1982], Lowery [1987], and Lyon & Werner [1987].)

In general, there appear to be two important processes that mediate the person-environment relationship. They are coping and cognitive appraisal. Coping is the individual's actions and activities taken to adapt to the situation as presented. Coping relates to the means or methods used to deal with or manage a perceived stressful event (Dietz, 1991). The other major mediator is cognitive appraisal. Cognitive appraisal is the individual's assessment or interpretation of the stressor or potential stressor. Cognitive appraisal relates to the individual's evaluation or perception of whether and to what degree any event or transaction is stressful (Dietz, 1991; Lowery, 1987). Denial and optimism (hope) are two other stress mediators (Lowery, 1987).

Nurses have studied a variety of stress reactions that occur as emotional and psychological manifestations of failed defense and coping. Chief among these are anxiety and depression. Often overlooked in research are the consequences or outcomes of exposure to stress. The outcomes can be either positive or negative. It is not known whether exposure to stress helps to immunize the individual against severe reactions to future stressors or whether the individual becomes worn down and more susceptible to being overwhelmed by the next stressor. Mastery of stress is advocated but not easily translated into simple techniques (Lowery, 1987). In nursing, hardiness and burnout have been investigated as stress outcomes.

Sources of Stress in Nursing

Stress is associated with the work of nursing. Individual nurses may experience internal tension, conflict, or stress. Occupational or job stress derives from the jobs and organizations that employ nurses. Stress is pervasive in work environments generally and appears to be intrinsic to nursing. Thus stress in nursing is an occupational and managerial concern (Huber, 1994). Individual nurse's health, job satisfaction, absenteeism, and turnover, along with client welfare, are thought to be affected by high levels of work-related stress (Norbeck, 1985). For a more in-depth background on stress in nursing, there are at least three articles that extensively analyze the theoretical and research literature (Hardy & Conway, 1988; Hinshaw & Atwood, 1983; Lyon & Werner, 1987).

There are a variety of sources of stress in nursing. In general, however, the sources of stress in nursing can be categorized into two broad types: sources that arise from the individual nurse and sources that arise from the work environment (Huber, 1994).

Sources of stress that arise from the individual nurse can be either internal or external in origin. For example, the individual nurse may bring to work internal personal emotional conflicts or the need to balance work and family roles. Similar to intrapersonal conflict and tensions in women's careers, the need to balance multiple roles in life may create an internal tension that is manifested by personal stress (Gardner, 1992; Greenhaus & Kopelman, 1981;

Huber, 1994). Stress on the individual nurse from an external source may be derived from the characteristics of an individual's personality. For example, the individual's personality may not fit in or match to a given work situation (Getzels, 1958). This is an external stress source in that the external work situation impinges on the individual.

Potential outcomes or consequences of the sources of stress that arise from the individual nurse include hardiness (McCranic, Lambert, & Lambert, 1987; Rich & Rich, 1987; Wagnild & Young, 1991), burnout (Bailey, 1980; Stehle, 1981), and reality shock (Kramer, 1974; Kramer & Schmalenberg, 1977; Schmalenberg & Kramer, 1979). Hardiness is a personality characteristic composed of commitment, control, and challenge. This outcome of withstanding high job stress is a variable that may reduce or buffer burnout. Buffering occurs because the higher the personal hardiness, the lower the burnout (Tarolli-Jager, 1994).

Burnout has been described as a syndrome of emotional exhaustion, negative attitudes, and cynicism toward clients that afflict individuals in the helping professions (Maslach & Jackson, 1981). Apathy, alienation, job dissatisfaction, and depersonalization of clients are associated with burnout (Tarolli-Jager, 1994). In the new graduate, the movement from school to active practice can create an incongruency or conflict in the values and behaviors of the two subcultures in nursing, termed "reality shock." Reality shock can create feelings of helplessness, powerlessness, frustration, and dissatisfaction. This crisis of role transformation may be resolved by adopting organizational values, returning to school, limiting personal involvement or commitment, becoming burned out, hopping among jobs, abandoning nursing, or becoming bicultural and working with the best of both worlds (Schmalenberg & Kramer, 1979).

RESEARCH NOTE

Source: Robinson, S., Roth, S., Keim, J., Levenson, M., Flentje, J., & Bashor, K. (1991). Nurse burnout: Work related and demographic factors as culprits. *Research in Nursing & Health, 14*(3), 223-228.

Purpose

Individual and organizational variables affect nurses' burnout phenomena. The purpose of this research was to examine perceptions of the work environment, selected demographics, and work related variables for their relationship to burnout in nurses working various work shifts. Nurse subjects (N = 314) from one southwestern metropolitan hospital were surveyed using the Maslach Burnout Inventory (MBI) and Moos' Work Environment Scale (WES).

Discussion

The three dimensions of burnout that were measured are emotional exhaustion, depersonalization, and personal accomplishment. Emotional exhaustion was predicted by high work pressure and low work involvement and low supervisor support. Depersonalization and personal accomplishment were predicted by task orientation, work pressure, work involvement, and age. There was a significant effect due to shift worked. No one single variable predicted burnout across all three shifts. Interpersonal dimensions were important for day and evening shift nurses. For night shift nurses, job clarity and involvement were important.

Application to Practice

Burnout is a personal and a professional concern to nurses. Understanding burnout contributes to knowledgeable strategies for decreasing or preventing burnout. Burnout consequences may include absenteeism, vague somatic complaints, work environment conflicts, and job withdrawal. High work pressure and low involvement need to be avoided. Work unit environments can be restructured to increase nurses' autonomy and involvement, reduce work pressure, and provide social support to help alleviate burnout-enhancing work environment stressors.

In contrast to the sources of stress generated within or from an individual, nurses experience stress that comes from the nature of nursing and the organizations that typically employ nurses. Sources of stress that arise from the job or occupational environment relate either to the intrinsic nature of the work itself or to a specific work environment. The intrinsic nature of nursing's work is recognized as stressful. This includes bedside nursing care delivery to ill or hospitalized clients (Mauksch, 1966; Volicer & Burns, 1977).

Work environments and organizations that employ nurses also generate stress for nurses. For example, the role of the nurse can be a source of stress and strain (Dewe, 1987). Further, organizations can generate multiple and conflicting demands on nurses (Gray-Toft & Anderson, 1981).

Role expectations sit at the interface of organizational structures and personal stress. The job experience generates numerous stressful situations. Energy and coping resources are devoted to the task of adapting and mastering the stress of role pressures and competing role expectations.

Hardy (1978) developed a role stress typology of seven sources of role stress: role ambiguity, role conflict, role incongruity, role overload, role underload, role overqualification, and role underqualification. Role theory (Thomas & Biddle, 1966) is a collection of concepts and hypotheses that predict how an individual will perform in a given role. Role theory indicates the circumstances under which certain types of behavior can be expected (Conway, 1988).

Role stress and role strain have been linked to stress in social systems (Hardy, 1978; Miller, 1971). Role expectations, location of the role in the social structure, inadequate resources, and the social context create role difficulties and stressors. Role stress arises from sources external to the role occupant. Role stress is a social structural condition that generates from role obligations that are vague, irritating, difficult, conflicting, or impossible to meet. Role strain is a subjective state of emotional arousal that occurs in response to external conditions of social stress (Hardy & Hardy, 1988; Huber, 1994). For nurses, the organizations that are the employers of nurses can create role ambiguity when role expectations are unclear, role conflict when role expectations are incompatible, role incongruity when the nurse's professional values conflict with role expectations, role overload when too much is expected in the time available, or role underload when advanced practice nurses are underutilized. Thus role stress and strain are common to nursing practice.

Specific work environments also generate stress in nursing. Specific characteristics present in healthcare organizations create stress. For example, the physical and technical environment, patterns of interpersonal relationships, professional-bureaucratic role conflict, multiple expectations, management, leadership style, communication patterns, staffing and workload, negative client outcomes, relationships with physicians, lack of participation in policy decisions, and inadequate knowledge and skills for role functions each can be a source of stress (Hinshaw & Atwood, 1983; McGrath, 1976). Leatt and Schneck (1980) categorized the organizational sources of stress as derived from either role-based or task-based situations. Hackabay and Jagla (1979) categorized ICU nursing stressors into the four categories of interpersonal communication problems, knowledge base stressors, environmental stressors, and patient care situations.

Hospitals and healthcare organizations have environmental contexts with elements that may help or hinder nursing's work (McClure, Poulin, Sovie, & Wandelt, 1983). Structural, procedural, and contextual factors cause stress and conflict (Landstrom, Biordi, & Gillies, 1989; McCloskey & McCain, 1987). Stress interrelates with other organizational variables such as organizational climate, group cohesion, job satisfaction, turnover, productivity, conflict, change, and organizational restructuring (Cleland, 1965; Hinshaw & Atwood, 1983; Hinshaw, Smeltzer, & Atwood, 1987; Huber, 1994).

Organizations form the context for stress and strain in nurse-physician relationships, sometimes called the "doctor-nurse game" (Hodes & Van Crombrugghe, 1990; Stein, Watts, & Howell, 1990). However, job satisfaction and turnover have been the major outcome variables of organizational stress that have been studied (Hinshaw, Smeltzer, & Atwood, 1987; Landstrom, Biordi, & Gillies, 1989; McCloskey & McCain, 1987; Price & Mueller, 1981; Weisman, Alexander, & Chase, 1981). Job satisfaction is a major predictor of anticipated turnover or intent to stay or leave. Anticipated turnover is a major predictor of actual turnover (Hinshaw, 1989). Job stress is an individual factor that influences job satisfaction, thereby having an indirect effect on anticipated turnover (Hinshaw, Smeltzer, & Atwood, 1987). In critical care envi ronments, perceived stress is related to job satisfaction and psychological symptoms (Norbeck, 1985).

Turbulence and organizational change create stress. Regionalization and integration transform simple organizations into complex networks of community healthcare systems. As healthcare organizations change due to social, consumer-related, governance, technology, and economic pressures, chaos and opportunities arise (Schumacher & Larson, 1993). With dramatic changes in the structures and functions of healthcare organizations, stress has become a constant, subtle, and unrelenting phenomenon perceived by staff (Woodhouse, 1993).

A sense of perceived control over related work pressures is critical to perceived stress and stress outcomes. External forces beyond a nurse's control that interfere with the ability to deliver quality care increase occupational stress. For example, some nursing stressors are lack of control over staffing patterns and staff mix, resource availability such as supplies and equipment, and lack of autonomy (Grant, 1993). Further, as organizations create and deploy work teams to deliver quality care, interpersonal stressors from the group dynamics of teams may create stress for both staff and managers (Keenan, Hurst, & Olnhausen, 1993).

Coping and Adaptation

Stressors are demands or threatening experiences from either the internal or external environment of an individual that create disequilibrium. Restoration and balance are sought as a result (Keenan, Hurst, & Olnhausen, 1993). Excessive occupational stress can lead to the undesirable outcome of burnout. Burnout in nurses undermines the nurse's helping relationship. Therefore, it is counterproductive for organizations to allow occupational stress to flourish without checks and balances. A preferable outcome goal is for nurses to function as self-dependent innovators who operate within realistic expectations and exercise control within a stressful work environment (Grant, 1993).

An individual's coping ability is the major variable modulating stress and its outcome. Coping strategies are key elements of nurses' stress reactions. The coping process is comprised of perception of stress, conditions and situational factors affecting cognitive appraisal, assessment of coping mechanisms, and the selection of a coping strategy (Harris, 1989). Nurses need to learn to manage or cope effectively with daily work life stressors by evaluating and moderating response patterns. For example, attitudes and skills, habits or typical approaches to problems, and specific actions for stress management all can be used to intervene between stress and the outcome. Effective coping actions reduce emotional distress, resolve or diminish problems, and maintain or enhance the sense of self (Woodhouse, 1993).

There have been a variety of recommendations for nurses for coping with and managing stress. For example, the development of an internal warning system to alert the individual to stress and provide a choice of responses has been recommended (Hartl, 1989). Nurses need to test the subjective and objective boundaries of stress and be willing to look after their own best interests. This may be a competing value to the concept of altruistic, unselfish service to others. However, guilt may be used by organizations to induce nurses to respond in ways that primarily serve the interests of the institution (Woodhouse, 1993).

Stress management techniques range from those focused on the individual to those focused on the organization. Some coping strategies used by nurse executives include spending time on non-work-related interests, using a personal support network, being active in the larger professional arena, identifying resources for problem solving, manifesting somatic symptoms, walking away from situations to gain perspective, considering resigning, rigid adherence to rules, complying, and participating in dysfunctional competition (Scalzi, 1988). Humor in communication can be used as a mechanism for coping with stress and thereby enhancing morale and productivity (Woodhouse, 1993).

A comprehensive stress management plan may be needed for organizations. This begins with a baseline stress assessment to determine levels and types of occupational stress. Department interactions and support systems availability can be analyzed in relationship to nursing stress levels. Educational programs can be developed around universal stress and coping themes such as overload, time management, decision making, prioritization skills, and change management. Thus individual and organization-wide stress assessments can be used to plan specific stress management sessions as a way of mitigating nursing occupational stress and enhancing nurses' coping (Grant, 1993). Narasi (1994) described the use of a needs-recognition graph by a group of hospice nurses who were struggling with the effects of restructuring and increased work hours. Stress management classes were used by the group to increase awareness of stressors, reveal feelings, assess reality, and transcend the present to an unknown future. The result was a refocusing toward hope, identity, health-directed behaviors, and a sense of the future.

Other methods of personal or organizational strategies for coping with stress include physical activity; nutritional control; environmental control; psychological strategies to improve attitudes, self-esteem, and self-mastery; and interpersonal strategies related to social support. Exercise, sports, hobbies, meditation, relaxation, and spiritual exercises are advocated. Stress audits can be personal assessments or organization-wide. Balancing an increase in personal control with coping with what is beyond control is a key strategy. Monitoring the effects of caffeine, nicotine, and rest are advocated to increase coping. Intervention techniques can be focused on filtering, buffering, and adapting to stress.

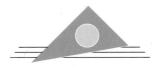

Leadership & Management Behaviors

LEADERSHIP BEHAVIORS	MANAGEMENT BEHAVIORS	OVERLAP AREAS
• enables followers to cope with stress	• uses humor	• uses humor
• models personal stress management	• manages personal stress	• manages personal stress
• uses humor	• plans for stress assessment	
• encourages adaptation and growth	• organizes the environment to decrease stress	
• mentors and provides social support	• evaluates individual and occupational stress	
• communicates ways of coping	• influences followers to cope with stress	
• envisions the future		
• inspires hope		
• influences greater personal and group control		

LEADERSHIP AND MANAGEMENT IMPLICATIONS

Stress is an important concern for leaders and managers in nursing. Stress is a pervasive fact of organizational operations. Both personal and occupational stress create consequences for leaders and managers that also may have an effect on meeting goals and levels of productivity. There is a long list of both work and non-work-related stressors. Leaders and managers will need to assess the levels and types of stress in individuals and in the environment in order to begin to moderate stress toward useful levels.

Stress at too high a level reduces nurses' coping and adaptive abilities and is counterproductive. Nurse leaders and managers may have a role to play in caring for the psychological needs of the staff. Personal hardiness may be augmented by increased awareness. Leaders and managers can provide counseling, support groups, team building activities, and stress management programs.

Nurse leaders and managers have a stake in assessing and diagnosing the sources of nursing occupational stress. This becomes the foundation for planning, implementing, and evaluating strategies to manage job stress. Within organizations, nurse productivity, job satisfaction, and retention are improved when occupational stress is managed. Some stressors can be modified, improved, or reduced by making structural or organizational changes. Adequate staffing, correcting problems in the physical environment, and facilitating positive communication are suggested strategies for nurse leaders and managers. Internal organizational systems may be malfunctioning and need correction. For example, organizational structures, client care variables, availability of support services, and nursing care delivery modalities may create stress and be amenable to modification for stress reduction. Organizational remedies should be founded on staff input and be directly related to improving the system (Huber, 1994; Norbeck, 1985). Further, nurses may need to have job-specific remedies like reasonable shift rotations and flexibility for child care.

Nurse leaders and managers may need to find strategies for nurses' coping with an environment that creates stress due to the threat of personal danger. For example, nurses who work in abortion clinics may be personally threatened with harm. Instances arise in which babies are kidnapped from hospital nurseries. Clients may physically assault caregivers. Caregivers may be involved in fistfights or throwing objects. Policies and procedures need to be in place for the protection of nurses and clients from physical injury and bodily harm.

Leaders can inspire hope and a vision for the future. They can communicate with humor and inspire others to adapt to stress. Managers can plan and organize the environment to modulate organizational stress. Leaders and managers can manage personal stress and influence others toward enhanced coping and support of one another. Thus both individual and occupational stress can be managed.

CURRENT ISSUES AND TRENDS

Healthcare reform and economics are creating stress and pressure for nurses. The turbulence and change as health delivery systems merge, integrate, regionalize, and restructure cause uncertainty, anxiety, role ambiguity, and stress. Pervasive stress is inevitable with such large-scale systems reforming processes. Nurses must cope with new ways of thinking and delivering care. Individual stress responses, turf battles, and conflicts occur as the friction surfaces among individuals. For example, teamwork and collaboration may ultimately provide a fertile ground for systems improvement, but teamwork may be a new mode of operating and, therefore, stressful. Individuals are likely to feel helpless, anxious, and out of control when faced with massive systems changes (Huber, 1994).

Leaders and managers may themselves be under sufficient stress and thereby have less energy to devote to helping their staff through difficult psychological transitions. Cost containment pressures may result in decisions to eliminate staff education for stress management. Institutional remedies may be substantially diminished.

It is difficult to prescribe methods for work-related stress management during high environmental turbulence. Educating and supporting staff nurses, reducing

JoEllen Koerner Envisions Nurturing the Self and Others

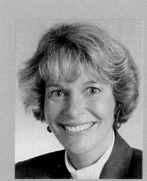

JoEllen Koerner

When a gardener plants seeds in fertile soil where sunlight and breeze grace the landscape, the work has just begun. Tending to the growth of what has been planted is the most critical labor in assuring a rich harvest. The caring leader who plants a compelling vision has a reversed image of life and leadership . . . it's not about me, but rather, about us. In order to transcend ourselves we must support, empower, and learn from others. It is in community that we, leader and community member alike, have the chance to become all that our potential holds. Thus, the leader's efforts are focused on building community with a nourishing environment while providing resources and experiences which foster personal and professional growth towards a shared vision.

Community membership requires that each is centered and rooted deeply in his or her unique way of being in the world. We must develop a reverence for the uniqueness of each individual, including ourselves. Understanding and honoring self and others is essential, leading to changes in attitudes and behaviors that radically transform outcomes for all. From the vantage point of mutual valuing we move out of a pattern of domination and control towards connection of the heart, soul and mind. Transformative leaders open the door to power, sharing it through creation of true partnership with mutual responsibility. This gives everyone's ideas a chance; the leader doesn't always have to be right. Recognizing others strengths frees us from our own weakness.

The caring leader establishes new order through shared dialogue with all involved. For individuals to move beyond maintenance mode behavior towards one of active design, an environment which honors and rewards risk-taking and innovation must be established. A transformational leader is in the practice of making heroes and creating legends so that new metaphors and models are held before the nursing practice. People grow when they are in the presence of someone who cares. There is an intimate link between our capacity for risk taking and our commitment to learning and growing. The nurturing leader doesn't push but rather, like a midwife, gently guides the birth of unique tales and gifts of the individual or group as they are ready to grow. This allows all to grow as they can from where they are . . . one size does not fit all. We quickly discover that the greatest risk in active growth is the risk of self-revelation, which paradoxically is also its greatest reward.

JoEllen Koerner has served as Vice President of Patient Services at Sioux Valley Hospital in Sioux Falls, South Dakota, for the past 11 years. Previous positions of leadership include Executive Secretary of the South Dakota Board of Nursing, Director of the Department of Nursing at Freeman Junior College, along with various clinical and management positions in acute care and rural medical clinic work. She is currently President of the American Organization of Nurse Executives.

paperwork, changing organizational climates, enhancing nurses' participation in decision making, and reducing workloads are positive strategies for nurses' stress that may not be implemented by organizations during unstable environmental conditions. Further, under healthcare reform initiatives there has been a major review of roles and tasks in nursing and healthcare. Role ambiguity has become a major source of stress, directly related to both advanced practice nurses and to unlicensed assistive personnel. With so many focal points for stress, nursing as a profession is challenged to create a vision for the future and strategies for today.

Stress and conflict also may create opportunities for nursing. Clarity of direction for the profession in carving out key nursing roles and responsibilities in a community-based, managed care environment is a key stress and coping strategy. Changes prompt the need to adapt. Building and nurturing teams, managing change, and strong leadership direction can create a climate for innovation and creativity as one productive response to uncertainty and stress. Conflicts and changes generate stress. Positive and proactive responses help nurses to cope and adapt to stress in a way that produces growth and productivity.

SUMMARY

- Stress is built into healing occupations.
- Stress needs to be neither too high nor too low.
- Stress is an individual response to a stressor.
- A stressor is an experience that is taxing or threatening.
- Occupational stress is a tension related to the job or role.
- Burnout is a response to chronic stress.
- Stress moves from potential stressor to outcomes and consequences.
- Coping and cognitive appraisal mediate stress.
- Stress consequences are either positive or negative.
- Sources of stress are individual or organizational.
- There are multiple factors causing stress in nursing.
- Stress outcomes take different forms from positive to negative.
- Coping modulates stress and its outcome.
- There are both individual and organizational stress management techniques.
- Leaders and managers can influence stress and stress management.
- The current healthcare environment is turbulent and stressful.

Study Questions

1. What sources of stress do you find to be the most important influences in your life and work?
2. What coping strategies are most useful for stress reduction? Why are they helpful?

3. To what extent should employers pay for stress management programs for nurses?
4. Why should nurses manage their own stress?
5. Why should nurses promote reality shock support for new graduates?
6. What can nurses do to manage stress in work teams?

Critical Thinking Exercise

Integrated Medical-Plex is an integrated healthcare network consisting of a tertiary teaching hospital, ambulatory clinics, a home health agency, and a long-term care facility. Integrated Medical-Plex is in the planning stage of opening up three new satellite community walk-in clinics. Nurse Catherine Ebinger, the Chief Nurse Executive, has been intimately involved in the planning for implementing the clinics. How to motivate or recruit RNs to work in the new clinics is a major concern. Meanwhile, Nurse Ebinger's attention has been diverted by the numerous "brush fires" that keep cropping up. For example, an OR nurse has been in to complain about a surgeon who shot the nurse with a staple gun "as a joke" (according to the surgeon). The nurse manager of the abortion clinic just faxed over an alert that a large group of hostile protesters were expected to picket tomorrow. The nurse manager wants to know how to protect the clinic staff's safety. On her desk this AM was a written complaint from the CRNAs on staff who allege that the group of anesthesiologists who practice at the hospital have conspired to bill Medicare and other third-party payors for the services actually performed by the nurses while the MDs were out of the house. Last, but not least, is the turmoil that is being fomented as other staff nurses hear about the bitter complaining of the trauma floor staff nurses who are angry at cuts in staffing and job insecurity. The RNs on the trauma floor contend that nurse to patient ratios of 1:9 are too high to be safe on PM shift. An incident report arrived from yesterday describing how a patient from room 41-10 had gone into the next room (41-12) to put the patient in 41-12 on a bedpan because the nurse was occupied with two admissions at once plus an epidural pump on another patient. Rumors are that the nurses are talking about forming a collective bargaining unit as protection against short staffing and layoffs.

1. *What is (are) the problem(s)?*

2. *Why is (are) this (these) a problem(s)?*

3. *What should Nurse Ebinger do first?*

4. *What factors should Nurse Ebinger assess and analyze?*

5. *What sources of stress are there?*

6. *What should Nurse Ebinger do about stress in the nurses?*

7. *What strategies could be employed to control stress and enhance coping?*

REFERENCES

Aurelio, J. (1993). An organizational culture that optimizes stress: Acceptable stress in nursing. *Nursing Administration Quarterly, 18*(1), 1-10.

Bailey, J. T. (1980). Stress and stress management: An overview. *Journal of Nursing Education, 19*(6), 5-8.

Benson, H., & Allen, R. L. (1980). How much stress is too much? *Harvard Business Review, 58*(5), 86-92.

Cleland, V. S. (1965). The effect of stress on performance. *Nursing Research, 14,* 292-298.

Conway, M. (1988). Theoretical approaches to the study of roles. In M. E. Hardy & M. E. Conway (Eds.), *Role theory: Perspectives for health professionals* (2nd ed.) (pp. 63-72). Norwalk, CT: Appleton & Lange.

Dewe, P. J. (1987). Identifying the causes of nurses' stress: A survey of New Zealand nurses. *Work and stress, 1*(1), 15-24.

Dietz, M. (1991). Stressors and coping mechanisms of older rural women. In A. Bushy (Ed.), *Rural nursing Vol. 1* (pp. 267-280). Newbury Park, CA: Sage.

Elliott, G., & Eisdorfer, C. (1982). *Stress and human health.* New York: Springer.

Fagin, C. (1987). Stress: Implications for nursing research. *Image, 19*(1), 38-41.

Gardner, D. L. (1992). Career commitment in nursing. *Journal of Professional Nursing, 8*(3), 155-160.

Getzels, J. W. (1958). Administration as a social process. In A. W. Halpin (Eds.), *Administrative theory in education* (pp. 150-165). Chicago: University of Chicago Press.

Grant, P. (1993). Manage nurse stress and increase potential at the bedside. *Nursing Administration Quarterly, 18*(1), 16-22.

Gray-Toft, P., & Anderson, J. G. (1981). Stress among hospital nursing staff: Its causes and effects. *Social Science and Medicine, 15A,* 539-647.

Greenhaus, J. H., & Kopelman, R. E. (1981). Conflict between work and nonwork roles: Implications for the career planning process. *Human Resource Planning, 4*(1), 1-10.

Hardy, M. E. (1978). Role stress and role strain. In M. E. Hardy & M. E. Conway (Eds.), *Role theory; Perspectives for health professionals* (2nd ed.). Norwalk, CT: Appleton-Century-Crofts.

Hardy, M. E., & Conway, M. E. (1988). *Role theory: Perspectives for health professionals* (2nd ed.). Norwalk, CT: Appleton & Lange.

Hardy, M. E., & Hardy, W. L. (1988). Role stress and role strain. In M. E. Hardy & M. E. Conway (Eds.), *Role theory: Perspectives for health professionals* (2nd ed.) (pp. 159-239). Norwalk, CT: Appleton & Lange.

Hartl, D. (1989). Stress management and the nurse. *Advances in Nursing Science, 11*(2), 91-100.

Harris, R. (1989). Review of nursing stress according to a proposed coping adaptation framework. *Advances in Nursing Science, 11*(2), 12-28.

Hinshaw, A. S. (1989). Programs of nursing research for nursing administration. In B. Henry, C. Arndt, M. Di Vincenti, & A. Marriner-Tomey (Eds.), *Dimensions of nursing administration* (pp. 251-266). Boston: Blackwell.

Hinshaw, A. S., & Atwood, J. R. (1983). Nursing staff turnover, stress, and satisfaction: Models, measures, and management. *Annual Review of Nursing Research, 1,* 133-153.

Hinshaw, A. S., Smeltzer, C. H., & Atwood, J. R. (1987). Innovative retention strategies for nursing staff. *Journal of Nursing Administration, 17*(6), 8-16.

Hodes, J. R., & Van Crombrugghe, P. (1990). Nurse-physician relationships. *Nursing Management, 21*(7), 73-75.

Huber, D. (1994). What are the sources of stress for nurses? In J. McCloskey & H. Grace (Eds.), *Current issues in nursing* (4th ed.) (pp. 623-631). St. Louis: Mosby.

Huckabay, L. M. D., & Jagla, B. (1979). Nurses' stress factors in the intensive care unit. *Journal of Nursing Administration, 9*(2), 21-26.

Keenan, M., Hurst, J., & Olnhausen, K. (1993). Polarity management for quality care: Self-direction and manager direction. *Nursing Administration Quarterly, 18*(1), 23-29.

Kramer, M. (1974). Reality shock: Why nurses leave nursing. St. Louis: Mosby.

Kramer, M., & Schmalenberg, C. (1977). *Path to biculturalism*. Wakefield, MA: Contemporary Publishing.

Landstrom, G. L., Biordi, D. L., & Gillies, D. A. (1989). The emotional and behavioral process of staff nurse turnover. *Journal of Nursing Administration, 19*(9), 23-28.

Lazarus, R., & Folkman, S. (1984). *Stress, appraisal and coping*. New York: Springer.

Leatt, P., & Schneck, R. (1980). Differences in stress perceived by head nurses across nursing specialties in hospitals. *Journal of Advanced Nursing, 5*, 31-46.

Lowery, B. (1987). Stress research: Some theoretical and methodological issues. *Image, 19*(1), 42-46.

Lyon, B. L., & Werner, J. S. (1987). Stress. *Annual Review of Nursing Research, 5*, 3-22.

Maslach, C., & Jackson, S. (1981). The measurement of experienced burnout. *Journal of Occupational Behaviour, 2*, 99-113.

Mauksch, H. O. (1966). The organizational context of nursing practice. In F. Davis (Eds.), *The nursing profession: Five sociological essays* (pp. 109-137). New York: John Wiley & Sons.

McCloskey, J. C., & McCain, B. E. (1987). Satisfaction, commitment, and professionalism of newly employed nurses. *Image, 19*, 20-24.

McClure, M., Poulin, M., Sovie, M., & Wandelt, M. (1983). *Magnet hospitals: Attraction and retention of professional nurses*. Kansas City, MO: American Nurses Association.

McCranie, E., Lambert, V., & Lambert, C. (1987). Work stress, hardiness, and burnout among hospital staff nurses. *Nursing Research, 36*, 374-378.

McGrath, J. E. (1976). Stress and behavior in organizations. In M. D. Dunnette (Ed.), *Handbook of industrial and organizational psychology* (pp. 1351-1395). Chicago: Rand McNally.

Miller, J. (1971). The nature of living systems. *Behavioral Science, 16*, 278.

Narasi, B. (1994). A tool for living through stress. *Nursing Management, 25*(9), 73-75.

Norbeck, J. S. (1985). Perceived job stress, job satisfaction, and psychological symp-toms in critical care nursing. *Research in Nursing & Health, 8*, 253-259.

Perlman, B., & Hartman, E. (1982). Burnout: Summary and future research. *Human Relations, 35*(4), 283-305.

Price, J. L., & Mueller, C. W. (1981). *Professional turnover: The case of nurses*. New York: Spectrum.

Rich, V. L., & Rich, A. R. (1987). Personality hardiness and burnout in female staff nurses. *Image, 19*, 63-66.

Scalzi, C. (1988). Role stress and coping strategies of nurse executives. *Journal of Nursing Administration, 18*(3), 34-38.

Schmalenberg, C., & Kramer, M. (1979). *Coping with reality shock: The voices of experience*. Wakefield, MA: Nursing Resources.

Schumacher, L., & Larson, K. (1993). Thriving and striving on the turbulence of rural health care. *Nursing Administration Quarterly, 18*(1), 11-15.

Selye, H. (1965). *The stress of life*. Toronto: McGraw-Hill.

Selye, H. (1976). *Stress in health and disease*. Boston: Butterworth.

Smythe, E. (1984). Burn-out: From caring to apathy. In E. Smythe (Ed.), *Surviving nursing* (pp. 46-57). Menlo Park, CA: Addison-Wesley.

Stehle, J. L. (1981). Critical care nursing stress: The findings revisited. *Nursing Research, 30*, 182-186.

Stein, L. I., Watts, D. T., & Howell, T. (1990). The doctor-nurse game revisited. *New England Journal of Medicine, 322*(8), 546-549.

Tarolli-Jager, K. (1994). Personal hardiness: Your buffer against burnout. *American Journal of Nursing, 94*(2), 71-72.

Thomas, E. J., & Biddle, B. J. (1966). Basic concepts for classifying the phenomena of role. In B. J. Biddle & E. J. Thomas (Eds.), *Role theory: Concepts and research* (pp. 23-45). New York: John Wiley & Sons.

Volicer, B. J., & Burns, M. W. (1977). Preexisting correlates of hospital stress. *Nursing Research, 26*(6), 408-415.

Wagnild, G., & Young, H. M. (1991). Another look at hardiness. *Image, 23*(4), 257-259.

Weisman, C. S., Alexander, C. S., & Chase, G. (1981). Determinants of hospital staff nurse turnover. *Medical Care, 19*(4), 431-443.

Woodhouse, D. (1993). The aspects of humor in dealing with stress. *Nursing Administration Quarterly, 18*(1), 80-89.

PART VII

Future Perspectives

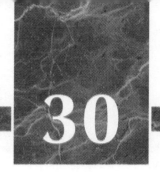

Health Policy and the Nurse

Chapter Objectives

∾

define and describe policy

∾

define and describe politics

∾

define and describe health policy

∾

explain policy-making

∾

analyze the public policy process

∾

explain how a bill becomes a law

∾

compare politics and power

∾

analyze health policy

∾

exercise critical thinking to conceptualize and analyze
possible solutions to a practical experience incident

*t*he forces of social, political, and economic change sweep nursing along in
times of rapid change. The healthcare delivery system has felt the strain of
cost pressures that led to national healthcare reform initiatives in the United
States. Central to the resultant debate about healthcare policy is the unresolved
issue as to whether everyone should be entitled to affordable basic healthcare.

As nursing has matured as a profession, nurses have become more cognizant of the need for activism in health policy and politics at all levels. As

the largest healthcare provider group, nurses need to be a visible and vocal presence in the healthcare reform debate. Nurses hold individual, personal perspectives as citizens and consumers of healthcare. Nurses as a professional group are integral to the delivery of healthcare services and need to be active as client advocates. Nurses as a provider group are a special interest lobby with identifiable skills, abilities, potential, and turf area. In order to have influence over legislation and other health policy decisions, nurses can organize, lobby, coordinate grassroots activities, serve on legislative staffs, or become elected officials. These and many other related activities provide avenues for nurses to be influential in the process of healthcare reform and enhance nursing's role as a major player in health policy and politics (Lescavage, 1995).

DEFINITIONS

There is a distinction between policy and politics. *Policy* is the formulation of value statements, the "shoulds" and "oughts" of larger and more important issues (see Chart 30.1). Policy tends to change in small increments. Policy is a result of setting goals and determining directions (Diers, 1985; Mason & Talbott, 1985).

Longest (1994, p. 3) defined public policies as "authoritative decisions made in the legislative, executive, or judicial branches of government intended to direct or influence the actions, behaviors, or decisions of others." Policies made in the public arena can be differentiated from policies made in the private sector. For example, decisions made by insurance companies or by the Joint Commission on the Accreditation of Healthcare Organizations (JCAHO) are non-governmental or private sector policies.

Politics is the process of influencing the allocation of scarce resources or the use of power for change. Politics occurs within the arenas of competition, legislation, elections, and government (Diers, 1985; Mason & Talbott, 1985). Nurses can have an effect on change in four major spheres of political influence: in the workplace, government, organizations, and the larger community (Mason & Talbott, 1985).

Health policy is the entire set of public policies that are related to or influence health and illness. The federal, state, and local levels of government all are involved in formulating health policy (Longest, 1994).

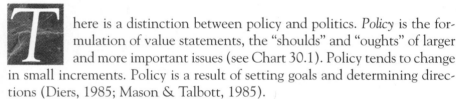

CHART 30.1
∽ DEFINITIONS

Policy
the formulation of value statements, a result of setting goals and determining directions.

Politics
the process of influencing the allocation of scarce resources or the use of power for change.

Health Policy
the entire set of public policies that are related to or influence health and illness.

Data from Diers (1985), Mason and Talbott (1985), and Longest (1994).

BACKGROUND

Policy-Making

Policy-making is an activity that goes on in many settings. At issue are values. Public policy occurs through the acts of government or governmental agencies. Policies occur as a result of national commissions, by legislation, by the judicial system, by state and local governments, in the private sector, and by regulatory agencies (Diers, 1985).

Policy-making is dependent on both values and analysis. This is because choices come from both values and analysis, and policy-making implies choice. For example, within the health policy arena there are numerous conflicts over values. One example is the criteria used to judge the healthcare system and thereby make resource allocation decisions. Analyses are done to provide data input into policy-making decisions. For example, detailed economic analyses may be conducted to explore the limitations of labor or capital costs (Fuchs, 1993).

Public Policy Process

The public policy-making process occurs in a cyclical fashion. It is an ongoing process, and one in which virtually all decisions are subject to modification or reversion. Thus there are numerous influences, often external from special interests, that buffet or impact the process. Clearly, policy-making resembles an open system, by virtue of the sensitive impact of the external environment (Longest, 1994).

There are three major phases to the policy-making process: policy formulation, policy implementation, and policy modification (see Fig. 30.1). The policy formulation phase is concerned with making decisions that lead to legislation. Activities of agenda setting and developing legislation occur in the policy formulation phase. These activities are distinct and sequential (Longest, 1994). The first step in any policy-making process is to bring the issue to the forefront or "get on the agenda" (Diers, 1985).

A window of opportunity is created for an issue to emerge on the public policy agenda when problems, possible solutions, and political circumstances come together in a favorable configuration. Problems may be serious but not emerge into policy issues. When they reach an unacceptable level, they may emerge into the public consciousness. For example, the number of people with AIDS and the number of people without healthcare coverage (uninsured) have launched into the public policy arena as national health problems. Problems tend to be noticed when they either are widespread and affect large numbers of people, impact a small but powerful group, strike the fancy of the nation via media coverage, or are linked closely to other well-accepted policy issues (Longest, 1994).

When a problem comes to the forefront, possible solutions help to trigger policy formulation. Differences or conflict may arise over the criteria to be used in evaluating alternative solutions to the problem. Policy-making may be slowed by the time it takes to critique and debate the relative merits of competing alternatives. Arguments may be generated over whether a solution will

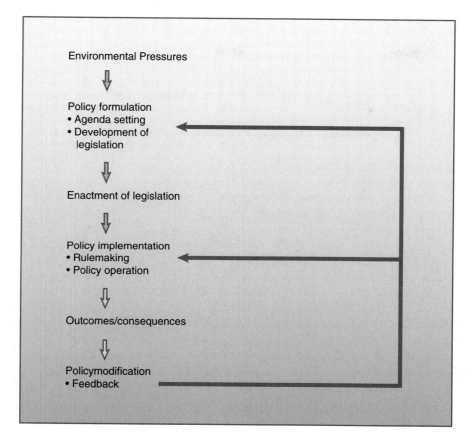

Environmental Pressures

Policy formulation
• Agenda setting
• Development of
  legislation

Enactment of legislation

Policy implementation
• Rulemaking
• Policy operation

Outcomes/consequences

Policymodification
• Feedback

Figure 30.1
Public policy process. (Adapted with permission from Longest, Jr., B. [1994]. *Health policy-making in the United States.* Ann Arbor, MI: AUPHA Press/ Health Administration Press.)

solve the problem, implementation timelines and feasibility, costs, benefits, and political considerations (Longest, 1994).

The political circumstances surrounding policy-making relate to the power necessary to launch substantive legislation initiatives. A political force may arise from a variety of sources. For example, public opinion or concern about an issue may initiate political forces. Special interest groups, key political leaders, and any other policy issues currently in focus may be powerful enough to create the window of policy-making opportunity (Longest, 1994).

Research and concept analysis are important tools for the policy formulation phase of the policy-making process. By analyzing data, providing documentation, providing an issues synthesis, or recommending a course of action (prescription), research can influence public policy (Brown, 1991). Sometimes a large and diverse set of policies result from the offering of solutions by multiple special interest groups armed with data (Longest, 1994).

The policy formulation phase concludes with the development of legislation. Formal enactment of legislation bridges the policy-making process into the

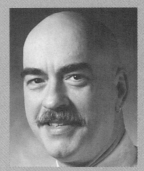

Peter Ungvarski

Peter Ungvarski Envisions the Importance of Nursing Research in Health Policy

The current climate of healthcare reform has brought nursing in the United States under close scrutiny. A question being asked more frequently is, what is nursing? Policy makers, legislators, and economists alike are demanding that we define the product of nursing, that is, our nursing care. They also want to know how much our product costs.

The future of nursing and the role nurses will play in the delivery of healthcare in the United States will be determined by our research efforts. A dramatic shift must take place from the preponderance of qualitative research to quantitative research.

The research sequence should begin with retrospective and prospective studies that identify the actual or potential problems that occur in specific client populations and settings, for example, clients with AIDS in acute care and clients with AIDS in home care. The research design should include dual identification of problems by the patient as well as the nurse and comparison of both findings. Studies have demonstrated significant differences in problem identification between the two groups. Identifying the prevalence of problems in specific populations provides an opportunity for establishing future research priorities.

Once problems are identified, the effectiveness of nursing interventions should be tested by simultaneously measuring patient outcomes and the costs of the interventions. It is no longer acceptable for nurses to say that nursing interventions work without being able to identify the associated costs. If the costs are expensive, then we must study strategies for care that are less expensive.

Multisite studies of the same problem and intervention are necessary for the results to be generalizable or to identify regional differences. For example, are there differences in how nurses manage dyspnea associated with chronic lung disease in Los Angeles and New York City and are the differences related to the environment and climate? Are there differences in host factors such as gender, age, race or ethnicity, income, and insurance status?

Finally, collaborative efforts should be increased with research designs that bring together experts in research and experts in clinical care. Clinical experts bring a wealth of experience to a study and insure that the question under study is relevant to practice.

If nurses are going to pull up a chair to the table of policy makers, legislators, and healthcare economists and planners, they must be prepared to identify the benefits and costs of "nursing care" and present quantifiable data. Concrete evidence can have a positive impact on policy making. The future of the healthcare of Americans and the benefits of professional nursing care depend on our research efforts.

Peter J. Ungvarski, MS, RN, FAAN, is Clinical Nurse Specialist, HIV Infection, and Clinical Director, AIDS Services, Visiting Nurse Service of New York. Ungvarski has been involved clinically in the nursing care of persons with human immunodeficiency virus (HIV) infection since 1981 and has done so in four major areas of practice: (1) critical care, (2) hospice, (3) the home, and (4) clinical research. He has written and published more than 40 articles on client care related to HIV infection and is an author and co-editor of the textbook *HIV/AIDS: a Guide to Nursing Care* (1995). He has testified before the United States Senate Labor and Human Resources Committee for improved education for health care workers regarding HIV infection and before the Presidential Commission on the HIV epidemic for increased resources for the home care of persons with AIDS. He has served as advisor to the Office of Technology Assessment, U.S. Congress, and to the National Institute of Nursing Research.

next phase of policy implementation. In the policy implementation phase, actions are taken and additional decisions are made about how to implement the legislation. Because laws tend to be vague about the details of implementation, early implementation efforts are targeted at making rules. Advisory committees may assist in rule-making, and a draft set of rules may be published for the purposes of notice and input reaction. As with other forms of decision making, power resides with those who are charged with the responsibility to implement legislation. For example, it is possible for those charged with implementing legislation to stall, alter, or subvert the intent of the law (Longest, 1994).

When the programs and activities that were designed by the legislation are up and running, the policy process is at the policy operation stage. Policies that are well written and have clear goals are more likely to be successfully implemented. Imprecise language and vague directives set up conditions under which those charged with implementation have greater difficulty in successfully completing their tasks (Longest, 1994).

The result of policy implementation is that outcomes occur along with consequences and individuals' perceptions of outcomes and consequences. Feedback can occur that modifies a policy at several points in the process: during agenda setting, during legislation development and formulation, during rule-making, and at policy operation stages. Policy modification occurs because problems become more sharply defined or better understood. A policy may impinge on other policies. Outcomes may not be desired. Political circumstances may change. Policies may become outmoded or inadequate. Policy modification may result in minor adjustments or reversals of the agenda.

Clearly, the policy-making process is political, cyclical, interactive, and heavily influenced by external forces (Longest, 1994).

The policy-making process is complex, dynamic, and creative. It does not always adhere to rational-logical ways of proceeding. In general, however, policy-making begins with agenda setting and then moves through stages that include specifying alternative solutions, decision making, implementation, and evaluation with feedback. Public policy comes to be reflected in a course of action or a course of inaction that governments, organizations, or individuals choose to achieve some goal or outcome.

How a Bill Becomes Law

Legislation in the United States is enacted by means of a multistage process. Although the process is complex, dynamic, and interactive, it can be outlined as to the basics of the path a bill takes in becoming enacted into law. The federal process follows an ordered set of steps (Longest, 1994).

The first step is a legislative proposal, called a bill or a resolution. Bills may be drafted by a variety of people, but only a member of Congress can officially sponsor the proposed legislation. The bill is then introduced by a member of Congress into his or her respective chamber (Senate or House of Representatives). The bill is given a number and referred to an appropriate standing committee. Hearings may be held to elicit viewpoints about the bill and its recommendations. After hearings the bill will be marked up, which is a process of line by line review, edit, or amendment. After mark up, the committee reports out the bill to the full committee with jurisdiction or to the floor of the House or Senate. The House or Senate places the bill on the legislative agenda for floor debate and action. The bill can be further amended in the debate that occurs as the bill is on the floor. Assuming all goes well, the bill is passed and sent on to the other chamber, where the committee referral process is repeated. This may entail hearings, mark up, and action by the other chamber. If both chambers pass different versions, joint conference committees are used to reconcile any differences. If the conference committee cannot reach agreement, the bill dies (Longest, 1994).

Assuming all goes well, the conference committee will iron out differences, and both chambers will accept their report. The bill is then sent to the President for signature, veto, or hold. If signed, the bill becomes law. If vetoed, the bill is returned to Congress, where a two-thirds vote of both houses will override the veto. A hold means that the bill will become law in ten days despite the President's disapproval by nonsignature (Longest, 1994).

The opportunities for nurses to be influential in the process of a bill becoming law occur at several stages. For example, nurses may help draft legislation or write letters in support of a bill during the formal introduction stage. Lobbying efforts by nurses can go on during the process of the bill's journey toward legislation and final action by the President. The key elements are the votes and final decisions in the process of passage. However, the precision and use of language in the multiple and final versions are extremely important for the implementation of the legislation. Nurses also may be influential in the executive branch of government's implementation of laws via specific rules and regulations. Communication and use of expertise are key strategies. Political power is the most effective method of influencing the passage and implementation of legislation. Nurses need to be taking a leadership role in political activism and advocacy.

Politics

The term politics often is associated with federal, state, and local government and the campaigning for and holding of political office by public officials. However, politics has been viewed more broadly as the pattern of interpersonal relationships and human dynamics among persons in a given setting. Politics has been described as raw human behavior or the art of who gets what, when, and how (Maraldo, 1985). Politics draws on power. Like the pervasiveness of power, politics also permeates all human interactions. Therefore, in order to understand the politics of a situation, it is necessary to analyze and understand the persons involved in the circumstances and the interrelationships among them (Maraldo, 1985). Power and politics are both integral to the processes involved with the allocation of scarce resources.

Politics may be discussed as activities that occur either in relationship to activities within organizations or in relationship to governmental or legislative actions. Scarce resources in organizational settings include money, personnel, and space. Politics become important in this context because of the contention for control over resources that is inherent in organizations.

Politics is important to nurses as they interact outside of their employing organization and seek to attain professional or personal goals. Nurses can exert influence for change in the governmental sphere of influence. The government determines a legal definition of nursing, formulates laws that impact on the practice of nursing, influences reimbursement for nursing services, and determines access to healthcare (Hanley, 1987; Mason & Talbott, 1985). Hanley (1987) identified four factors of political participation: voting, campaign activities, community activities, and protest. Thus nurses can become politically active by voting and encouraging voter turnout, participating in the activities of a candidate's campaign, communicating in the community, and being a part of protest activities. As a special interest group, nurses become involved in politics through contact with issues of licensure, self-regulation, and reimbursement. As caring healers, nurses become involved in politics through efforts to acquire public resources for client needs.

RESEARCH NOTE

Source: Hanley, B. (1987). Political participation: How do nurses compare with other professional women? *Nursing Economic$*, 5(4), 179-185, 188.

Purpose

All aspects of the healthcare industry are affected by political and policy decisions at the local, state, and national levels. Therefore, nurses' political participation is critical to nursing's attainment of professional goals and nurses' attainment of personal goals. The purpose of this research was to determine whether differences in political participation exist among women nurses, teachers, and engineers; the extent of any differences or similarities; and the relationship of predictor variables to behaviors exhibited. Membership lists from professional organizations of nurses, teachers, and engineers were used to draw randomly selected comparison samples of 450 nurses, 100 teachers, and 97 engineers. Subjects were surveyed by mail with telephone follow-up to assess their level of political activity. Political behaviors of voting, campaigning, community activity, and protest were assessed.

Discussion

The results showed intergroup similarities on religion, race, marital status, and age of youngest child. Nurses had the lowest educational attainment and were significantly less active in their professional organizations. Nurses belonged to significantly fewer professional organizations. Overall, women nurses, teachers, and engineers participated at approximately comparable rates in politics. Nurses had a significantly lower voting score. Nurses and teachers had equivalent scores on protest activities, both significantly higher than engineers. Analysis of predictor variables indicated that demographic variables of age, income, and religion; situational variables of unemployment and number of children; family socialization; and professional socialization were significantly related to political participation by nurses. This was less true for teachers and engineers. BSN-prepared nurses who were professional organization members were as active as teachers and social workers in all four modes of political behavior.

Application to Practice

Occupational gender segregation appeared to have only an indirect effect on political participation. BSN-prepared female nurses participated in politics similar to female teachers and engineers. Nurses can assume leadership in the political domain to advocate for clients and to protect and enhance their personal and professional interests. Professional organizations serve to monitor public and health policies as well as to politicize the members. Nursing education programs should include political education in both undergraduate and continuing education courses.

Health Policy

Health policy is a subset of public policy. It includes those public policies that are related to or influence health and illness. Health policies generally either affect a group or class of individuals or affect types of organizations. A complex and large number of decisions go into health policy formulation. Health policies emerge in the forms of laws, rules and regulations, judicial decisions, resource allocations, and broad "macro" policies such as global healthcare budgets. Health policies also may be categorized as either allocative or regulatory. Allocative policies provide subsidies to some group. Regulatory policies attempt to ensure that objectives are met by influencing or directing actions, behaviors, or decisions (Longest, 1994). Nurses may be involved in allocative health policies such as Medicaid assistance to children who qualify or who do not qualify. Nurses may become involved in regulatory policies when advanced practice nurses seek prescription privileges.

Ethical decisions may need to be analyzed and debated in relationship to health policy. Ethical principles outline a moral foundation for policy analysis. For example, abortion legality is a highly controversial health policy. The 1990 Patient Self-Determination Act (P.L. 101-508) was designed to enforce the client's right to make those decisions that concern medical care and intervention. Nurses' practice was impacted by this legislation in two ways: practically, as nurses had to ask about advanced directives; and ethically, as nurses learned to accept the range of decisions made by clients.

LEADERSHIP AND MANAGEMENT IMPLICATIONS

It is vital that nurses become involved in both politics and health policy. Nurses provide the caring element in the healthcare system. Nurses uphold a long and distinguished tradition in health promotion, wellness, and public health advocacy. Nurses remind the public that healthcare is more than medically-focused disease treatment and surgery. For example, nurses have taken the leadership to pressure state legislatures to pass motorcycle helmet laws for the purpose of primary prevention of head injuries.

Nurses also can take a leadership role at the local, state, and federal levels of health policy activities. For example, nurses can use their expertise to develop white papers and policy analysis data for key decision makers. Nurses can vote, lobby, campaign, and protest as activism methods to influence healthcare policy. Nurses can be locally active in communities by being involved in boards and commissions and by communicating about health policy issues.

Nurses can become involved in leadership and management roles within the politics of organizations. For example, professional nursing organizations

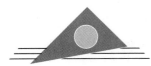 *Leadership & Management Behaviors*

LEADERSHIP BEHAVIORS	MANAGEMENT BEHAVIORS	OVERLAP AREAS
• envisions directions for health policy initiatives	• communicates about health policy needs	• communicates about health policies
• communicates about health policy issues	• gives testimony	
• acts to influence health policy and legislation	• writes letters to support a policy direction	
• enables followers to influence health policy	• bargains for scarce resources	
• lobbies influential decision makers	• implements laws and regulations affecting nursing practice	
• models supportive networking for information and influence		
• drafts legislation		
• encourages followers to be politically aware and active		

like the ANA develop position papers, debate health policy issues, and support candidates and positions. Nurses also may lobby or contribute money to lobbying efforts of political action committees (PACs). Nurses may choose to provide testimony to support a health policy effort.

At the individual level, nurses' leadership and management roles in client care management involve the use of influence at multiple levels. Nurses need to take the responsibility to keep informed about health policy and political issues. Awareness may be triggered and enhanced by sources such as professional organizations' position papers, reading professional journals, newspapers and other public media, or networking with colleagues in person or electronically. Nurses may contact their elected representatives for information or to express an opinion. Clearly, nurses need to be informed and aware of health policy issues. They need to be active in influence efforts. They need to communicate their positions to others. They need to support and lobby in conjunction with others as a group strategic action team. By taking these leadership actions, nurses can influence others to make changes needed to positively impact health care policy and politics.

CURRENT ISSUES AND TRENDS

The election of President Clinton saw the beginning of an era of intense focus on healthcare reform. Driven by concerns about cost, quality, and access,

President Clinton developed a healthcare reform proposal that centered around six key principles: security, simplicity, savings, choice, quality, and responsibility. These principles expanded on and departed from the prior health policy framework of access, quality, and cost (Donley, 1994).

The American Nurses Association (1991) formulated a position paper on healthcare reform called "Nursing's Agenda for Health Care Reform." It noted that nurses believe that the U.S. healthcare system needs to be restructured and decentralized to guarantee access to services, contain costs, and ensure quality of care. Nursing's plan was derived from consensus building processes within organized nursing. Nursing's plan shifts the healthcare system's emphasis from illness to wellness, envisions universal access, and presents a realistic approach to healthcare reform.

Financing and economics have dominated the present agenda of health policy. This has pressured nurses to understand economic and research knowledge in order to be credible in debates surrounding healthcare reform. Clearly, the control of healthcare costs is linked to economic recovery and deficit reductions at the federal level (Harrington & Estes, 1994).

Major research questions for health policy analysis and formulation in the 1990s include how to resolve issues related to access to healthcare, organization of health services, financing of health services, reimbursement of health services, costs of health services, quality of health services, special populations' needs, and ethical and legal issues (Longest, 1994).

Some key forces influencing the U.S. healthcare industry include the growing number of uninsured, demand for greater clinical and fiscal accountability, technology growth, changing demography of the population, changing professional labor supply, globalization of the economy, consolidation and mergers, and information management (Shortell & Reinhardt, 1992). Understanding these forces from the clients' perspective and the providers' perspective will help to focus health policy efforts in a way that translates concerns into effective political action.

Healthcare reform is an issue of today and the future. Organizational structures are changing in the healthcare delivery system in response to reform initiatives. Public policy debates continue over rationing, universal coverage, healthcare financing and regulation, and special populations' needs. Nurses have a contribution to make to the debates and a stake in the outcomes.

SUMMARY

* Nurses need to be visible and vocal in public policy and health policy debates.
* Policy is the formulation of value statements.
* Politics is the influencing of the allocation of scarce resources.

✤ Health policies are a set of public policies influencing health and illness.
✤ The public policy-making process is sequential and cyclical.
✤ Legislation is enacted following a multi-stage process.
✤ Politics is important in organizations and in governmental interactions.
✤ Health policies may be allocative or regulatory.
✤ Nurses have a leadership and management role in public and health policy.
✤ Financing, economics, and healthcare reform are current health policy issues.

Study Questions

1. What are nursing's major healthcare values?
2. Is caring a healthcare policy? Why or why not?
3. What kind of public policies govern your life? Govern nursing practice?
4. Which level of government is responsible for the health of the citizens?
5. Should illegal aliens be included in healthcare policy and benefits?
6. Why are nursing profession issues important enough to be on the public policy agenda? Which ones are?
7. Why is politics useful to nurses?
8. Why can nurses be influential in policy and politics? How does this happen?

Critical Thinking Exercise

Nurse Kelly Murrell has two years of experience in community health nursing, specializing in women's health care. She has become deeply involved in the many issues surrounding women's health care in community settings. She sees women disadvantaged by social circumstances and lack of financial resources. Nurse Murrell has read newspaper accounts of shifting funding priorities that are likely to dismantle state support for women's programs. This would directly affect her clients. Nurse Murrell has sought out her mentor, Nurse Linda Lopez, to discuss her concerns and also to explore whether to pursue an advanced degree as a family nurse practitioner. Nurse Murrell learns from Nurse Lopez that state legislators are considering bills to eliminate the funding streams and to restrict the practice of nurse practitioners and limit their prescriptive authority.

1. *What is (are) the problem(s)?*

2. *Why is (are) it (they) a problem(s)?*

3. *What should Nurse Murrell do?*

4. *What should Nurse Lopez do?*

5. *What public policy issues are involved?*

6. *What politics are involved?*

7. *What health policy issues are involved?*

8. *What actions can the two nurses take to affect public health policy?*

REFERENCES

American Nurses Association. (1991). *Nursing's agenda for health care reform: Executive summary.* Washington, D.C.: American Nurses Association.

Brown, L. (1991). Knowledge and power: Health services research as a political resource. In E. Ginsberg (Ed.), *Health services research: Key to health policy* (pp. 20-45). Cambridge, MA: Harvard University Press.

Diers, D. (1985). Policy and politics. In D. Mason & S. Talbott (Eds.), *Political action handbook for nurses* (pp. 53-59). Reading, MA: Addison-Wesley.

Donley, R. (1994). Health care reform: Implications for staff development. *Nursing Economic$, 12*(2), 71-74.

Fuchs, V. (1993). *The future of health policy.* Cambridge, MA: Harvard University Press.

Hanley, B. (1987). Political participation: How do nurses compare with other professional women? *Nursing Economic$, 5*(4), 179-185,188.

Harrington, C., & Estes. C. (1994). Introduction. In C. Harrington & C. Estes (Eds.), *Health policy and nursing: Crisis and reform* in the U.S. health care delivery system (pp. xi-xiv). Boston: Jones and Bartlett.

Lescavage, N. (1995). Nurses, make your presence felt: Taking off the rose-colored glasses. *Nursing Policy Forum, 1*(1), 18-21.

Longest, Jr., B. (1994). *Health policymaking in the United States.* Ann Arbor, MI: AUPHA Press/Health Administration Press.

Maraldo, P. (1985). Politics is people. In D. Mason & S. Talbott (Eds.), *Political action handbook for nurses* (pp. 81-87). Reading, MA: Addison-Wesley.

Mason, D., & Talbott, S. (1985). Introduction: A framework for political action. In D. Mason & S. Talbott (Eds.), *Political action handbook for nurses* (pp. 3-9). Reading, MA: Addison-Wesley.

Shortell, S., & Reinhardt, U. (1992). Creating and executing health policy in the 1990s. In S. Shortell & U. Reinhardt (Eds.), *Improving health policy and management: Nine critical research issues for the 1990s* (pp. 3-36). Ann Arbor, MI: Health Administration Press.

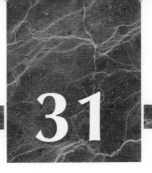

Career Development

Chapter Objectives

∾

define and describe a job

∾

define and describe a career

∾

relate adult developmental stages to careers

∾

distinguish among career anchors

∾

analyze careers and career planning in nursing

∾

analyze career styles and phases

∾

compare advanced practice nursing to nursing careers

∾

relate current issues to career development

∾

exercise critical thinking to conceptualize and analyze
possible solutions to a practical experience incident

*a*t some point, each nurse made the decision to enter the profession of nursing. This decision may have been made for a variety of reasons, including a desire to help people, a motivation toward healing, the role modeling by a significant person, or job security. For some nurses, nursing was an attractive occupation offering a variety of jobs. For other nurses, there was a strong motivation toward life-long work in a career. Each nurse responds to a unique composite of values, goals, interests, and aspirations on the path of work chosen over an adult life span.

The work of a professional extends over an anticipated lifetime of occupational service, encompassing activity, employment, and productivity. Career commitment is a nurse's attitude toward nursing as a profession or vocation and is the motivation to work in a chosen career role (Blau, 1985; Gardner, 1991; Hall, 1971). Commitment to a career is different from commitment to a job or to an organization. Commitment to a career is important in nursing because of its relationship to the development, satisfaction, and retention of staff nurses in organizations and to the overall profession (Barr & Desnoyer, 1988; Gardner, 1991; 1992).

DEFINITIONS

or a professional, there is a difference between a job and a career (Brink, 1988). A *job* is defined as an offered position (see Chart 31.1). A job is a contract with an employer for day-to-day employment. It is the work that is performed for pay. A career, on the other hand, is more than a succession of jobs. A *career* is defined as a chosen path or a contract made with the self for a satisfying pattern of professional contributions. A career encompasses a practical, self-directed, life-long plan for personal and professional growth. A career implies investment and involvement in a chosen field that extends beyond the concept of earning pay for an hour of work. *Career commitment* is defined as an individual's attitude toward a profession and the motivation to work in a chosen career role (Gardner, 1991).

RESEARCH NOTE

Source: Gardner, D. (1992). Career commitment in nursing. *Journal of Professional Nursing,* 8(3), 155-160.

Purpose

Careers in nursing have different patterns and styles. The purpose of this research was to measure career commitment in nurses and investigate the relationship of career commitment to turnover and work performance. A longitudinal descriptive survey using repeated measures was employed to study the attitudes and behaviors of 320 newly employed RNs from one tertiary care hospital. The Gardner Career Commitment Scale, Schwirian Six Dimension Scale of Nursing Performance, and turnover from hospital records were the instruments used to collect data.

Discussion

Measures were administered at 6 months and 12 months of employment. Career commitment scores were initially moderately high, but they dropped significantly over the first year of employment. Thus career commitment did not remain stable, perhaps due to job-specific frustrations. Career commitment was significantly and negatively correlated with turnover (higher career commit-

---

CHART 31.1
∾ DEFINITIONS

Job
an offered position.

Career
a chosen path or a contract made with the self for a satisfying pattern of professional contributions.

Career Commitment
an individual's attitude toward a profession and the motivation to work in a chosen career role.

Some data from Gardner (1991).

ment associated with lower turnover) and positively correlated with performance (higher career commitment associated with higher performance).

Application to Practice

If career commitment is not stable over the first year of employment, perhaps it is susceptible to the influence of organizational factors. Career commitment appears to interact with other professional variables such as performance and turnover. Organizations and nurses, through the policies and programs they implement, can use incentives and organizational structural components to encourage nurse career development and commitment. For example, promoting professionalism and autonomy may affect nurses' interpretation of work behaviors toward positive attitudes.

BACKGROUND

During their transition into adulthood, individuals face the task of identifying and pursuing a course of work and employment. An individual may take a job or embark on a career path. In a profession like nursing, a nurse may choose a haphazard succession of jobs that turn into a career or set out deliberately to build a career trajectory. A career may just happen, or it may be planned and structured. As a practical reality, planning a career is subject to uncertainty. This occurs because the process of implementing life goals is subject to interruptions. For each individual there is a reciprocal intertwining of work, self, and family roles. There appear to be different stages to a career and different styles used to balance the interactive needs of work, self, and family (Gardner, 1991). Therefore, both jobs and careers are best understood within the context of adult life stages.

Developmental theories highlight the reality of continual change because numerous changes take place during the lifetime of an individual. This dynamic process is referred to as growth and development and has been described in terms of ages and stages. For example, Piaget (1969) developed a comprehensive theory of childhood cognitive development that tracked the changes in cognitive development over time. Erikson (1963) developed a theory of personality development that covered the entire life span. His adult stages are early adulthood, young and middle adulthood, and later adulthood. The adult stages can be further broken down into eight phases (Henderson & McGettigan, 1994):

1. Transition to adulthood (18 to 22 years)
2. Young adulthood (23 to 30 years)
3. Adulthood (31 to 37 years)
4. Transition to mid-adulthood (38 to 45 years)
5. Mid-adulthood (46 to 53 years)
6. Transition to later adulthood (54 to 61 years)

7. Later adulthood (62 to 69 years)
8. Senior adulthood (70+ years)

Typical activities correspond to adult developmental stages and range from exploring identity (18 to 22), to balancing one's life (46 to 53), to doing what one is able and remembering (70+).

Clearly, as adults progress through predictable development stages, their needs, values, and inclinations will vary over time and in degree or strength. Thus for nurses, growth and development changes impact on the balance among work, self, and family needs and roles. This inevitably impacts on the work and career needs and decisions made by individuals. It can be predicted that needs related to a career will vary throughout the course of an adult's life. Changing career needs that parallel changing adult developmental stages appear to be normal and natural dynamics. However, many view careers as static, not dynamic.

Nurses can enhance their career development efforts through periodic self-analysis of their needs and goals (see Fig. 31.1). Centering within a career trajectory is enhanced by self-awareness and self-assessment activities. Self-assessment can be applied to career decision points, such as decisions about accepting a job, moving to a new job location, returning to school, sitting for certification in a specialization, or moving from full-time to part-time work. Nurses can explore and analyze the stage they are currently in and then pro-

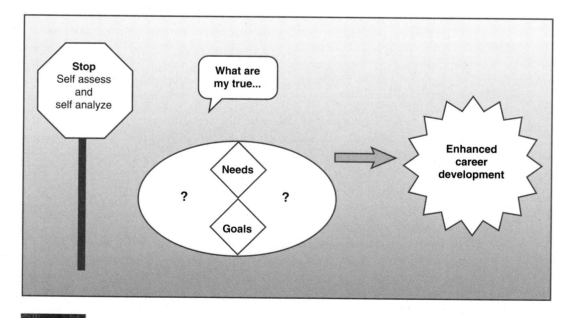

Figure 31.1
Centering within a career trajectory.

ject where they want to advance toward. One way to do this is to examine the concept of career anchors as it applies to an individual who has unique needs and talents and is in a specific developmental stage.

Career Anchors

Schein (1971, 1975, 1978) identified that career anchors can be used to explain individual values and motives as they apply to career decisions. Career anchors are a combination of personal needs, values, and talents that guide and constrain individual career decisions. People tend to have one primary anchor or a primary cluster of anchors. Anchors are a constellation or locus of features that the individual tends to prefer or is least likely to forego. Anchors are characteristics that the individual is likely to identify with or gravitate toward due to the individual's natural inclinations, values, and abilities. The eight career anchors are (Friss, 1989):

1. Service: concerned with helping others
2. Managerial competence: focused on interpersonal relationships and the ability to analyze problems
3. Autonomy: concerned with own sense of freedom
4. Technical-functional competence: motivated by the work itself; seeks job challenge and personal recognition
5. Security: concerned with long-term stability and benefits
6. Identity: guided by status and prestige
7. Variety: seeks many challenges; motivated by changing assignments
8. Creativity: needs to develop something of one's own

What this means is that nurses can analyze the career anchors and identify the one or ones that are most relevant to themselves. Since things change, career anchors may change over time in strength of need. Thus the nurse may benefit from periodic reanalysis. Theoretically, certain occupational groups subcluster around specific types of anchors. Sovie's (1982) review of nursing research identified the following three primary anchors as generally representative of nursing:

1. Professional recognition (identity)
2. Career mobility (security)
3. Advancement opportunities (technical/functional)

This research indicated that nurses are primarily interested in, concerned about, and therefore motivated by identity, security, and self-actualization needs.

Nursing as a Career

Nursing as a career offers many interesting possibilities for nurses. Nursing provides significantly more interesting part-time opportunities than most other occupations. For any individual, a career is a choice: a career can be structured or it may just happen without preplanning and is recognized in hindsight.

Table 31.1

Influences on Career Planning

SELF	REAL WORLD	WORKPLACE CHANGE	GOALS
Personal goals	Available options	Trends and issues in healthcare	Personal goals
Strengths and needs	Available opportunities	Trends and issues in nursing	Family goals
Anchors			Career goals
Desires for contribution to a practice area			

Opportunities do arise in nursing. Therefore, contemplation and planning steers an individual toward a pattern that is woven from among work, self, and family roles into a coherent whole with individual meaning. Planning for a career may be tough to do, but it is inevitable for helping the individual to capitalize on opportunities. For example, nurses can reflect on what they want to be doing at different points in their lives or where they want to be in 2, 5, or 10 years.

Certain information is helpful to know in planning a career (see Table 31.1). First, building self-awareness as a strategy for career growth suggests the discovery of such information about an individual as personal goals, strengths, needs, anchors, and desires for contribution to an area of practice. Second, the options and opportunities realistically available will color a career. They need to be evaluated. Third, trends and issues in healthcare and nursing might contribute to a career trajectory. For example, research has demonstrated that nurse practitioners are cost-effective, and legislation has been enacted to allow third party reimbursement for specialist nursing services. As opportunities within a reconfigured healthcare system open up for nurse practitioners, this becomes an attractive career path to many nurses. Changes occurring due to healthcare reform provide opportunities for nurses in new and creative career directions. Finally, nurses face issues of the relative timing of personal and family goals with career goals. Goals may mesh or create tension.

The First Job

The first professional job is thought to have an influence on personal satisfaction with nursing as a career. It also may influence future advancement.

The average work span for an RN is over 30 years. A nurse's career will involve an ongoing evaluation of potential employment opportunities. A nursing career is a process of setting career goals and continuous planning. If the first job shapes attitudes and has the potential to influence movement into a burnout cycle, as opposed to engendering excitement for a career in nursing, then a nurse needs to try to select the first job so that the nurse in effect is "planted where she or he will grow." For example, the nurse might assess the first job in terms of what it will offer in relation to specific needs and career goals and aspirations. As much as a nurse has control, the nurse should seek to structure the first job to derive opportunities to be mentored or precepted and to work in a positive milieu. This means that the nurse needs to look for an environment that will help him or her to succeed. A nurturing work environment may be as important as salary and benefits for coping and deriving satisfaction over longer lengths of time.

Bridging the gap from a nursing student to a new graduate includes a passage from a period of intensive investment in the focused goal of education to a transition phase into a whole other lifestyle. There is a potential crisis in the reforming of the identity from a student to a professional person. Career development perspectives take this into account by suggesting proactive career planning activities begin in the career preparation phase. Leadership and management principles suggest that the nurse manager envision an environment in which the "young" (i.e., new graduates) are nurtured through this transition. Units in a hospital and work groups in all settings can build programs to attract and retain new members by keeping in mind the importance of nurturing and mentoring the new and younger members of the profession.

Career Planning

Career planning builds on entry-level skills. Vogel (1990) said that career development is a lifelong process that links a nurse's unique personality, lifestyle, work style, goals, and aspirations to planned career growth. Vogel (1990) identified six stages of career development:

1. *Self-analysis:* This includes values clarification and personal goal setting. What is important to you?
2. *Career analysis:* This includes identifying career anchors, selecting valued skills, choosing career priorities, and setting career goals. What skills do you possess, and what do you want to achieve?
3. *Integration:* This is a reassessment point. As you review your career goals and progress, do you need to revise them?
4. *Planning:* This is a stage of reality testing, resource evaluation, and strategy selection. Are you on track to match your aspirations to accomplishments?
5. *Implementing:* This is a phase of putting the career plan to work. Are you committed to your goals? Are you actively pursuing them?
6. *Evaluation:* This is the assessment of progress toward specific goals and the level of general satisfaction with the career. Am I satisfied with my occupational role? Do I have a sense of achievement and productivity? Are my career priorities met? If not, what do I need to do to change this?

The new nurse needs to begin with self-analysis. McBride (1985) noted that those who are professionally alive realize that they constantly need to keep their knowledge current and learn new skills to do their jobs well. There are some specific steps that can be followed in making a career plan or in choosing a career goal (Henderson & McGettigan, 1994):

- Test goals.
- Weigh outcomes.
- Specify actions.
- Write a plan.
- Implement the plan.
- Evaluate progress.

Because of the phenomena of change and movement through developmental stages, nurses need to be aware of the value of periodic reevaluation of their nursing career and its ongoing development. For example, one useful exercise is to write down some career goals, then set them aside. At the end of a year, the goals can be evaluated for degree of accomplishment. This can become a personal annual review.

Transition or decision points occur periodically in any career trajectory. Societal influences, such as the knowledge explosion, changing demographics and economics, consumer demands, cost containment, and changes in the healthcare system may impact on nurses' career planning by slowing, modifying, or accelerating a career trajectory. External social forces and the needs of society shape the direction of nursing (Lynaugh & Fagin, 1988; Reverby, 1987). Therefore, nurses should:

- scan the environment
- set goals for themselves
- do career planning
- anticipate the future and be aware of trends

The best sources to keep informed include membership in professional organizations such as the American Nurses Association, use of networking, and reading professional journals. Some organizations encourage environment scanning and networking through attendance at professional meetings and participation in outside professional activities.

Career Styles

As a nurse moves on through time while working in nursing, a style will emerge in the nurse's career path. "A career is not necessarily a tidy progression of jobs with increasing responsibility that leads to a predetermined end" (Friss, 1989, p. 2). Careers often are not static. Friss (1989) identified five career styles found frequently in nursing:

1. Steady state: long work history; full-time lifetime commitment
2. Linear: hierarchical orientation; steady climb to jobs of increasing responsibility
3. Entrepreneurial: choose to go into business for themselves
4. Transient: hold a series of unrelated jobs of relatively short duration
5. Spiral: five to seven year period of employment that engages their talent, followed by other relatively long periods of work that provide new career challenges

These career styles are reflections of patterns that emerge in the careers of nurses. Nurses are a diverse group of workers. Organizations may benefit from constructing a vibrant mix of nurses with compatible career styles. Job classifications, policies, and promotional opportunities may need to be structured to capitalize on the creativity inherent in a diverse workforce. Leadership and management styles adopted by nurses can incorporate a recognition of nurses with diverse career orientations and styles.

Another way of looking at career styles is to explore the phases of nursing careers. The phases perspective suggests sequential growth in knowledge, experience, and leadership ability over time in a career. For example, McBride (1985) identified four career phases: preparation, contribution, administration, and advice. McBride's conceptualization explored an individual's progress across the continuum of a career span, from early entry to advanced maturity. Rather than tying career phases to developmental stages, McBride's four phases look at careers in a broad perspective. For example, some nurses enter the preparation phase of a nursing career after having obtained a degree or experience in another field or after devoting time to raising a family. For these nurses, linking a career phase to an adult developmental stage is less relevant or may not fit and make sense. Disconnecting ages and developmental stages from career phases may provide greater insight into second degree students or "nontraditional" nursing students and their subsequent careers. McBride's work is similar in tone to Benner's (1982) levels of proficiency that a staff nurse progresses through with increasing experience.

Benner's (1982) classic work on increments in skilled performance in nursing used the Dreyfus Model of Skill Acquisition to delineate five levels of proficiency:
1. Novice
2. Advanced beginner
3. Competent
4. Proficient
5. Expert

Benner noted that increments in skilled nursing performance are based on education and experience. Experience in a clinical area develops over time; therefore a nurse is not a nurse is not a nurse. What this means is that nurses and others need to recognize, value, and incorporate strategies to nurture nurses who are at different career stages or involved in different career phases. The result is a better utilization of the skills and abilities of nurses and greater nurse job satisfaction.

Some views of nurses within career paths take the organization's perspective rather than the perspective of the nurse within the profession of nursing. These frameworks examine nurses as they enter a new job in nursing, usually as a new graduate nurse in the first job. For example, one theory-based study (Seyboldt, 1983) outlined five distinct tenure categories:

1. *Entry:* under six months, "raw recruits"
2. *Early:* six months to one year, "young turks"
3. *Middle:* one to three years, "skeptics about supervisory expectations"
4. *Advanced:* three to six years, "burn-out candidates"
5. *Later:* over six years, "career-satisfied or old-guard"

The tenure-focused perspective is strongly pointed toward one related element of career commitment: a nurse's job satisfaction. Research has shown that job satisfaction, organizational commitment, and professionalism decrease over the first year of work (McCloskey & McCain, 1987). Further, career commitment does have a relationship to turnover and work performance and does decrease over the first year of work as well (Gardner, 1992). Tenure categories can be used to assess, track, and analyze nurses' career and job attitudes over time.

The complex, interactive, and dynamic factors affecting a nurse's professional development have been synthesized into a model that broadly categorizes career stages and phases into early, middle, and late. Bruhn and Cordova (1982) summarized the factors operating at different stages of career development into a model that displays factors affecting change and stability over the course of a professional career. This model identifies relevant factors and indicates possible outcomes. For example, in the early career stage, a nurse is influenced by factors such as influential role models and the motivation for nursing goals. The predominant theme is the forming of an identity as a nurse. One factor affecting situational adjustment is the work environment. Another factor affecting commitment or stability is employer support. If situational adjustment is positive and commitment is positive, then professional satisfaction is the outcome.

Mid-career factors include promotions, changing jobs, achieving balance in work and family, and productivity and creativity. The predominant theme in mid-career is contribution to nursing as a profession. One factor affecting situational adjustment is time demands. One factor affecting commitment or stability is monetary rewards. If the situational adjustment is negative but the commitment level is positive, burnout occurs (Bruhn & Cordova, 1982).

In late career, important factors include opportunities to change the profession and opportunities for leadership. Professional and personal maturity are predominant themes. Changes in institutional goals or managerial style affect situational adjustment. Status and degree of authority and responsibility affect commitment. If the situational adjustment is positive but commitment is negative, role conflict and ambiguity are possible professional outcomes (Bruhn & Cordova, 1982).

There appear to be distinct and different stages and phases to a nurse's career. It appears that a nurse's priorities may vary depending on the career stage and situational and commitment factors. Intervention strategies similarly may need to be adjusted to meet different nurses' needs at different stages.

LEADERSHIP AND MANAGEMENT IMPLICATIONS

Nurses and nurse managers can understand and use career concepts for selection, recruitment, and retention of RNs. Despite the continued practice of floating nurses without cross-training in times of low census, nurses are not interchangeable parts. Much of the work nurses do is complex, requiring a high level of skill and practice to acquire proficiency. Nurses are diverse and multi-tiered in relation to:

- level of education.
- level of experience.
- level of skill acquisition.
- time in the profession.

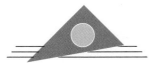 *Leadership & Management Behaviors*

LEADERSHIP BEHAVIORS

- influences followers to develop a professional career
- envisions a mentoring environment
- enables followers to pursue career opportunities
- communicates career values
- mentors new nurses
- is a role model of professionalism in nursing
- creates career growth opportunities
- challenges the system to promote opportunities for nurses

MANAGEMENT BEHAVIORS

- influences employees to develop skills and abilities
- manages employees with diverse career patterns
- plans for a career-diverse skill mix of staff
- organizes the work environment to facilitate career and professional development

OVERLAP AREAS

- influences others in career development

Increments in skill level of nursing performance develop over time. Thus being a novice, for example, is a normal and natural stage. Therefore, nurse leaders and managers need to envision a compatible mix of nurses and plan for the best integration and balance of skills and abilities.

If nurses are not all the same, who nurtures the novices? Are experts identified, rewarded, and praised? How many expert nurses are available in any work environment? Friss (1989) suggested that work groups benefit from having employees with differing career orientations. Does the incentive structure need to be modified to attract and retain a particular career type? Leaders enable followers to grow and attain high levels of productivity. Leaders can influence others to mentor and nurture each other. For example, Swanson (1994) suggested that leaders and managers might set up a program within the workplace to invite nurses to mutually develop plans to mentor and assist each other in professional development activities. Such plans could be formalized or informally mutually negotiated.

Career commitment is one aspect of nurse recruitment and retention. Staff development and inservice educators can use career commitment concepts to promote professional commitment and loyalty, and to reinforce nurses' career plans and goals (Gardner, 1991; 1992; Young, 1984).

Interest in the concept of reality shock, or the transition from school to work, stems from an in-depth study of the entry and early phases of a career. During these phases it is believed that group values and norms most influence a new member's behavior. In the transition time, the skills and values acquired in school or in other organizations are adjusted to the demands of the job and values and norms of the whole group. The concept developed and tested by Kramer (1974) is called "reality shock." Reality shock relates to the difficult transition of roles from student to RN employee. Roles as prescribed by educational settings and those prescribed by bureaucratic institutions employing nurses often result in conflict between the ideal and reality. Kramer's (1974) phases of reality shock are:

- honeymoon: a phase of initial good feeling while still new.
- shock: a clash of reality with ideal values.
- recovery: a period of beginning to learn to cope with the conflict in values.
- resolution of the conflict: a time of problem solution decisions and reintegration.

As nursing students transform their roles from student to staff nurse, a predictable process occurs in four phases. The honeymoon phase is a time of good feelings toward the job, exhilaration at a regular paycheck, and the mastery of skills and routines. Social integration into the work group and testing by others occurs. The second phase, shock, begins when the new graduate attempts to achieve a goal but the path is blocked by personal inadequacies or systems deterrents. Affective relations of moral outrage, rejection, fatigue, and perceptual distortion set in. Such strong reactions are energy-depleting. The third phase of recovery eventually occurs. In this phase, perspectives are put in balance and a sense of humor returns. Resolution happens when the nurse chooses a strategy to resolve the conflict between work and school values. The nurse may choose to adopt work values, adopt school values, limit commitment, burn out, hop jobs, completely withdraw by quitting, or become bicultural by working with the best of both worlds (Schmalenberg & Kramer, 1979).

New nurses can be supported during the emotional crisis stage of reality shock. Support groups of new nurses express the following areas of concern: competency, real-world reality, role expectations, floating, responsibility, boredom, feedback, friction, client care, physical labor, competing interests, change, death, fairness, the organizational system, and the nurse's self-concept. New graduates can be assisted in coping with reality shock through support groups and seminars. Organizational systems can be improved through structural and functional changes targeted at nurses' identified sources of stress (Schmalenberg & Kramer, 1979).

As a result of Kramer's work in the 1970s, internship and preceptorship programs have been developed to help new graduates adjust within the job environment. However, theories and research into career stages and phases indicate that coping and adjustment in a career may need to be nurtured throughout multiple stages or phases and not be confined to new graduates.

Strategies for career development and role transitions emphasize balancing ideal practice principles with real constraints of time and resources. For example, since the first six months of a new graduate's career are often quite intense, role models and preceptors can be used to help balance the tension. Nurses also can develop useful contacts, present their best side, and develop a portfolio of related documents that profile career development in a self-portrait. Some other strategies to cope with stress, counter "reality shock," and develop a career include building skills in networking, negotiation, marketing, and healthy self-interest.

Marketing oneself is a major career development strategy. An individual can consult texts and experts for advice about compiling a portfolio or dossier, using personnel placement or "headhunter" firms, interviewing skills, and resume or vitae preparation. For example, the preparation of a cover letter is an important self-marketing element for which advice might be sought. Mentors to help with such activities can be approached by building a network of colleagues and using networking skills to widen the pool of resources for personal career development.

Leadership and management influence can be brought to bear on the intersection between individuals' career needs and goals and the organization's responsibilities for ensuring that competent employees are delivering services.

For example, techniques of practice change as new knowledge develops. Professional preparation, whether formal education, continuing education workshops, or self-directed learning, will need to be continuous in order to stay current in practice. "Current" means, at minimum, practicing to the legal standard of a reasonable, prudent nurse. The future will demand another standard: that nursing interventions be based on research knowledge. Continuing education is one strategy for career development and is a major vehicle for professional enhancement of competence.

In approximately 12 states, continuing education is mandatory for relicensure. It is used as a mechanism for quality control and to address competency issues. Learning has to be life-long and continuous to keep current because society demands it, new techniques and the knowledge base change, there is a legal mandate to practice to current standards, and personal and professional development are enhanced. Employers are responsible for orientation and in-service at minimum. Organizations that value high performing professions will invest in their professional development. Professional employees are responsible for practicing to current standards and for personal and professional development. Both employers and employees can work together in ways that meet the employee's growth needs and the employer's competence responsibilities. Both nursing service and nursing education need to work with each other to enhance nursing career development by providing opportunities for career planning and progression. Efforts can be placed into portraying nursing more realistically and as more than a haphazard progression of jobs. Nursing is challenging, interesting, and demanding. Nurses can be helped to evaluate themselves and their development within a nursing career (Swanson, 1994).

CURRENT ISSUES AND TRENDS

Advanced Practice

In times of turbulent change, nurses may be confused about which career development options to chose to best advance themselves and their careers. For example, many advanced practitioners, especially clinical nurse specialists, have been targeted for reengineering and redesign because they are not direct caregivers and therefore are not considered to be cost effective (Ponte, Higgins, James, Fay, & Madden, 1993). On the other hand, there is some evidence that advanced practice nurses, including nurse practitioners (NPs) and clinical nurse specialists (CNSs), have not been deployed by organizations in a way to capitalize on their full skills and abilities. Legal scope of practice, delegation, and reimbursement policies may result in underutilization of NPs and CNSs (Nichols, 1992). The role of an advanced practice nurse is based on expert clinical knowledge and skill, yet the actual role varies by the context of the specific practice setting. Advanced practice nurses are positioned to play leading roles in managed care environments and within multidisciplinary cross-functional teams. Yet there is still pressure to justify the advanced practice nurse role. One way to approach this dilemma is to approach advanced practice as a portfolio of resources to be managed to the organization's advantage (Madden & Ponte, 1994).

The evolution of nursing in the U.S. has resulted in multiple levels of nursing practice. Certification, graduate education, and licensure for advanced practice are current issues facing nursing.

The American Nurses' Association's (ANA) (1980) *Nursing: A Social Policy Statement* delineates between generalist and specialist preparation. Advanced practice preparation occurs at the master's level. Expanding roles require education for independent or collaborative practice. Sophisticated technical and decision making aspects of care necessitate special education, certification, and advanced nursing degrees. Making decisions regarding educational advancement is a part of the career management process (Henderson & McGettigan, 1994).

Questions continue to arise about why nurses need an academic education at all. Is a baccalaureate in nursing worth it? Lowry (1992) used a net present value methodology for calculating educational costs and benefits. She found that an investment in a baccalaureate degree in nursing does yield additional monetary rewards beyond an investment in a diploma or associate degree. Education provides nurses with additional knowledge and skill as well as providing an additional source of legitimacy for expertise.

Career development may include obtaining additional education for advanced practice. Advanced nursing practice roles include nurse practitioners, nurse anesthetists, nurse midwives, and clinical nurse specialists. The skills and abilities identified as essential for safe and competent advanced nursing practice are beyond what is attained in a basic nursing education program. They are based on an academic degree at the graduate level with a major in nursing. The demand for nurses practicing in advanced roles with greater autonomy is increasing. Professional nursing organizations recognize advanced nursing practice through voluntary certification. Regulation of practice occurs on a continuum of least restrictive to most restrictive as follows: designation/recognition, registration, certification as title protection, and licensure. The National Council of State Boards of Nursing (NCSBN) has proposed the licensure of advanced nursing practice through the issuance of a second license for advanced practice (NCSBN, 1992). Although controversial, this proposal seeks to meet federal regulations requiring statutory recognition of advanced nursing for third party reimbursement.

Nursing certification is the recognition of expertise in a specialized area of practice. Certification is a credential for professionals to assure the public of their qualifications to provide specialized services to consumers. There are three ways this has been done:

1. By the professional organization. The ANA has been certifying nurses since 1973.
2. By individual states. This is a legal endorsement by a State Board of Nursing. About 40 states have advanced registered nurse practice acts.
3. By individual institutions. This is a statement issued by an agency to certify the ability for specialty practice.

In some states, eligibility for third party reimbursement depends on certification. In the ANA's *Nursing: A Social Policy Statement* (1980), the two criteria for a specialist are a master's degree and certification by the professional organization. The role of the states is controversial. The issues surrounding certification relate to control of practice by professionals and the scope of nursing practice (Bulechek & Maas, 1994). Certification may take the form of a gatekeeping function.

Graduate education is one avenue for career development. There are a large number of accredited master's programs in nursing. The National League for Nursing's (NLN) resource materials provide detailed information on graduate programs in nursing. Decisions regarding when and where to pursue graduate education are important career choices. There are both clinical and role preparation decisions for specialization. As part of an education-focused career decision, the admission requirements such as grade point average and entrance exams (usually graduate record exams [GREs]) need to be explored. Admission may take advanced planning, since submission deadlines may be nine months to one year in advance. Financial support may be available and come in different forms than what was available at the undergraduate level. Other areas to consider in a choice of graduate programs are the areas of study available, reputation of the school, philosophy of the graduate program, and opportunities for involvement in research. Ideally, the student will be able to match his or her career interests with the program's strengths.

SUMMARY

- Each nurse makes a decision, based on values, needs, and preferences, to become a nurse.
- Nurses' work extends over an anticipated lifetime of occupational activity.
- A job is day-to-day employment.
- A career is a chosen professional path.
- Career commitment is an attitude and motivation in a chosen role.
- Careers may intersect with adult developmental stages.
- Nurses balance work, self, and family roles.
- Career needs may vary over time.
- Career anchors explain individual career values and motives.
- Self-awareness is a career growth strategy.

- Nurturing and mentoring are needed for new graduates and all nurses in the work environment.
- Career development builds on entry skills and uses periodic evaluation.
- There are various career styles.
- Organizations analyze tenure categories for their relationship to turnover.
- Leadership and management strategies can be used to integrate individual career goals with organizational responsibilities.
- Certification, graduate education, and continuing education are strategies for career development.

Study Questions

1. Why should nurses plan a career? Why not just follow the available jobs?
2. Why are you motivated for a job or a career in nursing?
3. What developmental stage are you in? How does that affect your career planning?
4. How much should your employer contribute to your career development?
5. Is career planning encouraged in your employment setting? Why/why not?
6. Why do nurses pursue nurse practitioner certification or licensure?

Critical Thinking Exercise

It has been a monumentally bad day. Nurse Gloria Davis feels exhausted, discouraged, and frustrated. The recent resignation of two other nurses has shifted the already heavy workload toward impossible levels. Today several clients were in negative moods and barraged Nurse Davis with complaints about their needs not being met in a timely manner. Although Nurse Davis has three years of experience and really likes her job, the inability to provide the quality of care Nurse Davis believes is needed by the clients leaves her frustrated and angry. On the way home, Nurse Davis begins to mull over this situation, her feelings about it, and her options.

1. What is the problem?

2. Why is it a problem?

3. What should Nurse Davis do about the problem?

4. Is Nurse Davis more concerned about her job or her career?

5. Should Nurse Davis seek different options for her job, career, or both?

6. What career stages and phases apply to Nurse Davis?

7. What could Nurse Davis do to develop her career?

REFERENCES

American Nurses' Association. (1980). *Nursing: A social policy statement*. Kansas City, MO: American Nurses' Association.

Barr, N., & Desnoyer, J. (1988). Career development for the professional nurse: A working model. *The Journal of Continuing Education in Nursing, 19*(2), 68-72.

Benner, P. (1982). From novice to expert. *American Journal of Nursing, 82*(3), 402-407.

Blau, G. (1985). The measurement and prediction of career commitment. *Journal of Occupational Psychology, 58*, 277-288.

Brink, P. (1988). The difference between a job and a career. *Western Journal of Nursing Research, 10*(1), 5-6.

Bruhn, J. G., & Cordova, F. D. (1982). Coping with change: Professionally and personally. In: J. Lancaster & W. Lancaster (Eds.), *The nurse as a change agent: Concepts for advanced nursing practice* (pp. 429-441). St. Louis: Mosby.

Bulechek, G., & Maas, M. (1994). Nursing certification: A matter for the professional organization. In J. McCloskey and H. Grace (Eds.), *Current issues in nursing* (4th ed.) (pp. 327-335). St. Louis: Mosby.

Erikson, E. (1963). *Childhood and society* (2nd ed.). New York: W. W. Norton.

Friss, L. (1989). *Strategic management of nurses: A policy-oriented approach*. Owings Mills, MD: National Health Publishing.

Gardner, D. (1991). Assessing career commitment: The role of staff development. *Journal of Nursing Staff Development, 7*(6), 263-267.

Gardner, D. (1992). Career commitment in nursing. *Journal of Professional Nursing, 8*(3), 155-160.

Hall, D. (1971). A theoretical model of career subidentity development in organizational settings. *Organizational Behavior and Human Performance, 6*, 50-76.

Henderson, F.C., & McGettigan, B.O. (1994). *Managing your career in nursing* (2nd ed.). New York: National League for Nursing Press.

Kramer, M. (1974). *Reality shock: Why nurses leave nursing*. St. Louis: Mosby.

Lowry, L.W. (1992). Is a baccalaureate in nursing worth it? *Nursing Economics, 10*(1), 46-52.

Lynaugh, J.E., & Fagin, C.M. (1988). Nursing comes of age. *Image, 20*(4), 184-190.

Madden, M., & Ponte, P. (1994). Advanced practice roles in the managed care environment. *Journal of Nursing Administration, 24*(1), 56-62.

McBride, A.B. (1985). Orchestrating a career. *Nursing Outlook, 33*(5), 244-247.

McCloskey, J., & McCain, B. (1987). Satisfaction, commitment and professionalism of newly employed nurses. *Image, 19*(1), 20-24.

NCSBN (National Council of State Boards of Nursing). (1992). *Position paper on the licensure of advanced nursing practice*. Chicago: National Council of State Boards of Nursing.

Nichols, L. (1992). Estimating costs of underusing advanced practice nurses. *Nursing Economic$, 10*(5), 343-351.

Piaget, J. (1969). *The theory of stages in cognitive development*. New York: McGraw-Hill.

Ponte, P., Higgins, J., James, J., Fay, M., & Madden, M. (1993). Development needs of advance practice nurses in a managed care environment. *Journal of Nursing Administration, 23*(11), 13-19.

Reverby, S. (1987). *Ordered to care: The dilemma of American nursing, 1850-1945*. Cambridge: Cambridge University Press.

Schein, E. (1971). The individual, the organization and the career: A conceptual scheme. *Journal of Applied Behavioral Science, 7*, 401-426.

Schein, E. (1975). How career anchors hold executives to their career paths. *Personnel, 52*(3), 11-24.

Schein, E. (1978). *Career dynamics: Matching individuals and organizational needs*. Reading, MA: Addison-Wesley.

Schmalenberg, C., & Kramer, M. (1979). *Coping with reality shock: The voices of experience*. Wakefield, MA: Nursing Resources.

Seyboldt, J. (1983). Dealing with premature employee turnover. *California Management Review, 25*(3), 107-117.

Sovie, M. (1982). Fostering professional careers in hospitals: The role of staff development. Part 1. *Journal of Nursing Administration, 12*(12),5-10.

Swanson, E. (1994). Career development: Its status in nursing. In J. McCloskey and H. Grace (Eds.), *Current issues in nursing* (4th ed.) (pp. 549-558). St. Louis: Mosby.

Vogel, G. (1990). Career development: An integrated process. *Holistic Nursing Practice, 4*(4), 46-53.

Young, K. (1984). Professional commitment of women in nursing. *Western Journal of Nursing Research, 6*(1), 11-26.

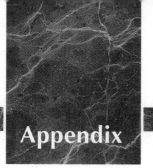

Appendix

Answers to Study Questions

Chapter 1: Overview of Nursing Administration

1. Does nursing administration differ from nursing practice? If so, how?

Nursing administration does differ from nursing practice. Nursing practice refers to the science and skills used to deliver patient care. Nursing administration is the use of nursing practice knowledge and leadership and management theories to organize care delivery, coordinate and manage client care, and create a positive work climate.

2. Are all nurses managers or is management more properly confined to levels above staff nurses?

Most nurses perform management tasks, but not every nurse is a nurse manager. Nurses in practice coordinate and manage direct care for a defined number of patients. The nurse manager's focus is on the administration of nursing service provided by a group of nurses, 24 hours a day. Orem (1989) defined nurse managers as "those who manage nursing services for organizations."

3. Are all nurses care coordinators? Is this the same as being a manager?

The nurse care provider focuses on the coordination of nursing care to individuals or groups. Activities of the nurse care provider include direct patient care, referrals, family support, and patient teaching. The nurse manager coordinates the nursing care providers and other health care workers to deliver cost-effective quality patient care. The nurse manager analyzes systems to increase productivity and decrease costs in care delivery.

4. Should a nurse follow a theory of administration as well as a theory of nursing?

There is no one accepted theory of nursing administration. The three primary sources of nursing administration knowledge are from nursing theory, management theory, and leadership theory. Theories that have been used with nursing administration include systems theory, bureaucratic theory, economic theory, management theory, organizational behavior theory, conflict theory, structural systems theory, and strategic choice theories. Administrative theories have also been used and include motivation, role, decision making, leadership, communication, and conflict.

CHAPTER 2: THE HEALTHCARE SYSTEM

1. What are the recent and projected developments in healthcare delivery? Are they changing?

The changes in healthcare center on cost containment and accessibility to healthcare for all citizens. The federal government, which pays for 42% of all healthcare expenditures, is demanding more accountability from healthcare professionals for quality outcomes within specified time frames in order to limit costs. Cost-based reimbursement and defined physician fees are trends in healthcare.

2. What developments will challenge nurse leaders and managers the most?

Nurse leaders and managers will be challenged to create new roles that meet the rapidly changing demands of a new healthcare delivery system. The shift of nursing care from the acute care hospital into the community will create dramatic changes for the professional nurse. Expanded nursing roles will require self-directed professionals to learn new skills in leadership, epidemiology, and clinical care. Reshaping nursing education curriculums, nursing care responsibilities, and reward structures will present new challenges for nurse leaders.

3. Where should nurses focus their vision and energy for the improvement of health services?

Nurses can improve health services by focusing on the care of special populations such as the elderly or those at highest risk in their community. Nurses are also in a pivotal position to control costs through case management, client advocacy, and expanded nursing roles.

4. Does the emphasis on cost containment overshadow nursing's role as a caring client advocate?

Cost containment is only one of the nurse's roles in client advocacy. Attention to costs is necessary when approximately 34 million Americans are uninsured and the cost of healthcare continues to rise. Nurses will continue to advocate for clients who are concerned about out-of-pocket costs and need guidance as to what services are available and at what costs.

5. **Should nursing control healthcare costs by slowing or halting nursing salary/benefit increases?**

The increase in the nurse's compensation is cited last in the list of reasons for increased healthcare expenditures. While the nursing profession has noted growth in starting salaries, there remains a lack of incentives for career longevity. A new graduate experiences maximum earning potential in less than seven years. Studies show a marginal salary increase of 26% to 30% across the span of a nurse's career.

CHAPTER 3: PROFESSIONAL NURSING PRACTICE

1. **On what basis can nursing argue that it is a profession?**

The three most commonly cited criteria of a profession include service, knowledge, and autonomy. Nursing meets the criterion for service based on the care provider role to clients. Meeting the criteria of knowledge and autonomy has been more problematic. Nurses are beginning to engage in autonomous practice through expanded nursing roles, which typically require a baccalaureate or master's degree preparation.

2. **How close to a true profession is nursing today? What elements are progressing the fastest?**

The process of professionalization is dynamic and evolving. The continuum can be visualized as moving from non-professional to semi-professional to professional. Nursing is in the process of moving from semi-professional to true professional status. Developments in nursing research are fueling the progress of nursing to a professional status. Also, progress has been made in educational standards, autonomy, and public policy influence.

3. **Should nurses put energy into activities of professionalization?**

Professionalization is the dynamic process where occupations such as nursing change in the direction of a true profession. Nursing must progress in the areas of knowledge and autonomy in order to achieve full professional status. A minimum of a baccalaureate degree is required to fulfill the educational component. To meet the autonomy requirement nurses must work on expanded roles to encourage self-organized groups and to gain control over their practice.

4. **What strategy or strategies can nursing use to move nursing's professionalization to full professional status?**

A strategy that can be used to move nursing to full professional status is strong leadership by nurses in healthcare. Effective nursing leaders can advocate for autonomous practice for nurses in expanded roles, can support healthcare reform, and can advocate for a minimum of a baccalaureate degree for entry into professional nursing practice. Rewarding and supporting nursing research that measures cost-effective client-centered outcomes will strengthen nursing's knowledge base.

5. Should nurses care about image and appearance, and if so, why?

Appearance is related to professionalism and gives an impression of competence. Appearance and dress is one nonverbal strategy to convey nursing professionalism.

6. What is the most prevalent media stereotype of nurses today? How could this be changed?

The most prevalent media stereotypes of nurses today ignore the work and achievements of the nursing profession. The public is unaware of nursing research, nursing advocacy, and the complexity of nursing care. The image of the nurse as a prostitute and alcoholic have hampered nursing's image. Nurses are working to improve the public image by demonstrating through research and policy making the effectiveness of nursing on the healthcare system.

7. Do nurses need to act and look professional to give a professional impression?

Appearance gives an impression of competence, ability, and power. A professional appearance is one way to communicate a positive nursing image. Other essential characteristics include adherence to a nursing code, theory-based practice, community service orientation, continuing education, research, self-regulation and autonomy, professional organization participation, publication, and communication.

8. Can you design the "ideal" nursing uniform: one that nurses like, find comfortable and practical, and yet clients can identify with?

Some elements to consider when designing the "ideal" nursing uniform are the public's preference for a white dress uniform and the nurse's preference of comfortable scrubs. Other factors such as safety concerns and infection control hazards must be considered.

CHAPTER 4: LEADERSHIP PRINCIPLES

1. How would you describe a leader? Identify one person who personifies leadership.

Leadership is the process of influencing people to accomplish goals. Leaders focus on people and innovation. This is different from managers, who are primarily focused on organizational goals and objectives. The manager focuses on systems, structures, and administration. Florence Nightingale was a leader in nursing. Her skill at leadership, risk taking, and vision helped to shape the profession of nursing. Who do you know that personifies leadership?

2. What are the important qualities of leadership?

Effective leaders create a vision and provide direction to the group. They exert influence, communicate clearly, and take calculated risks to accomplish goals. Followers perceive them as courageous, honest, trustworthy, and capable of mastering change.

3. What is the best way to learn leadership skills?

The best way to learn leadership skills is by education and practice. Nurses can improve their leadership ability by analyzing their interactions with others, diagnosing areas to improve, and then practicing the skills they need. Three important skills needed for leading a group are diagnosing problematic situations, adapting to new situations, and communicating clearly.

4. Who are the leaders in nursing?

Burns (1978) identified two types of leaders: transactional and transformational. Transactional nursing leaders work within the existing organizational culture. They maintain the status quo by coordinating and managing the environment, and focusing on day-to-day operations. In contrast, transformational leaders influence and change the organization's culture. They use innovation, charisma, individual consideration, and intellectual stimulation to effect change.

5. Can you be a leader in nursing?

Many leaders are needed in nursing. Nurses can learn and practice leadership skills that will enable them to be effective leaders. Exceptional leadership practices identified by Kouzes and Posner (1990) include challenging the process, inspiring a shared vision, enabling others, modeling the way, and encouraging the heart.

6. What leadership moments happen in groups?

Leaders must assess the group they are working with, match leadership behaviors to the environment, and adapt their style to the group's needs. Groups take on a personality, and a skilled leader will be able to ascertain the maturity and readiness level of the group. The leadership style will be different for a group that is knowledgeable, experienced, and mature compared to an inexperienced group in conflict. The experienced leader will be able to identify those moments when the group is ready for change and facilitate the process.

7. What is a good follower?

Followers are vital because they accept or reject the leader and determine the leader's personal power. Effective followers, as defined by Kelley (1988), have initiative and think for themselves. They are responsible, well-balanced, competent, committed, and contribute to the success of the organization.

8. What is your favored leadership style? Followership style?

Leadership styles are a combination of task and relationship behaviors used to influence others to accomplish goals. The three leadership styles are authoritarian, democratic, and laissez-faire. If you primarily give directive behaviors, then authoritarian is your style. A democratic style implies a relationship and person orientation, while laissez-faire promotes freedom for group or individual decisions. One style is not necessarily better than another. Each one has advantages and disadvantages, depending on the situation. Followership styles include the "sheep" who lack initiative, a sense of responsibility, and critical thinking; "yes-people" who lack enterprise and yield to the opinions of others; and "alienated" followers who are independent and critical but passively resist open opposition. Effective followers are those with initiative who are responsible and who think for themselves.

CHAPTER 5: MANAGEMENT PRINCIPLES

1. Which is more important: leadership or management?

Leadership and management are equally important processes. It is important to understand that their focus is different. How important one is over the other depends on what is needed at the time for the specific situation.

2. Why is management important to a nurse?

Management is important to a nurse because all nurses manage care. Nurses coordinate and deliver health services to clients. Nursing management is the coordination and integration of nursing resources by applying the management process in order to accomplish nursing care.

3. Are middle managers going to become obsolete?

The American Organization of Nurse Executives (AONE) (1992) defines a nurse manager as someone who holds 24-hour accountability for the management of a unit(s) or area(s) within a health care institution. The nurse manager's role is central to effective, quality client care. Many changes are occurring in health care today. The new managerial ideas of cross-functional, self-managed work groups and networked organizations necessitate a role change and a new challenge for managers. Senge (1990) stated that managers are really designers who create learning processes that make self-organization possible.

4. **How do Mintzberg's ten roles differ for nurses at different positions in a hierarchical bureaucracy?**

Mintzberg (1975) identified ten roles that describe a manager's job. The three interpersonal roles, figurehead, leader, and liaison, arise from the formal authority of the manager. Informational roles include monitor, disseminator, and spokesperson, and the decision making roles include entrepreneur, disturbance handler, resource allocator, and negotiator. Nurses at different positions in a hierarchical bureaucracy engage in the three role sets described by Mintzberg. The differences in the role use among the nurse care provider, nurse manager, and nurse executive are the amount of time they spend in each role and the individuals with whom they enact the role. For example, the nurse care provider provides direct care to clients, making clinical judgments by interactions with clients, physicians, and peers. The nurse manager focuses on the coordination of care delivery and manages interactions with employees, administrators, and to some degree clients. The nurse executive focuses on planning strategy, setting policy, and analyzing service delivery trends, and interacts most frequently with other administrators, managers, and board members.

5. **Is it easier for nurses to change to a new managerial role than it is for other types of healthcare workers?**

Nurses are positioned well to move easily and naturally into management because of the nurse's foundation in caring. Nurses blend care into management to effectively produce positive outcomes such as staff satisfaction and high productivity. Nurses serve as integrators and facilitators of client care.

CHAPTER 6: PROBLEM SOLVING

1. **How can problem solving be used in nursing practice?**

Problem solving can be linked to both the nursing process and the change process. Problems can be categorized by the level of complexity and framed as either an individual or a systems problem. The nursing process and the change process can be applied to the problem identified. The nursing process is a problem solving strategy widely applicable in nursing practice. Holzemer (1986) found that nurse practitioners adopt a common style of problem solving that focuses on management of the client.

2. **Identify a problem you are dealing with now. What is your feeling about this problem? How do you approach it psychologically?**

Your gut feeling about a problem is often associated with intuition. Intuitively, you may "feel" you know the answer, but this needs to be validated with a problem solving process. How you approach a problem may be influenced by your personality style. Kirton (1989) found that personality style relates to how an individual acquires, stores, retrieves, and transforms information. The Kirton Adaptation-Innovation Theory (Kirton, 1989) identified the two problem solving styles as adaptors and innovators. Adaptors are consistently methodical, reliable, and efficient in solving problems. On the other hand, innovators seek solutions in new and challenging ways, question current practice, and promote change.

3. Do you tend to respond emotionally or logically to a problem?

Steps of the problem solving process are logical. The six basic steps are: gathering information, defining the problem, developing solutions, considering the consequences, making a decision, and implementing and evaluating the solution. Emotional responses are often reactive and are not based on a process. What is your typical response to problem solving?

4. What strategy do you tend to use for problem solving? Are there other strategies to try?

Strategies for problem solving include direct intervention, indirect intervention, delegation, purposeful inaction, and consultation or collaboration. Examining the problem in terms of importance, priority, urgency, and commitment is necessary before selecting a strategy for problem solving. Depending on your energy level, interest, and time constraints you may choose strategies ranging from direct intervention to delegation to inaction. If you choose to be actively engaged, direct intervention may be the best strategy. If you feel the problem may go away you may choose purposeful inaction.

5. How does problem solving relate to leadership?

Both leaders and managers use problem solving skills. Nursing leaders are visionary and make decisions about new innovations, changes in organizational culture, and modifications in the work environment. Innovations require effective problem solving to garner needed resources to support change. The outcomes of their decisions not only affect nursing practice but client care as well.

6. How does problem solving relate to management?

The nurse manager uses problem solving in the work environment. Management entails solving the day-to-day problems in an organization, which include staffing the next shift, purchasing capital equipment, managing budgetary constraints, and allocating staff. These decisions have a direct and immediate effect on the work area.

CHAPTER 7: DECISION MAKING

1. What is your typical or preferred decision style?

You may choose decision styles ranging from an autocratic to a participative approach. The style you choose will be influenced by the type of problem and the individuals who are impacted by the situation. A careful analysis of the problem, the people, and the situation will assist you in choosing the best decision style to optimize positive outcomes.

2. How does clinical decision making differ from managerial decision making?

Both clinical nurses and nurse managers use three phases of decision making: deliberation, judgment, and choice. Clinical nurses use decision making to solve a client problem or select a specific nursing intervention. The sophistication of clinical decision making differentiates the professional nurse from the technical nurse. Managerial decision making entails selecting options that move to resolution of an organizational problem or achievement of an organizational goal. An example of a managerial decision is determining the best method to coordinate nursing care while controlling costs.

3. How are problem solving and decision making related in nursing?

Nursing uses problem solving and decision making for client care outcomes. Decision making is a subset of the problem solving process that involves selecting the single best course of action. This can be demonstrated through direct patient outcomes such as turning a client every two hours to prevent decubitus ulcers or budgeting the appropriate number of nurses to provide quality client care. Nurses make decisions daily in clinical and organizational situations. Using the steps in the problem solving and decision making processes tends to improve the desired outcome and meet organizational goals.

4. What important decisions do nurses make? Which ones do they collaborate on?

Nurses make clinical decisions about client care and the management of that care. Client care decisions range from when to turn a patient to which crisis intervention would be most effective. Nurses collaborate on areas of clinical decision making that overlap areas of practice. Medicine and nursing is an example of overlap. This gray area, combined with complex client care and team approaches, necessitates interdisciplinary collaboration for improved client outcomes. Nurse managers collaborate with other disciplines in situations where support is needed for a project, when interdisciplinary collaboration will improve client outcomes, and when there is adequate time to engage others in the decision making process.

5. What strategies work best for clinical decision making? For managerial decision making?

Nine formal decision strategies are trial and error, pilot projects, problem critique, creativity techniques, decision tree, fishbone or cause and effect chart, group problem solving and decision making, cost-benefit analysis, and worst-case scenario. Critical pathways are commonly used clinical tools that provide protocols describing activities that must occur to achieve a predictable outcome. Pilot projects and interdisciplinary decision making are often used to provide quality care in the clinical setting. In the management arena, the nurse manager uses a variety of strategies focusing on the one that best fits the specific situation. Trial and error is considered a poor solution to the problem and is rarely used by an effective manager.

6. How can information processing help nurse decision making?

Nurses make client care decisions based on data. How the information is collected, stored, retrieved, and analyzed (information processing) is critical to problem solving and decision making. The quality of the decision is directly related to the data gathered at the beginning of the problem solving process. Patient care outcomes are dependent on quality data.

7. What resources are available to assist with ethical decision making?

Research has identified the five most frequently reported ethical dilemmas in nursing practice to be inadequate staffing patterns, prolonged life with heroic measures, inappropriate resource allocation, colleagues' irresponsible activities, and inappropriate discussions of clients. While discussion most often has been centered around clinical issues, cost-cutting efforts in healthcare are increasing ethical concerns about unsafe work environments, inappropriate utilization of unlicensed assistive personnel, and chronic staffing shortages. Resources that are available to assist in ethical decision making include ethical decision making models such as the MORAL model; personal, professional, and organizational values; the ANA's code for nurses; multidisciplinary ethics committees; and the ethical principles of autonomy, beneficence, fidelity, justice, nonmalificence, and veracity.

8. What creative or innovative ideas do you have?

Creative ideas are central to innovations in healthcare. Nurses who are creative examine problems and opportunities differently and try new strategies in solving problems. Drucker (1986) identified seven sources of innovative opportunity: the unexpected; incongruity; innovation based on process need; changes in the industry or market structure; demographics; changes in perception, mood, or meaning; and new knowledge. Nurses can be creative in problem solving by taking basic knowledge, employing critical thinking, and seeking a new path to successful innovation.

Chapter 8: The Use of Groups, Committees, and Teams

1. Does nursing need to be structured into work groups for effective client care delivery?

In today's healthcare climate the coordination aspect of nursing practice is paramount, necessitating a collaborative approach to the provision of patient care in work groups. The nurse serves as the central coordinator of care and as such must work collaboratively with multiple disciplines to effectively and efficiently provide cost-effective, quality care. The work group provides the forum for nurses and other care providers to join together to formulate patient care decisions and to improve work processes.

2. What motivates an individual to join a group?

Groups provide an outlet for individuals to satisfy psychological drives and primary needs. The need for socialization, affiliation, and an opportunity for self-achievement often motivate group participation.

3. What are the significantly different elements between social groups and organizational groups? What elements are similar?

Organizational groups are established to create a sense of status and esteem, to test and establish reality, and to get work accomplished. The primary elements in social groups are opportunities for interaction with people and a sense of self-achievement. Both types of groups provide opportunities for social exchange.

4. How is leading a group like the nursing process? The management process?

The nursing process consists of the elements of data collection, diagnosis, planning, intervention, and evaluation. Leading a group parallels the nursing process. Assessment of the group's role and responsibility and an articulation of its purpose are essential functions of the leader. Planning functional and operational process components, facilitating the group's coming to agreement, and evaluating the work of the group are leader responsibilities necessary for an effective and efficient meeting.

The management process is also useful in leading a group and involves planning, diagnosing, coordinating the implementation of the single best solution, and evaluating and tracking outcomes. Planning and organizing the physical environment, preparing and motivating participants, preparing participants for productive participation, and facilitating the work of the group are essential components of the management process.

5. What team building strategies are used in nursing? How can this process be improved?

Interactive leadership, a leadership style which is prevalent in nursing, facilitates team building. It employs such strategies as participatory management, mutual respect, sharing power and information, and generating trust through shared ownership and decision making. Building team cohesion and performance can be enhanced by facilitating interdisciplinary collaboration, using conflict resolution skills, forming strong alliances with top decision makers, and enhancing collaboration and coordination skills.

CHAPTER 9: BUDGETING AND FINANCIAL MANAGEMENT

1. **How does budgeting relate to financial planning, control, and management in healthcare?**

   Budgeting is the planning function of financial management. The budget is a written financial plan aimed at controlling resource allocations and costs as well as an evaluation tool used to assess the effectiveness of the financial management process.

2. **Do nurses raise healthcare costs or lower them?**

   Nurses' salaries often are the single largest cost in a healthcare agency. Although nurses' salaries are substantial, nurses positively impact healthcare costs through responsible and educated decision making in the areas of care management, program development, and service delivery. Nevertheless, inattention to the judicious use of resources and ineffective coordination of patient care by nurses will increase healthcare costs.

3. **How would a nurse manager manage a revenue budget?**

   Operating revenues can be determined by multiplying the services provided by the charges for the services. Nurse managers can manage the revenue budget by making certain that all services are charged for and that all charges are appropriate.

4. **How can nursing institute costing out of nursing services for reimbursement? Should this be done?**

   Controversy exists as to whether costing out of nursing services is beneficial to nursing. Although there is a lack of standardization of definitions to compute direct and indirect nursing care costs that inhibits comparisons between settings and sites, it is important for nurses to cost out nursing services and capture incentives. McCloskey (1989) proposed a new model, amenable to comparison across sites, to cost out nursing services: amount of nursing time per nursing intervention × average nursing hourly salary and benefits + equipment costs = direct costs.

5. **What leadership roles and activities are important in budgeting and financial management?**

   Leaders envision what will be needed and creatively secure and allocate essential resources. Effective budgeting and financial leadership necessitates guiding workers toward goal accomplishment, justifying resource requests, and modeling cost-conscious financial planning and management.

6. **What activities of budgeting and financial management are appropriate at the staff nurse level?**

   Appropriate and necessary budgeting and financial activities for staff nurses include providing equipment and supply requests and evaluating usage, motivating clients toward recovery, completing jobs efficiently, and coordinating interdisciplinary teams to optimize positive patient outcomes and to minimize hospital stays.

7. **How can staff nurses best acquire knowledge and skills in budgeting and financial management?**

Nurse leaders often educate, model exemplary fiscally responsible behaviors, and provide opportunities for staff nurses to learn budgeting and financial management skills. Committee participation, small work groups, continuing education programs, and college courses will provide valuable knowledge in fiscal management.

8. **How are budgeting and financial management like balancing a personal checkbook?**

Consider your personal checkbook as your budget, or timetable, and financial plan. You have predetermined deposits (revenues) against which you draw expenditures (expenses). How you financially manage your expenditures will determine if you maintain a positive balance. Planning, organizing, acquiring, and controlling money and resources are essential elements that are inherent in personal and organizational budgeting and financial management.

CHAPTER 10: ORGANIZATIONAL CULTURE AND ENVIRONMENT

1. **What is the relationship between an organization and its values?**

Values are an integral component of what makes each organization unique. They form the basic patterns that are effective in completing work and they guide perceptions, thinking, feeling, and actions within the organization.

2. **To what extent does an organization's culture determine job satisfaction?**

Culture influences perception about the interpersonal milieu or environment of an organization. Work environments impact our job satisfaction. If the organization's beliefs, values, and assumptions are congruent with ours, job satisfaction will tend to be higher.

3. **How can you assess an organization's culture?**

Assessing an organization's history, traditions, social structure, values, rituals, and rules will provide an understanding of its culture. Assessment can occur at three levels: examination of the basic elements that make up a culture, analyzing the manifestations of the culture by level, and appraisal of the five critical cultural elements (mission statement, formal structure, informal structure, political structure, and financial structure).

4. How long does it take to really perceive the culture?

To examine all the cultural elements at the various levels requires time for observation and interaction. If you think about how long it takes to truly know another person, to understand their beliefs and values, it gives you some idea of how long it takes to understand the shared beliefs, values, and assumptions of an organization.

5. Is caring the central value for nursing?

Caring is at the heart of nursing and is a shared value which serves as a basis for nursing's work, and as such is considered nursing's central value. It is a core concept and "normative glue" in nursing.

6. What are the effects of leadership on culture?

Leaders can manage and modify an organization's culture by helping the group learn and accept new values and norms. Radical change requires leaders to design new products or work methods and to change organizational beliefs and values.

7. Does organizational culture reflect an individual's perception of the organization, or is it a relatively enduring characteristic?

Cultures are built over time and are slow to change. Beliefs, values, and assumptions, which are the elements of a culture, are deeply embedded core convictions that require examination, reflection, and a conscious determination to change. Shared beliefs and values are even more enduring because they are continually reinforced by the group.

8. How can you build a culture?

A strategy to build a desired culture is to fashion shared values. This can be accomplished by starting where the group is, establishing open discussions, identifying shared values and a mission, determining strategies, and taking planned action.

9. What is the best kind of organizational culture for nursing?

The culture that would provide the most effective support for nursing is one that is congruent with nursing's own beliefs, values, and assumptions. Organizational values that are similar to professional nursing values afford a work environment that provides a good "fit" for nurses. An example is the value of caring, which is reflected in how the organization treats employees.

10. What values are important in an entrepreneurial nursing environment?

Entrepreneurial activities are inspired in an environment that values trust, risk taking, open communication, access to information and resources, and employee worth. Organizations that support entrepreneurial activity encourage contributions and potential at all levels in the organization.

11. What nursing values create dilemmas?

Dilemmas are created when an individual's values and beliefs do not "fit" with organizational expectations. The disparity causes internal conflict, discomfort, and the dilemma of sacrificing expectations either to oneself or to the organization. When an organizational environment does not share the same values as the nurse, dilemmas will arise. Examples of nursing values that might conflict with those of the organization are caring, open communication, honesty, and issues of patient's rights.

CHAPTER 11: ORGANIZATIONS, MISSION STATEMENTS, POLICIES, AND PROCEDURES

1. How do previous employee experiences color perception and attitude? Why do these perceptions linger?

The way we perceive the world is formulated from our values and beliefs. Values and beliefs are molded by situations and persons who significantly touch our lives, causing us to reevaluate these core principles. Core principles of our personal, professional, and organizational culture are developed over time and are slow to change. The resistance to change is a stabilizing force and adds order to our lives. Employees enter new work environments with past perceptions and only over time will their behavior change.

2. Do nurses profess loyalty to the organization/job or to the profession/work of nursing? Can an individual have both?

Professional values are formulated during the formal educational process required for a profession. As a result, nurses, as professionals, begin their careers with loyalty to their profession. When nurses seek employment they are then faced with expectations of loyalty to the organization as well as the profession. When organizational and professional values differ, an underlying dynamic tension is created. Nurses will find that their decisions and actions will reflect continual adjustments between the professional and organizational pressures in an attempt to find the most comfortable "fit."

3. How do you use the change process to implement a new philosophy in a pre-established work group?

Leadership involves establishing a philosophy that will serve as the grounding principle upon which visions can be based and planning and actualization of the vision can occur. Leaders can move employees through the change process to create a new philosophy by first starting where the group is; motivating, educating, guiding, inspiring, and supporting employees in the process of relinquishing old beliefs and values; and molding a new philosophy.

4. What is the "philosophy in action"? Cite some examples. Describe why this makes a difference.

Subtle behaviors that demonstrate a lack of concern for people and an undermining of their success are described by Brown-Stewart (1987) as "philosophy in action." Examples of such contempt behaviors include lack of habitual courtesy, withholding of information, lack of education and orientation, and insufficient staffing. These behaviors decrease employee satisfaction, morale, and work performance and negatively impact client outcomes and organizational accomplishments.

5. What problems are solved by having policies and procedures?

Policies and procedures are standards in the form of written rules that guide decision making and performance. As such, they provide order and stability so that nursing functions in a coordinated fashion, decreasing the amount of random chaos in the work environment.

6. What decisions can nurses make without a written policy?

Some policies are unwritten, or implied, by patterns of decisions that have already been made within an organization. Professional nursing judgment is often used when making client care decisions. However, when managerial or client care problems arise outside of the nurse's scope of practice, the nurse must know who in the chain of command to contact.

CHAPTER 12: ORGANIZATIONAL STRUCTURE: CONCEPTS

1. What purposes for nursing does the structure of an organization serve?

The structure is built to accomplish goals by providing order, distinction, and a framework. The purposes for nursing are the same as for the rest of the organization: to control variations in behavior among individuals, avoid chaos, direct the flow of information, determine employee positions, and provide an efficient work flow.

2. What elements of organizational structure are found in nursing organizations?

The structural elements of an organization are division of labor, hierarchy of authority, rules and regulations that govern behavior, span of control, and lines of communication. All of these elements are found in nursing organizations.

3. What elements are most important for nursing practice?

It is important to think in terms of what elements of the structure facilitate the work of providing client care. Certainly having rules and regulations that govern behavior add functional order to work. The division of labor provides delegation of responsibilities, and the lines of communication provide line and staff reporting structures.

4. How are the structures of community agencies the same as or different from hospitals?

Hospitals, due to their size and complexity, often have complex bureaucratic structures. The services provided may be diverse, with multiple divisional lines and levels of authority. A board of directors heads the structure in hospital organizations as it does in community agencies. Historically, hospital organizations have been designed to be primarily internally focused, whereas community agencies have been structurally designed to be more externally focused. Community agencies that are linked with state and federal agencies are complex bureaucratic structures, whereas those linked to local government are structurally less complex.

5. What coordinating mechanisms are used in nursing and healthcare organizations?

The five basic coordinating functions used in nursing and healthcare organizations are mutual adjustment, direct supervision, standardization of work processes, standardization of work outputs, and standardization of worker skills.

6. How effective are the coordinating mechanisms used by nursing?

Nursing has used coordinating mechanisms with varying effectiveness. Mutual adjustment, peers relying on each other to effectively solve problems, has supported nursing since nursing's inception. Direct supervision, on the other hand, was effectively used before the advent of primary care nursing. During the decade of its popularity, delegation skills were lost, and nurses are only now developing them again through education and experience. Nursing has been slow to standardize processes, outputs, and worker skills. Standardization efforts within organizations and nationally through credential bodies are improving as demands for validation of skills, cost containment, and quality increase.

7. How have authority, responsibility, and accountability been used in nursing practice? What feelings do they create?

Organizational authority is used to fulfill a professional role in a specific job, while professional authority is used to practice professional nursing. Responsibility is accepted by each nurse who fulfills a position, while accountability is used to account for the quality and the quantity of the assigned work. These three elements of professional practice create mixed feelings. Authority may produce feelings of power and esteem, whereas responsibility and accountability may generate a degree of caution.

8. Is power in nursing centralized or decentralized?

Power in nursing is becoming increasingly decentralized as is the trend in many industries. Decentralized structures improve quality and lower costs by placing decision making closer to work processes. With increasing demands on healthcare to lower costs and improve quality, the trend is expected to continue.

Chapter 13: Organizational Structure: Types

1. Discuss the different types of organizational structures. Which best suit the practice of nursing?

Bureaucracy, matrix, and adhocracy are the three basic types of organizational structures. A bureaucracy is pyramidal, hierarchical, and centralized. A matrix is a complex combination of a centralized bureaucratic structure with a project team component. An adhocracy is a flat, decentralized structure with a project team or ad hoc committee component. Most nurses work in bureaucratic hospital structures, but adhocracy structures are expected to proliferate as healthcare moves into the community.

2. What factors need to be assessed prior to changing the organizational structure?

A thorough understanding of the existing structure is crucial before a plan for change is designed. Assessing the organization for the complexity of the organization, the level of specialization of the work force, the degree of centralization of services, and the degree of formalization of policies, procedures, rules and regulations is essential.

3. Why are organizations resistant to changing their structure?

An organizational structure is a significant element in the culture of an organization. Changing the structure tampers with the basic beliefs, values, and assumptions of the organization. Structural change will dictate system change, threatening an organization's identity and stability. When an organization changes the course of how business is accomplished, it risks the possibility that a new system may not function effectively, possibly jeopardizing the survival of the organization.

4. How do nurses foster or hinder restructuring?

Restructuring fundamentally changes jobs and positions in nursing and, in doing so, will elicit both opposition and support. Opposition to restructuring can be expected with downsizing of the RN work force and nursing management. Enhanced opportunities for nurses in expanded roles include case managers, coordinators across care settings, advanced practice nurses, and staff nurses with increased decision making opportunities and autonomy.

5. How do complex organizations adapt to their environment?

Adaptation in complex bureaucratic organizations is systematic and sluggish. Bureaucratic organizations are designed specifically for stability and survival over time and, as such, are not designed for a quick response to organizational change or to innovation. The very factor that has allowed bureaucracies to survive may be the factor that causes their demise in today's rapidly changing healthcare climate.

6. What changes are needed in nursing organizations? Why?

Nursing organizations tend to be bureaucratic. To meet healthcare reform demands they must change to become cost effective, efficient, and flexible structures with innovative cultures capable of responding quickly to the rapidly changing healthcare climate. Nursing organizations must change or risk becoming bureaucratic dinosaurs.

7. How are healthcare structures changing under healthcare reform? Why?

Healthcare structures are becoming decentralized and more fluid with the orientation on outcomes. Staff duties are being expanded, managers are assuming more accountability, staff costs are being reduced, services are being subcontracted, and there is a refocus on the core business. These changes are occurring to reduce cost and to increase flexibility to compete effectively in the turbulent healthcare environment.

Chapter 14: Decentralization and Shared Governance

1. What is the relationship between decentralization and shared governance?

Decentralization is the dispersal of decision making power to many points in the organization. Shared governance falls under the umbrella of decentralization. It is one form of a professional practice model which involves shared decision making by staff nurses and management.

2. How are shared governance and structure related?

Shared governance is an organizational structure. It legitimizes the staff nurses' influence in administrative decision making.

3. What conditions in the facility in which you are a student or employee would facilitate shared governance?

To answer this question, consider the conditions that facilitate the empowerment of staff nurses to make autonomous client care decisions. Possible conditions that you may consider include preparing staff for a new level of authority and accountability and providing education, information, and resources. Education on organizational systems and the budgeting process, strong administrative support, and interdisciplinary group team building are other conditions that facilitate the development of shared governance. What other conditions can you identify?

4. Are decentralization and shared governance characteristic of current hospital nursing organizations? Current community health and long-term care organizations?

The movement in hospital nursing organizations is toward decentralization and shared governance. Hospitals are the trend leaders among healthcare organizations in the movement toward more participative management structures. Many hospitals have implemented shared governance, but each will determine the level of nurse autonomy and peer control of functions and processes. With the advent of integrated networks, shared governance structures in community health and long-term care are emerging.

5. Does changing to a shared governance model change nurses' roles? If so, how?

Nurses' roles in a shared governance model are expanded to accept more responsibility and accountability for decision making. Nurses will not only be expected to provide professional care but will be instrumental in decision making affecting their work life and the provision of care. Decisions about acquisition of resources, educational opportunities, peer review, and quality monitoring and improvement are examples of additional responsibilities that are a part of a shared governance model.

6. What is the governance structure of the nursing organization you are most familiar with?

To answer this question, think about who makes decisions in your organization. Are staff nurses involved in making decisions that affect professional practice or their work lives? Is the decision making mutually shared with management, or is it exclusive to either management or staff? Are decisions limited to unit based decisions or are divisional level decision making opportunities available with input to the larger healthcare organization? If a shared governance model is identified, would it be classified as a councilar model, a congressional format, or an administrative shared governance model?

7. What questions should be asked to determine how decentralized an organization is in reality?

Some questions that will assist in the determination of where the decision making power lies include the following: Who has the authority to make resource allocation decisions? Who makes care management decisions? To what extent do nonmanagers have power over decision processes? What are the lines of communication in the organization?

CHAPTER 15: DELEGATION

1. What does your nurse practice act say about delegation and supervision?

Each state's Nurse Practice Act provides direction about delegation and supervision. It is important for you to know your state's specific requisites that govern nursing practice. You may obtain a copy of your state's Nurse Practice Act from your State Board of Nursing.

2. Should a nursing student delegate work?

It is important for nursing students to learn and practice delegation skills. These skills require advanced clinical judgment and for this reason are usually incorporated into role performance late in the curriculum in a structured practicum experience under the guidance of an instructor.

3. How extensively is delegating to non-RN personnel used in the work settings you have experienced?

You might want to consider not only how extensively but what tasks and in what situations delegation was used. Do you feel the delegation was appropriate?

4. How comfortable do you feel with delegation?

If you feel some reluctance or discomfort delegating, can you identify what is causing the discomfort? The basis of your discomfort may be a feeling that you could do it better yourself, a lack of ability to direct, a lack of confidence in subordinates, an aversion to taking a risk, a need to feel indispensable, or a fear of losing authority or personal satisfaction.

5. How do you delegate to assist others to further develop?

Delegating increasingly complex tasks that require responsible and reasonable risk taking after a foundation of knowledge and skills has been established is an excellent way for the delegate to grow. Providing responsible incremental growth experiences with adequate supervision will enhance job satisfaction and build trusting team relationships.

6. What criteria can be used to assess workers' competency?

The criteria used to assess competency must be pre-established and measurable and must be accomplished within a pre-determined time frame. It can include the following criteria: was the task or procedure completed correctly, completely, and within the time frame? Assessment should occur through periodic reviews.

7. **Do these criteria differ for RNs and UAPs? For nursing students?**

Competencies for RNs differ from those for UAPs. RNs are skilled in clinical judgment and complex decision making, necessitating cognitive and skill evaluation. Nursing students are evaluated by the same criteria as the RN, taking into consideration their evolving level of skills and knowledge. UAPs are evaluated according to the hospital's job description and policies that dictate their level of education and skill.

8. **What routine activities can RNs delegate to others?**

RNs can delegate tasks and procedures that are routine and standard. Examples include specimen collection, acquiring and recording of vital signs, bathing, and assisting with procedures. Activities involving assessment, evaluation, and nursing judgment cannot be delegated.

9. **When you delegate your work, what do *you* do?**

You will retain the professional functions of your role. An RN remains accountable and responsible and must supervise all those to whom nursing activities are delegated. The intensity of the supervision will depend on the experience and the expertise of the delegate. The nursing process is strictly a nursing function that cannot be delegated. Assessment, planning, and evaluation require significant time. Complex procedures, medication administration, and activities requiring nursing judgment are also limited to the RN care provider.

10. **What is a safe or minimum nurse to client ratio? Does this differ across care settings?**

A safe or minimum nurse to client ratio will depend on the setting, shift, skill mix, and circumstances. It can vary from 1:1 in a perioperative or critical care setting to 1:10 or more in a subacute care setting. The primary determinate of an appropriate ratio is that nurses must be able to provide safe care and adequately supervise those to whom they delegate. Staffing guidelines are often established by specialty nursing organizations and the Joint Commission on Accreditation of Healthcare Organizations.

11. **What is a nurse really responsible for when she or he is responsible for care coordination and delivery?**

The RN retains the responsibility and accountability for the provision of care to an assigned group of clients. It is the responsibility of the RN to assess clients. The RN may delegate aspects of care for clients whose care requirements are routine and standardized, whose outcomes are predictable, and whose reaction to illness and hospitalization is not threatening. The RN thus coordinates the care and delegates aspects as appropriate but remains accountable for care delivery.

CHAPTER 16: NURSING CARE DELIVERY SYSTEMS

1. Who has the authority to establish the nursing care delivery modality for the institution?

The chief nurse executive has the authority to establish the nursing care delivery model for the institution. Nurse leaders and managers within the institution play a key role in the development and selection of the care delivery model. Organizations using a shared governance model include staff nurses in the development and selection process.

2. How do nurses decide on which nursing care delivery system to use?

Nurses involved in the selection of a nursing care delivery system use a systematic assessment process that considers client characteristics, available nursing resources, and organizational support available to nursing. Current issues and trends such as cost containment pressures or rising client acuities are also considered. Prior to selecting a care delivery system, it is helpful for nurses to become clear on their philosophy for resource utilization, practice expectations, and the role of the registered nurse. Finally, a literature review of care delivery systems is essential to assure the best fit for the clients' unique needs in concert with the organizational goals.

3. Why are nursing care delivery systems being revised and restructured?

Care delivery systems are being revised and restructured in an effort to provide client care that is both quality and cost effective in a changing economic, technological, political, and social environment. Increased emphasis is being placed on cost containment, appropriate utilization of resources, professional nursing practice, seamless continuum of care, integration, multidisciplinary collaboration, and access to care. New or modified care delivery systems are emerging to better fit with the changing environment.

4. What issues arise when the care delivery system is changed?

Care delivery system changes may threaten the balance between meeting client needs and those of the organization. Important issues surface related to the quality and cost of services being rendered, client and care provider satisfaction, and the degree to which the needs of the client are being met. Other critical issues such as care provider role clarity, registered nurse preparation and delegation skills, a client-versus-task–focused perspective, and appropriate use of the registered nurse must be addressed.

5. What common themes emerge among the newest care delivery systems being developed? How do they compare to older modalities?

The newest care delivery systems seek to reconfigure nursing's work within resource constraints, care needs, and current ideas about professional nursing practice. They emphasize outcome management, collaboration, the use of a variety of caregivers with variable competency and preparation, and integrated practice. Common themes include accountability, cost containment, effectiveness, seamless continuum of care, multidisciplinary collaboration, and emerging roles. In contrast to the older modalities, they are more client centered with greater integration and multidisciplinary team collaboration. Newer care delivery models emphasize the professional role of the registered nurse within the context of a larger organization in which nurses must be concerned with both the quality and cost effectiveness of their care.

6. What care delivery system best fits a merger of hospital and community agencies, or are multiple care modalities needed?

It is not known which care delivery system is the best for each setting in which nursing is practiced; however, concepts from case management or managed care models seek to integrate services provided between the hospital and community agencies. Efforts are underway to develop a seamless continuum of care between multiple care providers in which services are client focused rather than hospital or agency focused. This requires a more cooperative, less competitive environment.

Chapter 17: Case Management and Managed Care

1. What are the goals of case management?

Case management strives to link, manage, or organize services to meet client needs. Essential goals are coordination and integration of a continuum of holistic care and promotion and preservation of health through periods of transition and risk. Conservation and allocation of scarce resources is also important. The provision of follow-up care that tracks and guides service delivery over the long term and across episodes and settings is another important goal.

2. What are the goals of managed care? How do they compare to those of case management?

Managed care strives to lower costs and maximize the value of services and the resources used. Managed care goals are similar to those of case management in that both seek to reduce costs and conserve resources. Managed care differs from case management in that managed care goals are broader and provide the structure and focus for managing the use, cost, quality, and effectiveness of health services targeted to 100% of clients. In contrast, case management goals focus on delivery of care for a targeted 10% to 20% of clients who are at high risk.

3. What are the outcomes anticipated by case management? By managed care?

Anticipated outcomes for case management are achievement of client outcomes within effective and appropriate timeframes and resources. Anticipated outcomes for managed care are similar but focus on the broader system in which costs are controlled or reduced through appropriate resource use while maintaining or improving quality services.

4. How is case management affecting the role of the nurse?

Case management shifts the balance between nurses' roles with some of the primary caregiving components exchanged for care coordination. The nurse will provide more coordination of services.

5. Who should be the case manager?

Nurses are skilled in the coordination of care and are well qualified to be case managers. Given the interdisciplinary nature of case management, the nurse is pivotal in coordinating services to clients. Client assessment, service integration, and follow-up are essential roles of the case manager. The nurse has the necessary knowledge and preparation to assess, plan, oversee critical paths, facilitate interventions, and evaluate outcomes.

6. Does the Public Health model apply to hospital settings? Why or why not?

The Public Health model, where case management and care coordination is the care delivery modality, has application for hospital case management. The model has direct applicability for use in the hospital, extended across the healthcare continuum, or linked to a population focus. The model may include some aspects of service provision or may be solely service coordination.

7. Do all clients need case management?

While all clients need coordinated care, case management serves the needs of targeted high-risk populations best. All clients do not need the close monitoring that case management provides, especially in an environment where case managers are a limited resource. Managed care may be a more appropriate modality for all clients as it provides structure and focus for managing the use, cost, quality, and effectiveness of health services.

CHAPTER 18: COMMUNICATION

1. What are the essential components of the communication process?

The communication process consists of verbal and nonverbal communication. Verbal communication is both written and spoken. Nonverbal communication is unspoken and is composed of affective or expressive behaviors. Four distinctions that have been made to characterize communication are formal/informal, vertical/horizontal, personal/impersonal, and instrumental/expressive.

2. What are the barriers to effective communication in organizations?

Barriers to effective communication in organizations include political and interpersonal subtleties and the complexity of communicating with multiple people. Organizations use various networks for communication such as hierarchical or democratic networks. Barriers in the hierarchical network may be associated with decreased opportunity for individuals to interact with their peers or people on other levels in the hierarchy. Barriers in the democratic network may be associated with communication inaccuracy and development of sub-hierarchies.

3. What problems of communication occur frequently in nursing?

Communication problems occurring frequently in nursing are related to being on the front lines, being the focus for displaced criticism, working with people who have health problems, and working in high-stress environments. Nonverbal communication problems exist when an unprofessional image of nursing is portrayed by the media.

4. Are superior-subordinate communication problems more common than peer-to-peer difficulties?

Communication problems are equally common in superior-subordinate and peer-to-peer communications. Problems associated with superior-subordinate communications may be the result of intimidation, lack of trust, lack of feedback, or inability to express needs. Problems associated with peer-to-peer communications may be the result of inability to give and receive constructive criticism, difficulty with need expression, turf issues, and lack of trust.

5. What solutions tend to help communication effectiveness?

Communication effectiveness can be enhanced by planning the message structure, delivery style, mode of communication, and method for feedback. Planning the message involves structuring it in such a way that it will be received positively and will engender the response preferred. Selection of delivery style includes careful selection of words to maximize impact. Mode of communication involves choices about timing and channel. Method for feedback includes a plan for checking out whether the delivered message was understood. Solutions for responding effectively to criticism are to ask for more information, agree with the critic, and use listening skills to uncover the real issue.

6. What is the relationship of communication skill to leadership effectiveness?

Communication skill is a key element of leadership effectiveness. Communication is a critical and important tool for effectiveness, in engaging and motivating people, and in getting the work done through others. Communication skills are essential in sharing the vision, in shaping values and norms to bond individuals and groups, and in implementing change.

7. What is the leader's role in helping others improve written and oral communication?

The leader plays an important role in mentoring others to improve their communication skills. This can be accomplished through a variety of methods, such as role modeling, soliciting and providing constructive criticism, and role playing. It is critical for the leader to model a communication style that is clear, direct, straightforward, respectful, empathetic, and timely.

8. How important is written communication skill in influencing an individual's image?

Written communication skill is an important job element impacting an individual's image. Written communication is common in organizations in such forms as fliers, memos, letters, faxes, e-mail, newsletters, and bulletin boards. Skill is required to structure a clear and concise written message that will be positively received. Written messages that are unclear or convey a negative tone may adversely impact an individual's image.

9. How do you personally communicate, both verbally and nonverbally?

It is important to be aware of your communication strengths and weaknesses and how your communications are received by others. What is your preferred mode, and is it effective with the receiver? It is critical for nurse leaders to be highly skilled communicators. One method of assessing your skills is to solicit feedback from your peers, employer, or subordinates.

10. How might you choose some other message or some other channel in order to increase personal effectiveness?

Consider your message structure. Are you consciously thinking about whether it will be received positively and engender the response you desire? Are your words clear and free of red flags, inflammatory language, and jargon? When selecting a channel, consider the advantages and disadvantages of written versus spoken communication. Are you aware of the nonverbals you project?

11. Do nurses, from the staff nurse to the chief nurse executive, present an image of nursing that you agree or disagree with?

Think about the image of nursing that you value. Would others agree with you? How would the public view the image of nursing in healthcare organizations you are familiar with? Do you have a different image for the staff nurse as compared with the chief nurse executive? Should there be a difference?

12. **What does the ideal nurses' uniform look like? Analyze your response.**

    Research has shown that the consumer prefers white uniforms with skirts and a cap as a nurse's uniform. In contrast, nurses think scrubs are practical and comfortable. How would you blend the two perspectives to meet the needs of both groups? Are the preferences of one group more important than the other?

13. **Why do nurses need to look professional?**

    Physical appearance and choice of clothing are forms of nonverbal communication that stimulate judgmental responses from others. They affect the amount of trust, confidence, and respect from the consumer. A professional appearance enhances the image of nursing and creates internal and external prestige.

CHAPTER 19: MOTIVATION

1. **How do you stay motivated to love nursing for the rest of your life?**

   It is important to be aware of what factors provide you with external and internal motivation. What are your values, beliefs, and assumptions that motivate you to love nursing? How will those change over time? Will the same factors still motivate you 10 years from now? How will your needs for growth and development, advancement, increased responsibility for work, challenging work, recognition, and achievement change?

2. **Does loving nursing guarantee quality care?**

   While loving nursing does not guarantee quality services, the nurse's motivation has a powerful influence on the provision of quality care. The love of nursing may serve as an internal driving force in motivating the nurse to provide excellent care, which in turn may generate external reinforcement from positive patient outcomes and satisfaction.

3. **What is the motivation to enter nursing as a career?**

   Nurses enter nursing for a variety of reasons. Examples of external motivators are the need for recognition and to be needed by others, acknowledgment, status, and economic compensation. Examples of internal motivators are the need for autonomy, a sense of doing important work, helping others, the need for competence, and self-actualization.

4. **What is the comparison of real-world nursing practice to what motivation theories say?**

   Many motivation theories can be readily applied to real-world nursing practice. The need satisfaction model is often used by nurses in the provision of care. For example, nurses use Maslow's Hierarchy of Needs to recognize that client teaching is ineffective if basic physiological needs are unmet. Herzberg's Motivation-Hygiene theory fits well in describing job satisfiers and dissatisfiers. Nurses do not appear to be highly motivated by the hygiene or maintenance factors, which include security, status, money, working conditions, and policies and administration. The motivators are related to the job itself and include growth and development, increased responsibility, challenging work, recognition, and achievement.

5. **What positive incentives are most important to nurses? To you personally?**

Positive incentives vary, depending on the needs of the individual nurse. The core of what motivates nurses to nurse is often the love of the work itself. One survey found nurses valued providing quality client care, caring about clients' best interests, being treated as a professional, having adequate staffing, and working in a safe environment (American Nurse, 1991).

6. **What are the elements of a motivating environment?**

Elements of a motivating environment include explicit goals, clear expectations, direct feedback and reinforcement, elimination of threats, individual responsibility, rewards, and trust. The nurse leader's job is to create an environment that fosters motivated behavior by identifying what nurses need to succeed, be satisfied, and feel what they do is an important service to clients.

7. **Is it manipulative or Machiavellian to deliberately plan and implement rewards and incentives to get other people to perform?**

The art of leading and managing groups of professionals requires creative, interesting, and continuous ways to make people feel good about what they are doing. While the use of rewards and incentives can be viewed as manipulative, it is a mutually beneficial relationship in which recognition is provided in exchange for quality performance. Personal, professional, and economic rewards have been shown to be powerful motivators in nursing.

8. **Under cost containment pressures, what is the effect on nurses of relying on recognition as the organizational motivation strategy?**

Cost containment pressures may create dissatisfaction in nurses who rely on economic rewards as an entitlement or as a motivator to perform. Productivity may decrease. Nurse leaders may need to develop and implement personal and professional recognition programs to compensate for the loss of economic rewards.

CHAPTER 20: POWER

1. **Pick a day in the past couple of weeks that you think of as average. Who were the people who had the most influence over you? Why were they influential?**

Whoever you identified as influential, think about them in the context of the eight mechanisms used as strategies to exert influence. What strategies were used by those individuals? Did they use assertiveness, exchange, upward appeal, blocking, or coalitions? Which strategies exert the most influence over you?

2. Do you view power as positive or negative? Give examples.

Understanding and analyzing power is a beginning strategy for knowing how to use power for positive and constructive ends. Many nurses perceive power as bad or negative. Power is not by definition negative. Positive power exerts influence on behalf of others while negative power exerts influence over others. What have your experiences been? How do you react to those exerting power over you?

3. Identify the kinds of power you use and the kinds of power others use on you.

What is your belief about your personal power? Do you believe you can influence events through personal effort? How about professional power? Do you get rewards from doing a job, acquiring expertise, being liked, and having charisma? Do you have the power to use your professional expertise and competence to make change, do something good for clients, advance the profession, or make a contribution? What are the strengths of power used by those you respect?

4. What types of power are you most comfortable with? Which would you consider trying?

Consider your comfort with sources of power, such as reward, coercive, expert, referent, legitimate, connection, information, or group decision making. In which situations might you use each? Which are you least comfortable with? What has led you to feel that way?

5. Think about yourself as acting with strength and power and feeling the most satisfied about it. What kind of things would you be doing?

It is important to analyze what gives you a sense of power. Nurses may be inclined to avoid an acknowledgment or analysis of power. However, to lead and manage, nurses need to acquire, possess, and use power. How closely did your actions with strength and power match your present environment? What will you need to acquire to feel the most satisfied?

6. What happens in situations in which you feel powerless?

What strategies do you employ when feeling powerless? Do you find yourself developing behaviors that may be counterproductive to the organization? When coming into direct conflict with the power others possess, do you fight, negotiate, collaborate, or do nothing? How effective has each strategy been for you?

7. Does a lack of power affect the way that you feel about situations?

Powerless positions demotivate workers, create powerless behaviors, increase dependence, and cause frustration or panic. How do you frame your attitude in powerless situations? How could you reframe your attitude to regain a sense of power?

8. When you are trying to control a situation, what makes you feel comfortable or uncomfortable?

Attempting to control a situation may evoke the use of power over others rather than on behalf of others. Which approach do you take in power conflicts? How a person acts when experiencing a power conflict is directly related to how they perceive the source, the nature, and the magnitude of other people's power.

9. How can power principles be structured to advance nursing's professional goals?

Nurses have the power to reinforce the image of nursing through the projection of enthusiasm, self-confidence, self-esteem, and quality care. For example, a perceptual image of competence enhances a power base of expertise. Power is also derived from the art and science of nursing practice. Nurses can use power to exert influence in making decisions about what will yield high-quality client care and be most cost effective. Another strategy is to develop and use the information power of nursing research.

10. What is the difference, if any, between power and manipulation?

Similarities exist between the concepts of power and manipulation. One view of power is the ability to get others to do what you want done. Manipulation is commonly viewed as controlling or playing upon others by artful, unfair, or insidious means.

11. How is organizational power used?

Organizational power is often seen as control over valuable resources. Sources of power in organizations are structural position, personal characteristics, expertise, and opportunity. Those with access to power and opportunity feel empowered to contribute to the organization, participate more actively, and exhibit higher morale. Organizational power implies the ability to mobilize support, information, and resources in order to meet organizational goals. Power is also used as a mechanism to resolve conflict.

CHAPTER 21: CONFLICT

1. What was the most recent conflict you experienced?

Consider the type of conflict you experienced. Was it intrapersonal, interpersonal, or intergroup? What were the antecedent conditions that led you to perceive and feel conflict? What was your manifest behavior? What was the conflict aftermath? Did you perceive the conflict to be positive or negative?

2. What types of conflict are common in nursing students?

An intrapersonal conflict example is role conflict in which the nursing student occupies many competing roles, such as working nurse, student, spouse, parent, and friend. Internal conflict may result as the student nurse attempts to fulfill more roles than time allows. An interpersonal conflict between a student and instructor may result over the due date for a paper or project as the student attempts to extend the deadline. An intergroup conflict may occur among a group of nursing students working on a group project when it is perceived that workload is not divided equally.

3. What sources of conflict are most common in nursing practice?

Nurses are prime candidates for conflict because of the need to work collaboratively with people of varying social, ethnic, and educational backgrounds. Conflicts may arise from differences in communication styles, goals, values, resources, roles, and personalities. Power distribution for nurses employed in a hierarchical system may lead to conflict as nurses attempt to meet the needs of their clients and advocate for scarce resources to provide the care.

4. What is your usual way of handling conflict?

Consider which mode you find yourself in when a conflict surfaces. Are you in the defensive mode? Do you tend to compromise? Do you use creative problem solving? Conflict resolution techniques include avoiding, withholding or withdrawing, smoothing over or reassuring, accommodating, forcing, competing, compromising, confronting, collaborating, bargaining and negotiating, and problem solving. Which are your preferred techniques? What others might you try?

5. What is the usual way nurses handle conflict?

Nurses use a variety of techniques, including avoiding, accommodating, compromising, competing, and collaborating. The degree of assertiveness and cooperativeness may vary, depending on the technique selected and the comfort level of the individual nurse or group. Conflict that occurs between nurses and physicians often is handled by nurses through compromise and accommodation rather than collaboration and problem solving due to power differences.

6. Does the way your immediate superior handles conflict help or hinder you?

Think about the conflict resolution outcomes your immediate superior achieves. Are they win-lose, lose-lose, or win-win? How is conflict framed? Is conflict viewed constructively as increasing group cohesion and morale, promoting creativity, producing change and growth, improving work relations, promoting more effective problem solving, and motivating group members? In contrast, is conflict viewed as a destructive force interfering with stability and harmony?

7. Is there one best way to handle the conflicts most common to nursing practice?

A variety of strategies can be used to handle conflicts in nursing. It is important to conduct an assessment of the conflict situation to identify the boundaries of the conflict, areas of agreement and disagreement, and the extent of each person's aims. The factors that limit the possibilities of managing the conflict constructively must be understood.

8. Do advanced practice nurses experience different conflicts? If so, what are they?

Nursing's role is not as clear as it used to be, and this can cause stress and frustrations. Advanced practice nurses face special challenges in defining and establishing their unique roles on the healthcare team. Healthcare reform and scarcity of resources may produce conflicts and resulting opportunities for advanced practice nurses. In addition, as nurses gain prestige and power, conflicts with physicians may result in collaboration rather than accommodation and compromise.

9. What organizational factors are related to unionization activity?

Organizational factors related to unionization activity center around work redesign with changes in staff mix, reductions in the work force, concern over the quality of services rendered, and job insecurity. Nurses are facing new challenges to provide care with fewer resources and increased levels of non-nurse assistive personnel. This has created conflict between nurses and administrators.

CHAPTER 22: PERSUASION AND NEGOTIATION

1. What persuades individuals to become nurses?

A variety of factors may influence an individual's decision to become a nurse. Those involved in the recruitment of nurses may emphasize the positive aspects, such as the opportunity to care for people, while downplaying the negative aspects, such as heavy workload and irregular hours.

2. What feelings are associated with interviewing for a nursing position?

An interview for a nursing position is a process in which applicants seeking employment attempt to persuade the interviewer that they are the best candidate. Applicants may be anxious, excited, and apprehensive when interviewing.

3. What was the last issue you negotiated?

Analyze your negotiation process. What was the central issue in the conflict? What were your goals? What were the goals of the competitor? How did the goals vary with respect to urgency and priority as the negotiation continued? Was it a win-win situation? What information was withheld to maintain a sense of negotiating power?

4. What behaviors contribute to cooperative and productive negotiation?

Cooperative and productive negotiation can only occur if the issue is negotiable, the negotiators are interested in both giving and taking, and the parties trust each other and the negotiating process. In a supportive environment, feelings are focused on the problem issue and strategies are sincere and problem-focused. Participants are well prepared for the negotiation, maintain a positive tone, encourage discussion throughout the process, and work toward a solution that everyone can support.

5. What words or actions indicate competitive negotiation?

A competitive negotiation process may have a defensive milieu in which there are feelings of superiority and strategies of controlling. Poor listening, inaccurate communication, strong reactions to stress, and failure to disclose information or feelings may be indications of a competitive negotiation. Information may be altered, filtered, given selectively, or withheld as a power gaining strategy. Questions may be framed so as to lead the other party to the competitor's point of view rather than to genuinely seek understanding.

6. What approaches or strategies of negotiation are most effective for nursing?

Negotiation approaches and strategies most effective for nursing include preparing for negotiation, communicating a general overview of what is to be accomplished, and reviewing why negotiation is required. The negotiation includes redefining the issue or issues, selecting when issues will be addressed, and encouraging discussion throughout the process. Final approaches include addressing the fall-back or compromise position for both parties, agreeing in principle during the settlement stage, and recapping and summarizing the agreement. After the negotiation process is complete, compliance with the agreement is monitored.

7. What factors are facilitators or barriers to collaboration among professionals?

Facilitators to collaboration among professionals include willingness to give and take, trust, mutual respect, good listening skills, willingness to work toward a solution that everyone can support, and mutual client-centered goals. Barriers to collaboration include competition, turf protection, win-lose strategy, arrogance, controlling, poor listening skills, self-interest focus, and defensiveness.

8. **Does collective bargaining increase professionalism in nursing?**

Some believe that collective bargaining increases professionalism in nursing by ensuring that nursing has a voice in decisions that impact client care. Collective bargaining exists to limit employers' ability to take unilateral action. Others believe that collective bargaining limits professionalism in nursing by creating a defensive environment between nurses and employers.

9. **What organizational factors are associated with unionization?**

Organizational factors associated with unionization include unilateral decisions made by employers to reduce cost by decreasing the labor force or replacing professional staff with lesser skilled workers. Threats to long-term job security and benefits, reduction in income, increased workload, and concerns over the quality of services rendered have created an increase in unionization activities.

10. **Is positional power eroding in nursing? With what forms of negotiation can nurses replace positional power?**

Positional power, or legitimate power, relates to the role or position held by nurses in organizations. When organizations make unilateral decisions about issues impacting nursing without the input of nurses, the nurses' positional power is eroded. Nurses may need to strengthen their expert and referent power to ensure that client advocacy occurs. Nurses may seek and use power to influence professional issues, ethical issues, or national health policy. Nurses can use negotiation to determine how nursing care is practiced and delivered in organizations by establishing a cooperative environment where the goals of all parties are valued.

CHAPTER 23: STAFFING AND SCHEDULING

1. **Should nursing services be staffed to the minimum, maximum, or mean? Why?**

Nursing service staffing varies, depending on the method of staffing used. Two general methods of nurse staffing are the traditional fixed staffing and controlled variable staffing methods. The traditional fixed staffing method is built around a fixed projected maximum workload requirement and is based on maximum workload conditions. The controlled variable staffing method is built below maximum workload conditions, and staff are supplemented as needed.

2. **What is the influence of the budget on staffing and scheduling?**

The budget plays a major role in the development of staffing and scheduling plans. Current economic constraints and limited financial resources have given rise to intense scrutiny of human resources. The nursing labor expense budget accounts for a large portion of the organizational budget. Cost reduction opportunities are being sought and implemented, including tighter staffing plans and the introduction of lower paid personnel.

3. To what extent should staff preferences determine staffing and scheduling?

Staffing and scheduling is a fine balance of competing interests and needs. Predetermined standards, budget constraints, personal preferences, and legal aspects must all be taken into consideration. Staff satisfaction with scheduling is important, especially with varied shift length and unusual work hours as nurses attempt to meet the demands of their personal lives. A negotiation process may occur to ensure that both organizational and personal needs are met.

4. What is the role of the patient classification system for staffing and scheduling? Does this vary by setting of care?

The patient classification system provides a quantified measure of nursing time and effort required to care for clients. It attempts to identify acuity, as a proxy for workload, that then becomes the basis for staffing and budgeting. The system used varies by setting of care and type of nursing unit. There are three broad types of patient classification systems: prototype, factor, and computerized real-time factor systems.

5. Should a manager do the schedule or should staff schedule themselves?

Scheduling methods vary, including manager scheduling, secretarial scheduling, computerized scheduling, self-scheduling, or a combination of some or all methods. A shared governance environment may value self-scheduling as an aspect of autonomy.

6. What is the "right" mix of RNs and assistive personnel?

It is not clear what the effective and efficient mix of RNs and unlicensed assistive personnel is or should be. Experimentation is occurring with changed configurations of staff mix and the roles and functions of each category of worker in nursing. Evaluative efforts have been sparse and not of sufficient rigor to document that the use of nurse extenders is justified on cost, satisfaction, and quality bases.

CHAPTER 24: COMPUTER APPLICATIONS IN NURSING ADMINISTRATION

1. What role do computers play in nursing care?

Computers play a vital role in facilitating nursing care. Nursing informatics is the manipulation of nursing data and information to support care delivery. The use of computerized technology to collect data, document, and retrieve critical information rapidly is essential in care delivery. As a nursing tool, informatics affords nursing the opportunity to collect, manipulate, and retrieve data to support the use of resources; optimizes patient outcomes; and provides comparative data.

2. Who uses nursing's data?

Nursing data are used by all healthcare providers for client care decisions. The data are used by administrators to determine patient census, acuity, type of nursing care, and required resources and to assist in strategic planning and quality management activities. As nursing data sets become standardized across settings, they will provide useful data for cost, outcome, and quality comparisons.

3. What are the data used for?

Data obtained are used to formulate decision support for the client, the healthcare provider, and the organization. Researchers use the data in their investigations to examine clinical, cost, quality, and effectiveness outcomes. Regulatory bodies review nursing data to determine compliance to rules and regulations.

4. What difference do nurses who manage healthcare services make and under what circumstances?

Nursing personnel constitute the largest number of healthcare providers in most healthcare organizations. Yet the role that nursing plays in managing healthcare services is often unrecognized and "invisible." Without standardized nursing informatics to collect and integrate nursing data, physicians and hospitals will continue to receive recognition and reimbursement for the services nurses perform.

5. What are the cost, quality, and satisfaction outcomes that nurses are mainly responsible for?

Nursing practice impacts all cost, quality, and client satisfaction outcomes. Examples of cost outcomes include length of stay, supply cost per unit of service, and labor costs by acuity level per client. Quality outcomes include medication errors, documentation compliance, and infection rates. Satisfaction outcomes may include patients', nurses', or physicians' ratings of patient care services.

6. Which data need to be client specific, nurse specific, or organization specific?

Client-specific data include clinical data related to the client, the client's plan of care, and evaluation of interventions. Nurse-specific data include licensure, certification and competencies, and employee satisfaction. Organization-specific data elements include human and fiscal resource statistics; recruitment and retention figures; quality and effectiveness measures; and variables reflecting access, availability, and utilization of healthcare services.

CHAPTER 25: QUALITY IMPROVEMENT AND RISK MANAGEMENT

1. Whose responsibility is quality management?

Quality management is the responsibility of the organization and the care providers. All levels of management and care providers are accountable for the knowledge of and adherence to standards of care. The professional nurse is responsible for monitoring her or his own practice.

2. What are the differences between institutional and professional responsibilities for quality? Why does this occur?

Institutional responsibilities for quality are directly linked to organizational efforts to provide a quality healthcare system. These responsibilities often include meeting external mandates for accreditation and reimbursement requirements. The professional responsibility for quality is more directly related to practice issues, client outcomes, and standards of care.

3. How is quality defined? How is it measured?

Quality can be defined as the characteristics manifested in the pursuit of excellence. Quality exists when outcomes compare favorably with standards and when effectiveness, efficiency, benefit, and appropriateness of service are demonstrated. Quality is measured by evaluating structure, process, and outcomes; relating outcomes to standards; and measuring performance. Structure looks at the internal characteristics of the organization, process evaluates the method of attaining the outcomes, and outcomes are measured by evaluating the services.

4. How is the implementation of TQM/CQI affected by healthcare reform?

The goal of reform is to provide accessible, affordable, client-centered healthcare services to all citizens. TQM/CQI methods can accomplish the goals of healthcare reform by incorporating multidisciplinary employee participation in service improvements, with an emphasis on customer satisfaction.

5. What components of CQI are easiest/hardest to implement? Why?

The easiest components of CQI to implement are identifying key processes in the organization in need of improvement, designating multidisciplinary teams, and scheduling meetings. The hardest CQI components to implement are shifting to a customer-oriented focus, involving all employees in decision making, and changing managerial performance expectations.

6. **How are research and quality management related? Can they be combined in one program?**

Research and quality management both focus on problem identification, measurement, and resolution. The focus of research is to generate knowledge, whereas quality management focuses on performance standards and integrates research findings into clinical practice. Incorporating research into quality management strengthens performance measures and the evaluation of care standards.

7. **What is the relationship of payment to level of quality?**

Maintaining a minimal level of quality in care delivery is mandated through accreditation by regulatory agencies. Without accreditation, reimbursement from federal agencies can be jeopardized or withheld.

CHAPTER 26: MANAGEMENT OF CHANGE

1. **How do individuals in organizations get the information resources that they need in order to effect change?**

Individuals in organizations obtain information resources through formal and informal networks, professional organizations, regulatory agencies, and professional associates. Internally, information flows upward and downward through formal networks in the organizational hierarchy. Informal networks are often called the "grapevine" and branch throughout the organization.

2. **How can informal leaders be used for successful change?**

The successful implementation of a change process cannot be achieved solely by management or formal leaders. Managers can use informal leaders to build coalitions and to enlist the remaining members to successfully implement change. Identification and collaboration with informal leaders minimizes resistance to change and maximizes staff involvement.

3. **What changes need to take place in nursing? Why?**

Several changes need to occur in nursing. The first change is to clearly articulate that nursing is a profession based on a solid body of knowledge. Clinical judgments are based in nursing science and involve the diagnosis and treatment of human responses. Nurses must assume accountability for their role in autonomous and interdisciplinary decision making in order to enjoy the financial and social rewards of a professional. Nursing also must implement a standardized nursing language, develop large data bases, and demand self-regulation to ensure professional control of nursing practice.

4. How does resistance manifest itself?

Resistance to change is often manifested in individuals by defensive and hostile behaviors because of the uncertainty and ambiguity in job requirements. Potential sources for resistance to change include misunderstanding of the purpose and need for the change, insufficient explanation or information concerning the change, inability or lack of involvement in the planning process, lack of trust between management and staff, and low tolerance for change.

5. How can nurses' perceptions be changed to result in empowerment? Why is this important?

Acknowledgment of nurses' perceptions, with inclusion of their ideas, feedback, and innovations, fosters autonomy, creativity, and active participation. If this is done consistently, nurses will readily perceive that their input into decision making is valuable. Individuals who feel empowered will be more apt to challenge the status quo and effect change.

6. How should nursing education change? Why?

Nursing education must provide nurses with leadership skills that include effective interpersonal skills, conflict management, team building, collegiality, and change. Nurses often react and adapt to changes, yet are not knowledgeable enough to initiate change. By educating novice nurses, the profession of nursing will be able to proactively and creatively take advantage of opportunities to effect change to improve nursing care, service delivery, and professional practice.

7. Do we have too much change? What can be done about this?

Change is inevitable. It is a constant process that can be planned or unplanned. The more unplanned change that occurs, the more out-of-control we feel. If we can move the change processes to the end of the planned-versus-haphazard continuum, we regain control and can actively plan the change, examine the potential results, involve the participants, and determine outcomes.

CHAPTER 27: PERFORMANCE APPRAISAL

1. What experiences have you had in the past with performance appraisals? Have those experiences been positive or negative? Why?

Experiences in the past with performance appraisals may be a combination of conducting and receiving. Recipients of performance appraisals that have been positive cite being given the opportunity to identify personal, professional, and system variables that either interfered with or enhanced performance. Goal setting done in collaboration with the manager results in a motivational process that could serve as a template for conducting one's own future employee performance appraisals.

2. **Why does the handling of the performance appraisal process leave an aftermath of feelings?**

A performance appraisal is an evaluative process that is very personal. You are being evaluated for your level of performance. The system used to quantify your performance is tied to both the evaluator's and your perceptions, biases, and values; therefore the evaluator's and your opinions may differ. This can result in a concern that the appraisal may not truly reflect your performance. If the evaluation is positive, you will probably feel rewarded and motivated to continue at a high level of excellence.

3. **Think about those times when you were evaluated in a positive and constructive manner. Why was that a good experience?**

Performance appraisals that have been positive and constructive are those that incorporated self-evaluation along with peer assessment and collaborative goal setting. The most important component of this type of evaluation is the self-assessment. The requirement of quantifying one's own accomplishments or identifying areas to grow assists in the individual's recognition of areas to improve or of capabilities to further develop. The collaborative goal setting process with the manager provides direction for future growth.

4. **How do you feel when you are expected to evaluate others? Why?**

Evaluating others is a process that one learns and is a skill that takes experience to develop. Objectivity must be maintained, with a focus on counseling, identification of resources for facilitating improvement, and negotiating for goal attainment. Developing the employee's potential for performance and stimulating growth and skill development is an on-going process that requires mentoring and continuous feedback.

5. **How are performance appraisals and quality improvement related?**

Performance appraisals and quality improvement share many of the same process steps. They share data collection, standards comparison, needs assessment, and mutual goal setting. Both processes measure outcomes.

6. **How should pay, promotions, and other rewards be tied to performance and its evaluation?**

Pay, promotions, and other rewards should be tied to the individual's performance and should be based on outcomes. Knowledge, skill, professional development, and the individual's accomplishment of goals should serve as the basis for the reward. Data should be collected, quantified, and documented throughout the evaluation period and should be presented objectively by the evaluator.

7. How do you evaluate the performance of a team?

Effective evaluation of the performance of a team is not without its system problems. A team evaluation should be based on *team* strengths, accomplishments, and demonstration of *team* motivation. The tendency is to evaluate the individual performance of the team members, but this does not appraise how those individuals worked together and problem solved *as a team*.

CHAPTER 28: PRODUCTIVITY AND COSTING OUT NURSING

1. Why would quality of care suffer when nursing care hours are reduced?

The quality of care is influenced by multiple factors, including the staff mix, the care delivery system, acuity levels, and the number of caregivers assigned to direct and indirect client care activities. When nursing care hours are reduced, there is less time to perform all of the required client care activities scheduled. The nurse is forced to work faster, streamline documentation, or decrease client-centered activities. When nursing care hours are cut drastically, the nurse may have to prioritize client care and complete the most urgent care first, leaving many client care activities undone.

2. Do more experienced nurses work more productively? Why or why not?

Productivity is based on many factors, including knowledge, experience, motivation, administrative support, and commitment to quality care. Experienced nurses are generally more productive than novice nurses because they have more experience and a strong knowledge base from which to make astute clinical judgments. If experienced nurses are not motivated, lack support from superiors, or have serious personal problems, their productivity level may decline. As novice nurses gain experience, speed in completing procedures accurately, and confidence in their clinical judgments, their productivity level increases.

3. Why should nurses worry about productivity?

Nurses comprise the single largest expenditure for healthcare organizations. When cost-cutting strategies are instituted, areas with large expenditures are targeted for reductions. If nurses are unable to show that they are productive members of the healthcare team—positively impacting patient outcomes—they will be targeted for reductions in force.

4. What issues in productivity are most urgent? Why?

It is important for nurses to standardize the measurement of productivity. Productivity measures are complex because quantifying nursing care outcomes is difficult, there are no clear relationships between care process and nursing outcomes, and the most efficient resources for performing care are unknown. Without a standardization of productivity measures, comparisons among units and facilities is meaningless.

5. How do nurses determine if their care is effective and efficient?

Effectiveness is doing the right things and achieving quality outcomes, whereas efficiency is how fast the service or product is completed in a cost-effective manner. Nurses have established quality improvement programs and monitor indicators of care for compliance. Quality programs determine how effective the care has been. Efficiency is usually monitored by productivity measures, and costs are tracked by examining actual costs compared to budgeted projections, adjusting for units of service or patient days.

6. Why should nurses cost out their services?

Costing out nursing services is important so nurses know the actual cost of services to clients. This knowledge is used for reimbursement decisions and to facilitate health policy. In order to obtain third party reimbursement, nurses must be able to cost out nursing care and clearly articulate the services nurses provide for a set fee. Armed with data, nurses will be able to negotiate contracts from a cost basis.

7. How can nurses control healthcare costs? Nursing costs?

There are many ways to contain costs. Skilled managers facilitate workers' efforts to collaborate efficiently and effectively in accomplishing organizational goals. Sibson (1976) identified four ways to increase employee productivity by substituting equipment for human labor, improving work methods, removing unproductive practices, and improving human resource management. Healthcare costs can be controlled by case management of those at highest risk, by providing community-based care, and by using nurse practitioners in primary care settings. Nursing costs can be controlled by evaluating skill mix, facilitating interdisciplinary collaboration, and using critical pathways.

8. What is the ideal ratio of nurses to clients?

There is no magic or ideal ratio of nurses to clients. The ratio of nurses to clients is dependent upon the acuity level of patients, the educational and experience level of the nurse, the technology required for client care, the work methods, the care delivery system, and the information system. Evaluating the standards of care, conducting time and motion studies, and evaluating client care requirements form the basis of tools necessary to determine the ratio of nurses to clients.

CHAPTER 29: MANAGING A STRESSFUL ENVIRONMENT

1. What sources of stress do you find to be the most important influences in your life and work?

Internal and external sources of stress occur concurrently in both personal and professional lives. Internal sources of stress can be attributed to emotional, psychological, or physical factors. On the other hand, external sources of stress may be a result of an individual's interaction with the environment. Work environment stressors can impact how an individual perceives his or her role and responsibilities.

2. What coping strategies are most useful for stress reduction? Why are they helpful?

The individual's personality characteristics and perceptions of the external environment, along with past experiences with similar stressors, will determine what coping mechanisms will be most useful. Coping mechanisms are used to maintain or regain equilibrium to adjust to perceived stressful situations. Effective coping mechanisms reduce emotional distress, enhance problem resolution, and facilitate self-esteem. Examples of coping strategies include humor, complying, resigning, using a personal support network, spending time on hobbies, and using relaxation techniques.

3. To what extent should employers pay for stress management programs for nurses?

Human resources are the largest fiscal expenditures for organizations. Work-related stress can lead to job dissatisfaction, poor performance, and high turnover rates. As a result of high turnover rates, personnel costs are increased because of recruitment and orientation of new staff. Employee-oriented organizations establish stress management programs to minimize occupational stress in order to foster job satisfaction, productivity, and retention.

4. Why should nurses manage their own stress?

The healthcare environment is stressful, with high patient acuity levels, staffing shortages, specialty care requirements, ethical dilemmas, and dangerous situations jeopardizing individual safety. In addition, each professional nurse has her or his own personal stressors. Taking steps to proactively manage and minimize the stress in your personal and professional roles enhances your level of productivity and satisfaction.

5. Why should nurses promote reality shock support for new graduates?

While trying to successfully make a transition from student to clinician, new graduate nurses experience personal and professional stressors. During this first year of reality shock, novice nurses gain experience. It is also within this first year that job satisfaction, organizational commitment, and professionalism are affected. Experienced nurses can assist, mentor, and coach new graduates to recognize stressors and to develop effective stress management strategies.

6. What can nurses do to manage stress in work teams?

Identification of stressors, effective communication, conflict resolution, and group support minimize stress in work teams. As the work team becomes more knowledgeable about stressors, collaboration occurs to design effective strategies to reduce stress in the work environment.

CHAPTER 30: HEALTH POLICY AND THE NURSE

1. What are nursing's major healthcare values?

There are numerous values that the profession of nursing maintains regarding healthcare. Access and availability of care, patient advocacy, and quality care are examples of the mainstay of nursing values.

2. Is caring a healthcare policy? Why or why not?

Policy making is dependent on values and analysis, therefore caring influences healthcare policy. As nursing advocates for healthcare reform, a central value, caring, guides initiatives to make services affordable, accessible, and client centered in order to optimize the health and welfare of the public.

3. What kind of public policies govern your life? Govern nursing practice?

Your life is governed by the judicial system, including taxes, laws, and legal judgments. Nursing practice is regulated by the state's Nurse Practice Act, licensure, standards of practice, and legalities. Organizational guidelines influence nursing practice as well as regulatory, governmental, and professional organizations such as the Joint Commission on Accreditation of Healthcare Organizations, the Centers for Disease Control and Prevention, and the World Health Organization.

4. Which level of government is responsible for the health of the citizens?

All levels of government (legislative, judicial, and executive) are responsible in some manner for the health of its citizens. The legislative branch creates bills to enact laws that affect healthcare. The judicial level oversees civil and criminal cases that influence the direction of healthcare. The executive level participates in policy development that impacts healthcare, such as universal healthcare and Medicare/Medicaid reimbursement.

5. **Should illegal aliens be included in healthcare policy and benefits?**

   The issue of healthcare benefits for illegal aliens is an ethical dilemma and as such requires a moral foundation for analysis. One may argue that healthcare should not be denied because of lack of citizenship. Another argument is that many health services are paid through government subsidies financially supported by taxpayers. If taxpayers cannot afford healthcare for all citizens, then they should not be expected to financially support healthcare services for illegal aliens.

6. **Why are nursing profession issues important enough to be on the public policy agenda? Which ones are?**

   Nurses introduce policy on public health and welfare. Nursing advocates for access to care for all citizens, which is a central issue in healthcare reform. Current nursing professional issues on the public policy agenda include continuing education for relicensure, reimbursement for advanced practice nurses, access to care, and the use of unlicensed assistive personnel.

7. **Why is politics useful to nurses?**

   Politics is influencing the allocation of resources or using power to implement change. The political system becomes an important tool that can be used by nurses to educate the public regarding accessibility and availability of healthcare services. Nurses can also use political agendas to effect public welfare and professional status.

8. **Why can nurses be influential in policy and politics? How does this happen?**

   Nurses have the knowledge of healthcare and political skills to effect public policy. Nursing is the largest group of healthcare providers and as a united group has a strong political voice. Nurses can be influential in politics by voting, encouraging others to vote, lobbying Congress, forming political action committees or coalitions, and, most importantly, running for political offices.

CHAPTER 31: CAREER DEVELOPMENT

1. **Why should nurses plan a career? Why not just follow the available jobs?**

   Individuals are motivated to study nursing for various reasons. Often, individuals seek nursing education to obtain an attractive position. However, frequently these individuals do not perceive nursing as a professional career precipitating role dissatisfaction, burn-out, and job turnover from haphazard job movement. Planning a career is indicative of commitment, investment, and active involvement in the profession.

2. Why are you motivated for a job or a career in nursing?

Identifying your reasons for attending nursing school will determine whether or not you perceive nursing as a job or a career. Examining your goals, strengths, and needs will help you identify your motivation for working and assist you in developing career goals.

3. What developmental stage are you in? How does that affect your career planning?

Individuals experience the dynamic process of growth and development as they continue through the life span. As adults progress through developmental stages, changes that are encountered often impact the balance between work, self, family needs, and roles. Adaptation or adjustment to these changes has an inevitable impact upon career needs and decisions. Identification of your current developmental stage through periodical self-analysis will enhance your career development.

4. How much should your employer contribute to your career development?

Regulatory organizations and the community at large expect quality, competent healthcare. In order to fulfill this expectation, professional preparation, continuing education, and/or self-directed learning must take place to remain current in professional practice. Employers and employees should collaborate to establish mechanisms to meet employees' professional growth needs. In order to fulfill the employer's obligation to hire and maintain competent practitioners, the employer should support career counseling and professional development through educational and fiscal contributions.

5. Is career planning encouraged in your employment setting? Why/why not?

Formal and informal continuing educational programs are frequently available for healthcare professionals. Most healthcare organizations provide some tuition or financial reimbursement for educational programs or continuing education. Managers may assist employees in developing professional goals in conjunction with performance appraisals, but often this does not include self-reflection, analysis, or career planning and development.

6. Why do nurses pursue nurse practitioner certification or licensure?

Nurses pursue advanced nursing education, certification, and/or licensure as strategies for career development and State Board of Nursing requirements. The demand for nurse clinicians practicing in advanced nursing roles with greater autonomy is increasing. As healthcare shifts from tertiary to primary care, advanced practice nurses will assume broader roles. Graduate level education, certification, and/or licensure are credentials to assure the public that clinicians have the qualifications to provide specialized services to consumers.

Index

Note: Page numbers in *italics* refer to illustrations; page numbers followed by t refer to tables.

A

Accommodation, in conflict management, 421
Accountability, definition of, 232
  personal, 291–292
Achievement need, 364
Activity, definition of, 358
Acuity, definition of, 449
Ad hoc committee, 156
Adaptors, 107
Adhocracy, 246–247, *247*, 249
  definition of, 242, *242*
Administrative model, of shared governance, 267, *269*
Adulthood, stages of, 594–595
Advance practice nursing, negotiations for, 443–444
Advanced practice nursing, 605–606
Advocacy power, 395
Affiliation need, 364, 365
AIDS unit, creation of, 511–512
Altruism, 41
Ambulatory care, quantification of, 456–457
Ambulatory Care Patient Classification Tool, 457
American Nurses' Association, 74
  Social Policy Statement of, 497
Analgesia, nursing labor costs for, 175–176
Anecdotal notes, for performance measurement, 536
Appearance, communicative content of, 341–342, *343*, 345
  professional, 44–45
Assertiveness, *385*
Assessment skills, 179
Assurance, definition of, 483
Attitudes, about motivation, 374–376
  about power, 383
  motivation and, 360, *361*
Audit, for quality assurance, 493–494

B

Authority, 388, 390, 391
  definition of, 232
Autonomy, in ethical decision making, 133
  in shared governance, 265–266
  professional, 424
Avoidance, in conflict management, 420–421

B

Bargaining, definition of, 436
  in conflict management, 422, 425
Base pay, 373
Behavior, change in, 512–513, *513*
  communicative content of, 341–342
Beneficence, in ethical decision making, 133
Bill, legislative, 584–585
Billing errors, 24–25, *25*
Blocking, 385
Bona Fide Occupational Qualification, 97
Brainstorming, 162
Budget(s), cost measure for, 175
  definition of, 168, 169
  performance, 174
  process for, 174–175
  traditional, 174
  types of, 170
  volume measure for, 175
  zero-based, 174
Bureaucracy, 242–244, *243*, 248. See also
  Shared governance.
  line and staff, 243–244, *243*
  pyramidal, 243, *243*
  vs. shared governance, 264
Burnout, 565–566
  definition of, 561, 562

C

Capital budget, 170
  definition of, 168
Capitated payment, 548

C

Cardiopulmonary resuscitation team, 246
Care modality, 300. See also *System of nursing care delivery.*
Care paths, evaluation of, 320
Career, definition of, 593
Career anchors, 596
Career commitment, 603
  definition of, 593–594
Career development, 592–608
  career anchors in, 596
  continuing education for, 605
  early stage of, 601
  first job in, 597–598
  graduate education for, 607
  late stage of, 601
  marketing for, 604
  middle stage of, 601
  planning for, 596–597, 597t, 598–599
  self-analysis for, 595–596, *595*
  skilled performance stages in, 600–601
  societal influences on, 599
  styles of, 599–602
  tenure categories in, 601
Career planning, 596–597, 597t, 598–599
Caregiver role, 458
Caring, concept of, 220
Case and effect chart, for decision making, 129–130
Case management, 307, 309–310
  care coordination role in, 325, 329
  client assessment in, 325–326
  definition of, 320–322
  development of, 326–327
  employment settings for, 327
  implementation of, 325–326
  models of, 324–325
  organizational assessment in, 325–326
  principles of, 325–326
  vs. managed care, 322
Case nursing, 302
Cash budget, 170
  definition of, 168

Central tendency effect, in performance appraisal, 540
Centralization, of power, 232, 260
Certification, 606–607
Change, 506–527
  adoption of, 515–516
    persuasion and, 437
  continuum of, 507–508
  definition of, 507
  in attitudes, 512, *513*
  in behavior, 512–513, *513*
  in group, 512
  in individual, 512
  in information systems, 508, 510
  in knowledge, 512, *513*
  in labor force, 508, *508*, 510
  in organizational structure, 508, *508*
  in reimbursement, 508, 510
  levels of, 512, *513*
  organizational culture in, 201, 203
  organizational structure in, 235–236
  planned, 510–513, 515t
    change agents in, 516–517
    definition of, 507
    effective, 522–523
    emotional responses to, 518
    individual response to, 525
    Lewin's force field analysis of, 513–518, *514*
    moving stage of, 514, *514*
    process of, 513–521, *514*, 516
    refreezing stage of, 514, *514*
    resistance to, 518, 520–521, *520*
    success of, 516, 522–523
    unfreezing stage of, 513–514, *514*
  power and, 390, *390*
  response to, 99
    groups in, 149–150
  stress of, 567, 571–573
  to shared governance, 271–272
  vs. innovation, 524
Change agents, 516–517
  definition of, 507
Change cycles, 522
Change theory, 513–521, *514*, 517t
Chaos, theory of, 99
Charge, definition of, 177
Charisma, 386
Checklists, for performance measurement, 536
Climate, organizational, definition of, 193

Clinical decision unit, development of, 519–520
Clinical indicators, 138
Clinical nurse specialists, 605–606
Clinical practice guidelines, 139
Coaching, 87, 534
Coalition, 385
Code blue review, 541
Code of Ethics, 39
Coercive power, 386, 398
Cognitive appraisal, of stressor, 564
Collaboration, 394
  in conflict management, 422, 425
Collective bargaining, 425, 426, 427, 438, 444
Commitment, career, 593–594, 603
  in persuasion, 433, *434*
Committee, definition of, 145, 155–156
Communication, 334–353
  assessment of, 347–349
  channel for, 339
  definition of, 335–336
  effectiveness of, 338–339, 342–343, 345
  emotional response to, 339
  feedback, 340–341
  formal/informal, 336, 344–345
  group, 337–338, *338*
    feedback during, 341
    types of, 338, *338*
  in conflict resolution, 423
  in leadership, 347–349
  instrumental/expressive, 336
  negative, 339–340
  nonverbal, 341–342
  of vision, 344–345
  organizational, 345
  personal/impersonal, 336, 348
  power and, 396
  problems in, 347–349
  sender-receiver model of, 336
  vertical/horizontal, 336
Community health nursing, quality assurance for, 488
Compensation, 20–25, *21*, 21t
  in motivation, 370, 373
  negotiation for, 442
Competition, economic, 445
  in conflict management, 422
Complex adaptive systems, 99
Compromise, in conflict management, 419–420, 422

Computer applications, 466–479
Computer-based Patient Record, 472
Computerized real-time factor patient classification system, 455t, 456
Conceptual acts, 3
Conflict, 406–428
  about professional autonomy, 424
  aftermath of, 410–411, *411*
  antecedent conditions of, 410, *411*
  collaborative work and, 415
  competitive, 410
  conceptualization of, 411, *412*
  constructive, 408
  definition of, 407–408
  dependency and, 415
  destructive, 408
  disruptive, 410, 417
  emotional cycle of, 411, *412*
  emotions and, 417
  felt, 410, *411*
  frustration in, 411, *412*
  interdependent relationships and, 392
  intergroup, 409, *409*
  interpersonal, 409, *409*, 415–416
  intrapersonal, 409, *409*
  job, 407
  management of, 413, 417–424, *419*. See also *Conflict management.*
  manifest, 410, *411*
  measurement of, 413
  miscommunication and, 414
  organizational, 407, 411–413
  perception of, 410, *411*
  personal behavior and, 416
  power divisions and, 414
  process of, 410–411, *411*
  role, 416
  sources of, 414–417
  staff retention and, 413–414
  stress of, 573
  types of, 408–410, *409*
  unresolvable, 414–415
Conflict management, 413, 417–424, *419*
  accommodating in, 421
  avoidance in, 420–421
  bargaining in, 422, 425
  collaboration in, 422, 425
  communication in, 423
  competing in, 422
  compromise in, 419–420, 422
  confrontation in, 422
  creative, 417, 420

Conflict management (*Continued*)
 defensive mode of, 418–419
 forcing in, 421–422
 inventories in, 422–423
 negotiation in, 422, 438. See also *Negotiation.*
 outcomes of, 423–424
 proactive, 425–426
 problem solving in, 422
 smoothing over in, 421
 team building and, 425–426
 withholding in, 421
Confrontation, 394
 in conflict management, 422
Congressional model, of shared governance, 267, *268*
Connection power, 388
Constructive criticism, 340–341
Contempt, for employees, 217
Continuous quality improvement (CQI), 74–75, 163–164, 485–486
 definition of, 483
Control, span of, 229, 256
Control chart, for quality assurance, 494
Controlling, definition of, 85
 in management, 87–88
Coordinating, definition of, 85
 in management, 86–87
Coping, 564, 568–569
Cosmopolitan-local construct, in professionalization research, 44
Cost(s), definition of, 170–171, 177
 of nursing services, 181, 183–185, *184,* 311–312, 552
Cost center, 176
Cost per unit of output, 551
Cost-benefit analysis, for decision making, 130, *130*
Cost-benefit model, 552
Cost-effectiveness model, 552
Costing out, 554
 definition of, 548, 549
 of nursing services, 183–185, *184*
Councilar model, of shared governance, 267, *268*
Courage, of leader, 55
Creativity techniques, in decision making, 128, 139–140
Critical incident description, for performance measurement, 536
Critical path, 307, 309
 definition of, 321–322

Critical path (*Continued*)
 for pneumonia, 322–323
 for quality improvement, 499–500
Critical pathways, for decision making, 138
Criticism, constructive, 340–341
Critiquing, in group communication, 341
Crossfunctional teams, 98–99
Cultural diversity, management of, 350–353
Culture, organizational, 193–200, *196*
 building of, 203, *203*
 definition of, 193–194
 explicit, 197
 human resources and, 204
 implicit, 197
 manifestations of, 197–198, 198t

D

Decentralization, horizontal, 261
 of power, 232
 vertical, 260–261
Decision making, 120–141
 about organizational structure, 234–236
 administrative, 125–126
 autocratic, 154
 clinical, *123,* 124
 consultative, 154
 continuum of control over, 126–128, *127*
 critical pathways for, 138
 decision trees for, 126, 128–129, *129*
 definition of, 121–122, *122*
 delegated, 154
 effective, 126
 ethical, 131–135, 134t
 executive, 137
 for delegation, 283–284
 for staffing, 450–452, 451t
 group, 153–154, *153*
  power of, 388–389
 in case management, 124–125
 information processing for, 131
 innovation in, 139–140
 joint, 154
 MORAL model of, 134
 organizational, *123,* 124
 participative, 265. See also *Shared governance.*
 perception in, 139–140

Decision making (*Continued*)
 personal, 123, *123*
 power over, 260, *261*
 prioritization for, 137
 problem identification for, 122
 situations for, 123–124, *123*
 steps in, 122–123
 strategies for, 128–131, *129, 130*
 styles of, 126
Decision tree, 126
 for decision making, 128–129, *129*
Defensive reaction, 341
 in conflict management, 418–419
Delegate, 281
 accountability of, 287–290
 definition of, 280
 resistance of, 286
Delegation, 229, 278–297
 barriers to, 284, 285–287
 definition of, 279–280
 feedback after, 340–341
 legal aspects of, 287–290
 pitfalls of, 285–287
 principles of, 281
 process of, 283–285
 style of, 286–287
 to unlicensed assistive personnel, 293
 tracking form for, 282
Delegator, accountability of, 287–290
 definition of, 280
Delphi survey technique, 162
Dependence, job-related, 392
Dependency, conflict and, 392, 415
Design group, 156
Diagnosis-related groups (DRG), in nursing productivity measures, 552–553, 554
Differentiated nursing practice, 457–459, *458*
Difficult people, management of, 90–92
Dilemma, 106, 195
Direct costs, definition of, 170–171
Discipline, by manager, 292
Disruptive conflict, 410
Distractions, in time management, 93
Division of labor, 229
Documentation, for performance appraisal, 540–541
DRG (Diagnosis-related group), in nursing productivity measures, 552–553, 554
Drugs, prescription, expenditures for, 20

E

Economic competition, 445
Economic rewards, in motivation, 373
Effectiveness, definition of, 548, 549
Effectiveness research, 467, 471–473, 474
Efficacy, definition of, 549
Efficiency, definition of, 548, 549
Ego needs, 362, *362*
Emotions, change and, 518
  conflict and, 417
Empathy, of leader, 55
Empowerment, 393, 399–402
  definition of, 52, 382–383
Environment, of social system, 210, *211*
  organizational, job satisfaction and,
    218–220, *219*
    stress and, 567
Equal Employment Opportunity Commission, 97
Errors, ethical issues of, 289–290
  nursing, 135–136, 138
Essay, for performance measurement, 536
Esteem needs, 362, *362*
Ethical issues, 132–135
  analysis of, 134
  code for, 39, 288
  contagious diseases and, 39
  decision making process for, 133–134,
    135, 183
  frequency of, 132–133
  in budgeting, 181–183
  in decision making, 131–135, 131–136
  in delegation, 293
  in health policy making, 587
  in staffing, 132–133, 135
  in stewardship, 182
  in unsafe situations, 289–290
  MORAL model for, 134
Exchange, *385*
Existence needs, 363
Expectancy theory, 361, 366
Expense, definition of, 168, 169
Expense budget, definition of, 168
Expert power, 386, 387–388, 391, 401
Expertise, of leader, 55

F

Factor patient classification system, 455t,
  456
Feedback, 340–341
Fidelity, in ethical decision making, 133
Fiedler's contingency theory, 62–64

Fight strategy, 394
Financial management, 173–176
  budgetary process in, 174–175
  cost awareness in, 178, 180–181
  definition of, 168
  ethical issues in, 181–183
  legal issues in, 181–183
  nursing billing in, 177–178
First impression, 342
Fishbone diagram, for decision making,
    129–130
  for quality assurance, 494
Float pool, 453
Flow chart, for quality assurance, 494
Followers, 53
  enlightened, 70
  maturity of, 66
Followership, 53, 69–71
  definition of, 52
  demographics of, 74
Forcing, in conflict management,
    421–422
Frustration, in motivation, 359–360
Function follows form model, 228
Functional nursing, 303–304

G

Governance, shared. See *Shared governance.*
Group(s), advantages of, 147–149
  behavior of, 160
  decision making by, 130, 153–154,
    153, 388–389
  definition of, 145–146
  disadvantages of, 151
  disruptive members of, 159–160
  leadership of, 157–158
  maintenance of, 158
  meetings of, 151–153
  members of, 158–159
  purposes of, 148–149
  reasons for, 147
  size of, 153
  stages of, 146–147
Group decision making, 130, 153–154,
  153
  power of, 388–389
Group nursing, 302–303
Growth needs, 363
Guessing errors, in performance appraisal,
    540
Guidance, of leader, 55

H

Halo effect, in performance appraisal,
    539
Hardiness, 565
  of leader, 400
Hawthorne Effect, 369
Healing power, 395
Health policy, 578–590, 587
  definition of, 579
  nursing leadership in, 587–589
  nursing research and, 582–583
Health services, definition of, 14
Healthcare expenditures, 17–20, *19*
  AIDS care in, 23
  billing errors and, 24–25, *25*
  diagnostic tests in, 23
  nursing compensation in, 20–22, *21*,
    21t
  payment for, 23
  per person, 19, *19*
  physician fees in, 20, *20*
  prescription drug costs in, 20
Healthcare system(s), 13–26
  definition of, 13–14, 16–17
  integrated, 15, 16
  leadership in, 23–24
  management in, 23–24
  structure of, 16–17, *16*
  types of, 14, 16–17, *16*
Hepatitis B, employee exposure to, 97
Herzberg's Motivation-Hygiene Theory,
    363–364, *363*
Home health agencies, perceptions of,
    192–193
Home health care, costs of, 172–173
  perceptions of, 199–200
Hours per patient day (HPPD), 452
Human development, stages of, 594–595
Human immunodeficiency virus (HIV),
    employee exposure to, 97
Human resources. See also *Performance
  appraisal.*
  legal aspects of, 97
  organizational culture and, 204

I

Image, of nursing, 342–343, 345
Imagination, in persuasion, 433, *434*
Incident report, in risk management pro-
    gram, 501
Incrementalism, 126
  for problem solving, 112–113

Indirect costs, definition of, 171
Indirect pay, 373
Individual, of social system, 210, *211*
Infection, employee exposure to, 97
Information power, 388, 398
Information systems, 466–479
  change in, *508*, 510
  engineering aspect of, 471
  for effectiveness research, 471–473
  for quality improvement, 470–471
  Nursing Management Minimum Data
    Set for, 475–477, 476t
  nursing's data needs for, 469–470,
    470t
  research aspect of, 471
Ingratiation, *385*
Innovation. See also *Change*.
  adoption of, 515–516
  benefit/cost analysis of, 517–518
  definition of, 523
  diffusion of, 524–525
  in decision making, 139–140
  sources of, 524
  vs. change, 524
Innovator, 107, 525
Input, definition of, 549
Inspiration power, 386
Integrated delivery networks, 15, 16
Integrative power, 395
Integrator role, 458–459
Intensity, of nursing services, 172, 185,
    450
Intensive care unit (ICU), restructuring
    of, 252–253, *252, 253*
  skill mix of, 294
Interactive model, of management,
    88–90
Intergroup conflict, 409, *409*
Internship, 604
Interpersonal conflict, 409, *409*
Interruptions, in time management, 93
Interview, job, 30-second hurdle of, 342
Intrapersonal conflict, 409, *409*
Iowa Model, 8, *8–9*

J
Job, conflicts of, 407
  definition of, 593
  redesign of, 236, 255–255
  satisfaction with, 218–220, *219,*
    373–374, 562–563
Job characteristics theory, 367–368

Joint Commission on Accreditation of
    Healthcare Organizations, quality
    assurance process of, 487–488
Justice, in ethical decision making, 133

K
Kanter's Structural Theory of Organiza-
    tional Power, 99–100

L
Labor, division of, 229
Language, in persuasion, 436
Leader, 52–53
  motive pattern of, 365
Leadership, 50–75
  behaviors of, 57, 71–73
  caring, 572
  change and, 521–523
  characteristics of, 55–58
  communication in, 54, 347–349
  competencies of, 57–58
  conflict and, 412–413
  conflict management and, 417–418, *419*
  definitions of, 4–5, 6–7, 51–52
  delegation in, 290–292
  exceptional, 71–73
  in career development, 602–605
  in health policy, 587–588
  management overlap with, 5–6, *7*
  motivation in, 375–376
  negotiating skills and, 441–442
  nurturing, 572
  optimizing behavior of, 57–58
  organizational goals in, 54
  persuasive skills in, 436–437
  power and, 389–390, *389,* 396–399
  power drive and, 383, *384*
  practices of, 71–73
  predispositions towards, 59–60
  productivity and, 59–60, 554–556
  situations of, 53–54, 60, 63–66, *64, 65*
  skills of, 54
  stress management and, 570–571
  styles of, 60–68
    authoritarian, 61
    definition of, 52
    democratic, 61
    effectiveness of, 64
    Fiedler's contingency theory of,
      62–64
    laissez-faire, 61–62
    productivity and, 59–60

Leadership (*Continued*)
  transactional, 66–68, *67*
  transformational, 66–69, *67*
  Tri-Dimensional Leader Effective-
    ness Model of, 64–66, *64, 65*
  theories of, 54–55
    attitudinal, 59–60
    characteristics, 55–58
    situational, 60, 63–66, *64, 66*
  transformative, 400, 572
  vision and, 400
  vs. management, 80
Legal issues, decision making process for,
    290
  in budgeting, 181–183
  in collective bargaining, 426–427, **444**
  in continuing education, 499
  in delegation, 287–290, 293
  in deployment, 183
  in employment, 183
  in licensure, 38, 39, 543, 606, 607
  in malpractice, 95–96, 289
  in management, 38–39, 95–98
  in negligence, 95–96, 289
  in policy making, 584–585
  in reimbursement, 606, 607
  in staffing, 116, 289–290
  in standard setting, 487–490, 497
  in supervision, 38–39, 287–290, 427,
    444
  in unsafe conditions, 290
  Medicaid, 18, 23
  Medicare, 18, 23
  Nurse Practice Act, 38, 288
  state code for, 288–289
Legislation, 584–585
Legitimate power, 388
Lewin's force field analysis, of planned
    change process, 513–518, *514*
Line and staff bureaucracy, 243–244, *243*
Line position, 229, 244
Long-range budget, 170
Lose-lose situation, in conflict manage-
    ment, 424

M
Magnet Hospital Study, 221–222
Malpractice, 95–96, 183
Managed care, 25–26, 307, 309–310
  definition of, 319
  evaluation of, 320
  vs. case management, 322

Management, 79–101
  as care, 83
  as cure, 83
  blended care, 84
  computerized information systems for, 473–475
  conflict, 417–424, *419. See also Conflict management.*
  conflict and, 412–413
  controlling in, 87–88
  coordinating in, 86–87
  definitions of, 5, 6–7, 52, 81–82, 94–95
  delegation in, 291–292
  four steps of, 82–83, *83*
  innovations in, 525
  interactive model of, 88–90
  leadership overlap with, 5–6, *7*
  legal aspects of, 87, 95–98
  negotiating skills and, 441–442
  of difficult people, 90–92
  of multicultural diversity, 350–353
  of organizational structure, 234–236
  organizing in, 86
  persuasive skills in, 437
  planning in, 84–85
  power and, 391
  productivity monitoring in, 554–556
  quality assurance by, 496–497
  roles of, 88–90, *89*
  stress management by, 570–571
  systems view of, 81–82, *82*
  time, 92–93
  training for, 95
  vs. leadership, 80
  work of, 88–90, *89*
Management by Objectives, 366–367
Management information system. See also *Information systems.*
  definition of, 467–468
Management theory, 5
Manager, 94
  discipline by, 292
  in motivation, 375–376
  performance appraisal by, 541–542
  personal accountability of, 291–292
Maslow's hierarchy of needs, 362–363, *362*
Matrix structures, 244–246, *245, 246*
  definition of, 242, *242*
Maturity, definition of, 64–65
Medicaid, 18

Medicare, 18
Meetings, group, 151–153
  leadership for, 153
  recorder of, 158
Mentoring, 371–372
Miscommunication, 337
Mission statement, 196, 212, 215
Mixed scanning, 126
Modular nursing, 305
Monitoring system, in risk management program, 501
MORAL model, of decision making, 134
Morale, problems of, 292
Motivation, 357–379
  attitudes about, 374–376
  attitudes and, 360, *361*
  definition of, 358
  economic rewards in, 373
  expectancy theories and, 366
  external, 360
  Hawthorne Effect in, 369
  Herzberg's Motivation-Hygiene Theory and, 363–364, *363*
  in nursing, 369–370
  in organizations, 368–369
  internal, 360
  job characteristics theory and, 367–368
  job satisfaction and, 364
  lack of, 530–531
  Management by Objectives and, 366–367
  Maslow's hierarchy of needs theory and, 362–363, *362*
  McClelland's theory and, 364–365
  mentoring and, 371–372
  Need Satisfaction Model and, *360, 361,* 459–361
  recognition in, 370, 372
  reinforcement theories and, 367
  rewards in, 370, 372, 376
  self-assessment of, 365
  structuring of, 377
  Theory X and, 368
  Theory Y and, 368
Motivation to work, definition of, 358
Motive, definition of, 358
Multicultural diversity, facilitation of, 351
  management of, 350–353
  guidelines for, 352

Multidisciplinary interdivisional committee, 156
Mutual adjustment, for work coordination, 231

N
National Labor Relations Act (1935), 425, 426, 444
"National Nursing Image Campaign," 343
National Practitioner Data Bank, 473
Need, definition of, 358
Need Satisfaction Model, *360, 361,* 459–361
Negligence, 95–96
Negotiation, 394, 436–446
  climate for, 441
  competitive, 438
  cooperative, 438
  definition of, 436
  for compensation, 442
  formal, 440
  in conflict management, 422
  maneuvering room in, 441
  process of, 439–341
  strategies for, 440–441
Networked organizations, 98–99
Nominal group technique, 162
Nonmaleficence, in ethical decision making, 133
Nonnursing tasks, definition of, 280
Nonverbal communication, 341–342
  definition of, 335
Non-violent restraint, 349–350
Nurse extenders, 292–293, 295, 460–462, *461*
  definition of, 450
Nurse manager. See also *Management.*
  definition of, 94
Nurse Practice Act, 38, 45–46
Nurse practitioners, 605–606
Nurse-managed clinic, group institution of, 149–150
Nurse-physician relationships, stress of, 567
Nursing, as career, 596–597, *597t. See also Career development.*
Nursing: A Social Policy Statement, 606, 607
Nursing activities, definition of, 280
Nursing administration, 1–10. See also *Leadership; Management.*

Nursing administration (*Continued*)
  definition of, 3–5
  Iowa Model of, 8, 8–9
  models for, 7–9, 8
  sources of, 5
  theoretical basis of, 5
Nursing assistant, evaluation of, 285
Nursing care delivery systems, definition of, 300
Nursing homes, environmental turbulence in, 272–273
  shared governance in, 273
Nursing hours per patient day (HPPD), 551
Nursing informatics, 471
  definition of, 467
Nursing Information System, 472
Nursing intensity, 172, 185, 450
Nursing management, 79–101, 81–82, 94–95. See also *Management*.
Nursing Management Minimum Data Set, 475–477, 476t
Nursing Organization's Liaison Forum, 163
Nursing practice, ANA standards of, 489–490, 490
  continuum of, 457–459, 458
Nursing profession, 28–46
  barriers to, 41–42
  criteria for, 32–34, 32t
  definition of, 31
  gender issues in, 42
  legal aspects of, 38
  nurses' attitudes toward, 42
  role behaviors in, 35–37
Nursing resources, definition of, 449
Nursing services, costing out of, 183–185, 184
  costs of, 181
  intensity of, 172, 185, 450
  physician practice style and, 185–186
  reimbursement for, 177–178, 475, 556
Nursing theory, 5
Nursing workload, definition of, 449
"Nursing's Agenda for Health Care Reform," 589

O
Objectives, of organization, 214
Open-ended essay, for performance measurement, 536
Operating budget, 170

Optimizing, in decision making, 126
Optimizing behavior, of leader, 57–58
Organization, communication in, 345
  definition of, 335
  conflict in, 407, 411–413
Organization(s), 209, 209
  accountability in, 232
  authority in, 232
  bureaucratic, 242–244, 243
  chart of, 249–251, 250
  climate of, audit of, 199
    definition of, 193
  culture of, 192, 193–200, 196
    building of, 203, 203
    definition of, 193–194
    explicit, 197
    human resources and, 204
    implicit, 197
    manifestations of, 197–198, 198t
  definition of, 209, 209
  environment of, job satisfaction and, 218–220, 219
  life cycle of, 230, 230
  middle line of, 244
  mission statements of, 212
  objectives of, 214
  operating core of, 244
  philosophy of, 217–219
  philosophy statements of, 212–213
  policies of, 214–216
  positions of, 232
  power in, 390–392, 390
  procedures of, 216–217
  purpose statements of, 214
  responsibility in, 232–233
  restructuring of, 254–255, 255
  staff of, 244
  strategic apex of, 244
  stress management plan of, 569
  stress of, 567
  structure of, 191–193, 191t, 230–231
    adhocratic, 246–247, 247, 249
    bureaucratic, 248
    change and, 235–237
    decentralized, 254. See also *Shared governance*.
    definition of, 226–227, 227
    divisional, 248–249
    horizontal, 250, 250
    matrix, 244–246, 245, 246
    simple, 248
    size in, 229

Organization(s) (*Continued*)
    social environment in, 229
    task factors in, 229–230
    technologic factors in, 229
    types of, 230–231, 247–249
    vertical, 250, 250
  support staff of, 244
  technostructure of, 244
  work coordination in, 230–231
Organizational chart, 249–251, 250
Organizational Climate Audit, 199
Organizational Culture Inventory, 199
Organizing, definition of, 85
  in management, 86
Outcome standards, for quality assurance, 492
Outcomes research, 471–473, 474, 497
Output, definition of, 549

P
Pain management, protocol for, 498–499
Paradox, 106, 195
Pareto chart, for quality assurance, 494–495
Participative/affirmative power, 395
Patient Care Specialty Technician, 462
Patient classification, 454, 455–456, 455t
Patient Self-Determination Act (1990), 587
Patient-centered care, 308–309
Peer review, definition of, 530
Perceived Conflict Scale, 413
Perception, in decision making, 139–140
Performance, 530–531
  categories of, 537
Performance appraisal, 529–546
  absolute standard in, 533
  anecdotal notes for, 536
  behavioral categories for, 537
  central tendency effect in, 540
  checklists for, 536
  comparative standard in, 533–534
  components of, 531
  conventional, 530
  critical incident descriptions for, 536
  definition of, 530
  developmental purpose of, 533
  documentation for, 540–541
  effective, 540–541
  evaluative purpose of, 533
  evaluator errors in, 539–540
  for professional accountability, 540–541

Performance appraisal (*Continued*)
  guessing errors in, 540
  halo effect in, 539
  informal aspects of, 534
  log notes for, 538
  mechanisms of, 532–533, *533*
  of teams, 543–544
  open-ended essays for, 536
  outcomes of, 535
  peer review for, 538
  performance categories in, 537
  performance measurement tools for,
    536–539
  principles of, 536
  problem distortion in, 539
  process of, 534–536, *534*
  purposes of, 532–534
  rater temperament effect in, 540
  rating scales for, 537
  recency effect in, 539
  self-evaluations for, 538
  standards for, 533–535
  subjectivity of, 531–532
  sunflower effect in, 539
  values and, 531–532
Personal accountability, 291–292
Personal power, 384–385, 391
Persuasion, 432–437
  categories of, 434
  definition of, 432
  effective, 433–434, *434*, 435–436
  language in, 436
  objective of, 432
  tactics of, 435, *435*
Philosophy, of organization, 217–219
Philosophy statement, 212–213
Physical acts, 3
Physician fees, 20, *20*
Physician's order, ethical issues and,
    289
Physiological needs, 362, *362*
Pilot projects, for decision making, 128
Planning, 168, *169*
  definition of, 85
  in management, 84–85
Pneumonia, critical path of, 322–323
Policy (policies), definition of, 215, 579
  formulation of, 580–581, *581*
  implementation of, *581*, 583
  modification of, *581*, 583–584
  of organization, 214–216
  vs. procedures, 216–217

Policy-making, 579–580
  process of, 580–584, *581*
Politics, 585
  definition of, 579
  participation in, 586
Position(s), definition of, 232
  of organization, 243–144
Position power, 391
Power, 381–403
  access to, 392
  advocacy, 395
  attitudes about, 383
  centralization of, 232, 260
  change and, 390, *390*
  coercive, 386, 398
  communication, 396
  connection, 388
  decentralization of, 260–262, *261*
    definition of, 232
  decision making, 260, *261*
  definition of, 100, 382
  effective use of, 394–396
  environmental enhancement of,
    401–402
  expert, 386, 387–388, 391, 401
  healing, 395
  in organizations, 390–392, *390*
  information, 388, 398
  integrative, 395
  leadership and, 389–390, *389*,
    396–399
  legitimate, 388
  mechanisms of, 385, *385*
  negative, 383
  of group decision making, 388–389
  of nurses, 395–396
  opportunities for, 398
  participative/affirmative, 395
  perception of, 395, 397
  personal, 384–385, 391
  position, 391
  positive, 383
  problem-solving, 395
  professional, 384, 385
  professional autonomy and, 399
  referent, 386
  resource control and, 391
  reward, 386
  sources of, 386–388, 391, 398–399
  transfer of, 401
  transformational, 395
Power moments, 394

Power need, 364, 365
Powerless job, 392
Preceptorship, 604
Primary nursing, 305–306, 324
Prioritizing, in decision making, 137
  in time management, 93
Private duty nursing, 302, 323, 324
Problem, definition of, 105
Problem critique, for decision making, 128
Problem distortion, in performance appraisal, 539
Problem solving, 104–117
  collaboration for, 114
  consequences of, 109
  consultation for, 114
  creative, in conflict management, 420
  decision making for, 109. See also *Decision making*.
  definition of, 105
  delegation for, 114
  direct intervention for, 114
  economic factors in, 116
  implementation of, 109–110, *111*
  in conflict management, 422
  indirect intervention for, 114
  information gathering for, 108
  prioritization in, 109–110, *111*
  problem definition for, 108–109
  purposeful inaction for, 114
  relentless incrementalism for, 112–113
  solution development in, 109,
    113–114, *113*
  steps of, 108–112
  styles of, 107–108
  teams for, 116–117
Problem-solving power, 395
Procedures, definition of, 216
  of organization, 216–217
  vs. policies, 216–217
Process standards, for quality assurance,
    492
Productivity, 554
  definition of, 548
  DRG-related measures of, 552–553,
    554
  in rural hospitals, 553–554
  increases in, 550
  leadership style and, 59–60
  measurement of, 550–553
Product-line budget, 170
Profession. See also *Nursing profession*.
  continuing education for, 499

Profession (*Continued*)
  definition of, 29–30
  self-monitoring of, 497
Professional, definition of, 30
Professional autonomy, conflict about, 424
Professional power, 384, 385
Professionalism, appearance in, 44–45
  behavioral inventory for, 40–41
  definition of, 30
Professionalization, autonomy criteria for, 32t, 37–39, 43
  barriers to, 41–42
  continuum of, 39–40
  cosmopolitan-local construct and, 44
  criteria for, 32–34, 32t, 37–39, 43
  definition of, 30
  ethics criteria for, 32t, 39
  knowledge criteria for, 32t, 34, 43
  research on, 42–44
  service criteria for, 32t, 34
Profit, definition of, 177
Program budget, 170
Prototype patient classification system, 455t, 456
Purpose statements, of organization, 214
Pygmalion effect, 70–71
Pyramidal bureaucracy, 243, *243*

Q
Quality, assessment of, 493–495
  definition of, 482–483, 489
  measurement of, 491–493
  monitoring for, 486–488, *486*
Quality assurance (QA), 484–485
  audit for, 493–494
  data analysis tools for, 494–495
  definition of, 483
  outcome standards for, 492
  process standards for, 492
  regulatory agency standards for, 487–488
  structure standards for, 491
  total quality management and, 488–489
Quality care, 210
Quality circles, 485
Quality control, clinical indicators for, 138
  clinical practice guidelines for, 139
Quality improvement, 481–503
  definition of, 483
  research studies and, 495–496

Quality of care, definition of, 482
Questions, in persuasion, 437

R
Rahim Organizational Conflict Inventory, 413, 422
Rapport, in persuasion, 435
Rater temperament effect, in performance appraisal, 540
Rating scales, for performance measurement, 537
Rationality, 385
Readiness, 389–390
Reality shock, 211, 565, 603–604
Reassurance, in conflict management, 421
Recency effect, in performance appraisal, 539
Recognition, in motivation, 370, 372
Reengineering, 236, 255, 273
Referent power, 386
Reimbursement, 177–178
  changes in, 237, 255, 508, 510
Reinforcement-based theories, 367
Relatedness needs, 363
Relentless incrementalism, for problem solving, 112–113
Research, quality improvement and, 495–496
Resistance, to change, 518, 520–521, *520*
Resolution, legislative, 584–585
Responsibility, definition of, 232–232
  zones of, 279, *279*
Restraint, non-violent, 349–350
Restructuring, 236, 254–255, *255*
  of intensive care unit, 252–253, *252, 253*
Revenues, definition of, 168, 169
Reward, in motivation, 370, 372, 373, 376
Reward power, 386
Risk management, 500–501
Role stress, 566–567
  conflict and, 416

S
Safety needs, 362, *362*
Salary, nursing, 20–22, *21*, 21t
Sanctions, 385
Satisficing, 126
Scalar process, definition of, 229
Scheduling, 92–93, 448–463. See also *Staffing*.
  definition of, 449

Schwirian Six-Dimension Scale of Nursing Performance, for performance measurement, 537
Security needs, 362, *362*
Self-actualization needs, 362, *362*
Self-assessment, of motivation, 365
Self-efficacy, 99–100, 401
Self-fulfilling prophecy, 70–71
Self-management, unit-based, 262–263
Semi-profession, 40
Sensitivity, power and, 383
Sexual harassment, 339–340
Shared governance, 263–271, *265*, 525
  administrative model of, 267, 269
  autonomy in, 265–266
  change towards, 271–272
  congressional model of, 267, 268
  cost-benefit analysis of, 266
  councilar model of, 267, 268
  definition of, 263
  effects of, 269, 271
  evolution of, 274
  models of, 266–271, *267, 268, 269*
  vs. bureaucracy, 264
Skilled performance levels, 600–601
Social system, components of, 210, *211*
Span of control, 256
  definition of, 229
Special purpose budget, 170
Staff, legal obligations to, 96–97
  scheduling of, 92–93, 448–463. See also *Staffing*.
Staff mix, definition of, 449
Staff position, 229, 244
Staffing, 448–463
  cost analysis of, 459–462, *461*
  decisions for, 450–452, 451t
  definition of, 449
  ethical issues in, 132–133, 134–135, 289
  fixed, 453
  hours per patient day (HPPD) in, 452
  legal issues in, 183
  methods of, 452–453
  nurse extenders in, 460–462, *461*
  organizational culture and, 204
  patterns for, 453–454
  standardized volume measures in, 451–452, 451t
  supplemental, 453
  variable, 453
Standardization, of work processes, 231

Standardized volume measures, in
  staffing, 451–452, 451t
Standards, for quality monitoring,
  486–488, 486
Standards of care, 489–490, 490
Standards of practice, 489–490, 490
Standing committee, 156
Stewardship, 182
Strategic planning, 169
  definition of, 168
Stress, 560–574
  adaptation to, 568–569
  change and, 567, 571–573
  conflict and, 573
  coping with, 564, 568–569
  definition of, 561
  general model of, 561, 563–564, 563
  nurse-physician relationships and, 567
  occupational, 561, 562
  outcomes of, 465
  role, 566–567
  sources of, 564–568
  work environment in, 567
Stressors, 564–568
  cognitive appraisal of, 564
  definition of, 561
Structure standards, for quality assurance,
  491
Sunflower effect, in performance appraisal, 539
Supervision, 282–283. See also
  Delegation.
  definition of, 280
  for work coordination, 231
  legal aspects of, 287–290
Supplies, cost of, 172, 180
SYMLOG (Systematic Multiple Level
  Observation of Groups) questionnaire, 160
System of nursing care delivery, 299–316
  case management as, 307, 309–310.
    See also *Case management*.
  case nursing as, 302
  costs of, 311–312

System of nursing care delivery (*Continued*)
  definition of, 300
  development of, 314
  functional nursing as, 303–304
  group nursing as, 302–303
  modular nursing as, 305
  patient-centered, 308–309
  practice environment and, 306–307
  primary nursing as, 305–306
  private duty nursing as, 302
  socioeconomic influences on, 312–313
  team nursing as, 304
  total patient care as, 303
  trends in, 312–313
System view model, 7

T
Task force, 156
Team(s), 161–162, 304
  building of, 161
    definition of, 145
  definition of, 161
  empowerment of, 56–57
  for problem solving, 116–117
  performance of, 161–162
Theory X, 361, 368
Theory Y, 361, 368
Thinly disguised contempt, 217
Thirty-second hurdle, 342
Thomas-Kilmann Conflict Mode Instru-
  ment, 422–423
Time management, 92–93
Time-motion study, 454
"To do" list, 377
Total patient care, 303
Total quality management (TQM),
  163–164, 485
  definition of, 483
  quality assurance and, 488–489
Total quality process (TQP), definition
  of, 483
Transactional leadership styles, 66–68, 67
Transformational leadership styles,
  66–69, 67

Transformational Model, 213–214
Transformational power, 395
Trial and error, for decision making, 128
Tri-Council, 162–163
Tri-Dimensional Leader Effectiveness
  Model, 64–66, 64, 65
Trust, in persuasion, 433, 434

U
Unionization, 460
Unlicensed assistive personnel, 292–293,
  295
Upward appeal, 385

V
Valence-instrumentality-expectancy the-
  ory, 366
Value, of service, 556
Values, in decision making, 131–135
Variable pay, 373
Veracity, in ethical decision making, 133
Verbal abuse, 339–340, 349
Verbal communication. See *Communica-
  tion*.
Vision, communication of, 344–345, 347
  of leader, 55, 400

W
Wellness care, 202
Win-win situation, in conflict manage-
  ment, 424
Withdrawal, in conflict management,
  421
Work Environment Scale, 199
Work groups, self-managed, 98–99
Work sampling, 455
Worst-case scenario, for decision making,
  130–131

X
X-Y Theory, 361, 368

Z
Zones of responsibility, 279, 279